Writing with Fire

BARBARA YOUNG WELKE

WRITING WITH FIRE

THE COWBOY SUIT TRAGEDY AND THE COURSE OF A LIFE

The University of Chicago Press
Chicago and London

The University of Chicago Press, Chicago 60637
The University of Chicago Press, Ltd., London

For more information, contact the University of Chicago Press, 1427 E. 60th St., Chicago, IL 60637.
Published 2026
Printed in the United States of America

35 34 33 32 31 30 29 28 27 26   1 2 3 4 5

ISBN-13: 978-0-226-85088-7 (cloth)
ISBN-13: 978-0-226-85089-4 (ebook)
DOI: https://doi.org/10.7208/chicago/9780226850894.001.0001

Library of Congress Cataloging-in-Publication Data

Names: Welke, Barbara Young, 1958– author
Title: Writing with fire : the cowboy suit tragedy and the course of a life / Barbara Young Welke.
Other titles: Cowboy suit tragedy and the course of a life
Description: Chicago : The University of Chicago Press, 2026. | Includes bibliographical references and index.
Identifiers: LCCN 2026009881 | ISBN 9780226850887 cloth | ISBN 9780226850894 ebook
Subjects: LCSH: Welke, Barbara Young, 1958– | Burns and scalds in children—United States—History—20th century | Flammable fabrics—United States—History—20th century | Children—Death | Wrongful death—United States | Personal injuries—United States | Résumés (Employment)—United States—History | Education, Higher—United States—History | Discrimination in higher education—United States—History | Sex discrimination in higher education—United States—History
Classification: LCC RD96.4 .W45 2026
LC record available at https://lccn.loc.gov/2026009881

♾ This paper meets the requirements of ANSI/NISO Z39.48-1992 (Permanence of Paper).

Authorized Representative for EU General Product Safety Regulation (GPSR) queries: **Easy Access System Europe**—Mustamäe tee 50, 10621 Tallinn, Estonia, gpsr.requests@easproject.com
Any other queries: https://press.uchicago.edu/press/contact.html

contents

preface

It was over twenty years ago, in February 2003, that I first read the long trial transcript in a case involving the death of a seven-year-old boy named Tommy McCormack whose cowboy playsuit had been consumed by flames. I am a legal historian and had found my way to this case through a published legal decision. The court's decision was brief: a single paragraph, devoid of factual detail. It was only in reading the transcript that I learned how this boy had died and began to see that he was one of many children across the United States who in the years of World War II and after were injured or died from burns when the fuzzy fabric simulated to look like fur on the chaps of the Gene Autry cowboy playsuit they were wearing exploded into flame.

I continued my search, discovering and reading case files in lawsuits involving other children, newspaper articles, and corporate and lawyers' records. But I hesitated in seeking out survivors and other family members of those burned in the cowboy playsuits, fearing I would be dredging up a long-past trauma for them.

In spring 2010, my teenage daughter, Frances, suddenly and unexpectedly suffered a series of strokes and died in a week's time. In the wake of her death, it was difficult to live; I could not imagine thinking. But as you will see, it was through Frances that I returned to the work of thinking.

I now questioned my sense that these other families' trauma could ever be past. The silencing of Frances's voice led me to see the importance of their having the opportunity to share their stories. I began a search to see if I might find survivors and other family members. The conversations I later had with some of them were powerful and transformative. Through them, I came to understand how fundamentally this event had shaped the course of their lives.

The course of life. *Curriculum vitae.*

The timing of Frances's death drew my attention to the curriculum vitae. She died between two major professional milestones in my life. They were things that I had worked hard for, things now drained of significance. They would appear on my curriculum vitae; Frances's death would not.

Today, most people see the curriculum vitae as only a professional form. But for centuries, the Latin phrase's literal meaning referred to the lived course of life. How was it that a phrase that had meant *the course of life* had been reduced to a form that claimed to represent a life, but from which so much of what gives life meaning was excluded? How does that exclusion of meanings shape what we know and how we know it, and who we understand ourselves to be?

My life tangled these two untold histories together. This book traces them both.

At first glance, telling these two stories, so apparently unalike and unlikely, together in one book may seem puzzling. In the foreground, a tale of heartrending wrong and loss. A history of a child's playsuit that exposes the dark side of "better things for better living through chemistry"; an age of businesses, celebrities, and the state promising consumer abundance on the cheap—an abundance that came at great cost to some. It is a history in which powerful actors failed to own their responsibility multiple times over: producing the harm, magnifying it in their efforts to maximize profits and escape liability, and, finally, working to minimize even what they paid in legal verdicts and settlements for the lives they had taken and transformed. This was the cowboy suit tragedy.

Against this history, the history of the curriculum vitae may seem a dry affair. And readers may find in some of its chapters a respite from the intensity and emotion of the cowboy suit tragedy. But the history of the curriculum vitae is no more simply a history of a form than the cowboy suit tragedy is a history of a product. This product and this form were made. How they were made and remade and by whom, and subject to what larger forces and structures, are central to the histories traced here. These two histories unfolded together over the course of the twentieth century. They were shaped as much by the global crucibles of depression and war as by other large-scale structures and forces. Their distinctness together with their commonalities cast into sharp relief: Life. Depression and War. Markets and Families. Law. Power. Precarity. This book is about the course of the lives this form and this product shaped.

Tracing these two histories together does other work as well. In history, as in so many fields, scholars are disciplined to separate the personal from the intellectual, to treat emotion and subjective experience as prejudicial. In its erasure of the personal from a life, the vita reinforces those norms. Including a history of the vita in a book that is most centrally about another history is then something like wearing a girdle on the outside of one's clothes to expose the girdle's construction and unnatural constraint.

Scholarly work, like all work, takes place in our lives. It is shaped as much by our lived experiences and the historical contexts in which we live, as by our training, which is itself shaped by larger institutions, structures, and forces. How could it be otherwise? In writing this book, I could not unknow my own experience of traumatic loss. I nonetheless might have left that loss and its shaping force unacknowledged or carefully segregated it in a preface such as this. I have instead, woven it through the narrative.

I began writing to Frances the month after she died, desperate to talk to her, to bridge a distance I could not understand or abide. I share excerpts from those letters here. Why? Weaving my experience of loss together with these two histories claims the personal knowledge I bring to this work. It challenges the boundary between the personal, intellectual, and professional that disciplinary training and institutional norms and values structure and reinforce.

But this is not all. The excerpts from my letters offer a sort of emotional bridge across time, enabling readers to more fully understand the grief and loss these other families experienced. They create a space in which we engage the world-erasing and world-making power of trauma and loss.

I explain my use of these letters more fully in a note on methods and sources at the end of this book. For now, perhaps, it is enough to say that I draw on excerpts from the letters I wrote to Frances in the first year and a half after her death. Each segment includes excerpts from letters written over multiple days, with a new paragraph signaling an excerpt from a new letter. "Dear Frances" was how I began each letter and is how I begin each segment here.

In what feels now like another lifetime, Frances asked me, "Why do you do this kind of work?" This book is at least the beginning of an answer. *Writing with Fire*. The cowboy suit tragedy wrote with fire on the lives of children, families, and communities. If we hope to even get close to understanding this history, we cannot stand apart from it. And so, I write here with what cultural anthropologist Ruth Behar described as "all the fire of feeling."[1] And in the challenge this book represents, there are both the destructive and generative properties of fire.

This book is a work of history. But it is also something more. It is a journey. And as with all journeys, meaning lies in the journey itself.

· PART I ·

Life

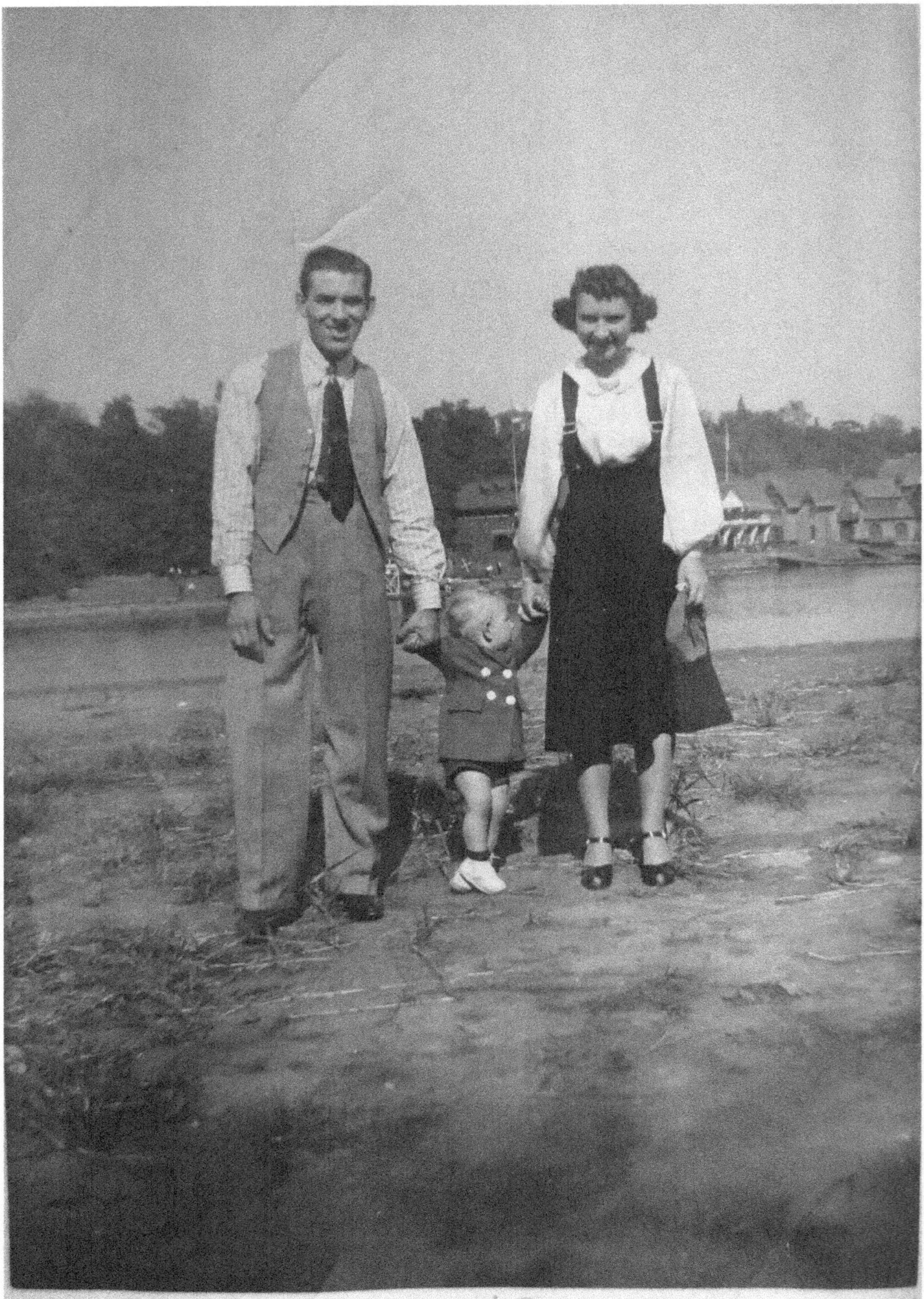

1940

chapter one · child's play

"What did you go by when you were a boy?" "They called me Tommy." Tom Habina was seventy-seven years old when I met him in December 2016. He had lived in Central Florida with his wife Dorothy for close to thirty years, but the accent of his Philadelphia boyhood remained clear. When Tom Habina's parents married in 1938, they rented a house on Spring Garden Street. The houses had stoops and tiny backyards with high wooden fences. He was born there on October 14, 1939. The streets were cobblestone. There was a little grocery store and next to it, a big empty lot. Much of the year, "trashmen" kept warm by a fire in that lot. "Kind of like a fire pit?" I asked. "Yes," he replied. "That was the days when they had the horse and wagon that they collected trash." "Do you have memories of playing in that neighborhood?" I asked. "Yeah, I had a lotta memories."[1]

"State your name and address." "Cecil D'Wayne Warnick, Potomac Park, Cumberland, Maryland." "How old are you?" "Ten." "Do you attend church?" "Yes ma'am." "Do you know the difference between right and wrong?" "Yes ma'am, when you do something wrong it's a sin." "Do you know the difference between telling the truth and telling a lie?" "Yes ma'am, when you tell the truth it is good, and when you tell a lie it's bad." "Do you know what happens to people who do not speak the truth?" "Yes ma'am, they are always punished." "Do you know what is meant by swearing to tell the truth?" "Yes ma'am, that's when you tell God it's the truth." "Do you remember wearing a cowboy suit that your mother bought for you around Christmas time in 1944?"[2]

The events that Cecil Warnick was being asked to remember in December 1948 had taken place close to four years earlier, when he was six years old. Far more years had passed for Tom Habina, searching his memories with me.

The differences in place and space in their childhoods are easy to see. Tommy was a child of the city. Cecil was a child of the country, born in that slender stretch of Maryland squeezed between Western Pennsylvania and West Virginia, in an unincorporated town of fewer than four hundred residents.[3]

The underlying commonalities in their lives are easily overlooked. Both were boys, born within a year of each other; both were white, firstborn sons of fathers who worked with their hands. Their early childhood were years lived against the backdrop of World War II.[4] Cecil Warnick's responses reflected the stark binaries offered children. There was truth and there were lies; there was good and there was evil; there was justice and injustice. The United States was on the side of truth, good, and justice. And justice would prevail. Lessons in knowing taught to children. And so, when Cecil was asked if he knew what happened to those who do not tell the truth, he responded, *if you don't tell the truth you don't go to Heaven*. People who do not speak the truth *are always punished*.[5]

The rhythm of daily life for children had been reshaped by child labor laws and compulsory-schooling laws. Children of working-class families in the 1930s and 1940s who in years past might have worked in mills and factories had hours on their own after school and on what we refer to as *weekends* without a thought of the revolution that term reflects.[6] Children's daily lives, moreover, were increasingly shaped by a popular culture that was national in its reach and a market in consumer goods that included playthings. Their radios carried the same nationally syndicated radio shows, their local movie theatres carried the same movies, the same newsreels and cartoons, and their stores carried many of the same brand names, down to toys and playsuits.[7]

Like hundreds, thousands of children, mostly boys, Cecil Warnick and Tommy Habina were both given Gene Autry cowboy suits in 1944. Tommy had gotten his cowboy suit for his birthday in October 1944. Cecil's mother bought his for Christmas from Lou's Auto Store in Cumberland, Maryland, that December. Most Gene Autry cowboy suits, like children's playthings more generally, were bought by women, mostly mothers, as gifts for special occasions for their children.[8] Tommy's mother had bought two—one for Tommy and one for his cousin Donald—from the McCrory store in Philadelphia. "They kinda almost dressed us up about the same," Tom Habina remembered. Their childhoods marked the emergence of what historian Viviana Zelizer describes as "the economically 'worthless' but emotionally 'priceless' child."[9]

Play became children's work.[10] Boys practiced for adulthood through

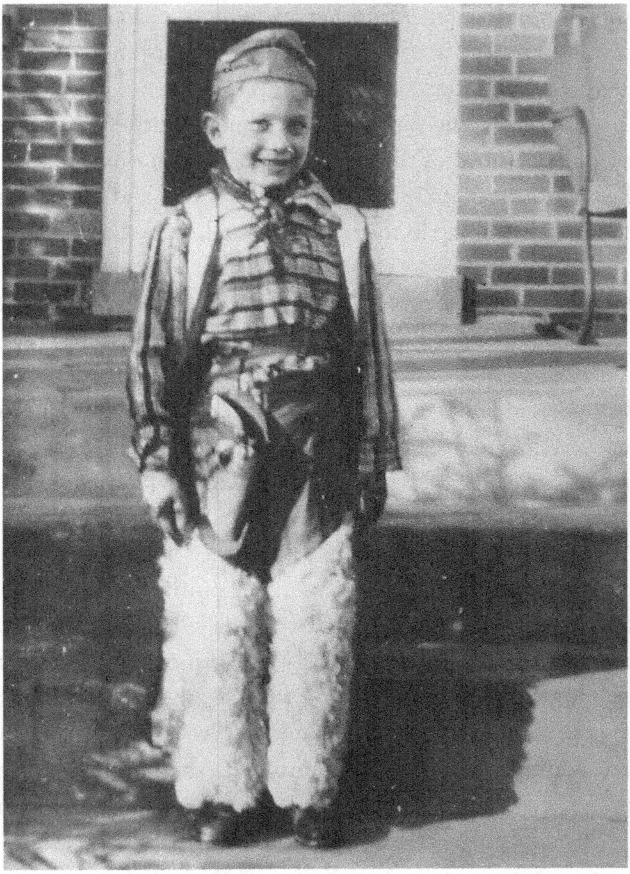

role-play in commercially made and sold playsuits that cast them as policemen, firemen, soldiers, and cowboys—male roles defined by independence, action, and the defense of social order and the republic. I wonder if anyone at the time thought about how central fire was to many of these roles.

The physical boundaries of their world were broad. "He more or less had the run of the yard and the neighborhood because he was old enough," Winifred Cunningham said of six-year-old Eddie Bradley. "He went to school by himself. He came back by himself."[11] Describing the paper mill town where he had grown up in north central Louisiana, Charles Baragona drew me a picture. Within two blocks of the mill house his family lived in were the elementary school, store, and movie theater; the paper mill where his father worked; and, most importantly, the Catholic church with a little clinic, convent, kindergarten, and playground.[12] For rural boys like Cecil Warnick, their playground might be the surrounding woods. Adult supervision was loose and shared by mothers, neighbors, older siblings, and—for Catholic children like Charles Baragona—the parish nuns. In his words, "Everybody's kids was like everybody's kids."

The pattern of play and supervision held more generally. As Mary Louise Cumberledge described of their daily life in Washington, DC, in the war years, she would check up on Toby, who was seven, and his siblings when they were outside playing in the neighborhood, if she "hadn't heard them around or wasn't sure where they were."[13] At age four, Kenneth Fox and his friend Roy Cizek, age three, went back and forth between each other's houses and yards in Terre Haute, Indiana, on their own.[14] "He was in the habit of playing right around our home," Kathryn Timberlake, of Kansas City, Missouri, said of her five-year-old son Scott. "He never went too far."[15] In Saginaw, Michigan, Jackie Izzo earned a quarter each week for "watching" her younger brother and sister.[16] Jackie Izzo was unusual: She was a girl who wanted a cowboy suit and she bought it herself, paid down at a quarter a week at Albosta's Hardware around the corner. The final payment came from a windfall. One night a woman in her mother's weekly Tunk Rum card group gave Jackie her winnings: two dollars.[17]

"Did your mother work?" I asked Jackie, immediately regretting the question.[18] Mothers' days were filled with work: shopping, cooking, cleaning, doing the wash, caring for babies and toddlers, caring for sick children, preparing and then sitting down for meals with their husbands before they went to work, taking an afternoon bath before he came home, burning the trash.[19] And many mothers also juggled outside jobs.[20] James McCormack worked days as a doorman in New York City; his wife Catherine took care of the household and their four boys, but in the evenings, she went to another job.[21] And in many families during the war years and after, the father was away in the service.[22] Eddie Bradley's father was in the Navy; his mother was a nurse; he lived with a woman who took in children.[23] This was the familial context of child's play.

Cecil Warnick was asked if he remembered wearing the Gene Autry cowboy suit. He described being in the woods near his home with other boys—Jackie Kochis, Muggsie Speelman, and Muggsie's brother—and having built a campfire to roast potatoes.[24] That ordinary part of Cecil's life was an equally ordinary part of other rural children's lives. So, on a cold January day in 1945, six-year-old Jimmy Detrick, who lived in Keyser, West Virginia, and other children built a bonfire to warm themselves while sledding. Like Cecil, Jimmy had gotten a Gene Autry cowboy suit for Christmas, purchased from the same auto supply store. He sat on his sled in his cowboy suit warming himself by the fire. Six-year-old John Russell built a fire near his home in Salt Lake City, Utah, with a seven-year-old playmate to roast wieners. For all these boys, building a fire with other boys was central to their play.

What fields and woods were to rural boys, open fields, alleys, and vacant lots were to boys who lived in towns, urban and suburban neighborhoods, and cities. The outdoors offered freedom.[25] Billy McMaster Jr. was born in Detroit in 1940, but with the war his family moved into defense workers' barracks-style housing in Center Line, Michigan. Out back: open field where children played.[26] Recalling his childhood in East Paterson, New Jersey, Gaither Bates Jr. described much the same. Behind the houses were open fields. "There was a lot of children my age," he remembered, "and it seemed like that's all we did was play."[27]

And as was true for boys in rural areas, fire was central to their play. Dennis McCarthy Jr. played with other children in a vacant lot near his home in Yonkers. The only thing unusual about five-year-old Joey Intelisano, his four-year-old neighborhood friend Gerry Sukinik, and other boys roasting marshmallows and playing around an open fire in a vacant lot near the boys' homes in Passaic, New Jersey, in June 1946 was that two of the boys were wearing Gene Autry cowboy suits. Billy McMaster, still recovering from polio, with a large brace on his leg, could not fully enter into a game with other boys, but he was nonetheless there, the chaps of his cowboy suit pulled over the brace, watching as the other boys ran around him in the field with a lighted torch.[28]

Although children played with fire, the fire they used in their play was often not their own.[29] Fire was a part of everyday life. Families burned trash, rubbish, and cardboard waste in metal tubs and barrels in their backyards, on the ground at the corners of lots, and in alley incinerators. There was nothing unusual in Mary Javinsky burning wastepaper in a backyard metal tub in Muskegon, Michigan. Or Evelyn Fox burning the cardboard crating from a new bedroom set in the backyard in Terre Haute, Indiana.

And in fall and spring, families burned leaves, brush, and grass. Sometimes children watched as adults worked. Three-year-old Andrew Javinsky played in his cowboy suit as his mother burned the trash. On a spring Sunday afternoon in Pennsville, New Jersey, four-year old Ron King went out to play in his cowboy suit and watch his neighbor burn grass while his parents finished a late lunch before his father left for work. On a Saturday in November in Louisville, Mississippi, his father away in the service, his mother away for a funeral, six-year-old William Augustus Strong III watched leaves being burned on his front lawn.[30] Sometimes they did not stop at watching. Four-year-old Gaither Bates Jr. one winter day was watching a neighbor burning trash. And then, as he put it, "being a normal boy, . . . I started throwing rocks into the fire."[31]

After Christmas, families burned their trees. Small wonder that older boys finding abandoned Christmas trees would think to burn them as younger children like five-year-old William Touhill in Philadelphia or four-year-old Marion Ormerod in Yonkers watched.[32] For children in industrial cities, rubbish fires in back lots were like magnets. It was a matter of happenstance that the Gene Autry cowboy suit five-year-old Wallace Tetla was wearing had been manufactured in the building behind which he played around a rubbish fire, near where his family lived in Passaic, New Jersey.[33]

The remains of fires were as interesting to children as fires themselves. "I used to play with a little Black kid," Tom Habina, explained to me. "I don't remember his name. I tried so many times to think of that and I'm unable to do it." But there was a fall day, Tommy's fifth birthday, when they were "playin' around" the trashmen's fire pit. Tommy had on the cowboy suit his parents had given him for his birthday. The other boy had this, "um, it was like a metal hook," and he "stirred it"—the remains of the trashmen's fire—"up a little bit."[34]

On an April Saturday afternoon, in Kansas City, Missouri, five-year-old Scott Timberlake rode his tricycle through a smoldering pile of leaves in a neighbor's driveway.[35] "He was chasing me and I ran through it," said Kenneth Fox, describing playing cowboy with Roy Cizek, running through the ashes from the cardboard crating Kenneth's mother had burned that morning. "And then we quit a minute because I was going to get a drink."[36] While Kenneth went inside, Roy sat down and waited. This was how child's play went: immersed in their imaginary world one moment, and in the next a child going inside to get a drink of water, like taking a break on a movie set.

Adults were mindful of the risks of fire to children. Mary Javinsky remembered staying with the trash she was burning until the fire was out and only later giving her three-year-old son Andrew a paper carton to put in the metal tub.[37] Evelyn Fox described staying with the fire from the cardboard crating until it had burned out. "There were several small children that played around there," including her son Kenneth, she noted, "and I couldn't leave a fire burning."[38] "I had warned my own children innumerable times," Mary Louise Cumberledge explained. Having learned through a neighbor of two local boys who had a reputation for playing with fire and matches, she had told her boys that she "would rather they didn't play with Jack Bontz and Bobbie Simpson."[39] "He was taught all the safety," Kathryn Timberlake said, explaining her warning of her five-year-old son Scott about the hazards of fire and matches.[40] Reflecting the shared character of

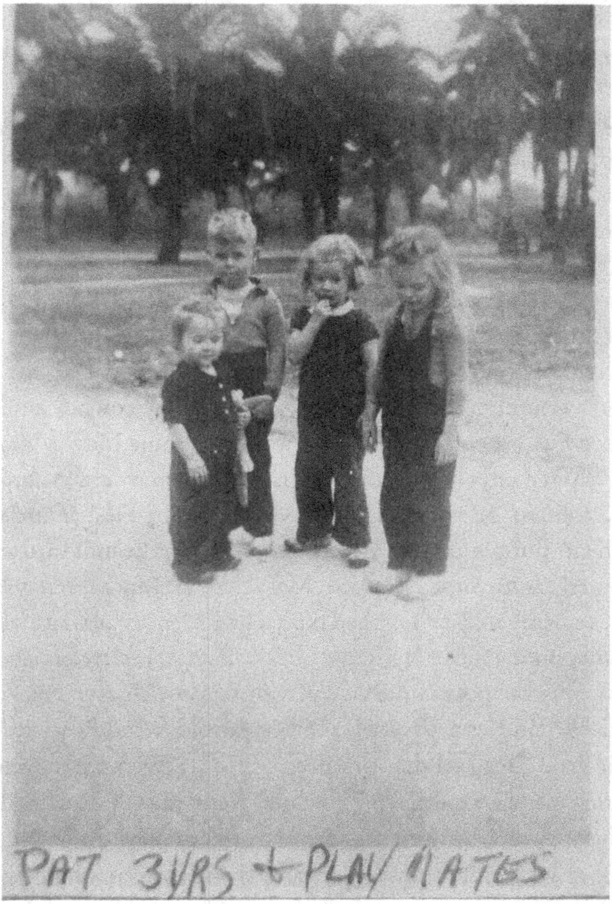

adult supervision of children in the 1940s, warnings were not limited to parents. Residents who saw six-year-old Richard Johnson and his friends having "a high time" with a fire they had started in an empty lot in Wilkes-Barre, Pennsylvania, warned them.[41]

Child's play was dynamic and organic; its storylines were unplanned. New participants changed the character of the play. On a cold January afternoon in 1944 in Royal Oak, Michigan, five-year-old Jackie Lockhart was outside, wearing the chaps of his Gene Autry cowboy suit, when a slightly older boy, Eddie Borkle, came over. As Jack Lockhart remembered, it was probably Eddie's idea to look through people's trash cans in the alley. The two boys found a bottle of lighter fluid that was not quite empty. Eddie suggested that they find a spot and light a fire. "There was a garage back in there on a dead end. Didn't face anything but the railroad tracks. So, we went back in that garage, and there was a log in there. And poured the fluid on it and lit matches and lit it up." And the day being cold, Jackie Lockhart got down close, "you know, to stay warm."[42]

A story that Charles Baragona Jr. told me about a day in September 1947, in Hodge, Louisiana, was not so different. He was six years old and playing on the swing sets at the playground by the convent with his little sister Theresa Mary, when a boy named Eddie Mischew, who was a year older, arrived. Eddie had some matches. Charles liked matches, but, as he put it, "I'd already had my butt tore up" for playing with matches. So, he crouched down by the stairs leading up into the convent, hidden from sight and protected from the wind by the angle of the steps, before striking the match.[43]

Parents who bought their children Gene Autry cowboy suits, or any kind of cowboy suit, probably imagined them as something to wear to play cowboy.[44] And many children did. "He had his cowboy suit on, and we were playing cowboys," Edward Alexander said of Bobby Flesher and what the two of them, along with Gay Miller, were doing in the junkyard in back of the Zimmerla Auto Shop in LaVale, Maryland, on Mother's Day in 1945.[45] As Eddie remembered it, "Gay had built a fire. After we played a while, Gay went home; Bobby started to stamp out the flames; I started to go home."[46] "They were just running in the field playing cowboy," Evelyn Fox said of her four-year-old son Kenneth and his three-year-old friend Roy Cizek. "They had their little guns and shooting each other."[47] "We were playing and he was chasing me, we were playing cowboy," Kenneth Fox explained.

But having a cowboy suit was not essential to playing cowboy, nor did wearing a cowboy suit necessarily mean playing cowboy. None of the boys Bobby Flesher was playing with had on a cowboy suit. Kenneth Fox wanted chaps like Roy Cizek had, but he did not have a cowboy suit.[48] Toby Cumberledge's brother whom he sometimes played cowboy with did not have a cowboy suit; none of his friends did; in fact, no kids he knew had a cowboy suit.[49]

Describing what her son Toby was doing on a day in March 1945, his mother, Mary Louise Cumberledge, said he had gone outside with his sister "to play in his cowboy suit."[50] Later asked about the things he did and the reasons why he wore his cowboy suit, Toby said to "play cowboys or something like that." But as he also said, "Sometimes, I would just like to wear it."[51] "On this particular day why did you put the suit on?" Toby was asked. "Just to wear it," he said.

That warm spring Sunday as Toby and Jane headed out to play, their mother was taking care of their brother, who was running a high fever. Their father was digging a flower bed. Toby and Jane wandered up the block to play with Bobbie Simpson, who was between their ages. Bobbie said he was going to do an experiment with his chemistry set. The experiment involved lighting a paper bag on fire and then putting it into a container to see if it would still burn. It was just a small brown paper bag, the size you might get when buying candy or a loaf of bread. And so, Toby and Jane watched as Bobbie lit the bag with a match and the fire took and the flames rose. "We thought the flames were getting too high," Jane later said. She did not want to stamp out the fire herself, afraid that her toes would get burned. And since Bobbie was barefoot, she asked Toby to stamp it out. And Toby, dressed in his cowboy suit, began stamping on the flaming paper bag.[52]

Many children wore their cowboy suits simply because they *would just like to wear them*. Just after Christmas 1945, in the basement of their house in Saginaw, Michigan, eight-year-old James Ikner Jr., with his younger sister watching, wore his Gene Autry cowboy suit as he did an experiment with his chemistry set—both gifts he had gotten for Christmas. On a Sunday afternoon in February 1945 in Pottsville, Pennsylvania, John Elwyn Jones, outfitted in the chaps of his Gene Autry cowboy suit, with holster and guns, piled up snow to build an igloo behind his family's apartment, and then he lit a match.[53] Maybe he had gone out to play cowboy and decided there was enough snow to build an igloo. Or maybe he put on his cowboy suit because he just liked it. Maybe he lit the match because he wanted to see if the flame would melt the snow. Or maybe he had just rediscovered that he had matches in his pocket and decided to strike one.

There was excitement in the forbidden. Michael Felton remembered wanting to show the cowboy suit he had gotten for Christmas to his friend Kingey Cole, who lived up the street from his maternal grandparents in Lewiston, Idaho. So, when they went to Lewiston for a Mother's Day weekend trip, he wore his cowboy suit. He wandered up to Kingey's; Kingey was home on his own. Michael was six, Kingey was five. There was some trash in the back and Kingey suggested that they burn it. "I had been taught not to play with fire," Mike Felton told me, "And so, I wasn't about to, uh, strike a match or set a fire." But Kingey was willing to. As Mike Felton remembered, "I stood there, mesmerized. I guess, knowing that I shouldn't be involved, but not touching anything, and so I watched him set the fire, and the fire started to blaze."[54]

Matches were a part of everyday American life used to light stovetop, oven, and furnace pilot lights and for burning trash. Children knew where to find them.[55] Nor were matches limited to the home. The development of nontoxic safety matches at the turn of the twentieth century and the free matchbook covered with advertising went hand-in-hand with the growth of the cigarette. As Allan Brandt notes, "the 'short smoke' of the cigarette, unlike other forms of tobacco consumption, was dependent on the 'quick light.'"[56] Fire safety manuals directed to children began with matches.[57] "I had a thing for matches," John Sansbury, born in May 1940, told me of his boyhood in Cedar Rapids, Iowa. "The folks," his parents, "didn't realize that, and I'd get packages of them, take them out and light 'em off."[58]

Playing with matches could be done by a boy alone as much as in a group. And for a boy on his own, at least part of the excitement was seeing how long he could hold the match as the flame got closer to his fingertips. Or for those playing with others, another boy's foot. Jackie Izzo first described the game of "hotfoot" to me. "Yeah, the records say that the kids gave me a hotfoot, right?" she said. "I think we seen a cowboy and Indian movie. And uh, white people gave the Indian—isn't it silly how they got a match in the moccasin?" Jackie laughed hard. "They said the cowboys gave the Indian a hotfoot, so one of the boys tried it on me. And put it in my shoe, a match, . . . They wanted to give me a hotfoot to see if I'd jump up and dance like the Indian."[59]

The quarter that Jackie Izzo received every week for looking after her younger brother and sister, included paying her for taking them to the neighborhood movie theater in Saginaw on Friday night. During the war years and after, children filled the seats of American movie theaters.[60] Charles Baragona Jr. remembered going to the movies with his little sister in Hodge, Louisiana. "My sister and I would get fifteen cents and go to a movie. The movie was nine cents, and we could get a penny piece of candy, and then one of us would get a nickel popcorn and the other would get a nickel Coke and we would share."[61] Saturday afternoon matinees, especially, were packed with children of all ages on their own.[62] Fire filled theater screens. In Westerns, a staple of those matinees, there was the glow and warmth of the cowboys' campfire; what was portrayed as the "good fun" of giving an Indian a hotfoot; and, more dramatically, scenes like a jailhouse set afire by a cowboy hoping to hide the evidence of his crime, or Indians on horseback with flaming torches setting ablaze covered wagons carrying settlers West, or US Army troops torching whole Indian villages in what was framed as "defense."[63] Children watched these scenes transfixed, alternately thrilled, excited, and, for some, gripped by fright and terror. But it was a delicious kind of fright because they took it in from a place of safety.[64] And they watched knowing that in the end, however dire the straits, the hero would come through and set things right.[65]

Movies provided plotlines for children's play. But they also could mis-

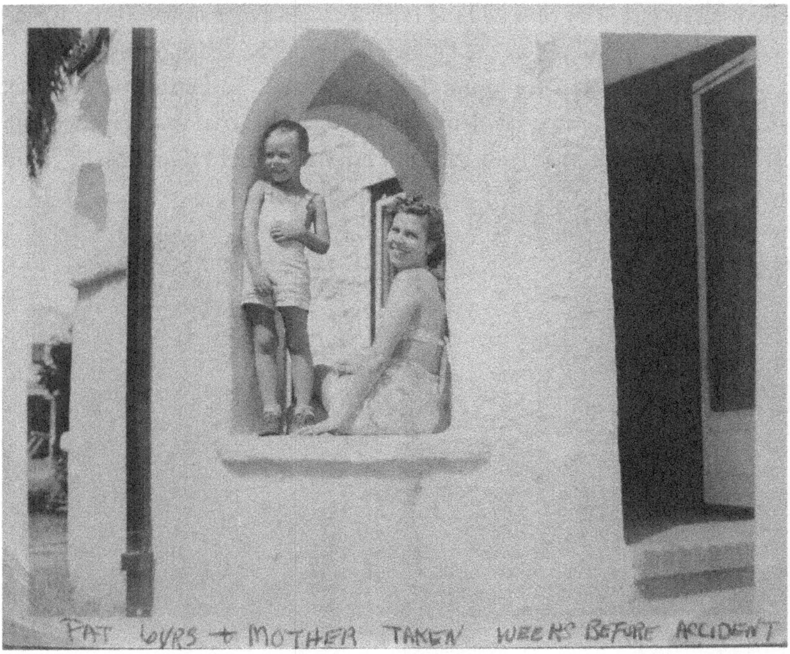

lead. As Jackie Izzo explained to me, that night in July 1944, the game wasn't hotfoot, it was "firecracker." It started with one of the cinders that covered the roads in their neighborhood. "They were kinda pretty," she remembered, "like a hunk of charcoal, with blue and green in 'em. . . . You take the tip of that match," and strike it against the cinder, "and it would go bang! Like a firecracker." On that Friday night, "the boys and I were goin' out, and we were gonna play firecracker."[66]

For all the independence that their world afforded, they were children, and the rhythms of their lives remained tied to those of home life. Marco Antonio DiTrapani and his friend played outside all morning while Marco's mother did her housework.[67] As noon approached, Searle Devens began stomping out the campfire he had built with a four-year-old playmate to go home for lunch.[68] Late in the afternoon, Billy McMaster watched other boys play with a paper torch in the open field behind his housing complex, knowing that he must be home at five o'clock for dinner. "We'd stay out until Mom called," recalled Gaither Bates Jr. "Mothers would just open a window and holler out your name and you just come running or," he chuckled, "pay the price."[69] And after dinner, the rituals of the end of the day. The McCormacks' oldest boy, Pat, was out. The three younger boys occupied themselves: Jackie lay on a bed in his pajamas reading comics; Tommy, having had his bath, played in the kitchen, wearing the chaps of his new cowboy suit; Jimmy was there too, still in the bathtub. Catherine McCormack had gone to her evening job. James McCormack relaxed in the front room of the family's four-room railroad-style apartment; if he'd looked, he could have seen back through the rooms from where he sat.[70]

graduation

Dear Frances,

Yesterday I cleaned out that nasty drawer in the kitchen—the one with all the pens and various other stuff that was so packed you couldn't get it open more than an inch or two. . . . Trying to create some order in a world that now feels without order or reason is about all I can do at the moment.

. . .

Today was graduation for the SPA Class of 2010. Wilder accepted your diploma. We lit a candle for you when we got home. It's a beautiful, green candle that Grandma Anzie brought us from Austria many years ago.

. . .

I had a dream this morning. Everyone had gone for a boat ride. I had stayed behind. I looked down this steep embankment to the other side of the lake. There was a boat—You were in it and smiling and waving at me. The dream woke me up. You were so real. And I woke up so ready to have you back only to come back to the crushing realization that you were gone and wouldn't be back. Oh, Frances. There are days when it just seems that you are away, that you will be back. And then there are days when I feel the full weight of your being truly gone and all I can do is cry.

. . .

How do I write about a day like today? I began it sad—wondering for the how manyeth time—why? Is there not some way to turn back time, to reverse events, to have you once again at the center of our lives. I long so to hear your laugh, to see you grab Sam in one of your full-body hugs, to say I love you to you, to hug you in a tight goodnight hug. But I can do none of these things, so I keep busy to keep the despair and sadness just an arm's length away. There is no peace.

chapter two · curriculum vitae

In classical Latin, *curriculum* was associated above all with movement: the movement of heavenly bodies; the change in the seasons; a racetrack or circuit; a chariot; the race of life, laps of life.[1] And *vita* meant life: biological existence, animation, possession.[2] Together, the two formed a flexible pair, word order meaning little in Latin: *curriculum vitae, vitae curriculum, vitae curriculo, curriculo vitae, curriculum vivendi*. The course of life.[3] Not a written statement. Not an academic form. The actual course of life. That meaning continued into the early modern world.

But in 1582, the Latin word *curriculum* appeared in the records of the University of Leiden denoting a course of academic study, perhaps the first such usage.[4] We are so accustomed to thinking of curriculum as a course of study that it is the earlier history of the word that sparks surprise, not what was in fact new in the sixteenth century. But if newly tied to education, *curriculum* remained in this moment not an anglicized word but a thoroughly Latin one, rooted in the word's earlier meanings. As historian William Clark notes, Latin was "how the medieval and early modern university presented itself. Traditional authority and academic charisma were as much vested in the charm of Latin as in elaborate costumes."[5]

The French Revolution and Napoleon's conquests devastated the university landscape in Europe.[6] But in the decades between 1789 and the 1830s, a new model of the university emerged, with German Protestant universities providing the model that would diffuse globally in the nineteenth and twentieth centuries. The modern research universities that emerged in Germany retained Latin as the language of knowledge. When the University of Berlin—the institution which epitomized the modern research university—opened in 1809–1810, it announced Latin as its official language. In this new university, the arts and sciences faculty would no longer be, as William Clark puts it, "the minion" of the faculties of law, medicine, and theology but instead the university's foundation, with a degree of its own: the doctorate in the arts and sciences: doctor of philosophy, PhD.

Supplanting in part the values and qualities that defined the medieval and early modern university were new values, new qualities: originality and creativity privileged over erudition; writing privileged over disputation; the individual scholar/teacher over the collective body of the faculty; education as a foundation for positions of state taking primacy over preparations for religious purposes. Reflecting these values, the defining requirement for the degree of doctor of philosophy in the research university was a dissertation, written by the candidate, based on his original research.

And at the University of Berlin and other German universities, appended to the dissertation was a document, written in Latin, on which the candidate's admission to examination depended: the candidate's curriculum vitae.[7] This, it seems, was the origin point of the curriculum vitae as a written narrative, an academic form. A bold harnessing of language, meaning, and history to buttress the authority of knowledge produced in this new research university with its own academic credential.

"To the Most Consequential and Honorable Order of Philosophers, with highest respect, George Bancroft submits this 'curriculum vitae.'"[8] George Bancroft was not quite twenty years old when he wrote his curriculum vitae. It began with his date and place of birth in Worcester, Massachusetts, on October 3, 1800, then detailed his sites of education and the subjects he had studied and expressed gratitude to those who had taught him. Handwritten in Latin on August 26, 1820, the brief narrative was the final requirement in preparation for his examination for the degree of Doctor of Philosophy from the University of Göttingen. A life reduced to a written form. Stripped of all details save birth and formal education. Written and submitted as a requirement for obtaining an academic degree.

George Bancroft had come to Göttingen after completing his BA at Harvard on his father's recommendation "for our ears had been filled with its fame." It was not just the University of Göttingen to which Americans flocked but German universities more generally: Göttingen, Halle, Berlin, Leipzig, Jena, Heidelberg, and others—and the leading scholars in philosophy, history, law, literature, ancient and modern languages, philology, mathematics, chemistry, medicine, economics, and other fields who were professors there.[9] The number of Americans studying in German universities in the nineteenth century peaked in the years between the mid-1870s and the early 1890s. As President Frederick A. P. Barnard of Columbia College wrote in 1886, "In past years it has seemed to be an impression almost universally prevailing among the young men graduating from American colleges with aspirations for making a career in a learned or scientific profession, or in the educational field, that a residence of one or more years at a German university was indispensable to anything like signal success."[10] All told, by the eve of the First World War, somewhere between nine and ten thousand Americans, overwhelmingly male, had attended German universities for advanced academic training.[11] Other Americans preceded Bancroft at Göttingen, but he was the first to earn a PhD from the university and so was the first to complete not only a dissertation but the rite of crafting in Latin his curriculum vitae.[12]

Americans traveled to Europe, especially Germany, for advanced education, not only because of the reputation of German universities but also because there was no alternative in the United States.[13] Noting this fact in a letter in July 1860, John A. Porter, dean of the faculty of the Scientific School at Yale, pressed the president and fellows of Yale College to institute the degree of Doctor of Philosophy.[14] One year later, Yale granted the first American PhD. Harvard established its Graduate School of Arts and Sciences in 1872 and granted its first PhD in 1873. Columbia University granted its first PhD in 1872. But graduate education and the research university, as such, only really began in the United States with the founding of Johns Hopkins University in 1876, which in its first decade awarded eighty-four PhDs.[15] The founding, in quick succession between 1890 and 1892, of Clark University, Stanford University, and the University of Chicago was like an accelerant. The flood of American students to Germany ebbed in the 1890s in significant part because there were now American alternatives.

Americans held German universities in awe and borrowed from them in creating the American university, but they did not simply copy form, structure, and aspiration. As Daniel Coit Gilman, the first president of Johns Hopkins University, noted, "We did not undertake to establish a German university, nor an English university, but an American university, based upon and applied to the existing institutions of this country."[16] Just as others have noted that research universities in the United States differed in important respects from German universities, so too did the forms related to the doctorate. The first doctoral dissertations in the United States did not include curricula vitae. No Columbia University dissertation, for example, awarded through the early 1890s included a curriculum vita or any similar document by a different name.[17] In its first decade, Johns Hopkins did not even retain candidates' theses.[18]

But as the pace of production of American PhDs quickened, so too did the formalization of requirements. In 1887, Hopkins revised its requirements for conferring the degree of Doctor of Philosophy adding, among others, three important new requirements. The first was that the dissertation's title page include specific language—the language that any twentieth or twenty-first century PhD in the United States would recognize: "This dissertation was completed in partial fulfillment of the degree of doctor of philosophy at . . ." The second was a requirement that the thesis include a "biographical sketch of the author." And the third mandated that within one year of conferral of the degree the author present 150 printed copies of his thesis, in whole or in part, to the university, including the author's biographical sketch. To ensure that this requirement was met, if the printed copies had not already been submitted to the university when the degree was conferred, the author was required to make a deposit of $50 to the university treasurer, to be returned to the author when the requirement was met.[19]

By the first decade of the twentieth century, though the exact required number of printed dissertation copies varied—150 at Johns Hopkins, 150 at Columbia, 100 at the University of Chicago, 200 at Catholic University, and so on—the requirement of printed copies was standard, though not universal, at the handful of research universities that granted the lion's share of American doctorates.[20] The printing requirement, a relic of the era before the microfilming of dissertations began in the late 1930s, was as breathtaking and burdensome to candidates at the time as it seems to us now.[21] At most institutions, the doctorate was not awarded until the required copies had been deposited, or legal or monetary assurance received that they would. The result was, in some cases, years of delay before a candidate who had completed all the other requirements for the doctorate actually received their degree.[22] But the point here is that by the late nineteenth or early twentieth century, all three requirements—title page with degree and institution, author biographical sketch, and printing—were standard for the doctoral degree.[23]

Johns Hopkins had not elaborated on what a candidate was to include in his biographical sketch or even noted the appropriate title for the document. In Hopkins's dissertations from the early 1890s, the required document is variously titled, where it was given a title at all, "Biography," "Autobiography," or "Life."[24] But even in its description of the required document as a "biographical sketch," Hopkins suggested not only an Americanization of the form but also an orientation distinct from that of the nineteenth-century German university curriculum vitae. Think back to George Bancroft's 1820 "curriculum vitae." It was a gateway form: a text written to document a man's course of study, submitted by him to the institution and faculty with whom he had trained, as part of the petition to be admitted to examination. It was, with the limited personal detail of place and date of birth, a narrative academic transcript with acknowledgments.

The American document, although similarly a degree requirement, had an altogether different orientation. Its focus was on an author's credentials, on the author as producer of an original work of knowledge. Together with the dissertation's title page and the requirement for the submission of hundreds of printed copies of the dissertation that could circulate to other institutions, other scholars—it spoke to the hunger of American universities to prove themselves as research universities. Columbia University offers a telling example. Columbia set out degree requirements in its first *Catalogue*, published in 1893. "There shall be appended to each dissertation a statement of the educational institutions that the author has attended, a list of the degrees and honors conferred upon him, as well as the titles of any previous publications."[25] Though the requirement did not call this statement a vita, many degree candidates did. "I, John Angus MacVannel, was born at St. Mary's, Ontario, October 5, 1871," began the author's statement appended at the end of his 1896 Columbia PhD dissertation. He titled the document, "Vita."[26] So did many other Columbia men.[27] MacVannel's 1896 dissertation was among the first at Columbia that included the new document. Others too completing dissertations under the faculties of philosophy and political science in 1896 and 1897 included the required document; it was another year before a student in the pure sciences did so.

Soon enough the vita was a taken-for-granted requirement of earning a doctorate. In 1910, Columbia amended the requirements that had been in place since 1893, requiring that the document "printed and appended to each dissertation" be "in the form of a Vita" and, in addition to the elements required since 1893, required "a statement of the place and date of birth of the author."[28] It was, to a significant extent, a case of requirements catching up with practice. From 1896 at least, many PhD candidates had not only titled the document, "Vita," they had also begun with their place and date of birth.[29]

Elements of the nineteenth-century German university curriculum vitae lingered in American vitae. In the vita that John Angus MacVannel wrote to append to his 1896 Columbia dissertation, he noted by name and field the professors whose lectures he had attended and concluded, "My major subject was with Prof. Butler, to whose guidance and continued kindness I owed the completion of this dissertation." So too Arthur Beatty concluded his 1897 Columbia vita, "To each of my teachers in English I feel great obligation, and especially to Professor Price, whose practical interest and patient sympathy have been freely given me in the preparation of this dissertation." Palmer Cobb closed his 1906 Columbia University vita with "especial thanks" to Professor Calvin Thomas "for proof reading, valuable criticism, and guidance in the preparation of this dissertation. More especially for that spirit of ready helpfulness and sympathetic interest which characterizes his relationship with those who are privileged to do work under his direction."[30] Prose and writing in the first person lent themselves to personal expressions of admiration and gratitude.

But if early American dissertation vitae included recitations of those with whom one had taken courses or expressions of gratitude, these elements became less and less frequent as more and more vitae were written in the third person.[31] And as these elements dropped out, not only at Columbia but more generally in dissertation vitae, the author emerged as a solitary figure.

By the end of the first decade of the twentieth century, most vitae appended to American dissertations, though still narratives, were written in the third person and were not personal at all. A statement of degrees awarded. A list of honors conferred. Other publications by the author. Vitae appended to Columbia University dissertations epitomized the American centering of the author as individual. A vita appended to the dissertation noting these items not only gave authority to the author's intellectual work in the dissertation but also increased the authority and prestige of the university where he had been trained. And, perhaps not surprisingly, with these changes too came the first shift from narrative to list. No personal data. No expressions of appreciation. A list in place of a narrative.[32]

The vita requirement in American dissertations, from the start, looked outward.[33] The purpose of requiring authors to submit hundreds of printed copies of their dissertation to the university was to promote the diffusion of knowledge. Every printed copy included the requisite title page and vita. And so, when a copy of a dissertation was purchased by another university for its library, shared through interlibrary loan, or checked out by a student or professor at the institution at which it had been completed, it included the author's vita.[34]

But the vita remained, nonetheless, a degree requirement. Few of the dissertations first published in scholarly journals included the author's vita in the original journal publication.[35] Searching Columbia dissertations from the first decades of the twentieth century that were reprinted from a journal, I found only one that included a vita in the original publication.[36] American universities could impose requirements on students as a condition of obtaining their degree, but even though university presses and academic journals were also creatures of the modern American research university, they did not operate under degree requirements.

The modern research university is celebrated for its innovation in research and publication, not for the curriculum vitae. But the curriculum vitae or, the vita, as it became more colloquially and generally referred to in the United States, appended to the dissertation, was crucial to what William Clark describes as a fundamental feature of the modern university: the "bureaucratic rationalization of the doctoral candidate."[37]

And so, words which from the ancient through the early modern world had meant the actual course of life were reduced to a form, a written narrative, and finally a list, in which the private self was severed from the public, like academic robes, part of the creation of the doctor of philosophy as "authorial persona."[38]

· PART II ·

Depression & War

longing

Dear Frances,

I didn't write yesterday, thinking that perhaps if I didn't I could avoid plunging into the desperate sadness that comes with every acknowledgment that you are truly gone. It didn't work. I went to bed feeling desperately sad, slept poorly, and when I finally did get to sleep woke up with a start from a dream that involved a child, a girl with a head injury being rushed into a hospital helicopter. And then I was awake crying and only escaped by getting out of the cabin into the early morning fog.

. . .

Oh, sweetheart, I miss you so. Tomorrow morning will be the two month anniversary of when you had your stroke. I'll never forget that awful morning—hearing your alarm clock ring for what seemed like a long time, feeling groggy and not much interested in beginning a new week myself, and then my own alarm clock going off, turning on the shower so it could start to get hot while I went to say good morning to you. And then discovering that you didn't seem to be up. And then trying to wake you. And then finally, me calling down to Dad, "Bill, you better get up here, something's wrong with Frances."

. . .

Dad said to me this morning we have to go on because you were so exuberant about life, that we have to go on because you were denied that right. And I can see this and believe it and yet I can't quite go on without you.

. . .

Every time I write I realize that at some point I need to stop writing, to say goodnight, to close this diary to you. I don't really know how. The hurt is so bad. The sense of longing for you is so great. Oh, Frances, I wish you were here so you could tell me how to go on. I need you now.

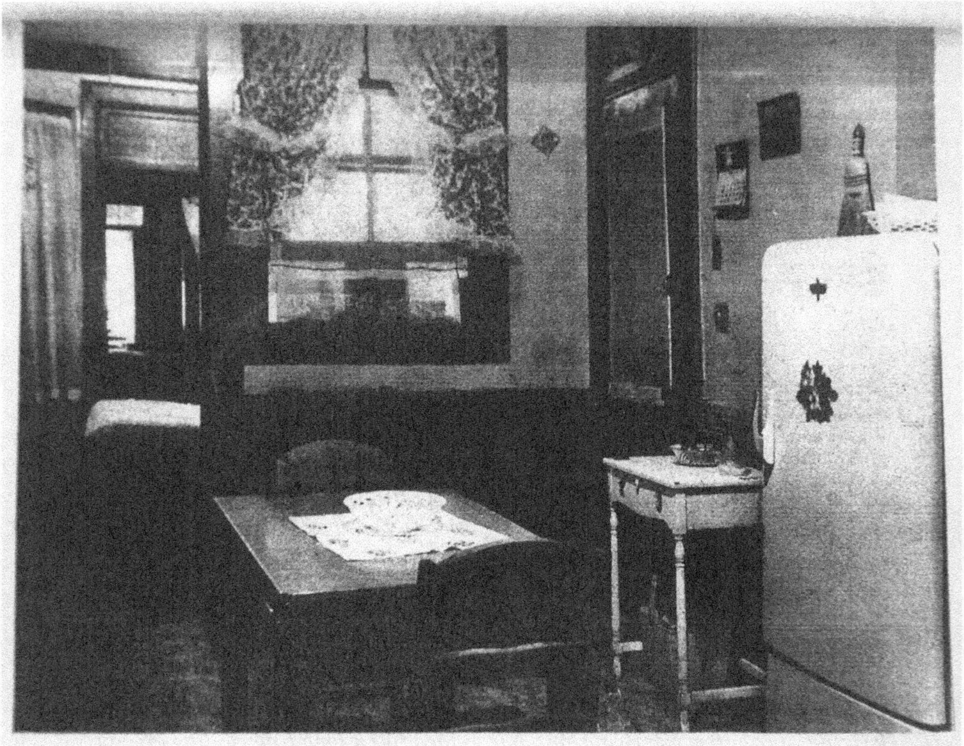

chapter three · "a circle of flame"

"I heard Tommy scream and I rushed out of the room, and Jackie was rushing out ahead of me. . . . Tommy was on fire. . . ." Tommy McCormack's older brother Jackie grabbed the bedspread he had been lying on to try to put out the fire. But he could not get close to Tommy, as he explained, "because he was in a circle of flame." "He was just all flames," Tommy's father James said of his seven-year-old son. "I can recall nothing, only he had his two hands up in the air . . . just flame."

James McCormack grabbed Tommy with his bare hands and plunged him into the bathtub, where his son Jimmy had been only moments before. Jimmy now stood, naked, watching. Water dripped on the kitchen floor. The flames extinguished, James left Tommy in the tub and rushed downstairs to the apartments below, calling to his neighbors to get a cab. Returning to the apartment, he pulled the rest of the blankets off the bed and wrapped Tommy in them and carried him down the stairs to a waiting cab and on to the emergency room at Mt. Sinai Hospital.[1] It was only in the emergency room that James McCormack realized that he himself had been burned. "Somebody called my attention to it. The skin had come off my hands."[2] It was 7:30 p.m. on Saturday, January 6, 1945.[3] It had all happened in a matter of seconds.

The McCormacks lived in a four-room railroad-style apartment on New York City's Upper East Side.[4] The apartment consisted of four rooms, each opening onto the next: a front living room, two small bedrooms, and a kitchen—the largest room in the apartment and, in winter, the warmest. James worked days as a doorman in an apartment building on the city's Upper West Side just off Central Park.[5] His wife Catherine worked evenings from 6:00 to 9:00, starting a half hour later on Saturdays. They had four children: Pat, age sixteen; Jackie, age thirteen; Jimmy, age ten; and Tommy, age seven. That evening James had gotten home from work around 4:45 or 5:00 p.m. Catherine had left for work at 6:30. She was gone when it happened. The McCormacks' oldest son, Pat, was out too. James had been sitting in a chair in the front room with his coat on because the room was cold. For that reason, the boys were not allowed in there after having their bath. Jackie was lying on his bed in his pajamas reading comics. Jimmy was in the tub. Tommy had had his bath too and was playing, dressed in an undershirt and the chaps of his new Gene Autry cowboy suit. James had seen him just a moment before. "I could see him all the time and hear him, because he come in—he wasn't allowed in the front room, it was cold in there. He was after having his bath. He wanted to come in for some reason, and I told him he was not allowed."[6]

Catherine McCormack learned of the accident when she got home from work that night. By the time she got to the hospital they were bandaging her husband's hands; he would be in the hospital for three days and out of work for a month.[7] It was 11:00 p.m. before she saw Tommy. He had been in shock when he arrived at the hospital, suffering third-degree burns over the greater part of his body, from his ankles to his stomach and his hands, burns of a type and extent that, as the doctor noted, generally resulted in death very quickly. He lay bandaged, sedated, and under an oxygen tent in a small glass-enclosed room next to a nurses' station.[8]

"Life changes in the instant," wrote Joan Didion. "The ordinary instant."[9]

Tommy McCormack was playing. Suddenly, instantly, he was in *a circle of flame*. Repeat. Sickeningly. A single airborne spark from trash burning in an alley trashcan; a dying ember in leaves burned at curbside earlier in the day; the spark from a "safety" match; the tiny flame of a dropped lit match; a fragment of burning paper fluttering out from a trash fire or dropped from a young boy's hand; the pop from sap in a burning Christmas tree; the wind catching the flames of a grass fire; the flame from a boy's brother's burning cowboy suit. Crouching down by the stairs protected from the wind and out of sight. Getting down close, you know, to stay warm. He was four or five feet away from the fire. Watching; doing a chemistry experiment; a game of hotfoot; roasting potatoes, marshmallows, wieners; trying to get warm; playing cowboy; hunting Indians; lighting a match to melt some solder to make something; swordplay with sticks from a fire; riding a tricycle; stamping out sparks from a fire in a back lot; stamping out the remains of a campfire; filling time; having a high time. "And, 'poof,' I went up," explained Jack Lockhart Jr., describing how he suddenly, terrifyingly, a five-year-old boy, found himself on fire.[10] His voice serious, Gaither

Bates Jr. remembered: A burning bit of paper flew out from the trash fire and landed on the chaps of his cowboy suit, and "it was like somebody lit a blowtorch."[11]

In the instant, the child or children were alone. There were no adults who saw the moment that was like someone lighting a blowtorch. Sometimes even the other children did not see it happen. Gay Miller had already gone home on the afternoon that he, Eddie Alexander, and Bobby Flesher built a fire in the junkyard behind the Zimmerla Auto Shop. And the last that Eddie Alexander had seen Bobby, he had "started to stamp out the flames." Eddie was leaving for home and "then I saw Bobby running up over the bank and his pants were on fire and the flames were up around his waist."[12]

Many of them in the terror of the moment, like Bobby, ran for home. From the junkyard, from a garage down the street, from a vacant lot, from the playground by the convent, from an alley or backyard, from a field, from the woods. All toward home. Toby Cumberledge had started to run, but his sister Jane, remembering what she had learned about fire safety, stopped him. And in that moment, a neighbor looking out her kitchen window saw Toby on fire and raced outside and ripped off his clothes.[13] Searle Devens's grandmother, along with another woman, had gone looking for Searle and his playmate when they did not come home for lunch. And, as they searched, they first heard Searle's screams, then saw him in a field in the distance, his chaps afire. They called out to him to roll on the ground.[14]

What was basic knowledge to adults was lost to most children in the panic and terror of the moment. "And, um, so at age five, I knew there was trouble, I knew I was on fire," Mike Felton explained to me. "And, uh, I didn't know that I should roll. And put out the fire. And so, I started to run."[15] "I remember running and screaming," recalled Gaither Bates. "I ran out of the garage," said Jack Lockhart Jr., and "I'm trying to get the flames out with my hands; hitting them." As he spoke, he furiously clapped his hands against his thighs, even though he was seated in a recliner, his legs stretched out in front of him, recovering from yet another skin graft operation from that injury over seventy years before.[16] "I remember trying to beat it out," John Sansbury told me of the flames, and he too slapped his legs wildly with his hands demonstrating, "and, and all of sudden it occurred to me that I couldn't."[17]

Sometimes one of the playmates they had been playing with ran with or ahead of them calling for help. Tommy Habina had not known where the boy he had been playing with went when it happened, but he clearly had run to his own house because in no time at all the boy's father appeared at the Habinas' door.[18] "Johnny, my buddy, ran ahead of me," Charles Baragona Jr. remembered, and he was calling out "'Mr. Berry, Charles' on fire.'"

And sometimes the playmates simply ran. When Jackie Lockhart ran out of the garage, aflame, the older boy he had been playing with "took off." "He just ditched you?" I asked, incredulous. "Yeah, he took off." There was no blame in Jack Lockhart's voice when he said this. He added, "He was scared."[19]

What terror and agony did a child afire experience? Seven-year-old James Hummel, afire, ran for home, tripped, and fell to the ground.[20] The detective who examined the yard where the Krzeczkowski brothers, Casimir, age seven, and Stanley, age five, were burned noted that the yard "showed that there were seven separate fires, some believed started when the boys ran around in agony with their clothes aflame."[21] When I had asked Tom Habina, "Do you remember that day?" There was a quiet sadness in his reply, as he said, "Yes," and told me about running into the house, his mother grabbing a leather coat and wrapping it around him to smother the flames, and her "hollering" for Tommy's father.[22] Gaither Bates Jr. had paused, steadying his voice to go on, before describing his legs to me: "The sight of my legs, it seemed like a baked potato that had got really burnt and crisp and yeller."[23] Mike Felton's voice too was choked with emotion when he described how he had run from Kingey Cole's house toward his grandparents' house; how his grandfather, who had recently had a hernia operation, vaulted a four-foot fence and put out the flames. And then he said, "I remember, like I know it, but probably I don't. And, you know, the mind gets rid of that stuff."[24]

Trauma erases memory. Jackie Izzo could remember events from earlier that night and from long after, but nothing of the terror or pain or what she did when her chaps caught fire. She had run, but her memories, not only of that evening but of the period in which she hovered between life and death, are the memories of what others told her happened. As in Christina Crosby's memoir *A Body, Undone*, so too might Jackie Izzo title the chapter of her life relating to when she was burned "The Event as It Was Told Me" and open, as Crosby does, "I will never know what happened."[25] The trauma of being burned as a child could even wipe out what came before it. "My memory starts with my getting burned. Okay?" Art Cumberledge Jr. told me. Whatever memories he might have had before that day of his early childhood were lost in that moment and never recovered.

Tommy McCormack's brother Jackie had said, "I heard screams." "I heard Tommy scream," said the boys' father. A child's screams were often what first alerted others. "I suddenly heard Jimmy scream," said Israel Edmund Detrick. He was outside helping a passing motorist whose car axle had broken. Just a moment before, he had seen his son Jimmy sitting on his sled four or five feet from the bonfire where the sledding children gathered to get warm. "I suddenly heard Jimmy scream, and when I looked up, his clothing was on fire and he was trying to put the fire out." Jimmy's father was only about fifty yards away. "I immediately ran up the hill, and on my way up Mrs. Leo Baker threw a plaited rug to me, and I picked it up and got to Jimmy as fast as I could," wrapping the rug around his son to put the fire out.[26] Tony DiTrapani must have screamed. He had been outside playing all morning with a friend. His mother was in the basement cleaning; there was no outside entrance to the basement. To get to him she had to go up through the basement, up the steps and through the kitchen, and onto the back porch. And only then did she see him there at the back of the lot, in flames. By the time she got across the lot to him, "he had nothing on from his waist down, it was all burned away. I just laid on him and smothered the flames."[27]

Sometimes the screams were from a mother seeing her child on fire. "I was not in the yard," Jackie Jones's father said, "but I was at home when it happened." He and his wife were in their apartment, a floor above street level. She had chanced to look out the window and "saw our boy in colored flames shooting up from and all around his legs." She screamed that Jackie was on fire. "I ran down the rear steps . . . to the yard," explained Jackie's father. "I ran out immediately but by the time I reached him . . . the cowboy trousers covering his legs were entirely burned off down to the woolen socks, which covered the lower portion of his legs and the wool-and-cotton underwear which he also had on and which was smoldering in tatters." I "picked my boy up in my arms and carried him up the stairs."[28]

It was often neighbors who first heard and responded to a child's screams. Jackie Lockhart, on fire, running for home, had gotten "about half a block away" when a lady, who had just gotten home with a new blanket she had bought for her baby, saw him. "She's got the baby in her arms. Saw me, put the baby down, grabbed the blanket, come over, and put me out." *Put me out*, as though he were a human torch. And then she "took me home. And the police came and all that and took me to the hospital up in Royal Oak."[29] The daughter in the family that shared the duplex with the Bates family was getting married the day that Gaither Bates Jr. was burned. Gaither had remembered running and screaming. The groom and ushers had been out front doing something with the car. "And the groom saw me, ran to me, took off his overcoat, and wrapped it around me. And they brought me into their house, and I remember laying on, you know, put me down on the couch."

Charles Baragona Jr.'s voice was choked with emotion as he described the scene, his friend Johnny running ahead of him calling out, "Charles' on fire." "So, um, his dad happened to be on the front porch and he grabbed me and they ripped my pants off, and Daddy come out about that time, and, uh, Henry, his dad had, uh, his car parked right there, and he says, 'Come on, I'll take you, we'll go in my car.' So Daddy held me, and," Charles Baragona's voice barely holding, he coughed, "Excuse me," he said, "and we went just around the block to the hospital was right there."[30] What was it he had said to me? *Everybody's kids were like everybody's kids.*

Sometimes it was strangers, passersby, who witnessed and responded to what was happening. A patrolman driving toward City Hall noticing a group of boys around a bonfire in a vacant lot, when suddenly one of the boys runs from the lot with his clothes ablaze. The officer stops, grabs a blanket from his car and, grabbing the boy, wraps it around him, beating out the flames with his hands before rushing the child to the hospital.[31]

Or a man returning with a friend from a round of golf when he passes a woman crossing the street who says to them, "'Isn't that a horrible thing? A boy is over there burning to death.'" And when he looks, he sees this child "spread-eagled" in "flames to his waist." He drops his golf bag, rushes to the boy, and tackles him, rolling him on the ground, trying to cover him with his own body, to put out the flames. "Did you know the boy?" the man was asked. "No, I didn't know him."[32]

A shipyard worker standing at the corner of a block hearing children's screams of terror, rushing into the yard where the screams were coming from and discovering two boys in flames, catching one of them and rolling him on the ground to smother the flames. A truck driver making a delivery of scrap iron at a metal company hearing the same screams and scaling a seven-foot brick wall and four-foot wire fence on top of it to reach the boys, seizing the other boy and rolling him on the ground. Both men's hands burned. Joined by a third man who had heard the boys' screams from his own backyard down the street.[33] Stella Krzeczkowski had been just across the street at the store when it happened. Before leaving for the store, she had looked out the apartment window to check on her sons Stanley and Casimir Jr. playing in the yard below behind the apartment building.[34]

"When it happened, we were not at home," Frances Flesher said. "It happened on Mothers' Day. . . . We were visiting in Ridgley." A neighbor called to tell them. When they reached the hospital, "we found Robert was terribly burned and screaming with pain."[35] Billy Strong's mother was returning to Louisville, Mississippi, from her sister's funeral in Pensacola, Florida, the day it happened. His father was in the service, stationed in Guam, and Billy's paternal grandparents, who also lived in Louisville, were away as well, en route home from the hospital in Jackson, Tennessee.[36] "I was not present," Laura Bradley had to answer to one question after the next, about where exactly her son Eddie Bradley had been when it happened, whether there was fire or heat present, and if so, what kind of fire, how close he had been to it, which part of his clothing caught on fire first, what he had been doing immediately before his cowboy suit caught on fire.[37] She was a registered nurse; Eddie's father was in the service. Eddie was living with a woman who took in children. "I had him in 1944, nearly a year," Mrs. Winifred Cunningham said. "Then he went back with his mother"—perhaps an extended visit for Christmas when his mother gave him the cowboy suit?—"and he came back with me again the last of January 1945."[38] Eddie was burned the next month.

Was it different, did it feel different for those who were just upstairs, in the basement, at the kitchen table when it happened? Was it different for mothers, who had primary responsibility for children and the household, than for fathers?[39]

Tommy McCormack's mother, Catherine, had not seen, not been there when it happened. It was several days before she could ask Tommy about that night. Whatever it was he told her—a child of seven, heavily sedated, hovering between life and death—she told the hospital staff, and they recorded it in Tommy's hospital record, a record long since gone.[40] On the night it happened, she had only her husband's and two other sons' stories of the events of the evening, none of whom had seen the moment in which the cowboy chaps Tommy was wearing took fire. When she got back from the hospital late that night, she took what remained of the Gene Autry cowboy suits that Milton Henry had given her husband for their youngest sons and threw them in the trash.[41] One can feel her anger and anguish. Jimmy had never worn the cowboy suit meant for him. It went into the trash. Tommy had first put on the chaps of his cowboy suit that night after his bath. The fire had consumed the chaps, but she threw everything else in the trash.

Her actions suggested that something made her think or feel that the cowboy suit was perhaps, in some way, at least in part the cause of what had happened. She wanted every piece, every reminder, any future threat of the cowboy suits gone from her household. In so doing, she acted out an ancient legal principle: A thing or animal that caused a person's death was "deodand," meaning it was forfeited to the crown or given to God. If a man died in a fall from a tree, the tree was cut down; if he drowned in a well, the well was to be filled up.[42]

Though in that moment Catherine McCormack did not know whether her son Tommy would live or die, she wanted the cowboy suits gone. Did she imagine, could she not have imagined, was it in particular a mother who would imagine what the course of events would have been had she been there? On a witness stand three years later, before a jury, she had to say that she had not been there, that she had been at work, and he, her husband, James McCormack had to say that he had been there, when this thing had happened.[43] And in the fact of her absence and his presence they bore as parents an impossible burden. It was an unjust burden.

guilt

Dear Frances,

You are everywhere—your backpack sitting on the chair next to me at the kitchen table all packed up for school; in the tea cabinet when I go to make a cup of tea—your flavors; in the laundry room—your soccer bag . . . and then there is, of course, your room with the smell of sweet pea body mist which I keep spraying because it helps me feel like I might just yet, even yet be able to hug you one more time and this time never let you go.

. . .

Last night we drove back to the cabin. It was cold (low 50s) with a strong, steady wind blowing from the North so that the waves lapped along the shoreline of the lake. I've never liked big wind. It leaves me feeling disturbed and uneasy. I know you never liked big wind either. I remember the time in Evanston when you were about three and the wind caught your tricycle and blew you along faster and faster, until finally your little legs simply couldn't keep up and you stuck your feet out only to discover that you had effectively been a brake on the wind and your tricycle whipped ahead until we caught you and made it all okay.

. . .

Today is the two-month anniversary of when we had to come home from the hospital without you to the silence of a house without your laughter, without your smile. All week I have been reliving that short week (5 days—a work week, a school week) from the time of your stroke, through the days in Intensive Care at Children's Hospital. For some reason that I don't fully understand I have been rooted in those 5 days at the hospital, desperately trying to bring the story to a different close.

. . .

I force myself again and again to face the fact that you are gone, but I just can't make it stick because I so desperately want it not to be true. My whole life, especially growing up my mom would say if I wanted something enough and worked hard enough at it, I could make it happen. But try as I might, I can't seem to change the ending of this story. I can't get you back. Oh sweetheart, I hope you didn't have to know that the end was coming. If I can't have you back, that is my one wish. Oh, please let it be so.

. . .

I am more and more lonely for you. Last night was a wrenching night. It is an awful weight to have failed in the most fundamental obligation of a parent: to save and hold safe from harm your child. I asked Dad last night if you would have thought that we failed you, if you would've been angry at us for somehow not knowing and making you safe.

. . .

I am finding it hard to have any desire to live without you, Frances. I wonder that most people, even those who lose a child live on. How? Why?

chapter four · letters from strangers

That haunting, profoundly individuating phrase: *Life changes in the instant. The ordinary instant.* But as we know, not only in the ordinary instant. Many of the children whose Gene Autry cowboy suits exploded into flame as they played—their play *the ordinary instant*—were born during what Americans often refer to as the "Great Depression." The global depression of the 1930s was not an ordinary instant. The desperate search of so many Americans for employment—livelihood, identity, dignity—in the 1930s was not the ordinary instant. In Germany, Hitler's and the Nazis' rise to power, the passage of laws stripping individuals of their positions, targeting them because of their religion or religious ancestry, forcing them into a desperate search to escape not only to secure a livelihood, but life itself, was not the ordinary instant. It was in, a product of, this moment that was neither ordinary nor instant, this moment that set so many in search of security, that the vita, a profoundly individuating form, began to circulate in American academic life.

The AAUP, American Association of University Professors, first noted the "increasingly numerous letters of application from strangers for appointments" in 1929.[1] The increase in the numbers of American graduate students and PhDs in a saturated market, by the end of the 1920s, had driven growing numbers to strike out on their own in pursuit of academic positions.[2] The structure of academic employment in the United States in the early twentieth century was almost bound to produce letters from strangers in an economic downturn. Positions were not openly advertised. News of vacancies and recommendations for appointments circulated through an elaborate, closed patronage network of department chairs, leading men, college presidents, and deans, a gatekeeping system in which a man's reputation rested in significant measure on the reputation of the men who recommended him. Moreover, there was no system of permanent tenure. The bulk of the teaching staff in academia were employed on a year-to-year basis. For graduate students, research universities had a limited number of fellowships and in-house teaching appointments, saved for their "best men." Most graduate students made up an itinerant academic labor force.[3] And so, unsought letters of inquiry and applications for teaching positions, letters from strangers, grew more numerous in university departmental files.

Embedded in or attached to those letters were a new kind of form, individual self-fashionings of qualifications, with odd titles like "Brief Historical Sketch," "Data Concerning My Qualifications," "Information Sheet," and "Personal Data."[4] They came from men at every career stage, including those struggling to find a teaching appointment that would enable them to continue to work toward their degree and those with years of teaching or industrial research experience. There were letters from women, too, but they were fewer—reflecting the structured exclusion from and marginalization of women within academia. "There are so few openings," as a woman wrote to her former advisor at the University of Minnesota in 1934, "and for most of those that do exist, it seems that men are almost invariably preferred." She added, "I should like a teaching position, but would take industrial laboratory work or almost anything."[5]

The first place colleges and universities had sought to economize in the 1930s was by eliminating positions at the bottom of the ranks, leaving those who had barely gotten a foothold suddenly facing joblessness. "If there is to be an opening in your Physics Department this coming year, will you please consider me an applicant for such a position?" wrote an assistant professor in the Department of Physics at NYU. As he explained, "Because of financial conditions in the department, it is necessary to reduce the staff and that is why I am trying to locate elsewhere."[6] Chemistry and physics were fields in which industry had offered an alternate career path for some. In less than a decade's time, war would leave the nation scrambling to find enough qualified men and women in these fields. But in the 1930s, just as the number of positions in academia shrank, so too industry suddenly found the need for the research skills of those with advanced degrees a luxury many businesses could no longer afford.[7]

The absence of postings for academic vacancies meant that those seeking positions searched, in a sense, in the dark. A letter to the University of Pennsylvania in May 1930 from a man expecting his PhD from the University of Pittsburgh that summer was typical: "I will receive my Ph.D. in Chemistry this summer, and am interested in knowing if there is an opening in your chemistry faculty."[8] Flip through any department file in any discipline from a year in the 1930s and you will find such letters. They wrote letter after letter not knowing whether there might be a vacancy at all. "I have written to about sixty of the larger schools and commercial research laboratories about the possibility of a teaching or research position," a recent University of Minnesota PhD wrote to the director of the School of Chemistry in September 1931. "It seems as though I have tried everything I can think of, apparently without any success."[9]

It was one thing to voice desperation to a former advisor or department head, another to voice it to a stranger—and yet it was almost inevitable that their desperation would come through. "I beg to acknowledge your very courteous reply to my inquiry concerning a position in physics," began a February 1933 letter to the chairman of physics at Princeton. "I have sent out eighty-five inquiries, and have so far received fifty replies, all negative, so I shall be grateful to be considered, if any vacancy should develop."[10]

Department chairmen and leading scholars in the profession more generally were agonizingly aware of the shortfall in positions. In fall 1933, the AAUP reported to its members that colleges and universities had dropped more than two thousand faculty since June 1930.[11] They understood its consequences: insecurity and embitterment. Though department chairmen were uniformly courteous in responding to letters from strangers, they held out little or more often no hope for an appointment.[12] "There is no vacancy on our staff" was the common, repeating refrain.[13]

Universities had been concerned about the placement of the holders of their highest degrees almost from the start of granting PhDs.[14] Columbia University established an Appointments Committee in 1898. Others followed: The Appointments Office at Harvard, the Bureau of Recommendations at Chicago, the Department of Personnel at Princeton, and so on.[15] With the Depression, the number of universities with appointments offices grew.[16] Professional societies too were eager to systematize academic employment to assist those at the beginning of their careers or those facing unemployment.[17] From its founding in 1915, the AAUP, the first collective organization of professional scholars, prioritized employment and the pipeline of PhDs. But it was only in 1929 that the AAUP, and in the 1930s that discipline-specific professional societies in fields such as sociology, political science, and economics, made their first attempts to encourage colleges and universities to advertise positions, offered individuals the ability to advertise their need for a position, or circulated professional bios of new PhDs.[18]

None of these efforts, though, was intended to create an open market for academic positions or to encourage candidates to write unsolicited employment inquiries. University appointment offices faced faculty resistance from professors and department chairs who jealously guarded their prerogative in selecting and recommending suitable candidates for positions.[19] Resistance too was the response to services established by discipline-specific societies—resistance grounded in the fear that advertising vacancies would produce an onslaught of unqualified applicants, lead to a loss of institutional prestige, and be useless in any event for its lack of the personal knowledge of a man provided by patronage networks through which news of vacancies and recommendations flowed. And even with the protection of anonymity, few candidates advertised their search for a position in the 1930s, so difficult was it to overcome the widely held sense that it was unbecoming of a professional man to advertise himself.[20]

But though university placement offices and professional-society appointment services failed miserably in these early decades, their forms for registration—and the example of those advertising in situation-wanted columns—provided desperate job seekers an unintended sort of professional training in the details about the course of a life—personal, professional, educational—considered relevant to a teaching appointment. University placement office registration forms and professional-society forms and advertisements uniformly began with personal data.[21] And so, as though completing a form from which the lines had been erased, those desperate for employment writing to introduce themselves offered their qualifications beginning with "personal data."[22] The format, content, and opening details of the document Wilmond Warner Parker enclosed with his letter to the Department of History at the University of Chicago on December 1, 1930, was representative.

> Personal:
> Full name – Wilmond Warner Parker.
> Age – 22.
> Height – 5' 11".
> Weight – 150 lbs.
> Health – good.
> Religion – Congregational (but not a church member).
> Unmarried.[23]

To a modern reader, it seems a strange list of details as a foundation for a teaching appointment. But Parker's enclosure addressed standard questions on early university placement office registration forms. Other forms, in letters from strangers, included additional personal details that again were standard on university placement registration forms, things like date and place of birth, use of tobacco or alcohol, and military service.[24] Following personal data, they noted degrees, institutions, and teaching experience.

But it is the personal data in their opening that marks these makeshift forms, that gives away, as it were, the models that men relied on in creating their own forms. In part, the personal details capture data that was considered relevant in collegiate-level teaching appointments and so highlight the era as a different time. But the kinds of personal data included also reflected the structure of university appointment offices, which had a single, all-purpose registration form that every candidate completed, regardless of their educational standing or type of employment sought. Princeton was unusual in having, early on, a separate "Department of Teaching Appointments" with its own form, but that department handled teaching placements at all levels, from primary and high schools through colleges and universities.[25] Many men, again following the model provided by university appointment office registration blanks, enclosed a photograph of themselves. As one man put it, "the enclosed snapshot will give you some idea of what I am like on the outside."[26]

Strikingly, even those who graduated from institutions that required PhD candidates to attach a vita at the end of their dissertation did not title these strange documents of their own fashioning in search of a teaching position "curriculum vitae" or "vita." And equally strikingly, department chairs replying to these letters did not seem to recognize this document crafted in pursuit of a teaching appointment as being like that other.[27]

It was a second stream of letters from strangers—German scholars and scientists terminated from their appointments in universities and institutes under the Third Reich's racial laws—that gave this new form a name.[28]

In early spring 1933, two months after Hitler became chancellor, news began to circulate in England and the United States of scholars in Germany dismissed from their academic appointments under a new law, the law for the "Restoration of the Professional Civil Service."[29] Under the law, those who were Jewish or of Jewish descent as well as those with views unacceptable politically to the new regime were removed from their positions.[30] The efficiency of terminations, first in Germany, and later in the decade across continental Europe, rested on the fact that in Germany, as was true through most of Europe, universities were state institutions.[31]

The response in the United States was a complex mix of concern and mobilization of support; excitement and a sense of opportunity at the unexpected availability of some of the world's most eminent scholars and scientists; gatekeeping to ensure that displaced scholars not take positions from American candidates in a depressed market; and antisemitism.[32] By the end of May 1933, less than two months after the law's passage, the first aid organizations—in the United States and Europe—had been established to assist displaced scholars in finding emergency, temporary academic positions.[33]

From the start, the ability to leave Germany or to enter other countries was not simply a matter of their own desires. Legal exits required a passport; admission required a visa. Laura Fermi chose 1930 as the starting date for her study *Illustrious Immigrants* because the United States' new, restrictive immigration regime, the National Origins Act of 1924, went into effect on July 1, 1929.[34] Thereafter immigration was limited by strict national quotas, which in the European crisis of the 1930s quickly became exhausted.[35] The law included exceptions that in turn further fundamentally shaped the character of the migration. One of those exceptions was for professors, their spouses, and their unmarried children under the age of eighteen.[36] To qualify under the exception for such a "non-quota visa," an individual must have held an appointment as a professor in the preceding two years and have accepted an offer of an academic appointment in the United States.[37]

The question was who would receive such offers. Many German scholars—and, later in the decade, other scholars in continental Europe—who lost their positions or were likely to be targeted were known in the United States or England through their work and through extensive ties they already had with scholars and foundations abroad. In other words, many were not strangers. Some of these men's names were at the top of lists of scholars whom university presidents, chancellors, and leading scholars in the US and England hoped to recruit. Offers came to them without asking.[38] But a far larger group did not have international reputations and contacts. Some who would go on to distinction were unknown at the time; some were in fields or specialties where there was little demand; some were of an age (over fifty-five) where it was deemed they had already produced their best work; and some, on investigation, were not regarded as "first-rate men."[39] And so, while many were not strangers, far more were.

Whereas Americans searching for appointments on their own groped toward a form to introduce themselves and summarize their qualifications, German scholars had one: the curriculum vitae. The curriculum vitae, or *lebenslauf*, was a fundamental component of German academic life; it was the origin of the degree requirement in many American universities that PhD candidates attach vitae at the end of their dissertations. It mattered in this sense that the scholars first presenting curricula vitae in search of teaching appointments came from Germany, the acknowledged birthplace of the modern university. Unlike in the United States, where in 1930 the vita remained solely a degree requirement appended to a dissertation, in Germany it had become a standard professional form, which scholars and scientists revised and updated over the course of their professional lives.[40] But though the vita was an established professional form in Germany, the European crisis raised its stakes a hundredfold.

Letters enclosing qualifications began soon after the first dismissals.[41] In the single year from 1935 to 1936, well before the crisis reached its climax, Alvin Johnson reported that the New School for Social Research received more than five thousand letters requesting support.[42] As Johnson's report highlights, German scholars sent their vitae in letters not only to friends and professional colleagues abroad but also to strangers: university presidents, organizations assisting displaced scholars, foundations, other émigré scholars, and individuals whom they had heard provided support for others. Anyone who themselves might have a position to offer, know of a position, or know someone who might, or who could offer them advice or put in a good word for them. Letter after letter closed, "May I submit to you my curriculum vitae," or "For your further information, I beg to enclose my curriculum vitae . . . ."[43] As one man advised an acquaintance, "You send a curriculum vitae to 500 universities, colleges, etc. . . . translated quite clearly into American, without false modesty. That often leads to something."[44]

And those who received the letters—whether friends, strangers, or aid organizations—in turn circulated copies of the curriculum vitae on to others. "I am enclosing seven copies of his life history which speaks for itself" noted one such letter, referring to the scholar's vita.[45] There was no need for him to explain why he sent multiple copies; the reason was obvious: These were to be circulated to others. Or as a letter to presidents of leading colleges and universities from the National Coordinating Committee for Aid to Refugees and Emigrants Coming from Germany in February 1938 began, "One of the leading Foundations in the country has recently issued a Confidential List of Displaced German Scholars . . . in the fields of Archaeology, Biology, Chemistry, Engineering, Law, Mathematics, Philosophy, Medicine, the Social and Economic Sciences. In fact, there is hardly a branch of intellectual activity which is not represented. . . . They are eager to obtain academic positions. . . . Should your institution require the services of someone on any of your faculties, we hope you will write us and we will cheerfully send you the curriculum vitae of such a scholar."[46] And so, driven by intolerance and hatred, by the restrictive regime of US immigration law, and by the pursuit of academic freedom, livelihood, and life, the curriculum vitae circulated broadly in the United States in the 1930s.

From the start, the various aid organizations supporting displaced German scholars did not arrange appointments or provide direct financial support at the request of individual scholars. Rather, they made grants at the request of a university or college that had identified a scholar they would like to hire.[47] Accordingly, being known or becoming known by universities and colleges in the United States was essential. The size and scale of the higher-education landscape made the prospect both promising and daunting. There were over a thousand colleges and universities in the United States in 1930 scattered across the nation. The curriculum vitae was well suited to introducing oneself from a distance, critical in a context in which most of those seeking a position were not even in the United States and where securing a visa depended on first securing an academic appointment. Moreover, its character—that is, the fact that it was a form—meant an applicant could be, in a sense, in multiple places at the same time. In a context where time was of the essence, this mattered.

A form. A written, autobiographical narrative of a professional and intellectual life. "Career of Life," as one German scholar who had been stripped of his academic post because he was a Jew translated "curriculum vitae."[48] No life is captured in a single telling or has only one version. Audience, purpose, context fundamentally shape the narrative of a life. German scholars wrote and rewrote their vitae acting on advice both intimate and impersonal—family, friends, acquaintances, other scholars, aid organizations—and reflecting their own experience and changes in their circumstances.[49]

Those who stayed in Germany following their dismissals avoided direct statements on their vitae relating to their termination. They could not have done otherwise.[50] But in seeking appointments in England or the United States, the limited supply of funding, the large number of those competing for that support, and the straitened economic circumstances of universities and colleges made candid disclosure on vitae of the fact and basis of termination a necessity.[51] German scholars also suddenly found that their fate depended on their work being considered significant and original to English, and even more important, American scholars. And this too meant revising how they described not only their past work but also their future plans. Even as their access to archives and publication narrowed and then closed entirely, the importance of demonstrating continued productivity grew. And suddenly, too, details of effective teaching took on new importance, and so statements about the numbers of students taught and the reception of their lectures appeared on vitae.

Perhaps the most fundamental transformation was also the one most visibly apparent: the language a vita was written in. An appointment in the

United States or England required the ability to teach and publish in English. And so, all who could do so rewrote their vitae in English, providing tangible preliminary evidence of that skill.[52] A vita might moreover augment that basic point in its description of publications in English and experience teaching in English.

Finally, vitae became documents supporting a visa. And this purpose too required its own, distinct telling of a life.

Ernst Kantorowicz's path to a life and teaching appointment in the United States illustrates all these transformations.[53] Born in 1895 into a wealthy Jewish manufacturing family in Posen in present-day Poland, Kantorowicz earned his PhD at the University of Heidelberg in 1921, was appointed professor without salary in 1930 at the University of Frankfurt, and in 1932 was appointed ordinary professor at the University of Frankfurt.[54] He had held his professorship for only one full term when the Nazis came to power in 1933. In November 1934, he was forced to resign.[55] Though urged to leave Germany by friends who had left earlier, like fellow medievalist Theodor Mommsen, Kantorowicz remained, believing, against all evidence to the contrary, that if needed he could escape to England.[56] With the *Anschluss* in March 1938, the final doors to travel, access to archives, and publishing in German closed. With a chance query in July 1938, asking if he would be willing to have his name submitted for a possible appointment at a "prestigious California university," Kantorowicz began in earnest to seek a way out.[57]

In his July 1938 query, Fritz Demuth had directed that if Kantorowicz was interested in being considered, he should send "a 'curriculum vitae' (three copies) to be forwarded." Demuth wrote from London; any documents he received he would pass along to others. Two days after Demuth's letter, Kantorowicz replied, "I am only too willing to have you suggest me for the lovely professorship." He enclosed copies of a vita dated July 29, 1938.[58] It was the first of at least four times he would rewrite his vita over the next year as he sought the required offer of a position necessary for gaining a non-quota visa and a foothold in the United States.

The two-page, single-spaced, typed narrative with the heading "Curriculum vitae" that Kantorowicz sent to Fritz Demuth clearly drew heavily on his German vita. It began traditionally: "I, the undersigned ERNST HARTWIG KANTOROWICZ, was born in 1895 May 5 at Posen, capital then of a prussian [*sic*] province, where my father owned a well-known factory, founded by his grandfather in 1823 . . ." But a whole series of elements reflected Kantorowicz's understanding that this narrative of his professional life and scholarly work must do particular things for him to secure an offer of a teaching appointment in the United States. It was, firstly, written in English and included a peculiar paragraph at the end: "As to my knowledge of English I may add, that I had an English governess for the first twelve years of my life and that I had no difficulty at Oxford either in lecturing or in teaching." He listed no German references; only four from England, three of which were from Oxford. In contrast to many, he did not note that he was Jewish or refer specifically to Germany's new race laws, but he did specifically note the loss of his position. He noted the editions, translations, and sales of his 1927 book on Frederick the Second (1194–1250). Describing successive changes in his research agenda as avenues of research and publication closed to him, he worked to link his scholarship to that of distinguished American scholars. And he made clear that there was no longer a possibility of his working as a scholar in Germany. "The slight chance of publishing books or papers in German language has vanished almost completely, since Vienna . . . became german by the 'Anschlus.' Unfortunately, therefore, I have no possibilities of working productively at present."[59]

Subsequent versions of Kantorowicz's vita in 1938–1939 highlighted his newly developed American credentials, the impact of his Jewish identity on his ability to publish in Germany, and his desire for an appointment in the United States. In a vita from March 1939, he dropped the reference to having had an English governess and added reference to a series of lectures that he had given at Harvard, Columbia, Yale, and Smith College while on a temporary visa in the United States in early 1939. He revised, as well, his intellectual biography, deleting the narrative describing the series of dramatic shifts in focus in his scholarship pressed upon him by circumstance and presenting instead a narrative of continuity, prevented from publishing by the German state. In a final paragraph in that vita, he described his efforts and commitment to emigrate permanently to the United States.[60]

Kantorowicz's experience highlights, as well, a broader fact of the intellectual migration: A scholar's biography alone did not secure a man an appointment. As soon as he sent his vita to Demuth in July 1938, Kantorowicz began desperately reaching out to those he knew personally or who had complimented his book on Frederick the Second though never having met him, seeking their recommendations.[61] In August 1938, Fritz Demuth, having received one personal recommendation for Kantorowicz, urged him in a PS: "It would advisable to let us have as many more testimonials as possible." Letters speaking to the caliber of his work were important, but so were "personal opinions."[62] Having long resisted Theodor Mommsen's pleas that he consider at least a temporary visit to the United States, Kantorowicz had secured a temporary visa for a six-week visit to the United States, sought Mommsen's assistance in lining up lectures for him to deliver, and while in the United States eagerly made as many personal contacts as he could. As Mommsen had written to Kantorowicz, "A necessary precondition is personal acquaintanceship."[63]

Like so many others, Kantorowicz had entered the United States initially on a temporary visa. Under US immigration law, securing a permanent visa required that he leave the United States to apply for one. He had hoped to do so from Canada, but Canadian officials refused to make commitments in the absence of an individual being in Canada, so ultimately, Ernst Kantorowicz went to Havana. This was the context for a final vita, distinct from all the others, reflecting the particular work it had to do to qualify Kantorowicz for a non-quota visa under US immigration law. Drafted in July 1939, this vita became "Document 1" in Kantorowicz's case for a non-quota visa. The remaining documents in his application were keyed to it. Kantorowicz had been forced to retire in November 1934 and had not taught since that point. By others taking up his case, he had been offered a one-year appointment at Johns Hopkins, funded by grants from the Oberlander Trust and the Emergency Fund. At the last minute, an appointment at the University of California–Berkeley finally came through, but it too was an appointment of one year, and at the time that he was seeking the permanent visa, the salary terms of that appointment had not yet been set. So, it was the Hopkins appointment, with no reference to its limited term, that appeared on what I will call Kantorowicz's visa vita. On that vita, as well, was a statement that Kantorowicz had lectured at Oxford in 1936–1937, a fiction presented as documented fact, a ploy necessitated by the strictures of the non-quota visa exception requiring an applicant to have taught in the preceding two years. It, like the term of the teaching appointment in the United States, went unquestioned. At the end of that vita, as important as any other detail, and through which all its statements of fact were likely read, was a distinguished list of American references beginning with former American Ambassador William E. Dodd and Supreme Court Justice Felix Frankfurter.[64] Granted a non-quota permanent visa two days after his arrival in Havana, Kantorowicz traveled to Miami and on from there to Berkeley, where he would spend the next eleven years of his life.

Even apart from the strict numerical restrictions under US immigration law in place in the 1930s, the crisis in Europe would have brought European scholars seeking academic appointments to the United States and with them the vita as a job placement form. A visa was required of all immigrants, and quota immigrants too had to prove that they had a means of support in the United States. But the strict numerical national quotas on immigration, coupled with the narrowly tailored non-quota exception for professors, gave the vita an outsized role, one bound to produce instances of self-refashioning.

"Sigmund, didn't you say you were a kind of lecturer or academic lecturer at the University of Genoa?" The query was in a letter from Sigmund Cohn's cousin Ludwig Hamburger in September 1938.[65] Cohn had been a judge in Germany, not a professor, but having lost his position in 1933 under the Civil Service Restoration Act, he and his wife and two daughters had immigrated to Italy. In the nearly five years they had lived in Genoa, he had cobbled together a new livelihood and identity. He had earned a doctorate in law at the University of Genoa and had passed a state examination and certification to teach Italian and German. He had worked as a sworn translator, had taught German in private schools and as a substitute at the local university, and for three years he had been "a kind of assistant" working mostly on translations for the professor of national economy at the University of Genoa.[66]

In September 1938, Italy passed a race law that required Jews who had migrated to Italy after 1919 to leave the country in six months or face forced deportation. For Sigmund Cohn's family, such a deportation would mean being sent back to Germany. Understanding that the quota for immigrating to the United States was exhausted, Ludwig Hamburger described to Cohn the non-quota exception for professors.[67] It is unclear from their correspondence whether Cohn had had a vita before, but the one he now drafted in English claimed a new professional identity. "As you may see from the enclosed curriculum vitae I am an assistant professor in the university of Genoa (Italy), a city I moved to with my family in 1933 after having lost, being a Jew, my position as a judge in Germany."[68] Over the next four months, as one door of possible escape after another—Colombia, Argentina, Portugal, Cuba—closed in their faces, Cohn, his friend Rudi Hearns in the United States, and his cousin Ludwig Hamburger in Geneva, Switzerland, sent letter after letter and with each enclosed Cohn's vita. Letters from strangers.

One day, December 15, 1938, a telegram from his friend Rudi Hearns arrived with word of an academic appointment. "Your telegram," Cohn wrote in reply "was like a dream to us." A few days later, a letter from the New York City–based National Coordinating Committee for Aid to Refugees and Emigrants Coming from Germany confirmed the appointment on the staff of the University of Georgia.[69] Cohn had no idea how the appointment had come about. He had had no contact with anyone at the university, did not know what he would be teaching, the term of the appointment, or the salary. But he knew the most important thing: With this appointment he could secure non-quota visas for himself, his wife, and their two daughters.

The circuitous, fortuitous path by which Sigmund Cohn's vita produced an academic appointment and a path of safety out of Europe showed the complex networks through which vita traveled in the crisis and the possibility that, through a vita, one might present a professional self that, though a stranger, would provide the foundation for an appointment. Among those to whom Ludwig Hamburger had sent Sigmund Cohn's curriculum vitae had been a woman in New York City named Mrs. Sylvia Wubnig. Hamburger knew Wubnig through her husband, who had held a position in the International Labor Office in Geneva. She, in turn, passed Cohn's curriculum vitae to her personal friend Cecilia Rasovsky, who was secretary and executive director of the National Coordinating Committee for Aid to Refugees and Emigrants Coming from Germany, urging the committee to assist him. Through this committee, Cohn's vita and urgent need reached Harold Hirsch, a prominent Jewish German American lawyer and philanthropist in Atlanta. Cohn's doctoral training both in Germany and Italy in law and his background as a judge was likely appealing to Hirsch. In any event, Hirsch was a graduate of the University of Georgia, had a long record as a major benefactor of the university, and had close relations with the university's president.[70] It was through Harold Hirsch's intervention that the president of the University of Georgia offered an appointment, funded by Harold Hirsch, to Sigmund Cohn.[71]

For all those for whom a vita provided a lifeline, there were many more for whom it did not. As historian Laurel Leff notes, discrimination against women in European universities meant that they were far less likely to hold the kind of appointments that the State Department conditioned visas on, or to have achieved the kind of scholarly recognition—that is, as "world-class" scholars—on which aid organizations, foundations, and institutions like the New School conditioned financial support. Visas for non-quota immigrants were conditioned both on having held a teaching, not a research, appointment and on having received an offer of a teaching appointment in the United States. Both conditions were less likely for women. And so, discrimination became the foundation of exclusion.[72]

Lucie Adelsberger was a doctor and research scientist, an immunologist and pioneering allergist, with a long list of publications in prominent medical journals.[73] She had lost her scientific position at the Robert Koch Institute for Infectious Diseases in Berlin in 1933 under the Civil Service Restoration Act and was denied, like other Jewish doctors, the license to treat patients covered by public health insurance. For the next five years, she independently wrote scientific articles while also practicing medicine in the Jewish community in Germany until the Nazis passed a law stripping doctors who were Jewish of their medical licenses. Urged in fall 1938 to come to the United States on a temporary visa if she hoped to secure an offer of an academic appointment—"it is very difficult to get any sort of commitment on paper about a position if the applicant is not personally known"—she did so and received an offer of an instructorship in bacteriology at Harvard.[74] An executive order issued by President Roosevelt while Adelsberger was in the US in the wake of *Kristallnacht* might have enabled her to remain despite having entered the US on a temporary visa. But her concern for her elderly mother led her to return to Berlin. All her efforts to secure their mutual safety were stymied.[75] On her return to Berlin, Adelsberger was told by the US consular service that she did not qualify for a non-quota visa because she had engaged only in scientific work, not teaching.[76]

"My great fear," Walter Benjamin wrote his friend Theodor Adorno on August 2, 1940, "is that we have much less time at our disposal than we imagined." Adorno understood the magnitude of the danger as much as anyone. In a letter two weeks earlier, he had pressed Benjamin on the urgency of sending his curriculum vitae. Benjamin assured him that the vita and list of publications were coming; his bibliography would be incorporated into the vita given the press of time.[77] Like so many others, Benjamin had become versed in the intricacies of American immigration law. He wrote of quotas exhausted, of the necessity of an offer of a teaching appointment in the US, of the increasing emphasis the consulate in France was placing on the visa requirement of proof of teaching within the last two years—a requirement he could not meet—of the necessity of requirements being eased to make possible his immigration.[78]

Facing the threat of deportation to Germany if he remained in France and was captured, yet lacking an exit visa legally permitting him to leave France, on September 23, Benjamin crossed the border into Spain illegally. In a final note written two days later, facing what he called "a situation with no escape," Benjamin ended his life.[79]

Over the course of his adult life, Walter Benjamin wrote six *lebenslauf* and curriculum vitae.[80] Each tailored to the purpose for which it was written.[81] His last—the one written in response to Adorno's urgent pleading—was titled "Curriculum Vitae Dr. Walter Benjamin."[82] None of Benjamin's vitae achieved the goals for which they were written. To the extent that they have been a focus of scholarly attention, it has been as fragments of his intellectual biography, not as markers of his pursuit of the elusive security offered by an academic livelihood. Benjamin's vitae were modern in that they were written narratives, crafted to gain academic positions or funding. But they were anomalous in an equally important sense: Whether by virtue of personality or his lack of an institutional career path, or both, Benjamin's vitae traced the course of his life in ideas rather than milestones of a career. His vitae stood, in this sense, like Benjamin himself, apart.

Lucie Adelsberger's last letter to the Emergency Committee in Aid of Displaced Foreign Medical Scientists was dated January 5, 1941, a few months after Walter Benjamin's death. She had heard that the State Department was creating a special visa for scientists.[83] "And for me it all depends on getting such a visa," she wrote. Some six months later, an interoffice memorandum from July 1941, from the physicians' committee to the migration department, noted, "Some time ago, Dr. Libman, Chairman of our Medical Scientists Committee, received word from the above mentioned scientist who sought to obtain a non-quota visa. In as much as she has had no previous teaching experience, I am convinced that she would not be eligible for a non-quota visa—but I am merely calling this to your attention in case efforts to obtain a regular quota-visa for her should be made. Her Curriculum Vitae and other documents are on file with us." A month later, on August 12, 1941, the National Refugee Service replied, saying, "Upon examination of this material we feel that nothing can be done in this matter at the present time." The quota, they noted, was exhausted; there was no point in seeking affidavits, even if they had known whom to approach.[84]

Having failed to find a path of escape for herself and her mother, Lucie Adelsberger continued to provide medical care for Berlin's Jewish community. In May 1943, she was deported to Auschwitz. At war's end, she numbered among the survivors of the German death camps. She arrived in the United States on October 29, 1946, a stateless refugee. A set of notes by a caseworker for the physicians' committee from a few weeks after her arrival noted that she had already managed to secure a residency at Manhattan General Hospital for the remainder of that year.

Rather than acknowledging the US's restrictive immigration regime, the caseworker's notes placed the onus of her failure to escape on events in Europe. "The timing of her return to Germany in 1938, was such that she found herself caught in European events, unable to get out. . . . Even there," the notes went on, "she continued her medical work, but under primitive conditions and was, of course, removed from research developments. Because of this gap, Harvard is unable to utilize her services now, but has been told that there may again be opening for her after she has brought herself up to date." The file closed in 1947 with a note that Adelsberger was working at the Bedford Hills Sanitarium, one of the limited kinds of positions that émigré physicians, especially women, found open to them. A position at Harvard never materialized, but by at least 1951 she had returned to medical research, employed by the Laboratory Division of Montefiore Hospital in New York City, where she would remain for the rest of her career.[85]

night sky

Dear Frances,

I picked raspberries today along the road to our cabin. . . . The raspberries reminded me of when we were first looking at the cabin and you had fallen in love with it and the realtor picked raspberries along the driveway and gave them to you and you were so excited about the idea of our having a cabin that had raspberry bushes.

. . .

Oh, Frances, is your spirit out there somewhere that I can reach? Each day I try to grasp what has happened, but it just seems so unreal. I don't know how to go on.

. . .

I woke up again this morning in the morning that you had your stroke. I remembered your expression. I remembered the medics. And then, once again, my body was yours—lying in the bed, heavy, unable to move. And I needed then urgently to get up, to open the curtains and let the day in.

. . .

Every night when I go from the main cabin to our cabin, I look up and, if the sky is clear, I see the Big Dipper high above the main cabin. I remember the two of us trying to find the Big Dipper in the night sky in St. Paul for your space science class last winter. Me telling you it was the easy one and then my lying on the sidewalk searching the sky wondering aloud whether the sky could have changed since my childhood, but simply not being able to see it. The sky is so dark up here. You can see millions of stars. I think of you every night in that one quick glance upward.

. . .

I'm back to the start. Why did you die? Did you have to die? I'm back to the day of your stroke, the days in the hospital. . . . I am haunted. I feel lost.

. . .

How can it be August without you? We are broken. The three of us try to function, try to support each other, try not to get upset about things—a leaking roof, a driveway draining into the lake, a stopped-up toilet—that in the broader scheme of things are just not a big deal, but we are trying to deal with them in a fragile state, as we deal with the one thing that really does matter and that is that we don't have you. It's raining again. The roof is leaking. I'm exhausted. I'm going to bed.

. . .

Dad and I are home. The house feels like a place we used to live in a former life. Your [school] backpack is still sitting here on your chair [in the kitchen] where you'd packed it up on Sunday to be ready for school on Monday. Your purse is hanging on the back of the chair. Your cell phone is on the table.

. . .

Today I have felt an ache in my chest all day and an unshakeable sadness that I have given into with tears when I tried to speak and so I go quiet. I find myself thinking that we have done this long enough can't we have you back now. I no longer cry out, "I want her back," but the feeling remains deep and persistent. I cannot imagine that we must live the rest of our lives without you, and that in doing so the gap between us will grow—we will grow old, while you remain.

chapter five · "made to man's order"

You would not know it from a black-and-white photograph, but the Gene Autry Official Ranch Outfit, made by the M. A. Henry Co., was awash with color and texture. There was the plaid shirt (orange, black, red, and white); a short blue-and-khaki vest with an image of Gene Autry on the lower front of both sides; a red, white, and blue lariat; and the chaps, red, green and khaki in color at the top with "Gene Autry" emblazoned across the waistband and a creamy white, furry fabric running down the front and side of the legs from mid-thigh to the bottom. The playsuit was sold in a box with a large picture of Gene Autry on his horse, Champion, on the front.[1]

In its first season on the market in 1941, the fabric on the chaps of the Gene Autry cowboy playsuit was a goat fur from China. But even before Pearl Harbor, war in the Pacific cut off the Henry Company's supply and led the company's president, Milton A. Henry, to search for a new fabric on the US market, something cheap, with a dependable supply. The Gene Autry Official Ranch Outfit that Tommy McCormack and other children played in had that new fabric on the chaps.

Like most consumer products, it was a composite of the work of a number of enterprises and individuals. The fabric was made from a rayon fiber by Du Pont, a company that only a few decades before had made nothing other than explosives, woven into a high-pile fluffy fabric with the appearance of fur by the Woonsocket Falls Mill, marketed to the "trade" by E. F. Timme & Son, purchased by the M. A. Henry Co., and used on the chaps of its cowboy playsuit, bearing the name Gene Autry under a license with the "singing cowboy," purchased by retailers and jobbers for sale across the United States.

The commercialized market of playthings for children was a central element of the "land of desire" that historian William Leach describes taking shape in the opening decades of the twentieth century. At the heart of that world were department and chain stores and dry-goods houses committed, in Leach's words, to selling goods "cheaply in constantly growing volume and at higher profit levels."[2] But the observation relating to cheap goods and the search for profit never applied only to retailers. As the Gene Autry cowboy suit illustrates, it applied equally all the way up and down the manufacturing, distribution, and sales chain.

The American toy industry had taken shape in the opening decades of the twentieth century.[3] The first New York Toy Fair was held in 1903, the same year the inaugural issue of the industry trade magazine *Playthings* was published. Tariffs and the First World War played their role in the development of the industry, protecting US manufacturers and crushing the German toy business, such that by the 1920s, it was not a boast to claim the United States as the "real toy center of the world."[4] Buffalo Bill's Wild West shows at the end of the nineteenth century had first created a market for cowboy playsuits for boys. Radio shows and "talkies" expanded the market in children's playsuits in the 1920s and 1930s.[5] Toy buyers found their way to manufacturers through *The Playthings Directory*, which by the mid-1930s included over two dozen manufacturers of playsuits, including cowboy suits. But even with the expansion of the market in fantasy toys, playsuits represented a tiny fraction of the market in children's playthings.[6]

Milton Henry's company first appeared in *The Playthings Directory* in 1934.[7] Henry had worked his way into the novelty business, beginning as a salesman likely for the same company that by 1933 bore his name. Born in 1905, the youngest of eight children, only five of whom survived childhood, Henry's formal education ended at age fifteen. Henry's parents, Jews from Russia or Poland, had immigrated to the US in 1890 or 1891, part of the massive wave of immigrants from Eastern Europe that fed rising anti-immigrant hostility and led to increasingly restrictive immigration laws, culminating in the 1924 Immigration Act that—as the European crisis unfolded in the 1930s—narrowed the path of escape to a trickle. By 1938, the Henry Company had relocated its showroom to the heart of New York's toy district at 1107 Broadway.[8]

That same year, Gene Autry signed a contract with Mitchell J. Hamilburg to act as licensor for Gene Autry products. I suspect that it was Milton Henry who approached Hamilburg and Autry, leading in late 1940 to a licensing contract to produce a Gene Autry cowboy suit.[9] Under the contract, Autry received 5 percent of the wholesale price on the sale of every suit. For Milton Henry and his company, the license was a branding opportunity, setting its cowboy suit apart from others on the market, with the benefit of what amounted to free advertising that came with every new Autry recording, movie, appearance, and weekly radio broadcast of Autry's *Melody Ranch* show.[10]

On the eve of the first anniversary of his contract with Autry, just as Henry hoped for renewal of the contract, he lost his supply source for the cheap imported fur he was using on the chaps. Henry could afford no delay. The New York Toy Fair began in February. Toy buyers for department stores, hardware and auto chains, jobbers who resold goods across the country, and even small-scale store owners descended on New York for the fair to look at the goods and place orders. Merchandise, showrooms, and salesmen had to be ready. Orders in the weeks of the toy fair then had to be filled in time for retailers to get them on store shelves for the Christmas season beginning in November. Not being ready for the Toy Fair put Henry at risk of losing both a season and the Autry contract. It was a salesman in the plush toy business who suggested that Henry talk with someone at E. F. Timme & Son and likewise mentioned to a Timme salesman that Henry was in the market for a plush fabric.[11]

By the end of the 1930s, E. F. Timme & Son, based in New York City, had been in the plush fabric business for close to half a century. In 1897, Edward Timme, in his forties and already in the plush fabric business, established the partnership with his only son, Otto.[12] In 1913, the partnership had established the Woonsocket Falls Mill in Woonsocket, Rhode Island, acting as its sole agent.[13] By the end of the 1920s, Timme & Son's trademark plush fabric "Timme Tufts"—a fabric made from alpaca fur and used as lining in children's coats—had made Timme, pronounced "Timmy," a national name in the textile and clothing business and had made the business a source of family wealth.[14]

It was a family business. When the founder Edward Timme died in 1919, ownership and control of the business passed down through his children.[15] When Edward's son Otto died in 1937 and for five years after his death, his executors operated the business, including Edward Timme's grandson, William E. Roschen, who by that point had twenty years' experience in the business.[16] Roschen had worked summers at the firm while in textile school and been a stockholder and director of the Woonsocket Falls Mill. Returning from service in the US Navy in World War I in 1919, he joined Timme as an employee. In 1928, he became treasurer of Woonsocket, and in 1942, when E. F. Timme & Son was reorganized as a limited partnership, Roschen became the sole general partner; his aunt Martha E. Sultan and his cousins Ilse Bischoff and Carola Terwilliger became limited partners.[17]

The extended Timme family owned a majority of the stock in the Woonsocket Falls Mill. Other than a few unrelated small stockholders, the only non–family members to own stock in the mill were Arthur Robertshaw and his son Arthur Robertshaw Jr., who had been with the family business and had managed the mill throughout its history—Arthur Jr. taking over from his father—under a board of directors led and dominated by the Timme family.[18] E. F. Timme & Son purchased the raw materials the mill used, made design decisions, had exclusive contact with customers, handled all invoicing and collections for sales, and kept Woonsocket's books in its offices in New York, with Woonsocket paying a share of Timme's expenses, including for insurance.[19]

When William E. Roschen and Arthur Robertshaw Jr. began work in the business, "textiles" still largely meant fabrics created from animal, insect, and vegetable fibers: wool, fur, silk, cotton, and linen. But a revolution in the world of textiles resting on the modern science of chemistry and fed by war, depression, and growing mass-consumer markets was already in motion. The first man-made fiber—what would come, in the early 1920s, to be rebranded as "rayon"—was initially known as artificial silk. Pioneered in France in the 1890s from nitrocellulose, at about the same time in Britain it was discovered that treating cellulose with various chemicals transformed it into a yellow viscous liquid that they called "viscose," which could then be regenerated as threads by immersing the viscose in an acid bath. By the late 1920s, rayon was a $2 billion global industry, and the United States was the largest rayon producer in the world.[20]

The major producers of rayon in the United States at the start of the 1920s were controlled by British and German companies.[21] But a US company was in the process of making the United States a major site not just of rayon production but also of its control. As early as 1908, Du Pont, the American explosives giant, driven by the threat of excess capacity, had begun searching for alternative industries where it could generate profit from its expertise in nitrocellulose chemistry.[22] Beginning from a joint venture with a French company following World War I, in less than a decade Du Pont took over sole control of the enterprise and production of Du Pont rayon. The 1920s were the boom years for the rayon industry. From 1925 to 1929, Du Pont enjoyed an annual 33 percent return on investment. Although rayon sales continued to grow in the 1930s, the "rayon profit bonanza" ended with the Depression because of the dramatic increases in productive capacity that had accompanied the boom years. Du Pont's return on investment in the 1930s on rayon dropped to 7 percent per year, well below company expectation for its ventures.[23]

E. F. Timme & Son and the mills for which it acted as exclusive buying and sales agent, including Woonsocket Falls Mill, had been among the first customers for "Du Pont Rayon," as it was trademarked in 1925.[24] Timme's textile markets made it a cradle-to-grave firm, selling to trades ranging from the slipper to the outer-clothing trade, from the carpet to the home upholstery trade, from children's plush toys (stuffed animals) to the casket trade. The search for new customers and new markets was never-ending.[25] Initially, Timme's fabrics had been made entirely from vegetable and animal fibers: cotton velours, alpaca pile fabrics; mohair plushes, wool plushes, frieze (wool) velours.[26] These fibers did not disappear from its lines in the 1930s, but as was true in the textile field more generally, the lower cost of rayon meant that rayon or blends that included rayon claimed an increasing share of their fabric lines. By 1940, E. F. Timme & Son was buying hundreds of thousands of pounds of viscose rayon thread from Du Pont every year.[27]

What made rayon a magical fiber was not just its low cost but also that, as a product produced through chemistry, it could be made not only to mimic far more expensive natural fibers like silk but also to do things that traditional fibers could not. As a 1939 article in *Harper's Bazaar* titled "This Magic Called Rayon" put it, "It is as if you were able to dictate your own instructions to a spider: make your web coarse as horsehair—or make it a hundred times as fine; make it soft and spongy, like soft yarn; make it with a knot every three inches; make it shine like money—or make it dull as chalk."[28] The process began from wood pulp or cotton linters, the short, fuzzy fibers left on a cotton boll after the spinnable material had been removed. This was the "cellulosic" foundation of rayon. As the article described, the process "is controlled every step of the way; it is carefully planned in advance and the thread which emerges is one that has been made to man's order."[29]

By the point that "This Magic Called Rayon" was published, the early problems in producing rayon had been worked out, including things as basic as producing a fiber of uniform quality and one that did not dissolve when wet. In 1924, the company established a technical division and four years later spent half a million dollars building a new laboratory for the division.[30] And in 1927, within the Technical Division, Du Pont established a laboratory committed to Pioneering Research, under the directorship of a twenty-seven-year-old PhD chemist named William Hale Charch. In 1936, Du Pont merged its rayon company into the parent company as the "Rayon Department."[31]

In all its corporate R&D programs, Du Pont recruited chemists with PhDs from top university graduate programs, establishing pipelines of students through leading research scholars, funding graduate fellowships at top institutions, and hiring graduate students for summer employment. They were looking for Anglo-Saxon, Protestant men. Getting the right man depended on personal contacts. As the head of Du Pont's chemical department put it, "the matter of getting a reliable opinion about a prospect is very largely a personal matter, and not one which can be reduced to a formula."[32]

From the outset, science and profit were tightly interconnected at Du Pont. As the head of the Chemistry Department was regularly heard to say at the end of presentations, "This is very interesting chemistry, but somehow I don't hear the tinkle of the cash register."[33] Creating viscose rayon fibers *made to man's order* was fundamentally a collaborative process. Du Pont scientists worked closely with those in the trades that they hoped to enter. Research and development intertwined.[34] Within the Rayon Department, men in the Research and Development divisions visited department stores to see what merchandise currently made out of other fibers might be replaced by rayon, noting manufacturers' names for the purpose of introducing them to Du Pont Rayon fibers.[35] Working in the labs in the Pioneering Research and Technical divisions, Du Pont scientists created and adapted fibers, ran fabric trial runs, and tested the fibers and fabrics for properties seen as important to market success. And even as the Research Division tested a new fiber, the Development Division worked closely with manufacturers so that fibers could be created that would meet demand, sending them samples of fibers that were being pioneered in the lab for testing in the field. Manufacturers, in turn, sent back reports of the fiber's performance. Men from the Development Division visited customers at their factories and offices to see their operations and conduct interviews intended to assess the strengths and shortcomings of a fiber in its current stage of development.[36]

William E. Roschen was the man at Timme who worked with Du Pont. He exchanged phone calls, fabric samples, reports, and visits with men from the Development Division based in Wilmington, Delaware, who in turn reported to the Pioneering Research Division in Buffalo, New York, who in turn reported back to the Development Division in Wilmington, who in turn reported back to Roschen at Timme in New York City.[37] Every step in a fiber's development, in other words, was collaborative.

Among those collaborations were exchanges, beginning in 1938, related to the effort to create a fiber that could be woven into high-pile plush fabrics with a woolly appearance, the kind of fabric that Milton Henry would be looking for two years later for the Gene Autry cowboy suit. As the Development Department reported to Church in a 1939 memo, Roschen saw "a substantial market" for such a fabric.[38]

The effect Timme was looking for when it passed along to Du Pont a sample of curly mohair related to its texture and appearance, not fur's natural resistance to flame. They all knew—that is, William Roschen, Arthur Robertshaw Jr., the chemists at Woonsocket Falls Mill, the chemists in the Rayon Department at Du Pont—that rayon fibers manufactured to produce pile fabrics were inflammable; that is, they readily burned. Inflammability was a byproduct of this rayon thread *made to man's order* to become a fabric that looked like fur, even though it lacked one of fur's most important properties. As the director of Du Pont's Viscose Rayon Research Section would later note, the inflammability of viscose rayon yarn had been a matter of consideration by Du Pont from as early as the mid-1930s. But their various attempts to make the yarn flameproof had failed because other properties of the yarn, such as "running performance," "strength and durability" had been, as he put it, "very adversely affected."[39]

The threat fire posed to public safety had made regulation of fire hazards among the earliest sites of municipal and state regulation, beginning with wooden buildings and gunpowder manufacturers like Du Pont.[40] In the early twentieth century, horrific fires claiming hundreds of lives, like the Iroquois Theatre Fire in Chicago in 1903 and the Triangle Shirtwaist Fire in 1911, expanded the scope of fire regulation, leading to municipal ordinances and state laws regulating everything from air vents to fire escapes, and on to requiring that furnishings in public buildings, including theater curtains and scenery, be flame-resistant.[41] But there were no state, much less federal, laws banning the sale of inflammable fabrics, whether for home furnishings, clothing, or children's playsuits.[42]

New personal habits like the dramatic growth of cigarette smoking, including in bed and while driving, the increased use of fibers like rayon that lacked the natural flame-resistance of wool and other fibers of animal origin, the alarming increase—to retailers, manufacturers, and insurers—by the mid-1930s of "product liability" claims, and, most dramatically, World War II made the question of how and whether fibers and fabrics could be made flame-resistant or flameproof a matter of increasing attention.[43] In May 1936, the National Bureau of Standards published a circular on "Flameproofing of Textiles," noting that the circular was prepared in response to "[t]he widespread public interest in the flameproofing of textiles, as evidenced by the numerous requests for information on the subject."[44] In 1940, *The American Dyestuff Reporter* published a comprehensive bibliography with 208 entries and abstracts.[45] The publication dates on the entries highlighted for just how long the question of inflammability had concerned scholars and scientists in a broad range of fields.

What that 1940 article also made clear was that questions of inflammability, flameproofing, and testing were matters not just of human safety, property loss, or scientific inquiry, but also of profit. There was profit to be made in the market in developing an effective, patentable, water-resistant, flameproofing treatment. It was the hope of gaining access to the theater curtain trade and securing a patent on a flameproofing process that underlay Timme's and Woonsocket's attempts at flameproofing the pile fabrics they made from Du Pont rayon. But everything they tried failed. As Arthur Robertshaw Jr. would later note, the treatments "spoiled" the fabric.[46] As was true of every element of their relationship, Roschen shared their results with his contacts at Du Pont.[47]

Knowing the rayons it was producing for pile fabrics were inflammable, Du Pont nonetheless treated the issue as a matter that might be addressed at a later point.[48] In late April 1939, in a letter to Dr. Charch, Manfred Keller of the Development Division raised the concern that "wool is definitely less inflammable than viscose rayon. As a matter of fact, in England fire insurance companies ask woolen mills for higher rates if they use rayon in their plants." Although at this point, Keller noted, only one of their contacts in the carpet industry had inquired about "fire-proofness," he continued, "I could visualize where the degree of fireproofing might be of quite some importance in our carpet fiber development." He closed, "It might be well if some preliminary thoughts would be given to ways and means of fireproofing viscose rayon carpet fibers, in case this problem should become of major importance."[49] Charch's reply a few days later was short and to the point. To be effective, any such treatment would have to be water insoluble and would raise the price of the fiber. "If this subject ever gets to be of importance," he noted, they would address it then. "I believe, however, that our attitude on this subject should be one where we will delay consideration of it until some form of our synthetic fibers has found rather general acceptance in the carpet field."[50]

In 1941, Charch's Viscose Rayon Research Section finally began an investigation of the burning properties of rayon sparked by "certain brushed rayon fabrics hav[ing] apparently given a bad account of themselves." And they found that "brushed cotton and viscose fabrics flash very badly when flame is applied." But it was close to four years later, mid-March 1945, before an internal report was about to be issued.[51] And, in the meantime, as was true at Timme and Woonsocket, Du Pont continued production and sales.

The process that had begun at Du Pont with the chemical degeneration and reconstitution of wood pulp and cotton linters to make rayon was completed at Woonsocket Falls Mill where the Du Pont rayon fiber was woven into a high-pile fabric *made to man's order*.[52] In turn, at the Henry Company, in a sort of fabric disassembly and reassembly line, Henry's employees cut the yards of fabric woven by the Woonsocket Falls Mill into pieces and sewed them – roughly a third of a yard of fabric per cowboy suit – to make the front of the chaps of the Gene Autry Official Ranch Outfit. At the Henry Company factory in Passaic, New Jersey, Henry had two hundred employees. Any number of those employees bought the Gene Autry cowboy suit for their own children or for a relative's or friend's child.

What Milton Henry knew about the high-pile fabric he purchased through E. F. Timme & Son would only become a point of contention later. The Woonsocket Falls Mill and E. F. Timme & Son replaced the Du Pont Rayon trademark with their own tradenames and advertising that were intended to and in practice created the impression of fabric woven from natural fibers. What Du Pont shipped to one of Timme's mills as rayon left the mills with invoices listing a fabric with names like "Peachfox," "Chamois," "lambs wool." These names were representations of color, not fiber content, Timme would later say. All the fabric that the Henry Company purchased from Timme and Woonsocket was high-pile rayon with a cotton backing, but it was only in December 1944, after Timme and Woonsocket signed a cease-and-desist order with the FTC, that Timme began stamping the invoices it sent to the Henry Company "rayon and cotton."[53]

Later, when the harm their actions produced threatened their reputations and profits, all three entities and their principals put everything they had into deflecting responsibility onto others in the manufacturing and sales chain. But that was only later. Through the war years, their focus was on sales.

When Henry went looking for a fabric to take the place of the goat fur on the chaps of the Gene Autry cowboy suit, what he cared about was appearance, cost, and reliability of supply. E. F. Timme & Son could offer him all three. "Peachfox Fluffy," the Timme fabric Henry settled on, had a fluffy fur-like appearance and a cotton backing; except for the cotton backing, it resembled the fur that Henry had been using. It had the advantage of being cheap, especially in comparison to the alternatives: $2.10 a yard rather than $4.00 a yard for a high-pile fabric that was a blend of wool and rayon. And it was available in a secure supply.[54] In March 1942, Henry signed a contract with Timme and over the next three years purchased thousands of yards of its plush pile fabric.[55]

Gene Autry had seen a sample of the first suits Henry made under the contract in 1941, the ones with the goat fur on the chaps, but what they were made from was not what concerned him. Looks, style, and quality—that is, whether the suits were similar in quality to the suits endorsed by other personalities—were what he cared about. By the time the new suits came off the line, the ones with the fabric from Woonsocket Falls Mill, Autry was in the military. Autry's agent, Mitch Hamilburg, saw one of the new suits, but like Autry, his concern was looks and style, not fabric content.[56]

The only other major change the Henry Company made in the Gene Autry Official Ranch Outfit in these years stemmed directly from Autry joining the US Army Air Corps in summer 1942. Henry replaced the cowboy hat in the Gene Autry cowboy suit with an army-style khaki hat. The change was a savvy business move promoting wartime sales by drawing on Autry's own carefully calculated image as a patriot. Autry's enlistment was itself a move to protect his brand. With other stars going into the service—Jimmy Stewart, Clark Gable, Ty Powers—Autry thought asking for a deferment would hurt his image. So, he maneuvered his way into the army air corps and made his induction a media event on his own radio show.[57]

Henry had the first Gene Autry Official Ranch Outfits featuring the new fuzzy fabric on the chaps on models in his New York showroom in time for the spring 1942 Toy Fair. "A lot of customers were in the market very early," he explained, "on account of the shortage of goods."[58] He might have completed the statement: the shortage of goods on account of the war. By late spring he was filling the first orders. The new suits would be on the shelves of department stores, chain stores, variety and five-and-dime stores, hardware and auto accessory stores, and local mom-and-pop stores for the 1942 Christmas season beginning in November. Depending on the components the suit included, it sold for between $3.49 and $4.95.[59]

In their very inconsequence, Gene Autry cowboy suits reflected a basic fact of the manufacturing and retail world. "The general public seldom realizes," Ralph Hower noted in his monumental study of Macy's of New York, "the extraordinary extent to which a large store devotes its staff and resources to buying rather than selling."[60] On the eve of World War II, Macy's stocked over 394,000 different types of merchandise, not counting different sizes and colors.[61] Macy's did not sell the Gene Autry Official Ranch Outfit, but other department stores did.[62] And the point Hower made about Macy's held true not only for them, but also for the variety, five-and-dime, and hardware and auto accessory stores that sold the Gene Autry cowboy suit.

The Gene Autry cowboy suit reflected another basic fact of the American manufacturing and retail world by the mid-twentieth century: national distribution. As Milton Henry would note, "Oh, we sold them to McCrory's Stores Corporation, H. L. Green Company . . . Sears Roebuck—and various department stores throughout the country, as well as the large jobbing houses throughout the country."[63] And so cowboy suits made in Passaic, New Jersey, and the Bronx by a New York company were distributed and sold across the United States.

Chain stores often bought centrally, whether collecting orders from individual stores or deciding centrally which stores would sell particular merchandise and how many articles.[64] McCrory's, a variety chain store established in 1881 with the first store in Scottsdale, Pennsylvania, by 1942 had 202 stores.[65] The buyer for McCrory's had offices in the same building at 1107 Broadway in New York City where the Henry Company showroom was located. In 1942, McCrory's ordered 41½ dozen Gene Autry cowboy suits, just shy of five hundred suits, and sold the suit in forty-six towns and cities across sixteen states and the District of Columbia. The quantity for any given McCrory store reflected the size of the market and ranged from six dozen for McCrory's Brooklyn store down to one-quarter dozen, a mere three suits, for the McCrory's in Chambersburg, Pennsylvania. In 1943, McCrory's more than doubled its purchase of Gene Autry cowboy suits, buying 1,170 suits from the Henry Company and expanded the number of stores it sold the suit in as well, from forty-six to sixty-seven in twenty states and the District of Columbia.[66]

Regionally based chains like McCrory's, and other chains like Hecht's, by virtue of their store locations concentrated sales of the Gene Autry cowboy suit in the eastern half of the United States. But national retailers like Goodyear Tire and Rubber Company and national jobbers and purchases by smaller stores meant Gene Autry cowboy suits were sold across the nation.

A point that *The Playthings Directory* had made about toys in 1925—namely, that for stores that were not in the toy business, toys could nonetheless be an important draw, "attracting the juveniles and their parents"—held as true during the war as it had in earlier years.[67] And this truth was compounded by the fact that, during the war, many goods that stores had sold for children—metal toys, "wheel goods"—were harder to come by because of rationing and materials diverted for war needs. So, one could find the Gene Autry cowboy suit at hardware stores like Albosta Hardware in Saginaw, Michigan; Burton's Hardware in Westbrook, Maine; and City Hall Hardware in Providence, Rhode Island. Goodyear sold the suits in its own stores and catalog as well as acting as a jobber selling to small, independent auto accessory stores like the five stores Louis Lutz and his wife owned in a partnership: Lou's Auto Stores.

The Lutzes' main store was in Cumberland, Maryland, with smaller stores in Frostburg, Maryland; Bedford, Pennsylvania; and Piedmont and Kaiser, West Virginia. They sold auto accessories, radio supplies, and tires. It was during the war, likely pressed by the shortage of goods in his regular lines, that Louis Lutz added toys, including playsuits and sporting goods.[68] In early March 1944, Louis Lutz went into New York City for the Toy Fair.[69] As a Henry Co. salesman told Lutz, "all the other auto accessory stores who were handling toys were selling the same type merchandise." He ordered six dozen Gene Autry cowboy suits that day. They arrived in July. He put them in his stores in October or November for the 1944 Christmas season. That first season, they sold one and a half dozen cowboy suits, carrying over the remaining suits for the next year. In 1945, they sold most of the remaining suits, left with only half a dozen to sell in 1946.[70]

The Henry Company made its last major sales of the Gene Autry Official Ranch Outfit with the fuzzy, fur-like fabric on it in spring 1945. In one sale in early April 1945, the Henry Company sold five thousand Gene Autry cowboy suits to Goodyear, which Goodyear distributed, in turn, to its Tire and Auto Accessory Stores across the United States, sold through its 1945 holiday catalog, and sold as a jobber to other tire and auto accessory stores.

Well after the Henry Company stopped selling the Gene Autry cowboy suit with the fuzzy, fur-like fabric on the chaps, the suits continued to circulate in the marketplace, and in this regard the Gene Autry cowboy suit reflected another basic fact of the retail world. Having sold the Gene Autry cowboy suit to national jobbing houses, the suits continued to find their way into stores for sale. Ben Sayre, the manager and salesman at a bicycle and sporting goods store in Terre Haute, Indiana, bought a dozen of the Gene Autry cowboy suits in the fall of 1945 for the holiday season from "a traveling man" who came by the store. The store did not generally handle cowboy suits and toys, but it was the first season after the end of the war and "our other lines were hard to get . . . we had to have something to sell, see."[71] Well after the 1945 Christmas season, the suit appeared on store shelves far from New York. Namie's five-and-dime in Jonesboro, Louisiana, was selling the suit with the fur-like chaps in August 1947, when Charles Baragona Jr.'s mother went shopping for a birthday present for her son.

There were also all those retailers who, like Louis Lutz at his Lou's Auto Store, had bought the suit for sale in one season only to find they had suits remaining, so that even though the Henry Company was no longer selling the Gene Autry cowboy suit with the fuzzy fur-like fiber on the chaps, the Gene Autry cowboy suit was still being sold.[72] And so families like Richard Szumita's parents in Pawtucket, Rhode Island, could buy the Gene Autry cowboy suit from City Hall Hardware in December 1947 for their youngest son for Christmas.

And beyond sales, there were hand-me-downs. Verne Wilhelm, an auditor for Goodyear, had bought the Gene Autry cowboy suit for his son from a Goodyear outlet store in Parsons, Kansas in October 1945. He liked to buy his children something on his road trips. In fall 1947, the Wilhelms passed the suit down to their neighbors, the Timberlakes, for their son Scott. The two families had been friends since the Timberlakes first moved into the neighborhood; their girls started in kindergarten together.[73] There were hand-me-downs for Halloween and suits long since put away in the attic brought out when a younger child came of playsuit age.[74] All of which meant that even as the Henry Company in 1947 introduced a redesigned Gene Autry Official Ranch Outfit, no longer featuring fur or something that looked like fur on the chaps, the suits the company had made from spring 1942 to spring 1945 continued to circulate in the market.

magical imaginings

Dear Frances,

The summer is coming to an end. It hurts so badly to see/know that your classmates are all preparing to head off to college, to know that you too would have been excitedly planning.

. . .

Dad and I paddled for several hours tonight. It is our only way of coping with evening and nightfall—time we almost always spent with you. The night was calm after a later afternoon rain. It is supposed to get very hot here in the next day or two. Grieving is made harder in the heat.

. . .

I used to wake in the mornings and had to remind myself that you were gone. Forever. Now I know and a deep, penetrating sadness has settled in. I miss you, sweetheart, so desperately. Even as we, or maybe now especially as we move into what would have been your final weeks at home before starting your freshman year, I feel the ache of you being gone more deeply. It's almost as though I feel like these are my last few weeks with you.

. . .

How is it that I can reach a point where I think I fully know you are gone only to be ambushed later in the day, caught afresh all over again as one who has just been told the news.

. . .

Dad and I took a very short paddle today. As we paddled a small aluminum boat passed us with the sort of motor at the rear where the driver steers by holding a tiller. It's the second time we've seen this pair: a young college age guy at the tiller and sitting at the front of the boat, a college age girl with long blonde hair. They look like they could be a couple. Each time it has caught me—today the girl had on a green jacket. I imagined that this could have been you at some point on this lake with a boyfriend at the tiller. I could see you in such a boat, with your hair streaming out behind you and it has left me feeling so sad that it can never be so.

...

The signs of fall are clear: pants and long sleeves all day, sunny, but cool, and the darkness earlier each night. 8:20 p.m. tonight. It means that the part of the awake evening in the dark—time that can no longer be escaped by paddling—is getting longer. The darkness presses in on us and we ward it off with lights.

...

I find my thoughts returning to that young 'couple' in the small alumacraft boat with the tiller. This morning while Dad and I were paddling, I found myself excitedly thinking that you might have liked such a boat. I thought about you zipping around the lake in your little boat, laughing, hair streaming out behind you. It fills me with a sort of contentment to imagine it. It is not the kind of boat I would have ever imagined getting, but I see now it would have been perfect. You would have loved the freedom of that little boat. I mentioned it to Dad and he tried to ruin it for me—saying it would be the worst kind of boat for a big lake like this, that they are inherently unstable with the tiller and driver both at the back. He would have gone on, but I stopped him. I said, "Humor me. It can't be in any event, so just let me have my beautiful dream."

...

The strange peace I felt yesterday imagining the boat you might have had and visions of you, blonde hair streaming, Sam happily on board, tooling about the lake is gone. I would be happy, whole in an instant if you suddenly, magically reappeared.

chapter six · global war

The beginnings of a transformation of the vita into a job placement form that began from the margins in the 1930s, fed by the search of American scholars for jobs in a depressed market and the desperate search of Jewish scholars and others at risk in Nazi-occupied Europe for escape and even survival, was fed in turn by global war. For it was in the years of World War II that curricula vitae began to appear with regularity in American academic life.

War shapes the course of lives. There was the continued, if vastly diminished, stream of émigré scholars fleeing Nazi-occupied Europe, the continued search for job security of those who had come earlier, and displaced and stateless scholars after the war. There was the urgent need for thousands of highly trained men and women in government and for secret war projects and other war research. And while war projects secured many hundreds of men in graduate programs draft deferrals, their time was nonetheless not their own, their research, training, and lives diverted. Then there were the returning US servicemen who had been unceremoniously pulled out of college, graduate programs, and teaching by the draft, who with the war's end were equally unceremoniously dropped back into civilian life.

Though the term *curriculum vitae* continued in these years to be used primarily by émigré scholars, the vita became a fundamental introductory form for all these men and others whose timelines and networks had been disrupted by war. In other words, the vita, introduced as a placement form in American academic life in the 1930s by the forced flight of European émigré scholars, gained a deeper footing in response to the displacements of a violent, global, disordered world. But even as it did, the form itself was transformed.

There were, no doubt, a range of forces at work in the proliferation and

Americanization of the vita. But the war itself was high among them. In the late 1920s, when the phenomenon first emerged of men and women shifting for themselves, fashioning their own letters and supplementary documents of introduction in search of teaching appointments it was remarked as strange, new, and anomalous. The scale of unemployment among PhDs and the tide of letters from strangers through the years of the Depression had provoked concern and discussion and led to the first attempts, however limited and ineffective, to systematize placement. But war disrupts established ways of doing things. War has the capacity to render the anomalous unremarkable.

The war did not come to American colleges and universities all at once. It came, as you might say it did to the nation more generally, in stages. There was first the steady stream of émigré scholars, beginning with Hitler's rise to power and increasing dramatically by decade's end as the German war machine rolled across Europe. Through the war years and after, one could find vitae of émigré scholars in departmental placement files in any field.[1] "Years of wandering" was how geographer Eric Fischer titled the section of his unpublished memoir following the German takeover of Austria in March 1938 and the effort to find safety.[2] Only in February 1941 did Fischer arrive in the United States, together with his wife Irene and young daughter. They had found safety but not security. As Fischer described, "During the first two years, I must have written several dozens of application letters, documented with curricula vitae and lists of publications. Some were not answered at all, most brought negative form letters, some writers showed human interest; a very few came with, however unacceptable, offers."[3]

German and Austrian vitae had been narratives of a life written in complete sentences in paragraph form. They were documents to be read, not taken in at a glance. Life in the United States changed their vitae. The one-page "Autobiographical Statement" that Eric Fischer sent to Bernadotte Schmitt and William T. Hutchinson in the Department of History at the University of Chicago in spring 1944, three years after arriving in the US, was in the form of a list, organized by category: personal status, education, professional experience and achievement, foreign languages, travels, memberships, references.[4] He listed his publications on a separate page. But publications too now regularly appeared as an integral component, one category on, a scholar's vita.[5]

The processes by which individuals learn and become acculturated to professional norms and forms, and the significance of forms for identity and knowledge, are rarely the subject of discussion, much less retrospective scholarly inquiry. What was it that led émigré scholars to refashion their vitae as lists? War placed a premium upon time. Bard College Dean Charles Harold Grey, as Fischer explained, advised him "not to overload my curriculum and list of publications, rather prepare several different ones, aimed at the presumed interests of the addressee: people are inclined to glance superficially over lengthy papers, but not actually read them."[6] What Cornelia Visman has noted of files applied equally to the vita.[7] The vita structured as a list facilitated economy of reading, broke not just time but life into discrete units, allowed the reader to skim, focusing on what most interested them, imposing as little as possible on a reader's time to which the author had no claim, and yet simultaneously materialized key elements of one's identity. In the context of the war, moreover, a narrative vita positioned a scholar in the past, in the old world. By contrast, a vita formulated as a list, divided into categories, signaled something both modern and American, suggesting that its author had transitioned successfully to American professional life.

Both the vita Fischer addressed to faculty in the History Department at the University of Chicago in 1944 and a vita he sent to Harold Sprout in the Department of Politics at Princeton in September 1945 began with "Personal Status." But in form and content this section of the two vitae differed in meaningful ways. The opening of the 1944 vita read,

> I was born in Vienna, Austria, January 13, 1898.
> I am married to Irene Fischer, graduate of Vienna University and Institute of Technology (mathematics and descriptive geometry), presently working with Professor John T. Rule, Mass. Inst. of Tech. We have a daughter 7 years of age. We came to America in February 1941, and took our First Papers in June 1941. My draft status is 4A.

In the 1945 vita, phrases stripped of verbs replaced full sentences. Much of the personal detail was gone:

> Born Vienna, Austria, January 13, 1898.
> Married to Irene Fischer, graduate of Vienna University and Institute of Technology (mathematics and descriptive geometry).

The differences reflected in part the different work he needed the two documents to do. From the time of their arrival in the US, the Fischers were dependent on both their incomes for their survival. His vita might lead to not only a position for him but one for her as well.[8] By September 1945, their family circumstances and the larger context had changed. The war was over; his wife Irene had found a teaching position in Washington, DC, where they had settled.

But the difference in the two vitae was not just one of detail. Perhaps it seems a small difference—the stripping of subject and verb from statements about place and date of birth and marital status; the disappearance altogether of the fact that they had a child. After all, Eric Fischer's name appeared at the top of the document. And yet. The shift from narrative to list, the erasure of first person, the conversion of a life to data made it easier to ignore the life, the humanity of the subject of this document.

And there was another significant difference in the two vitae. In the 1944 vita, Fischer had divided his professional experience and achievements into two categories:

"a. abroad"
"b. In the United States."

Within each the listings were chronological. In contrast, in the 1945 vita, "Professional Experience and Achievements" was a single category organized in reverse chronological order. In other words, the section began in the present, in the United States. Eric Fischer's life was now here, and his vita—in form and substance—made that clear.

When Eric Fischer had arrived in the United States in spring 1941, a more general uncertainty reigned. Though the United States was not yet formally at war, the draft had begun, and many faculty, especially in the sciences, were already engaged in war-related research on government contracts—absorbing as well, in many cases, their graduate students' research time.[9] Spring was ordinarily when teaching and research appointments were made for the next year. But departments and universities knew neither how many students nor how many faculty they would have in the fall.

In March 1941, reflecting the particular demand that the war already was placing on those with advanced training in physics, but also the more general uncertainty of the moment and the demands of total war, the Physics Department at Princeton circulated a form for all graduate students to complete. "Because of the defense situation it is very difficult to know exactly what members of our staff will be here during the coming year and how many of them will be devoting most of their research time to defense." Noting that "much of the defense research is of real scientific interest and the Department plans to consider work on such projects equivalent to ordinary research in graduate training," the text continued, "Would you be willing, should the need arise, to substitute for the research ordinarily expected of you either," and then there were two blanks for "teaching" or "work on defense projects."[10] I expect that most responded affirmatively to filling either role as the department needed. But that choice was made easier by the fact that many of their professors were or would be engaged in applied research for the war, the explanation relating to the "scientific interest" of the research, and that it would count toward a man's degree. As would become clear only with time, the moment marked a sea change in elite universities' attitudes toward applied research and government contracts.[11] The shift extended well beyond physics and the sciences more generally.

The scale and urgency of the need, new structures of employment at newly created laboratories and war projects on and away from university campuses, funded under contracts with the federal government, led to new hiring models with implications for how men saw, understood, and marketed themselves. The Metallurgical Laboratory at the University of Chicago offers a case in point. Established in February 1942 for the secret study and use of the newly discovered chemical element plutonium, the laboratory, at its peak in July 1944, had a staff of over two thousand. Filling that staff required recruiting on a wholesale scale by men who wrote to other men they did not know. "Dear Sir," began a December 1943 letter addressed to the "Head, Department of Chemistry" at the University of Pennsylvania, and signed by the "Assistant Personnel Director" of the Metallurgical Laboratory. A letter most certainly repeated to other "Heads" at major chemistry departments across the country. "This letter is a request for assistance from you. I realize full well the extra burden that has been placed on your shoulders during these trying times. . . . However, the work we are doing here at the University of Chicago Metallurgical Laboratory is of such vital importance to the war effort, and our needs for well-qualified men have grown so greatly that we are no longer able to meet the demands through ordinary channels." They needed a large number of men at every level of training in chemistry and chemical engineering: bachelor's, master's, doctorates. "I am enclosing a supply of blanks which you may use to furnish us the names of such men. . . . Secrecy requirements" made it impossible to divulge details of the lab's work beyond saying that the work "will have a decided effect on the war's outcome."[12]

Reflecting the long-standing division between original and applied research, the Department of Chemistry at Penn neatly divided their placement files between positions in academia and industry. The letter from the Met Lab was filed in the placement file for academic positions: the Met Lab was at the University of Chicago under the supervision of University of Chicago faculty. The war blurred the distinction between industry and academic positions. Men in both contexts during the war worked on applied research under government contracts. And as was true for the positions at the Met Lab, so too for industry research positions—applicants completed forms.[13]

A blank. Translation: a form. Industry qualification blanks included not only education, experience, publications, references, and so forth but an extensive list of personal details: place and date of birth, marital status and other dependents, citizenship, height, weight, hair color, physical disabilities and so on. Completing a form, one answers the questions asked. Constructing a form of one's own, men looked to forms they knew as models. And so, just as those desperately searching for academic employment in the 1930s had used teacher placement registration forms as their model in fashioning documents for their own introduction, so too here men duplicated to some extent the forms they knew. The scale of the need, the stakes of the endeavor, the urgency of the event meant that far more men than ever were completing industry qualification or application "blanks," or research lab blanks, and at the same time—or, years later, when with war's end they were released to return to their first hope of an academic position—fashioning their own forms.[14]

The proliferation of forms more generally—itself accelerated by war—contributed to the transformation of vitae from narrative to list divided by categories. In 1940, the American Council for Émigrés in the Professions (ACEP) began giving registrants a form to complete, titled "Outline of Curriculum Vitae."[15] The form was divided into categories: personal data, education, medical training, publications, licensure and preparation for medical practice in the United States, First Papers. Each had a set of questions with blanks for responses. So, for example, under personal data: name, religion, age, date of application, married, single, divorced, children or number of dependents. At the bottom of the form: a request for six photographs, suggesting that while the form itself would be copied to circulate for potential positions, original photographs would accompany the form. The ACEP's focus was émigré professionals—doctors and lawyers—including medical scientists and legal academics, not academics more generally. But it highlights the role the vita was coming to have as a placement form in professional life and advanced that role.[16]

Universities too in faculty appointments expanded their use of forms. The University of Minnesota had first adopted a "Request for Information" blank from candidates for faculty positions at the university in the 1920s, the same context in which university placement offices adopted Teacher

Placement blanks as a tool in placing their students. The original form does not, though, seem to have been systematically used. But in 1945, the School of Chemistry turned to a revised version of the form in its consideration of candidates for faculty appointments. So, for example, writing in October 1945 to a young chemist who had spent the war years working on the Manhattan Project at Oak Ridge, Tennessee, Dean S. C. Lind wrote, "If you would be interested in considering a position with us, I should like to hear more about your plans. I enclose one of our forms for request for information. If you are interested I trust it will not be too much trouble to fill it out and return it to me in the near future."[17]

The "Request for Information" blank was one example of a form that played a role in training candidates in the information relevant to a university making a faculty appointment. It expressed an interest in formulaic descriptions of one's life, training, and experience. The 1945 version of the Minnesota form differed in important respects from the form first adopted in the 1920s. The original form, in keeping with the belief that handwriting offered the measure of a man, asked the "informant" to complete it in their "own handwriting." The revised form specified that answers be typed. While applicants were still asked to submit a photograph, there was no longer a question asking for "church affiliation, if any." Instead of asking whether the individual was "in good health," the form now asked candidates to "indicate any physical or health disabilities." The 1920s form had asked whether the individual was married but had not asked about children. The 1945 form had blanks for both marital and parental status, including number of children. And whereas the 1920 form had not asked about citizenship, the 1945 form did. The bulk of questions on both versions of the form related to education, honors, teaching experience, publications, and references.

Although both forms were numbered lists of questions, the two had a dramatically different feel. The 1920s form had a conversational quality. Most of the questions were framed explicitly as questions. The 1945 form no longer had this quality. With very few exceptions, verbs, question marks, complete sentences were gone. The shift in format had not made for a shorter form. There were now twenty-nine questions rather than the original twenty, and the form was a page longer. But it felt more direct. And expectations had risen. The 1920s-era form asked, "Have you written for publication? What?" The 1945 form assumed faculty candidates would have publications: "Attach your bibliography." The title of the form was itself important: Request for Information. What was sought here was not a life story but selected facts of a life.

One can see the appeal of standardized application forms for universities and individual departments. They offered a standardized set of metrics and the same categories of information from each candidate. Forms enabled one to quickly scan a candidate's qualifications and return to any particular qualification, because that element appeared always at a particular spot on a particular page of the form. Forms did not take the place of the kinds of personal exchanges that had long defined academic placements. The School of Chemistry's files at the University of Minnesota, like those of others, in the 1940s were thick with correspondence related to a handful of young men who had spent the formative years of their early careers in the Manhattan Project. The School of Chemistry asked these men, just as they did men seeking positions who wrote with no introduction (letters from strangers), to complete the university form. No one questioned the request.[18] They had become acculturated to forms. The war had continued their education in this most important respect.

"No longer able to meet the demands through ordinary channels." This is what the query from the Met Lab had said. The point was repeated in different ways through the war years. Before the war, leading men fielded queries about potential candidates for a position. In letters and in conversations, as at annual professional meetings, they responded with suggestions, describing a man's qualifications and, when offering multiple men's names, describing their relative strengths and weaknesses.[19] This system did not disappear with the war; in fact, the state's war research machine was built through it.[20] But the demand for technical brainpower outstripped the capacity of the system. Total war required the skills of large numbers of highly trained individuals in every field.[21] Not only chemistry, physics, and engineering, but also agriculture, economics, geography, psychology, sociology, history, anthropology, languages. And so with growing frequency, those in search of a man, whether for a teaching appointment or research under a government war contract—and most often, they did use the language "man"—asked "any man who is available and may be interested" to write for themselves.

Such requests were not limited to projects on the scale of the Metallurgical Laboratory or Manhattan Project. "Dear Sir," opened a letter dated April 30, 1943, from the executive officer of the NDRC-funded Explosives Research Laboratory at Carnegie Institute of Technology in Pittsburgh to Dean Lind at the School of Chemistry at the University of Minnesota. The laboratory in Pittsburgh was adequately staffed at the moment, but the related laboratory at Woods Hole, Massachusetts, "under the direction of Dr. E. Bright Wilson of Harvard University," was in "urgent need" of five or six men in physical chemistry or physics training, two or three of whom needed to be men "with Ph.D.'s. . . . If you know of any man who is available and who may be interested in such a position, will you please ask him to forward me, as soon as possible, a brief resumé of his career with any other information that may be pertinent. A photograph should be included as well as a transcript of his academic record. Please ask him to request several of the professors under whom he has studied and who know him best to write me letters of recommendation."[22] The recommendations of advisors, as this query suggested, remained important, but the process of finding a man would not begin from them or rest as exclusively on them.

The scale and urgency of the need for those with advanced training was itself an engine for the curriculum vitae, but equally so was the uncertainty of life produced by total war. Uncertainty about the future was the most certain fact of the war years. Eric Fischer's letters and enclosed vitae ("autobiographical statements") to faculty in the History Department at Chicago and the Department of Politics at Princeton in 1944 and 1945 reflected a precarity of academic life not limited to émigré scholars in the war years. Fischer arrived in the United States in February 1941. By necessity, he initially focused his energies on learning English. It was the war and its urgent need for individuals with advanced training in geography that provided a serial security for him through the war years. He secured his first real academic appointment in 1943: a yearlong contract to teach geography in an Army Services Training Program at Bard College.[23]

By the fall of 1943, more than 30 percent of the students in American colleges and universities were there by virtue of military training programs for the Army, Navy, and Air Force.[24] The programs provided not only essential training but also employment for teachers, the war having cut deeply into college and university enrollments, and it provided as well funding for institutions. But Fischer's appointment, like the programs more generally, was temporary, ending altogether in 1944. As Fischer explained, "I share the fate with many others to have to look for another position because of the reduction of the ASTP and the complete uncertainty about the fate of Bard College under the curtailed program." He added, "Being a rather recent immigrant I have not the connections of born Americans."

A year and a half later, in September 1945, Fischer's vita to Professor Harold Sprout in the Political Science Department at Princeton made it clear where he had found his next temporary foothold: "Present Position: Research analyst, Office of Strategic Services, Washington, D.C."—and, handwritten in pen, "geographer, P-4." But as Fischer explained in the accompanying letter, this position too was about to end. The war was over "and as this organization"—the Office of Strategic Services (OSS)—"will liquidate within a few months, I try to find some other adequate position." Again, his fate was a shared one. Hundreds of scholars from a broad range of academic disciplines had been drawn into war work with the OSS.[25] While some held tenured positions to which they could return, many others had no such security.[26]

The postwar release of men from their wartime positions became another force in the proliferation of vitae not only from men in search of positions but on their behalf by those who had so recently depended on their skills. Within a matter of days following the Japanese surrender, Francis Wheeler Loomis, who before the war had been chair of the Department of Physics at the University of Illinois and who through the war held the position of associate director of the Radiation Laboratory at MIT, circulated an announcement of the imminent availability "of the largest block of physicists, electronic engineers and the like which has ever been gathered together for group research."

Men had long gained new supporters through the structure of academic placement and appointments, as a man trained at one institution was appointed as an instructor at another and, a few years later, recommended for an appointment at a third institution with the support of both the men who had trained him and men at the institution where he had held an instructorship or other teaching appointment. What was new here was, in part, the scale. I mean not just the numbers, although they were important, but what those numbers meant or had allowed. War projects like the Radiation Laboratory at MIT; the Metallurgical Laboratory at the University of Chicago; the Manhattan Project at Los Alamos, New Mexico, and Oak Ridge, Tennessee; and so on had gathered all the talent in a few places and, under the pressures of war, tested it. There was no equivalent in the disaggregated academic placement system that had existed before the war. As Loomis's announcement from the Radiation Lab noted, the men and women to be released accounted for "a large fraction of the physicists and electronic engineers available for staffing academic departments."

What was also new was the demand and the scale of the market for their skills. "Industrial companies," Loomis noted, "are very interested in employing large numbers and will begin recruiting them" as soon as they can be released. "In my opinion," he closed, "it would be unfortunate for the country, and for industry itself, if so many of them were absorbed by industry that it became impossible adequately to staff the universities and colleges." The group included individuals qualified for appointments at every rank: assistant, associate, and full professorships. "If you wish to be put in touch with possible candidates and will describe your needs to me, I shall be glad to assist you."[27]

In hardly over a month's time, in a process that must have been repeated at one institution after another, Dean S. C. Lind of the Institute of Technology at the University of Minnesota had in hand from Loomis a list of four men to consider for openings in the Chemistry Department at Minnesota, their qualifications briefly and neatly summarized. On a page with the heading "Assistant Professorship at the University of Minnesota." Loomis noted each man's name and age, and beneath each:

PhD granting institution and date
thesis title
teaching experience
Radiation Laboratory work

It was clear. It was concise. Like a vita, the list could be quickly and easily digested.[28]

A set of vita-like documents sent in early November 1945 to University of Minnesota Professor L. H. Reyerson by George B. Kistiakowsky were equally to the point. Kistiakowsky, Harvard Professor of physical chemistry, had headed the explosives section of the National Defense Research Committee and served as technical director of the Explosives Research Laboratory at Harvard before joining the Manhattan Project in 1943. "Attached to this letter," he wrote, "you will find a number of sheets"—there were nine in all—"each a brief life history and technical experience of a chemist selected by Dr. J. Kennedy and myself from the list of our most outstanding staff members as possibly of interest to you as a member of your teaching staff." Running across the top of each sheet was what he had termed "a brief life history": name, age, marital status, and number of dependents. Beneath that came a series of headings and supporting detail: "Education," then "Technical Experience," "Preferred Field of Employment," "References" and "Publications."[29] The list from the Radiation Lab, the individual sheets of Manhattan Project men, were produced not by the men whose qualifications were described on them but by the men recommending them. What they show is how the war itself had been a force for economy and systematization, producing new ways of summarizing men's qualifications and perhaps new expectations for how men seeking appointments would describe themselves. They were, after all, written by leading academics, men who would themselves read and assess applications of men for positions in the months and years to come.

Men also wrote their own vitae, variously titled, that their superiors in war research, PhD advisors, or former military commanders then sent with letters of recommendation on their behalf. Writing in late October 1945 in support of a member of his staff for a teaching position in chemistry at the University of Minnesota, the research director of the Underwater Explosives Research Laboratory at Woods Hole, Massachusetts, closed his letter, "For your convenience I am enclosing an outline of his training and experience."[30] The man who was the focus of the letter—Paul M. Fye—had completed his PhD at Columbia in 1939, taught for two years as an assistant professor of chemistry at Hofstra, and then in 1941 joined the Underwater Explosives Research Laboratory in Pittsburgh, moving to the lab at Woods Hole in 1942 where he became research supervisor and deputy research director. As was true for the research work of many during the war years, Fye's superior was not at liberty to describe the character of the work in detail, but he noted Fye's supervisory and organizational skills, his mature judgment "in the appraisal of the meaning and significance of scientific data," and capped his recommendation with the names of other highly regarded research scientists: "Think you will find him very well thought of by Dr. E. B. Wilson, Jr., and by Prof. G. B. Kistiakowsky."[31]

The enclosed three-page document, which began, "Information concerning:" would look and sound familiar to an academic today. It began with Fye's name and current position, date and place of birth, and religion, and then was divided into a series of categories with headings in all caps and underlined so that they stood out: Training; Teaching Experience; Research Experience; Scientific Publications; Scientific Societies, Honors, Prizes, etc.; Foreign Languages; and, finally, References. With the exception of the inclusion of religion and the absence of the title "Curriculum Vitae," it was a thoroughly modern document.[32] Fye's "qualifications"—coming as they did with Dr. Cross's recommendation—were interesting enough to Minnesota that Dean Lind sent Fye a "Request for Information" blank.[33]

While many of those who were drafted or came to work in war research had completed their PhDs, many others had just begun or were in the midst of graduate training when the war caught them up. Many were specifically recruited into war research by their graduate advisors.[34] Before the war, advisors had often made the first introduction for a student and then encouraged that student to write. What was different now was the way in which some advisors began to advise their students to write. Earl Spaeth began work on a PhD in chemistry at UCLA in fall 1942 and from his second semester in the program through the completion of his degree worked on the antimalarial war project in which his advisor was engaged. With that project coming to a close in the next two months and his degree in hand, his advisor noted in a letter to Lee Irvin Smith in chemistry at Minnesota, "I have suggested that Dr. Spaeth write to you . . . and submit an outline of his qualifications." Writing to Smith a few days later, Spaeth enclosed "a statement of my personal qualifications."[35]

But war service provided many others advocates who were not academics, and that fact too played a role in their drafting vitae. James Macgregor Burns was a 1939 graduate of Williams College and had begun work in 1940 on a PhD in public administration at Harvard. Then came the war. His first year of war service was with the National War Labor Board, but from 1943 to 1945 he served in the US Army writing a history of the Guam invasion (published by the War Department) and co-authoring a history of the Okinawa invasion. I suspect that in the absence of his war service, acquiring a nonacademic but well-connected Princeton University booster in a commanding officer, Burns would not have written a vita. In a context where vitae were not yet expected accoutrements of professional academic life, Burns had no need of a vita. He was a Williams and a Harvard man, had already taught at Williams with the prospect of returning, and there was interest in him at Harvard. It was likely at the request of his commanding officer that he wrote the "biographical sketch" his commander sent to Princeton University President Harold W. Dodds with a note saying, "I am extremely enthusiastic about getting him to Princeton and hope that a way can be found to do it."[36] As it turned out, the chairman of Princeton's Department of Politics was also enthusiastic. The war had depleted junior faculty ranks at universities, and George Graham was glad to receive word of Burns.[37]

What Stevens called a "biographical sketch" and Burns called a "personal history," we would call a curriculum vitae. In reply to a letter from Graham, Burns sent a "personal history," saying "I'm not sure from your letter whether or not you have the 'personal history' that I sent John Stevens, so I am enclosing another copy."[38] The "personal history" Burns sent differed slightly in format and substance from the version his commanding officer had sent. Burns had reformatted the document by centering its headings. It was a small change, but the headings now stood out in a way they had not before. And rather than indenting each entry under a heading, he now placed each entry flush with the left margin, all words in the title capitalized, followed by the dates of the position ("Instructor in Political Science, Williams College, 1941–42"). He then indented slightly subsequent lines describing each position, further highlighting each distinct element of his experience. It was a far more polished, easier to digest, document. There was one final significant change: Just below his name, he added, "Married, one child." Having read his "personal history," Graham invited Burns to "spend a day with us at Princeton" and from there made him an offer of an assistant professorship.

In the event, Burns's case offers a more important example for my inquiry than it did for the course of his life. His "personal history"—this document on which he recorded his field of study, his academic record, his range of professional experiences, his publications—offered a tool for Burns's former commanding officer and "friend" of Princeton University to bring Burns to Princeton's attention. It allowed Princeton to take the measure of the man, in the sense of qualifications, with limited investment on its part. But having met that bar, it was not Burns's vita but his personal connections—the conversations with Burns, the enthusiasm of highly regarded scholars—in other words, coming to know Burns, that led Princeton to offer him a three-year appointment at the rank of assistant professor. Burns turned down Princeton's offer to go to Williams because, as he wrote to Graham, the "chance to do 'creative' teaching with advanced students proved irresistible."[39]

Burns, Spaeth, Fye, and many other men like them drafted vitae that an influential booster, advisor, or academic-turned-war-researcher sent along with or following up on their own recommendation. But while war brought new intellectual opportunities and professional connections for many men, it set others adrift. Drafted into the Army, Navy, or other service, military service represented a profound rupture from their intellectual life. These men on their release and resumption of intellectual life too crafted what were, I imagine, their first vitae, and they sent them along with their own letters of introduction. "I am writing to place my qualifications before you for consideration in case there is a vacancy in History at the University of Chicago," wrote one such man in early April 1946. "For your convenience I am enclosing an outline of my personal and professional record." He had spent the last four years in the Coast Guard and was now completing his PhD at Columbia, where he noted, his "complete papers" were on file with the Columbia University Appointments Office. The one-page "Outline of Record" he enclosed organized by categories—present address, permanent address, personal, academic training, honors received, publications, experience—lacked only a list of references.[40] "I would like to apply for a position as Instructor in the field of American History," began another letter. He had graduated cum laude from Harvard in 1939 and was working toward his master's degree there when he was drafted and "then spent four and a half years in the Army." Released in February 1946, he had begun work on his PhD at Columbia. "I have appended a summary of qualifications and experience."[41] Like letters from strangers in the years of the Depression, they were far less likely to receive a positive response, but in a way that had not been true in the 1930s, these men seemed to know how to craft a vita even if they did not yet call it that.[42]

The outcome of the war depended on the fighting force, and so it is not surprising that the fighting force itself was made a subject of study. In summer 1941, a Special Services Division was established within the War Department, and within it a Research Branch. Their task was to provide the Army with "facts about the attitudes of soldiers" that the army command could use in formulating policy. Their research, leading to some three hundred reports, covered issues ranging from the particular—which of two kinds of huts men preferred in Alaska; the laundry situation in Panama; preferences for winter clothing of frontline troops in Belgium, Luxemburg, and Germany—to the global—how the fighting force in World War II differed from that in World War I; why men believed they were fighting; the order of demobilization; and the postwar plans of soldiers, including how many would go back to college if there were federal aid for veterans.[43]

But no one studied the staff of the War Research Branch itself and the thousands of other men and women whose training and careers were interrupted, requisitioned, and redirected by the war into applied research for the war effort. Their numbers were, of course, far smaller, and for the most part they were not formally in military service; they could be understood as having been "called" to the task.[44] Had there been such a research branch, its reports would have revealed how dramatically here, too, war transformed men and institutions. In his first letter to George Graham in the Department of Politics at Princeton, James Burns had said, "Although I'm interested in doing some writing, I feel that the main business of a teacher is to teach."[45] And so it had been. And teaching would remain the main business at many institutions.

But for many scholars as well as institutions, the war marked a turning point in the balance between teaching and research. The immersive research experience that defined so many men's (and, though in far smaller numbers, women's) war service profoundly impacted not only their research interests but also their self-understanding and their expectations of an academic life. This too would shape the subsequent history of the vita. In spring 1941, the Princeton Physics Department had told its graduate students that "much of the defense research is of real scientific interest." And it had been during the war and would continue to be after. The point was true not just in physics and related fields but more broadly.

Sociologist John A. Clausen noted, of his and others' experience who had been drawn into the War Research Branch as graduate students or early career scholars, "We acquired more hands-on research experience than most of our predecessors had in a lifetime."[46] With the publication in 1949 and 1950 of the four-volume series *Studies in Social Psychology in World War II*, a large share of the intellectual work of the War Research Branch acquired a larger audience, further advancing the scholarly reputations of the three most senior scholars in the branch.

But perhaps even more importantly, the research conducted in support of the war effort now served a second purpose: advancing the careers of the young scholars whose names the volumes included as authors, many of whom had been students when they were pulled into the Research Branch.[47] In an article titled "Research on the American Soldier as a Career Contingency," published as part of a retrospective on "*The American Soldier* and Social Psychology," Clausen focused not on authorship in the volumes but on membership in the group of social scientists who made up the War Research Branch. "The concept of identity is difficult to define at all precisely and even more difficult to assess," he reflected. "It entails our sense of who we are and what we stand for, or are committed to. It reflects our feelings of continuity with our past histories and potentialities for change—what we can become. It is at the same time a sense of personal uniqueness and the incorporation of a feeling of belonging with others. It reflects our implicit beliefs as to our efficacy and the respects in which we matter to others." He acknowledged that none of the former fellow War Research Branch colleagues he surveyed had used the word "identity" but argued that "there is considerable agreement among social psychologists that the most salient social roles provide the core of one's sense of identity, and if ever a role was salient, that of the research analyst in the Research Branch was. . . . Identities inevitably change over the years," he continued, "but for many of us I believe that the Research Branch has left strong residues in our current identities."[48]

I read his words and thought of the relationship between identity and the vita. And I thought, too, of the identities of the children burned during the war years and immediately after in Gene Autry cowboy suits.

summer's end

Dear Frances,

Will Dad and I spend the rest of our lives never having talked to each other about what it means to have lost you?

. . .

The summer is coming to an end. People have been asking me for some time when we are going to come back to St. Paul and I look blankly at them and say, "I have no idea."

. . .

I said to Wilder last night that I miss your lists. Right now you would have a list of things that needed to be bought or done before you headed off to Carleton and you would be happily, busily working your way down that list—all of which would be written in & crossed out in gloriously colored pens.

. . .

I spent several hours this afternoon going through my drawers & closet, piling things on the bed to give away. Each cleaning task feels like preparation, a sort of getting closer and closer to your room and the project that awaits me there. I can't imagine that task yet and so your room is just as it was when you went to bed on April 25th almost 4 months ago.

. . .

I talked with a student today. She asked if I had any fun stories to share from the summer. I said no, that it was just a hard summer. She then said something about 'firsts' being hard. I wonder about people. Every day without you is a first, every day you don't get to live is a first. I grieve not just for myself, but for you, for all the things you would've done, tried, thought about, lived, and now don't get to.

...

It's still this morning and totally quiet. The lake is almost like glass. The sun has come up and the sky is clear. With the cool nights, the buzz of the insects from earlier in the summer is gone—at least first thing in the morning. There's an occasional chatter from birds, but otherwise it is completely quiet, just the sound of my pen on the paper. You would've been still sleeping, cozy under a mountain of covers and at least half a dozen pillows.

...

It's the time of night on a school night when you'd come up and gather Sam in your arms and hug him and pet him and then I'd get down on the floor and we'd pet him together and talk. . . . The house is so quiet without you here—your music when you showered, your laughter, your enthusiastic hugs of Sam, your visits (when I was upstairs working) brought this house to life. It would've been quiet when you left for Carleton, but then you would have been home now, over Winter break, next summer. It's knowing that I'll never hear your laughter again that makes the quiet so hard.

...

I have days when I remember us as a happy family. What will we become?

chapter seven · "playing with fire"

Readers of *The Cincinnati Enquirer* might easily have missed the short news story with the headline "Burns Fatal" in the middle of page 18, bounded on all sides by war news.[1] With the war, the space given to "local" news declined dramatically as costs of publication rose, labor was scarce and paper in short supply, and advertising revenues declined as major advertisers diverted to war work. To say the story was four paragraphs would mis-convey its length. It was only ninety words. It began: "David Lonneman, 5 years old, 1935 Garden Lane, died last night of burns suffered four hours earlier when his clothing was ignited in the basement of his home." The second paragraph noted that the child was the son of Herbert R. Lonneman, treasurer of the Wittenborg Toy Company. A police report was the source for the details that filled out the story. The child had been "dressed in a cowboy suit." He and several neighboring boys "were playing with matches in the basement." He was burned "over his entire body." Other Ohio cities reprinted a clipped forty-word UP story straight off the wire with slight variations in title: "Youth Dies of Burns Wednesday," "Burns Fatal to Boy," "Boy, 5, Dies of Burns," "Burns Are Fatal."[2]

The importance of the question of what subscribers read was magnified in cities that had more than one daily and where a story did not appear in all the papers. *The Cincinnati Enquirer* came out in the morning; Cincinnati's other two papers, *The Cincinnati Post* and *The Cincinnati Times-Star*, were evening papers. Morning dailies competed with getting to work, evening dailies with exhaustion and family time. And then there was the question of who got the paper at all. *The Cincinnati Enquirer*'s weekday circulation in 1942 was 127,329 households.[3] How many of those subscribers got to page 18 on November 5, 1942? The history of the press focuses on the main event—the biggest papers, the most distinguished editors, long-term trends, coverage of history-defining news. But most news stories, even in the war years, were one day's news. Missing that day meant missing the story.

Had the police not been called, David Lonneman's death likely never would have become news. In major American cities, an unending series of incidents might be news. But first, they had to be known. A child burned while playing with other children in the basement of his family's home was not public. The incident became public with the call to the police. But in major cities, calls to the police came in "almost every minute of the day and night." The work of a reporter involved, as a first step, going through "the bare facts outlined in a police slip, generally in about ten words" and determining in a matter of minutes whether it was worth looking into or not. "Mainly," as Walter Arm, a police reporter for the *New York Herald Tribune* in the 1940s, explained, "he weighs these stories and finds them wanting in interest other than routine."[4]

David Lonneman's death made the event "other than routine." Between the 1870s and the 1930s in the United States, as Viviana Zelizer describes, there was a "profound transformation in the economic and sentimental value of children." Reducing infant mortality became a national priority; children's hospitals were established; a federal children's bureau was established; child labor was banned; a national safety campaign was launched to protect children against accidental death. By the 1920s, as Zelizer describes, "children's accidental death emerged as a 'serious, fundamental national problem.'"[5] David Lonneman's death was news. But of what? A five-year-old boy had died. He had been playing with matches. His clothing had caught fire. Every story that reported his death mentioned these details. The stories also noted that the boy had been playing with others. They, presumably, were not harmed; there were no details about them or their clothing. All the reports also mentioned that he had been wearing a cowboy suit. The UP wire story described it as "wolly [*sic*]." It noted that the boy had received the cowboy suit for his birthday the day before the incident.

Just over a month later, on Monday, December 28, 1942, a headline on page 25 of the Rochester *Democrat and Chronicle* read, "Yule Gift Brings Tragedy to Boy, 11." The story was from Geneva, New York, roughly fifty miles southeast of Rochester. The opening paragraph read: "A Christmas present in the form of a cowboy suit, of which he was very proud, turned the holiday into tragedy for Fred Yerkes, 11, Saturday night."[6] The next paragraph noted the boy's parents' names, their address, and the hospital where the boy's condition was reported as "serious," with third-degree burns on his legs, abdomen, and arms. It was only in the third paragraph that the story got to what had happened. The family was preparing to move and the boy's mother had "sent the lad into the backyard to dispose of some rubbish." When he set fire to it, "the flames apparently caught on the fluffy imitation fur of his cowboy pants." He had run screaming into the house where his younger sister "tried to beat out the flames with her hands."

When the Rochester paper had gone to press on Sunday, December 27, Fred Yerkes was still alive. By the time the story appeared the next morning, he had died. The Rochester daily ran a second story reporting his death. Identified in the first story by the name his family called him, he was now identified by his full name. Death is an official event.[7] *The Ithaca Journal* also published two stories about the incident, "Boy's Burns Fatal" and "Gift Causes Tragedy."[8] While the story of the Yerkes boy's death was likely front-page news in Geneva, it was tucked far back in the papers in Ithaca and Rochester.

Donald Frederick Yerkes and David Lonneman were both likely wearing Gene Autry cowboy suits. All the signs are there. The cowboy suits with the high-pile viscose rayon made to look like fur had gone on the market in 1942. The families bought the suits in November and December that year. The chaps were what had taken fire. They were "wolly"; they had "imitation fur" on them. There were enough details in both stories to suggest the chaps of the cowboy suit took fire readily and burned rapidly. The boys had hardly had them for more than a day before they were burned. But Geneva, New York, and Cincinnati, Ohio, were over five hundred miles apart. Though newspapers had brought the news of each boy's injury and death to readers in other cities in New York and Ohio, there was likely not a single person who read both stories. And even had there been such a reader, that both boys had been wearing cowboy suits was hardly a clue to anything. In the early 1940s, across the US, hundreds of thousands of boys wore cowboy suits.

"RED TANKS RACE INTO CRIMEA; FIFTH ARMY CRACKS NAZI LINE": The headline—all caps, the font larger than the paper's masthead—shouted from the front page of the Passaic *Herald-News* on November 2, 1943. The *Herald-News* subscribed to both the AP and UP, and most of the stories on the paper's front page—that day and every day in the war years—were from a wire service. But any reader of the *Herald-News* on November 2, 1943, would have seen the headline: "Playing with Fire Costs Boy His Life." And the subhead "Eastside Brothers Set Grass Ablaze—Both Become Human Torches."[9] *The Cincinnati Enquirer* had given David Lonneman's death ninety words. The *Herald-News* gave the story of five-year-old Stanley Krzeczkowski and his seven-year-old brother Casimir Jr. most of a column on page 1 and continued onto page 2. What made one death worth so many more words than the other? Here was a heartrending story about two young brothers. One of them had died; the other was left in critical condition. The incident happened outside in the middle of a weekday in an industrial city. There were multiple adult witnesses. Heroic attempts at rescue. The drama and horror were palpable. The witnesses had heard the boys' screams. Seen the boys on fire. The police had been called. Detectives had examined the scene, interviewed witnesses, made a full report.

But if the question was how this tragedy had happened, the events were seen in strikingly similar terms. One needed read no further than the headline: "Playing with Fire Costs Boy His Life." The opening sentence of the story told readers the boys were "playing with matches." The matches set fire to dry grass in the yard, trapping the boys in the flames. "Both boys were dressed in flimsy cowboy suits, made of material that was quickly consumed by the flames." Here were cowboy suits again. Clothing had played a role. But the key, the story suggested, was children playing with matches. The detectives, as the *Herald-News* reported, had found six burned matches near the house and a paper book of matches, one of which was removed.

Milton Henry's factory—where he made the Gene Autry cowboy suit and employed two hundred workers—was located in Passaic. Henry lived in New York City, but it is impossible not to wonder whether he might have seen or heard about the story in the *Herald-News*. Did he know that some employees bought Gene Autry cowboy suits directly from the factory? Would he have known or remembered that Stella Krzeczkowski, the boys' mother, had been one of his employees in the Passaic factory? Whatever he knew, there must have been employees in the factory who had worked with Stella—whether she was still employed there at the time or not—who read the story and knew that she had bought cowboy suits for her boys there. Other Passaic families who had had a child burned when their cowboy suit caught fire—incidents that had not become news—must have read the story of the Krzeczkowski brothers.[10] News reads differently to those it touches directly.

The only other coverage of the event was an article that same day in the *News*, in nearby Paterson, New Jersey, and a follow-up report on November 3 in Passaic's *Herald-News* on Casimir Jr.'s condition.[11] In both stories, important details dropped out, which meant that clues to a different reading of what had happened were lost. The first story in the *Herald-News* had drawn on a detective's investigation of the fire, in which he noted that there were seven separate fires, "some believed started when the boys ran around in agony with their clothes aflame."[12] In other words, these fires had been started not by matches but by the children's flaming cowboy suits. The opening sentence of the story in the *News* read, "Trapped in the center of a patch of dried grass they fired with matches, two small Passaic brothers were so badly burned yesterday one died a few hours after being admitted to Beth Israel Hospital and the other is in critical condition."[13] The follow-up report on November 3 in the *Herald-News*, noting Casimir Jr.'s condition as critical, described the boy as having been "badly burned . . . while playing with matches" and noted, "Matches lit by the boys set fire to tall, dry grass in the backyard and they were trapped in the flames."[14] Neither of these stories mentioned what the boys had been wearing; the role of the cowboy suits in the tragedy dropped out.

If a person wanted to trace how American newspapers covered incidents of children burned "playing with fire" in the 1940s, new commercial databases that have digitized hundreds of newspapers, especially from small and mid-size cities across the United States, would be all one needed. Newspapers in the 1940s were filled with brief stories of children, mostly boys, seriously and fatally burned at play.[15] But if the goal was to find every incident in which a child was burned wearing a Gene Autry cowboy suit, even digitized newspaper databases fall short. Some absolute number of children were burned in these cowboy suits. We will never know it. Consider that in two years, as far as I can judge, there had been news reports of only four children burned, three of whom died, in what seem certainly to have been Gene Autry cowboy suits. The cowboy suit with the high-pile viscose rayon on the chaps was sold across the United States from 1942 through 1945, and in some places much later. Long after it was sold in stores, it continued to be worn by children. In 1944, to take one year in that time frame as exemplary, there were 1,754 English-language dailies published in the US. There were 11,474 weekly papers. There were hundreds of daily, weekly, and monthly newspapers in languages other than English.[16] Most newspapers from the 1940s remain undigitized. Many no longer exist in any form.

It is one thing to identify broad patterns, to trace change over time; it is altogether another to uncover the full scope of a tragedy that played out across a nation over more than a decade that no one at the time knew was happening. Many Gene Autry cowboy suit incidents never made the news.[17] Many that did did not identify the clothing a child was wearing.[18] Any number that identified the clothing misidentified some important element of it: mistaking a cowboy suit for an Indian play suit, fur for fringes, suggesting it was not the same kind that others had been wearing.[19] To undertake a search thinking one might find even every reported instance in this dramatically incomplete database is like asking an archive to be organized by the categories salient to the researcher who knows something that was not apparent at the time.

But what can be gleaned is nonetheless important to understanding how it was that despite many incidents making the news, the press and in turn its public continued to see these events as like all those other incidents of children burned at play that they knew about from life experience or read about in the paper. News reports reflected and reinforced the narrative of a serious national problem. That problem was children and fire. The lesson was one that public fire-safety campaigns had been teaching since at least the 1920s: Matches should be kept away from small children; playing with fire costs property and lives.[20]

I continue searching. "Boy," "Child," "Girl," "Play," "Matches," "Fire," "Clothes," "Cowboy Suit," "Gene Autry," "Play Suit" . . . working my way systematically through combinations of search terms . . . "Burned," "Injured," "Severely Injured," "Died," "Fatal." And I continue to find events I had not known about before. The research is emotionally exhausting. So many children burned. Each time I discover a story—new to me—with the hallmarks of a Gene Autry cowboy suit incident, I have a terrible sinking feeling. Why should one of these incidents be any more devastating to find than other stories of children burned? It is at least in part because there was a cause here that was beyond their ken. I know something they did not. This was not an accident. This was not their fault. The sinking feeling also relates to knowing that I will never know every child who was burned in a Gene Autry cowboy suit. There is a way in which knowing—even retrospective knowing, identifying, naming, remembering—provides a sort of historical redress of a wrong.

Through 1944 and the first months of 1945, there were more newspaper stories of children burned across the United States when the cowboy suit they were wearing caught fire. The hazardous character of the children's play remained the focus of most stories. On January 14, 1944, the *Daily Tribune* in Royal Oak, Michigan, reported the story of a five-year-old local boy, John Lockhart, whose "cowboy play suit trousers caught fire" after he and another boy lit some lighter fluid they had found.[21] The lesson to be learned from the incident related to proper disposal of hazardous materials. As the article reporting on the boy's condition the following day explained, "The burning resulted in a warning to Royal Oakers against placing unemptied bottles of cleaning fluid, other liquids and medicines in junk baskets for rubbish collection."[22]

Then there was the four-and-a-half-year-old boy, William Kingston, from Freehold, New Jersey, fatally burned when, playing with a friend in the kitchen, he decided to light the rope he was using as a lariat from a gas jet on the stove. Many small towns like Freehold, a town of just under seven thousand residents, had a weekly newspaper or no newspaper at all. The story of William Kingston's fatal burns in May 1944 first appeared in dailies in nearby cities. Each of the papers noted that the boy was wearing a cowboy suit, but the hazard, they suggested, lay in the child's play. One story hinted at another element: Perhaps the child was poorly supervised. His mother was gone when the incident happened; he had fractured his skull a year before in a fall from the porch.[23] One paper's coverage held clues, if one had known how to read them. The child's "trousers were burned off" but his underwear only "charred." No mention of the rest of his clothing taking fire at all.[24]

The day after Jackie Izzo was burned in Saginaw, Michigan, in July 1944, the headline of the front-page story in *The Saginaw News* read "Playmates Take Turns Applying The 'Hotfoot': Girl, Six, Badly Burned." The article mentioned that the girl was wearing cowboy pants and described "the fringe" as having taken fire, but the focus was on the children's play.[25] When *The Saginaw News* reported in August that doctors, in their battle to save the girl's life, had amputated both her legs, *The Detroit Times*, unable to resist a catchy headline, reported "'Hot Foot' Costs 2 Legs."[26] And each report repeated the original inaccuracy in the description of the cowboy pants. That same month, *The Philadelphia Inquirer* reported on an incident in Philadelphia without mentioning that the burned boy, Joseph Moore, was wearing a cowboy suit. "Clothing Ablaze, Boy Badly Hurt," read the headline. The focus: child's play. A patrolman driving toward City Hall "noticed a group of boys around a bonfire in a vacant lot at 18th and Bristol sts [*sic*]. As he drove past the spot, the Moore boy ran from the lot with his clothes ablaze."[27]

The individual, serial character of the incidents involving children wearing cowboy suits obscured their underlying shared or collective character. News coverage reflected and conveyed the sense that these were accidents, individual family tragedies, local news. Several weeks before Jackie Izzo was burned in Saginaw, Michigan, 167 people lost their lives, with seven hundred more injured and thousands of others imperiled in a matter of minutes when the Big Top of the Ringling Brothers and Barnum and Bailey circus went up in flames in Hartford, Connecticut.[28] The Hartford circus fire was the kind of mass public event that was front-page news in newspapers across the United States. It remained in the news as the death toll rose. It was understood from the moment it happened as national news. "Big Top Bursts into Flame," read the headline in *The Cincinnati Enquirer*. "5 Accused of

Manslaughter as Circus Deaths Reach 139," read the headline of the Passaic *Herald-News*. "Death Toll is 145 in Big Circus Fire," reported Royal Oak's *Daily Tribune*.[29] The circus itself was the kind of public event that would have been reported on in local papers, the rare public entertainment that garnered both AP and UP coverage, and so reporters were on the scene and captured pictures of terrified women and children running, with the flaming big top burning behind them.[30] The big top was a single piece of fabric; a protection against the elements; a way of assuring that those who saw the show had paid for admission. Fire was as integral to the circus as the tigers and the trapeze. Public safety required that the covering be in some manner flameproofed. The scale of the human loss demanded investigation, immediately triggered criminal charges, and as quickly individual lawsuits for injury and death.[31]

In contrast, even where one incident involving a child burned in a cowboy suit in the same town or city followed closely on another that made the news, the connection went unexamined, unrecognized. In March 1945, the Yonkers *Herald Statesman* reported: "Two Young Boys Suffer Burns as Bonfires Set Clothing Afire." The boys—five-year-old William Wetherell and four-year-old Guy Tortenson—had been injured in separate incidents, one day apart, in different parts of the borough. The common thread highlighted in the police report of the two incidents was boys and bonfires.[32] The story and headline noted that their clothing caught fire; it did not note that both boys were wearing cowboy suits.

Part of the failure to see what was right before them was that other information in the scene loomed larger: the frequent incidence of children being burned by fire; the nature of the children's play. The headline in *The Alexandria Gazette* on March 14, 1945, reporting on a local boy, five-year-old Tony DiTrapani, having been burned the preceding afternoon, read, "Trash Fire Play Burns Boy Badly." The story noted that the boy was wearing a cowboy suit and that the "fur front" of the suit had "burst into flames," but it was the boys' play that was the focus of the police report and in turn the news story: DiTrapani and a playmate had been "gesturing with sticks taken from a trash fire." The story closed, "This is the third injury this week by fire to a youngster."[33] With this as the closing note of the story about Tony DiTrapani, it hardly seems surprising that the newspaper did not question whether there might be some other connection to the Engleside boy, five-year-old Elwood Leary Jr., whose death the paper had reported the preceding October.[34] Leary too had been playing around a trash fire. The Fairfax County police report on that incident noted that his "clothes became aflame," but apparently did not note what he was wearing.[35]

And then there was the immediacy, the unceasing urgency, of the war itself. The headline on page 1 of the *Florence (SC) Morning News* on January 7, 1945, read in large, thick bold letters, "AMERICAN TROOPS TAKE FRAITURE." From well before December 1941, American newspapers had closely followed the war, but with the bombing of Pearl Harbor, the US declaration of war, and American troops on land and sea in Europe, Africa, and Asia, the war never lost its place on the front page of American newspapers. That may have been truest of newspapers that relied most heavily on the wire services for their news, but there was hardly a community that did not have some local boy or boy whose parents were residents "over there," and so news of the war was itself local news.

News reports of a local boy who had been burned competed with war news. The brief story of six-year-old Frank Johnson having been seriously burned was sandwiched between a story with the headline "Carrier Planes Make Heavy Raids on Japs" and another reading "Selective Service Orders Induction of Deferred Men."[36] Three months later, a brief notice about another local boy—"little Mitchell Gray Lee, five-year-old son of Mr. and Mrs. E. C. Lee"—who had been burned while playing in his backyard was printed in the *Morning News* "Seen About Town" column. The story noted that he was in Saunders Memorial Hospital and gave a brief recounting of the accident. "According to reports he got hold of some matches and struck one, lighting a piece of paper which set his cowboy suit afire."[37] The report made no connection to the story about Frank Johnson from three months earlier.

Fire held complicated, competing meanings in the war years. On the same page as the story about Mitchell Gray Lee was a two-column AP story describing the American and British firebombing of Berlin, Dresden, and other German cities. "It is estimated unofficially," the story noted of Berlin, "that more than 65,000 persons died in the flaming ruins of the Nazi capital and that 400,000 were made homeless."[38]

Most incidents of children burned in Gene Autry cowboy suits never made the news, and of those that did, a very small number became AP or UP stories. In becoming news, death retained greater currency than injury. But equally important was proximity to a major city with wire service reporters. A UP or AP story went out over the wire, where it in turn could be picked up by member newspapers to fill one of those tiny spots that required a story of under fifty words. Howard Diable's death might never have been reported at all beyond his hometown of Pitcairn had he not been rushed to a hospital in Pittsburgh where he died. Pitcairn had only a weekly published on Fridays. Pittsburgh was a major industrial city of close to seven hundred thousand people with three dailies. Both *The Pittsburgh Sun-Telegraph* and *The Pittsburgh Press* reported the boy's death. Their coverage was short and to the point, captured in their headlines "Child Fatally Burned" and "Boy, 5, Dies of Burns." Neither paper noted what he was wearing beyond saying his "clothing ignited" from a bonfire.[39]

Had an AP reporter not picked up the story, that the boy was wearing a cowboy suit when he was burned would not have been part of the news coverage at all. With this addition and that he and other boys had been playing follow-the-leader, the story appeared in small-town newspapers across the state of Pennsylvania. Their reportage mirrored that of papers in smaller newspaper markets across the US: At least on the page where the story reporting Howard Diable's death appeared, the news all came from the AP. The only thing local was the advertising.[40]

AP and UP reports gave news from places like Pitcairn, a city of just over six thousand in southeastern Pennsylvania, a broader orbit. There were thousands of Pitcairns, in this sense, across the United States. Every town that picked up the AP story about Howard Diable was one. But even as the orbit of the news was amplified, something was lost. "The best editor is the man with an insatiable desire to know the facts of a matter," Joseph G. Herzberg, the famed editor of the *New York Herald Tribune*, wrote in 1947. He dwelt on the importance of "the reporter's curiosity."[41] The story of Howard Diable's injury and death, treated as obvious, reflected a failure of curiosity. News-wire memberships were not just a means of news-sharing; they also reduced the need for reporters of one's own who might take an AP or UP report and use it as the foundation for a local investigation. What exactly was the child wearing? Had it played a role in his injury? Is this item being sold here? Has any child here been burned in similar circumstances?

On Sunday, April 8, 1945, a double headline spanned the columns of page 1 of the Washington, DC, *Times-Herald*: "Patton Seizes Nazi Gold Hoard" and "Yanks Smash Japs Naval Power." But just beneath these headlines, in columns 2 and 3, was an investigative report by *Times-Herald* reporters Roland Nicholson and Spence Drummond: "D.C. Parents Warned: Inflammable Cowboy Suits Kill One Child Here, Burn 7" and "Fuzzy 'Chaps' Flare Like Torches; Stores Are Notified, Probe Launched."[42] Here was what for so long had been lacking: a story clearly identifying the danger. The opening sentence of the article noted that the chaps on the suit were "highly inflammable and capable in a split second of turning children into flaming torches."[43] Each of the children had been wearing the same outfit: a cowboy suit made by a New York firm, M. A. Henry Co., and sold under the trade name of Gene Autry. Tests by the DC deputy fire marshal, Capt. R. A. Warfield, had determined the "woolly material designed to simulate fur" to be highly inflammable. The article identified the children by age and by when they were burned, and their parents by name and address: Tony DiTrapani, five, from Alexandria, who had died just a week ago; Arthur "Toby" Cumberledge, eight, burned on March 25; Lawrence Gates, seven, burned on February 11; Edward Bradley, six, burned six weeks ago; and Willie Wilks Jr., nine, "Negro," burned on January 23, all being treated in Children's Hospital; William "Billy" Greatorex, four, burned a year ago and still being treated twice weekly at the same hospital. It included pictures of several of the boys in the hospital and a family photo of Tony DiTrapani, who had died. The article also noted that the fire marshals' investigation had begun "on the strength of an anonymous phone call in the latter part of March." Both the *Times-Herald* reporters and the fire marshal had interviewed hospital officials and parents of the burned boys and in so doing alerted them that the tragedy that had befallen them was not just an accident.

The news report was more important because notice was all they could give. As the DC deputy fire marshal noted in the article, "the District has no laws governing inflammable clothing." They could investigate, alert parents, retailers, and the manufacturer—and they had. As the article noted, the store had immediately withdrawn the suits from sale. The Merchants and Manufacturers Association had notified local retailers and the National Association of Retail Credit Stores. Recalling the "circus tragedy" of a year ago, the paper suggested its reporting would add pressure to the demand for fireproofing of materials. But as the story noted, the danger likely was not confined to Washington, DC. "Because their trade name is that of a famous screen cowboy, it is likely that they are sold all over the country and that tragic experiences here have been duplicated many times over."

For five straight days, the tragedy was major news in the nation's capital. *The Washington Post* and the *Washington Evening Star* joined in covering the story, but it was the *Times-Herald*'s investigative reporting that really broke the story.[44] Each day there were new details. More boys in the DC area had been injured; more boys had died. The potential scale of the tragedy grew as the *Times-Herald* revealed that the Henry Company claimed to have sold "some 200,000 of the suits to stores throughout the country."

The *Times-Herald* called Gene Autry in Houston, where he was in the Air Transport Command. With headlines proclaiming, "Autry to Probe Fabric of Togs Bearing Name" and "Gene Autry, Movie Star, Will Join in Probe," the *Times-Herald* reported that Autry had "expressed genuine distress," said he would get in touch with Mr. Henry, and that he would do "'anything I can for the children burned here." He said things that were not true: that he was paid a flat fee for the use of his name. And he began to spin the evidence. "Even if it appears that those suits aren't to blame, I want to come to Washington and see those boys. . . . Hell," he said, "I like children."

It mattered that the news had broken in the capital. The Bureau of Standards was based in Washington, DC, and S. H. Ingberg, chief of the fire resistance section, tested the "fur" chaps and confirmed Deputy Fire Marshal Warfield's assessment. The Merchants and Manufacturers Association and the American Retail Federation were based in Washington, DC. In its April 11 coverage, the *Times-Herald* reported that the associations' warnings about the suits had gone out to retailers across the nation.[45] And it mattered that the news had broken in Washington, DC. because US Congressmen were there and responded to the news. On the second day of the *Times-Herald*'s coverage, Representative John E. Rankin of Mississippi, on the floor of the US Congress, demanded an investigation, legislation, and possibly criminal action against the manufacturer.[46] His words and demand for legislation too became part of the coverage.[47]

Milton Henry "damned Rankin's outburst, with a remark that the source of the criticism should be considered." And the *Times-Herald* reported that too. When asked what action he planned to take, the paper reported Henry said, "'Why wave a red flag and scare everyone to death, when we aren't sure what the trouble is?'" A reporter asked, "Not even to prevent recurrence of what has happened in Washington?'" Describing Henry as "about 40, tall, polished, and well dressed," the article noted, he "threw up his hands in a helpless gesture. 'This is the first instance of this sort that we've had since I began making the suits more than four years ago. I'm anxious to do whatever I can to correct matters. After all, this is my business. I've got a good name and I've got to protect it.'"

And it mattered that the news broke in Washington, DC, because the Depression and then the war had trained the nation's eyes and ears on the capital. Spurred by Rankin's demand that whoever was responsible for the inflammable material used in the Gene Autry cowboy suit chaps be sent "to the penitentiary," *Times-Herald* reporter Roland Nicholson, reporting from New York, told his DC readers on April 10 that New York City's fire marshal, Thomas P. Brophy, would conduct tests the next day of the suit.[48] On April 11, the *Times-Herald*'s headline read, "LaGuardia Asks Full Report on Cowboy Suits Made in N.Y." Reporting from New York, Nicholson described a test of the suit's inflammability that newsmen made. They mounted a Gene Autry cowboy suit on a frame near the East River and then took a match to the lower edge of one leg of the chaps. With stop watches and cameras they captured the event. "Death Wears a Child's Cowboy Suit . . . In Only 82 Seconds!" read the caption to the photo sequence of the burning suit. As Nicholson wrote, "It was not difficult to see that a child inside the suit would have been hopelessly trapped." Spectators had gathered to watch. As the "intense flame totally consumed the garment," Nicholson wrote, "a tenant woman . . . muttered 'My God!'"[49]

Timing is everything in what becomes news. And news or its absence in turn shapes the course of events, the course of lives. Late on the afternoon of April 12, 1945, President Franklin Delano Roosevelt died. He was in Warm Springs, Georgia. The news was out on the wires by early evening, and radio programs interrupted their broadcasts to announce the president's death, but it wasn't until the next day that the news appeared in print.[50] The front page of the *Times-Herald* was a full-page photograph of Franklin Delano Roosevelt.[51] It is impossible to know how news coverage and in turn the hazard itself would have developed had Roosevelt not died when he did. It seems possible, in at least some news markets, that other papers would have undertaken their own investigative reports on the cowboy suit hazard.

As it was, they did not. *The Philadelphia Inquirer* had run a front-page story on April 12 reporting on the hazard, noting one boy in nearby Conshohocken, five-year-old David Speaker, who had died in January, and listing two New Jersey boys whom the *Times-Herald*'s coverage had highlighted as having been injured in Gene Autry cowboy suits. The *Inquirer*'s story alerted citizens of Philadelphia to the hazard, identifying the cowboy suit by name and describing it. But the story was not an investigative report. There was no follow-up. Had reporters for the *Inquirer* surveyed Philadelphia-area hospitals, they would have found at least four boys seriously burned in the last seven months in Gene Autry cowboy suit incidents who were still hospitalized. Only one of those incidents—Joseph Moore, burned in August 1944—had made the news when it happened.

The New York City fire marshal's investigation, announced just three days earlier, was also completed and submitted to Mayor LaGuardia on April 12.[52] There clearly had been pressure to work quickly. The report was just over a page, less without its heading. It identified the M. A. Henry Co., with a showroom on Broadway in Manhattan and a factory in Passaic, New Jersey, as the manufacturer of the suit and the Woonsocket Falls Mill in Rhode Island as the source of the fabric, E. F. Timme & Son acting as sales agent. It confirmed the inflammability of the fabric: "It is a highly combustible material, easily ignited by an open flame or spark from a bonfire and it is particularly dangerous for children to wear cowboy or play suits trimmed with it. When this material is ignited, the flames spread with great rapidity." As was true in Washington, DC, the fire marshal reported that "there is no City Ordinance or law prohibiting the manufacture, use or sale of this product." The report included material misstatements of fact which could only have come from the principals themselves that downplayed the scale of the hazard.[53] It stated that the Henry Co. had only used the rayon pile "for a brief period" and that it was "now using a material known as 'Timme Tufts,' a combination of alpaca and cotton, which is slow-burning." The Henry Company never used Timme's trademark fabric.[54]

But perhaps most shocking of all was the confidently expressed statement, "There is no record of any death or injury by fire to a child in this City while wearing the subject play suit." One wonders where the fire marshal expected to find such a record. In 1940, the US census reported the population of New York City as almost 7.5 million people. Four of the five boroughs in the city, with populations of between one and three million, had more people than many US states.[55] In such a context, the fire marshal's office must have known that its own records dramatically understated the number of deaths and injuries in fires.[56] One wonders whether the fire marshal's investigators in fact looked beyond their own records. They certainly had not checked area hospitals. Tommy McCormack lay at that moment hovering between life and death at Mt. Sinai Hospital. A boy named Michael Blessington had died in a New York City hospital less than two weeks before. Arnold Weinstein, a Brooklyn boy, remained in Long Island College Hospital, and William Wetherell, a Yonkers boy, was in St. John's Hospital. And there were others.

But in a city the size of New York, even where the police or fire department were called, these incidents hardly had a chance of being "other than routine." William Wetherell's injuries, along with those of another boy, Guy Tortenson, had been reported in the *Herald Statesman*, but the report had not mentioned that the boys were wearing cowboy suits, and in any event, I suppose, Yonkers fell outside the fire marshal's jurisdiction.[57] Neither the *New York Herald Tribune* nor any other daily in the city had reported the incidents in which Tommy McCormack, Michael Blessington, Arnold Weinstein, Dennis Duffy, or any of the other boys I know to have been injured in Gene Autry cowboy suits in the city were hurt.[58]

Had President Roosevelt not died when he did, Mayor LaGuardia might have commented to the press on the report, and families of children who had been injured or died might have contacted the fire marshal or mayor's office or a newspaper. But as it was, the report did not make the news. The day after receiving it, Mayor LaGuardia wrote to Representative Rankin sharing the substance of the investigation and noting that though there was no local law which would prohibit the sale of the cowboy suit in the city, "We have had no similar experience in New York City at any time."[59]

Reading the coverage in the *Times-Herald* from April 8 through April 12, it would be easy to believe that now everyone knew. And it seems likely that most adult residents of Washington, DC, did. Perhaps more so than in any other place in the United States, the adult population in the capital was attuned to the news.[60] The *Times-Herald* had the highest circulation numbers of the four Washington, DC, dailies and broke the story on a Sunday, a day on which newspaper circulations were highest.[61] Moreover, the *Times-Herald*'s investigative reporting expanded news coverage of the hazard beyond the capital. Its coverage was what had led to attention to the issue in Congress with a demand for investigation and legislation; it had triggered an investigation in Virginia; it had triggered Mayor LaGuardia's demand for an investigation in New York City; it had triggered the warnings of national retailer organizations to their members. And because the news broke in Washington, DC, it was taken up by major newspapers that had their own news bureaus in the capital and by the AP and UP and reprinted in newspapers scattered across the US. The warnings by national retailer associations to their members undoubtedly saved many children's lives as the outfits were taken off store shelves. Here was an instance where chains were a positive good. News, in this respect at least, reached into small markets it otherwise might not have reached. It was extended further by local chambers of commerce.[62]

But despite all these things, outside Washington, DC, the news did not break for the vast majority of Americans in April 1945. Gene Autry cowboy suits never sold in the higher-end department stores, those most likely to be members of retailer associations. And if one means by "breaking news" a clear exposition of the hazard, the news did not break even in many towns and cities where there was some news coverage. The AP and UP wire services differed materially in their reporting. The first UP stories appeared in newspapers on April 9, 1945. They identified the hazardous cowboy suit by name, describing the chaps, "covered in front with a wool-like substitute resembling fur," as dangerously inflammable, and repeating Deputy Fire Marshal Warfield's advice to parents to "get rid of them immediately." Residents of cities where the UP story appeared had a chance at least of knowing of the danger.[63] The AP story, by contrast, included none of the details from the *Times-Herald*'s investigative reporting. Strikingly, in more papers that ran the UP story, the story was front-page news; in newspapers that ran the AP story, the story was more likely buried deep in the inner pages of the paper.[64]

In the wake of President Roosevelt's death, newspaper coverage of the hazard changed. But the reasons for that change went beyond Roosevelt's death. The scope of the hazard itself changed. A week after the president's death, the first hearing on inflammable fabrics, what would come to be called "flammable fabrics," was held in the office of Representative J. Leroy Johnson (R–CA). In January, California had become the first state to consider and pass a state law making it unlawful to sell inflammable wearing apparel.[65] The California law—spurred by an incident in the state's capital, Sacramento, involving brushed rayon—targeted items made from synthetic fabrics: things like children's bathrobes, shower curtains, and women's evening gowns.[66]

The California law had spurred organizing in the textile industry, so that by the time news of the cowboy suit broke in April 1945 in Washington, DC, the industry was ready.[67] The headline in the *Times-Herald* on Friday, April 20, 1945, read "3 Groups Study Law to Ban Sale of Unsafe Cloth."[68] The word went out on the AP wire: Tests in Congressman Johnson's office had shown that the hazard was not just a particular cowboy suit; "the entire clothing field" required investigation.[69] And just like that, the hazard of the Gene Autry cowboy suit was absorbed into a more generalized hazard, a broad field of inquiry that would require study and testing, the development of standards and testing equipment, all by experts in the textile field. A generalized inquiry was less attention-grabbing than headlines of burned children. Coverage would slip further back into newspapers, the sort of thing that might appear as a small item on a business page or not at all. The effect was something like that of an individual slipping into a crowd and disappearing.

Gene Autry tapped into that shift. Ever conscious of his image, Autry made good on his promise to visit the burned boys in DC. It seems hardly a matter of chance that his visit to the capital came on the same day as the demonstration in Rep. Johnson's office of the burning properties of the cowboy suit bearing his name. Autry had notified Spence Drummond of the *Times-Herald* that he was coming. Alongside the story with the headline "Priest Wants Law to Insure Against Inflammable Textile," was a photo, three columns square, of Autry handsomely dressed in his military uniform, with his characteristic warm smile, bending over the hospital bed of Eddie Bradley, the boy's hand in his. The accompanying article, with the headline "Victims of Autry Playsuits Shake Hands with Their Hero," explained that

Autry was only in the capital for the day but had made visiting the hospital the "first order of business."[70] Discovering that Toby Cumberledge had been released from the hospital, Autry made an "unannounced"—that is, to the family, not the press—visit to the Cumberledge home. His words were for a larger audience. "I'm sorry you were burned," he told Toby. "Hurry and get well." And to Mrs. Cumberledge, "I just can't figure it. I just don't know. The manufacturer's been making these suits for five years, and this is the first time anything like this has happened." And to Spence Drummond, words that he also knew would be printed: "If the kids hadn't been burned while wearing one of my suits, it might have been while wearing another kind."[71]

The limits of the breaking news became apparent the next day: Sunday, April 22, 1945. Donald, James, and Joseph Powell lived in East Liverpool, Ohio, a city of roughly twenty-three thousand people, forty-seven miles south of Youngstown. They had been to church that morning. That afternoon, the three brothers were playing cowboy and Indian on a hillside near their home, wearing identical cowboy suits they had gotten for Christmas, when Donald, age seven, seeing a small fire started by some other boys, attempted to stomp it out. His fuzzy cowboy suit ignited, and in fright he ran to his older brother, James Wesley, who was nine, whose suit also caught fire. Joseph, who was six, seeing his brothers in trouble, attempted to help them, and his own cowboy suit ignited. A woman and her son, who lived nearby, heard the boys' screams and rushed to their aid. Their hands were burned beating out the flames, but their clothes did not take fire.

The banner headline on the front page of the *East Liverpool Review* the next day read, "REDS DRIVE FOR HEART OF BERLIN" and beneath that "Yanks Advance 28 Miles; Link-Up Still Not Announced," with a large map of the city of Berlin centered at the top of the page. But the local story in column 1 was "2 Boys Burned Fatally While at Grass Fire." Donald Clark Powell, age seven, died in City Hospital at 5:45 p.m. two hours after being burned; his brother James Wesley Powell, age nine, died at 11:55 p.m.; their brother Joseph Robert, age six, in City Hospital, was "expected to recover."[72] It was not until a month later, the character of the hazard now understood, that the *East Liverpool Review* reported that the coroner had joined the drive to ban inflammable clothing. "Prevention is a lot better than inquests."[73]

Even in the midst of breaking news coverage, events suggested how little protection a single story buried in the inside pages of a newspaper might provide. On April 11, 1945, in the midst of the breaking story in Washington, DC, the *Cumberland Evening Times* published a specific warning directed to mothers about the Gene Autry cowboy suit. The article—"'Juvenile Booby Traps': Mothers Warned Cowboy Suits May Cause Death of Children"—identified the cowboy suit by name, described what it looked like, explained what element of it was highly inflammable, and noted that it had been sold nationally and that one DC-area boy had been killed and eight others injured. But the article appeared well into the paper, printed at the bottom of a densely packed page of news. And its opening paragraph almost made light of the danger: "Cumberland children who prefer to be 'cowboys' instead of playing the role of brave marines battling the Japs are in actual danger of losing their lives—if they happened to receive Gene Autry outfits from Santa Claus."[74] A month later, two local boys were burned in independent incidents on Mother's Day. The newspaper immediately recognized the incidents for what they were: "Booby Traps: Child Burned When Cowboy Pants Ignite." But the earlier coverage had not protected the boys from being burned.[75]

One might have expected that AP and UP reporters, having picked up the story as it broke in Washington, DC, would read subsequent incidences through a new lens. But reporters for the wire services had their "beats" just like reporters for local dailies did, and so—as more children were burned in Gene Autry cowboy suits—the old narrative held and was picked up in turn by papers that relied on the wire services for news. "Boy Dies of Burns," read the headline of the AP story out of Birmingham in early May 1945, published in the *Tampa Bay Times*. The short article would have been familiar to anyone who had read news reports of children fatally burned in 1942 or 1943 or 1944.[76] And as was true during the war years, most incidents never made the news at all.[77] There was no news story about six-year-old George Baker in Toronto, Ohio, or six-year-old Robert Smith in Dubuque, Iowa, or eight-year-old Ralph Krau in Depew, New York, whose cowboy suit exploded in a blinding flash of flame when he ventured too close to a bonfire built by adults celebrating V-J Day near his home. It was almost as though the tragedy was a part of the war, something that, like the war, was now past.

The end of the war did not change reporting. Incidents of boys fatally burned when their cowboy suits caught fire, for the most part, remained local news, the substance no different than reporting on such tragedies before the news of the Gene Autry cowboy suits had broken. "Funeral Today Chesley Johnson," read the headline on August 22, 1945, in Florence, South Carolina's *Morning News*.[78] "Burns Fatal to Son of Coach," read the headline on August 27, 1945, in the *Wilkes-Barre Record*, reporting on the death of Richard Johnson.[79] "William Augustus Strong III" led the obituary in the *Winston County Journal* in Louisville, Mississippi, on November 9, 1945.[80] "Hospital Treats 3 For Serious Burns," read the headline in a Tampa, Florida, paper in early January 1946, lumping the news of six-year-old Patrick Peterson being burned when his cowboy chaps caught fire as he played in the yard, with two other unrelated instances of burns.[81]

There were moments in 1946 when the danger of the Gene Autry cowboy suit reclaimed a limited public attention. But they were few, their impact fleeting.[82] A double tragedy in Baltimore in late February 1946, in which two brothers were burned wearing identical cowboy suits—four-year-old Larry Meisner, who died the same day, and his two-year-old brother, Wayne, who died two days later—was picked up by the AP and in turn by newspapers in both cities close to Baltimore and those with no connection to it. The stories were the same; only the headlines differed. "Boy Dies, Brother Badly Burned in Cowboy Suit Fire," read the headline in *The Washington Post*; "'Cowboy' Game Ends In Tragedy for Boys," read the headline in the *Charleston (WV) Daily Mail*; and "'Cowboy-Indian' Game Ends In Death of Youth," read the headline in the *Kingsport (Tenn.) News*.[83] The stories read just like stories of boys burned during the war years. The next day came a second AP story out of Baltimore noting that the fire department was making a canvas of retail stores in the city to determine if the suit was still being sold. The story described the suit—"The suits were described as having fuzzy wool chaps, which Fire Department officials said were highly inflammable"—without identifying it by name. And this story was carried by a different set of newspapers, all in Maryland. It was as though the story of boys being burned was universal, whereas the story of stores canvassed for cowboy suits was local or only as broad as the state. All that differed, again, was the headline. "Check Stores for Cowboy Suits After Second Child Dies," read the February 28 headline in Hagerstown, Maryland's *The Daily Mail*, "Parents Warned on Cowboy Suits" and "Hundreds of Children Are Endangered; Two More Boys Die of Burns," read the headline in the *Cumberland Evening Times*; and "Cowboy Suit Sales Probed as Second Victim Succumbs," read the headline in *The Washington Post* the next day.[84] *The Washington Post* carried a second AP story out of Baltimore with a warning to parents from the state insurance commissioner and fire marshal, Lawrence Ensor, that "all cowboy suits should be investigated for inflammability before children are allowed to wear them."[85] Other papers did not pick up this story.

In June 1946, the cowboy suit hazard became "breaking news" once again. In early June, the Passaic *Herald-News* reported the story of two neighbor boys in Passaic, New Jersey, roasting marshmallows with other boys: five-year-old Gerald Sukinik, who was burned to death, and four-year-old Joseph Intelisano, who was burned but expected to survive.[86] The initial news story on the tragedy read like the story in the *Herald-News* from close to three years earlier of Casimir Jr. and Stanley Krzeczkowski. The only difference being that the story about the Krzeczkowski brothers had mentioned that the boys were wearing cowboy suits.

Two weeks after the initial story about Joseph Intelisano and Gerald Sukinik, the *Herald-News* carried its own investigative report, written by staff writer Stanley E. Gusty: "Death Lurks in Boys' Play Suits."[87] The opening paragraph of the story noted that within the last three years, at least six area boys had been burned when the Gene Autry cowboy suits they were wearing burst into flame. And accompanying the front-page story was a photo of Joseph Intelisano in Passaic General Hospital, his bandaged legs suspended in the air, with a caption that began "He's in Pain." The article included coverage of six boys—Casimir Jr. and Stanley Krzeczkowski, burned in November 1943; John Zibor and Freddy Piechota, burned in October 1944; and Joseph Intelisano and Gerald Sukinik, burned in June 1946. Of the earlier incidents, only that involving the Krzeczkowski brothers had made the news—reported as a story about children playing with fire. Reporters for the *Herald-News*—as had been done in April 1945, tested the suit to see how quickly it would burn, capturing the test in a four-sequence photo: "The torch is lit"; "Chaps aflame"; "In 30 seconds"; "One minute—it's all over."[88] The article noted that legislation was now pending in Congress to curb hazards of this sort and cited a pending federal court case by a woman against a retailer for a robe that burned in a fashion similar to the cowboy suits.

But what the *Times-Herald*'s 1946 coverage also made clear was how little ground had been gained. Despite breaking news and national retail association warnings, the suits were still for sale in some local stores. A follow-up story noted that Passaic area merchants were halting sales of the dangerous suits.[89] A second article that day noted that the flammable-fabrics bill in Congress was "bottled up" in the Committee on Interstate and Foreign Commerce and that there was no likelihood of action in the current session.[90] The *Herald-News* sustained the coverage for a few more days, but then the news moved on.[91] In early October, the *Herald-News* reported, "Another Passaic Boy Burned When Cowboy Suit Ignites." As five-year-old Wallace Tetla's mother told the paper, the suit had been purchased by a friend of the family employed at the M. A. Henry Company. The paper did not note whether the Tetlas took the *Herald-News* or had seen the investigative report warning parents of the hazard.[92]

Moved by the incidents in New Jersey, in January 1947, Congressman Gordon Canfield introduced his own bill in Congress to ban inflammable fabrics from interstate commerce.[93] And in March 1947, the *Herald-News* shared Gerald Sukinik's father's letter to Representative Canfield: "We lost our little boy last June through one of the cowboy suits that you are trying to outlaw. We thank you for your efforts to spare other parents the pain we endured. If I can do anything in any way to further the bill please let me know."[94] It would be seven more years, 1953, before a flammable-fabrics bill became federal law.

During the war years, the circulation of newspapers had been at an all-time high. The total daily circulation of English-language daily newspapers in 1943 was well over forty-four million.[95] Circulation numbers remained high after the war. But circulation is not the same thing as reading. Reading did not mean every story. Then, as now, readers focused on different parts of the paper. And even as everyday life remained profoundly rooted in the local, news increasingly came from and was about somewhere else.

Knowing, too, is a complicated thing. A story about a boy fatally burned in a distant city or even a stranger in one's own was tragic. It could call forth donations of money, blood, or even skin from strangers. But it was a story about an accident to one child. I suspect that even among those who may have read or heard something about some cowboy suit that had led to injuries, their knowing dimmed with the passage of time. Or with the belief that it had been a wartime thing of shoddy merchandise. Or with the assumption that the hazard had been addressed. Or with the notion that this is simply what happens when children play with fire. Readers did not have the opportunity you have had to see how coverage of this tragedy played out over time. There were no search engines. Nothing that collated news relating to particular topics. The newspaper went out with the trash. It was itself an ideal fire-starter.

The news broke in a limited way, at a point when thousands, maybe several hundred thousand, of the suits had been sold. And in most places, there never was news at all about the hazard the Gene Autry cowboy suit posed. And so, it is unsurprising that long after April 1945, more children were burned in Gene Autry cowboy suits, and when those incidents were reported at all, they were stories of a tragedy to a local child and his family or some child in a distant city.[96]

But another kind of news began to circulate as early as 1946, and that was of lawsuits being filed—and while news of a lawsuit was local, news of a verdict or a settlement would have a far larger orbit.

fall

Dear Frances,

Dad & I spent the day on a long, long paddle . . . It felt good to be on the lake again in a canoe, quietly paddling with Dad. I felt like you were along with us. Sometimes I have that feeling and there's a certain contentment that comes with it. But as we were heading back, I found that sort of desperation coming over me, a sort of panic like I just had to get out of there. But there's no getting out of a canoe when you're 9 miles from your cabin. And so I just had to paddle with tears locked in, my chest aching.

. . .

I hadn't anticipated how sad I would feel to be here. The last/only time you were at the cabin was in the fall. . . . As Dad and I were cooking tonight and the sun was setting, I remember the three of us—you, me, and Dad—sitting outside in October 2009, watching the sunset, talking to Wilder on a cell phone. We imagined then that we had forever together as a family. We were so caught up in the moment. I am so thankful for that time, grateful even that we could have been so carefree, so confident of our future together. I could not have dreamed that none of our plans would come to be, that Dad and I would be here alone, talking on the phone to Wilder at school, and you gone. I am sick with loss. How I wish you were here.

. . .

I dreamt about you last night. It was at Burntside Lake and you were all dressed up in this white dress and you were beautiful and happy and you were working to get the Queen to give an island to be used for a girl's camp. I woke up from the dream and wanted to go back into it. It was so wonderful to see you so happy, so free, so confident, so full of life.

. . .

I find myself thinking of your week at the hospital sometimes when I first wake up, sometimes when I lay down to go to sleep. These are hard times because I want so much to know that you didn't suffer, that you weren't in pain, that you were not afraid, that you did not know what had happened. I want so desperately for you to have left this world happy, excited for your future, and knowing how deeply we loved you. I want you to have left this world feeling safe in our love.

. . .

Today has been a struggle. I meet people and they ask what I teach & I don't know how to answer because I don't feel like I know anything or teach anything. Yet the demands are there—letters for this student for grad school, letters for 2 more students for jobs, . . . I simply don't feel like I have any energy or desire to do anything. I want to quit, to escape. I want this nightmare to end. I want you back. But I know I can't have that.

chapter eight · "falling out of time"

Seven-year-old James Hummel, his cowboy suit afire, ran for home. He tripped and fell. Adults, alerted by his screams, reached the boy, extinguished the flames, and took him to the hospital.[1] He survived for one hour.

James La Rue Hummel was born in Berwick, Pennsylvania, on April 2, 1939.[2] He died at 6:20 p.m. on September 16, 1946. His death certificate noted his age as seven years, five months, fourteen days. He was Albert and Alverda Hummel's only child. The coroner certified the cause of death based on a "view" of the boy's body. He noted the "immediate cause of death" as "internal burns of lungs and skin on outside burned to a crisp." Where the "certificate of death" asked "due to," the coroner noted "clothing ketching fire." He did not note what the child had been wearing, a Gene Autry cowboy suit his parents had bought in December 1945 and given their son for Christmas. The coroner ruled the death an "accident." There was no inquest.[3]

The certificate of death for James Hummel would be one of the only official documents that registered the fact of his life. Birth certificates, death certificates, a Social Security card, the US decennial census, and, for men beginning with World War II, mandatory selective service registration at age eighteen: the ways in which the modern state makes a nation by knowing its population.[4] But the Social Security Act was still new when James was born, and, in any event, his parents had not registered him. That his name appeared in the US census was a matter of the happenstance that his short life straddled a census year.[5] Now, with this document that represented the public-facing side of death, James Hummel's life was part of the nation's vital statistics.

We can know elements of a life through documents, but forms are not, do not capture, a life. "We come into the world alone, unlike all who have gone before us," Elizabeth Cady Stanton wrote in 1892. "No mortal ever has been, no mortal ever will be like the soul just launched on the sea of life. There can never again be just such a combination of prenatal influences; never again just such environments as make up the infancy, youth and manhood of this one. Nature never repeats herself, and the possibilities of one human soul will never be found in another. No one has ever found two blades of ribbon grass alike, and no one will ever find two human beings alike."[6]

David Lonneman, age five
Donald Frederick Yerkes, age ten
Daniel Fogarty, age seven
Stanley Krzeczkowski, age five
Albert Thatcher, age nine
Dennis Duffy Jr., age four
Stanley Janes, age five
Lee Scott Campbell, age six
William Kingston, age four
Howard Diable Jr., age five
Elwood Athey Leary Jr., age five
Thomas James Hizny, age seven
Ernest Bell, age nine
Richard E. Furmanski, age six
Michael Blessington Jr., age seven
Arthur Lunsford, age six
Chesley Franklin Johnson, age six
Thomas McCormack, age seven
David Speaker, age five
Willie B. Wilks Jr., age nine
Marco Antonio DiTrapani, age five
Richard Johnson, age six
Donald Clark Powell, age seven
James Wesley Powell, age nine
Robert Henry Flesher, age eight
Daniel Marszalek, age six
William Augustus Strong III, age six
Larry E. Meisner, age four
Wayne A. Meisner, age two
Gerald Sukinik, age five

James Hummel, age seven
Robert Swalwell Jr., age five
Nelson Hoxie, age six
Paul Johnson, age five
Thomas Purcell, age four

They were only children, only sons, firstborn sons carrying a father's name, youngest children, oldest children, one of two, one of five, two of three, the only two.[7] They were from towns with fewer than two thousand residents and cities of over seven million. They would have started school the next year or had started school that year, were in the first or second or third grade. After being burned, they had survived one hour, three hours, four hours, seven hours, nine hours, eleven hours, one day, eighteen hours, two days, three days, four days, nineteen days, one month and twenty-seven days, three months and one day, four months and six days, four months and fifteen days, four months and twenty-five days, seven months and fourteen days, eight years and twenty-three days.

Elaine Scarry writes that "for the person in pain, so incontestably and unnegotiably present is it that 'having pain' may come to be thought of as the most vibrant example of what it is to 'have certainty,' while for the other person it is so elusive that 'hearing about pain' may exist as the primary model of what it is 'to have doubt.' . . . Whatever pain achieves," she insists, "it achieves in part through its unsharability, and it ensures this unsharability through its resistance to language."[8] However true Elaine Scarry's observations are generally, they do not represent the bond between parent and child. James McCormack's hands were burned when he grabbed his flaming son, Tommy, and plunged him into the bathtub filled with water for Saturday evening baths. The next day, making his way to the glass-enclosed room next to the nurses' station, he heard screaming and knew it was Tommy, knew the meaning of his son's screams to the core of his being through the most elemental language that binds parent and child. Long before children have spoken language, they communicate their most basic needs with adults through their cries, the register in the cries of hunger, pain, fear, and terror distinct. For James McCormack, for the parents more generally whose children were burned, hearing their child's cries and screams, there was no doubt, only unbearable certainty.

The four-month hospital record for Tommy McCormack included 130 pages of nurses' reports. They noted the child's "blood curdling screams" and periods of terrible despondency. The doctors experimented with placing the child in a plaster cast, thinking that if they could immobilize him, "keep his extremities at rest, that he might have less pain." It did not work. Then, too, there was the special bed with a hole for his buttocks, making it easier to keep him clean when he urinated and moved his bowels—because when the linen was soiled, changing it required rolling him from one side of the bed to the other. "Most severe burns of this type, as we know, are fatal," the doctor would later explain. "That is, they result in death very quickly. . . . This boy lived for some time." When he was asked why the boy was sometimes taken off the critical list, he explained that it was to spare the parents. "Every time a patient is on the critical list, it means that he can be seen day and night by his family, and it isn't a good thing because the parents naturally will stay around as much as possible, and with a boy who is suffering so much, they would themselves feel so badly that it would have a very bad effect on them."[9]

Tommy McCormack was burned on January 6, 1945. For the next four months, his parents, though they had three other children, would be with Tommy as much as the hospital allowed. Catherine McCormack quit her evening job. James McCormack too spent hours at the hospital. There were times when Tommy would ask for some little thing, a comic book or something, and they would go out and get it. But when they got back, he did not want it anymore. Once or twice, the nurses put Tommy in a little wagon and took him up to the roof of the hospital to be in the sun. And "I would entertain him as best I could," said James McCormack. They worked unsuccessfully to get him to eat, and so his only nourishment came intravenously, never enough because the burns in a sense ate up the food. The doctors never attempted grafts, sure the child would die in the attempt.[10] After four months and six days, Tommy McCormack died on May 12, 1945, four days after the nation celebrated V-E Day.

Through the war, service flags hung in the windows of homes and apartments across the nation with blue and gold stars, blue signifying a family member in the service, gold, a family member—son, brother, husband, father—killed. The flags acknowledged the sacrifice not just of the men themselves but of their families and their communities. A grade-school-age girl from Davenport, Iowa, counting blue and gold stars in the windows on her side of the street on the walk to school: sixteen blocks, eighty-six flags, 183 stars, four gold. Then one day, she sees a woman sitting on a porch with a gold star in the window. She stops, looking up at the woman on her porch. She wants to say she is sorry. But the most she can manage is a little wave. To the "gold star mother," as the mothers of sons who died were known. After that day, the girl no longer counts the flags in the windows of the homes she passes on her way to school.[11] Here is the shared sacrifice of war—a sacrifice that is, all the same, borne alone.

Studs Terkel talks with an Iowa farmer and his wife years after the war. There was, first, the Depression, the farmer says, "and what it did to the farmers: foreclosures the norm; grain burned; corn at minus three cents a bushel; rural despair. Oh yes, it changed with the war. 'That's when the real boost came. The war—'" As Terkel notes, "There is a catch in his voice. He slumps in his rocker. His wife stares at the wallpaper. It is a long silence, save for the tick-tock of the grandfather's clock." And then the man's voice picks up again, the war "'—it does something to your country. It does something to the individual. I had a neighbor just as the war was beginning. We had a boy ready to go to service. This neighbor told me what we needed was a damn good war, and we'd solve our agricultural problems. And I said, "Yes, but I'd hate to pay with the price of my son." Which we did.' He weeps. 'It's too much of a price to pay.'"[12] 405,399 American deaths in World War II. If deaths that had some larger purpose in them were, nonetheless, "too much of a price to pay," what of deaths that had no larger purpose?

But the war was not only context. Edward Johnson was at sea with the navy when his six-year-old son Richard, wearing his Gene Autry cowboy suit and playing with other boys, was burned in Wilkes-Barre, Pennsylvania. He survived for almost five months, dying on August 25, 1945.[13] William Augustus Strong Jr. was still stationed in Guam when his son, William Augustus Strong III, was burned on November 3, 1945, on the front lawn of the family's home in Louisville, Mississippi. By the time news reached him, his son was dead. By the time he arrived home a week later, the funeral service was past, his only son buried.[14] Some parents lost "boys" both to war and to this seemingly senseless death. Nine-year-old Ernie Bell's father, older brother, and stepbrother were all in the service when Ernie was burned and died on December 3, 1944. Less than a year later, Ernie's parents lost their oldest son, Ernie's half-brother Clifford, in an aircraft accident on base in Weatherford, Texas.[15] Six-year-old Arthur Lunsford, the youngest child of Lester and Belle Lunsford, was burned in a Gene Autry cowboy suit in Seat Pleasant, Maryland, on December 29, 1944; he died on February 27, 1945. Later that year, the Lunsfords lost their only other son, their eldest child, killed in action in Germany.[16]

There was also simply time lost that could never be recovered. Robert Swalwell, of McKeesport, Pennsylvania, had gone into the service when his son, named after him, was twenty-two months old. His son was four years old when he got out of the service in March 1946. Less than two years later, on November 1, 1947, Robert Swalwell Jr. was burned, surviving one day. He was five years and ten months old.[17]

They came from many faiths: Baptist, Catholic, Christian Scientist, Jewish, Latter-Day Saint, Lutheran, Methodist, Presbyterian, Seventh-Day Adventist. Faith meant one thing in life. It meant another in the shadow of death. Joseph Intelisano Jr. was born into an Italian Catholic family in Passaic, New Jersey, in which religion structured everyday life and meaning. His father was named after Joseph of Mary and Joseph; his mother, Epiphania, was born on the Epiphany, the Christian feast day that celebrates the revelation of God incarnate as Jesus Christ. They christened their firstborn child Joseph Jr. As his sisters later remembered, the story in their family was that their father had taken their brother as a newborn to the parish church and held him up at the altar, saying, "If he is not to do good in the world, Lord, take him now."[18] Joseph Intelisano Jr. was four years old when he was burned in June 1946. In the weeks that followed, his mother spent her days in the hospital with her son; his father went to their parish church to pray.[19] William Augustus Strong III's obituary in the Louisville, Mississippi, *Winston County Journal* read, "Early in life he was dedicated to God in the Methodist church." He was "a regular and faithful attendant at Sunday School, where not long ago he named the Twenty-Third Psalm as his favorite scripture."[20] The Sunday morning of the day in April 1945 that Donald Clark Powell (age seven) and his brothers James Wesley (age nine) and Joseph Robert (age six) were burned in East Liverpool, Ohio, they had been to church, where they were "members" of the Sunday school at the Second United Presbyterian Church. By 5:45 that evening, Donald Clark was dead; his brother James Wesley died at 11:55 p.m. Clyde and Hattie Powell's youngest child, six-year-old Joseph Robert, was in the hospital in critical condition.[21]

Six-year-old Charles Baragona Jr.'s chaps caught fire as he played with matches in the shadow of the stairs of the parish school in Hodge, Louisiana, in September 1947. His life hung in the balance. In the months that he was in the Shriners Hospital in Shreveport, the nuns who had taught him at the parish school in Hodge and from St. Mary's Convent in Shreveport were his regular visitors, seeing to his religious devotions and keeping his mother, Theresa, abreast of his spiritual and physical well-being. "Dear Theresa," began a letter from Sister Celeste, describing her most recent visit with Charles, "Charles sang his 'Angel of God' song and said the Hail Mary and Our Father for me and even remembered the Act of Contrition I taught them."[22] "My God, I am sorry for my sins with all my heart," a children's version of the Act of Contrition, begins. "In choosing to do wrong and failing to do good, I have sinned against You whom I should love above all things. I firmly intend, with Your help, to do penance, to sin no more, and to avoid whatever leads me to sin. Our Savior Jesus Christ suffered and died for us. In His Name, My God, have mercy. Amen."[23]

In another letter, Sister Mary Hyacinth focused on the question of how God could have allowed this thing to happen. "Today, I went to see your little boy Charles with Sister Celeste," she began. After describing Charles saying his prayers with them, she turned to his mother's certain anguish.

> Oh! Theresa, you must <u>have suffered terribly</u> when this awful accident happened to your darling little boy. This was a heavy cross to bear. But God will bring out some good from this big trial. One day, we will found out, the reason why our dear Lord allowed this to happen. Let us trust in Him always. Let us pray to Him in all confidence for He loves us. Let us ask Him to cure your darling little one. Oh! I believe in prayer. We must pray hard and wait patiently for God's answer. Take courage, Theresa, God is watching over your little Charles.[24]

As Robert Orsi notes, "Physical distress of all sorts, from congenital conditions . . . to the unexpected agonies of accidents and illness, was understood by American Catholics in the middle years of [the twentieth] century as an individual's main opportunity for spiritual growth." The "ethos" or "theology" of "sanctification through suffering . . . was pervasive."[25] The prayers of the sisters and of Charles Baragona Jr.'s mother and Joseph Intelisano Jr.'s father were answered. Their boys survived. But there were other children from Catholic families who did not, boys like David Lonneman, in Cincinnati, Ohio; Daniel Fogarty, in Baltimore, Maryland; Thomas Enoch Purcell, in Minersville, Pennsylvania; and Michael Blessington Jr. and Tommy McCormack, in New York City.

The children's bodies "reposed" at home and at funeral "homes."[26] Funeral rites and burials took place within a matter of days. The announcement of seven-year-old Michael Blessington's death read simply: "Blessington—Michael, on March 28, beloved son of Michael and Agnes. Reposing at his residence, 134–38 174th St., Springfield Gardens, L. I., until Friday, 9:30 A. M. Interment St. John's Cemetery."[27] A double funeral was held for Donald Clark and James Wesley Powell at the United Presbyterian Church in East Liverpool, Ohio, three days after they were burned and died.[28] Richard Crull Johnson's family were members of the Baugham Memorial Methodist Church in Wilkes-Barre, Pennsylvania. Richard died five months after being burned; a private service and his burial took place two days later.[29]

Robert Henry Flesher's family were members of the Trinity Evangelical Lutheran Church in New Cumberland, Maryland. He had been eight years old when he was burned. He was ten when he died of a heart attack one year and eight months later, never having left the hospital. "Rites" and his burial took place three days later.[30]

The services ranged from private services at the family's, a grandparent's, or a minister's home, to services at funeral homes and elaborate church services with pallbearers, music, and flower bearers. For six-year-old Daniel Marszalek, the youngest of ten children, a full article detailed "the mass of the angels" at St. Stanislaus Polish National Church in Scranton. The article noted the priest who had "celebrated" the mass and conducted the "committal" service at the cemetery; the children's choir that sang; the names of the pallbearers and flower bearers.[31] The announcement of the service at the First Baptist Church in Florence, South Carolina, for six-year-old Chesley Franklin Johnson included the pastor's name who would conduct the "rites," the names of pallbearers, the choir that would sing under whose direction, the organist who would play, and the name of the Bible class that would be in charge of flowers.[32]

These children were "survived" by their parents. Many were also "survived" by siblings. And most were "survived" by grandparents. "In addition to his parents," the announcement of five-year-old Elwood Athey Leary Jr.'s death noted, "the child is survived by four sisters," listing them by name.[33] The announcement of six-year-old Richard Crull Johnson's death read, "In addition to his parents, he is survived by his sister, Ann Johnson; his paternal grandmother, Mrs. Anna Johnson, Wilkes-Barre, and his maternal grandparents, Mr. and Mrs. Martin Crull, Lewisberry."[34]

Through the nineteenth century, that many children would not survive infancy and early childhood had been a given. There was suffering for their families, nonetheless. One has only to consider the abundance of child elegies in nineteenth-century American poetry; the practice of families having lovingly arranged memorial photographs taken of their dead child; and more individual, intimate expressions of loss like Ralph Waldo Emerson's letters and journal entries in the days after his son Waldo died.[35] But by the mid-twentieth century in the United States, that a parent would have to bury a child in any circumstance other than war had become unnatural.[36] And so child death, rather than being something that many families would experience and that was broadly part of the culture, became private, the burden of the few.

"I have to go," says the character identified only as "Man"—and, later, "Walking Man"—in David Grossman's prose poem of mourning, written after his own son's death. The man's wife—identified as "Woman"—responds, "Where?" "To him," says the man, referring to their dead son.[37] When the book opens, it has been five years since they received news of their son's death, years in which they have fallen silent. The man sets out and is joined by others who have also each lost a child and who are also lost in grief. As they walk, they speak. Walking Man, speaking to his son, says,

> I seem to understand
> only things inside time.
> The way I miss you
> is trapped in time as well. Grief
> ages with the years, and there are days
> when it is new, fresh.
> So, too, the fury at all that was robbed
> from you. But you are
> no longer
> You are outside
> of time.
> How can I explain
> to you, for even the reason is
> captured in time. A man from far away
> once told me that in his language
> they say of one who dies in war,
> he "fell."
> And that is you: fallen
> out of time,
> while the time
> in which I abide
> passes you by
> . . . .
> I see you
> but I do not touch
> I do not feel you
> with my probes of time.[38]

The nuns had said to Charles Baragona Jr.'s mother, "One day, we will found out, the reason why our dear Lord allowed this to happen." I wonder what she and others who were told similar things heard or took from such statements. Whatever it meant to Charles Baragona Jr.'s mother in the moment, that it did not mean inaction or unquestioning acceptance was suggested by the fact that she repeatedly sought a lawyer to bring suit on their behalf. But in the moment of their loss, the parents did not know of any reason for it. When at least some of those whose child or children had died learned the reason behind their children's deaths, the only comfort that knowledge could bring them was perhaps some allaying of guilt, but along with that allaying came "fury at all that was robbed" from their children.

Burns are to pain what the loss of a child is to death. These children died and were buried before their parents could have any understanding of the pain and anguish that awaited them. For many, their child just that morning had been full of life. And now he was gone, fallen out of time, in a death that they knew had brought their child or children blinding pain and terror.

Six-year-old Billy Strong was remembered as having picked the 23rd Psalm as his favorite scripture. "Surely goodness and mercy shall follow me all the days of my life," the psalm closes. "And I will dwell in the house of the Lord forever."[39] Did that memory or the psalm itself comfort his parents? Some parents may have found comfort there, while others questioned or rejected a faith that told them their "dear Lord allowed this to happen," that this was their "cross to bear," that "God will bring out some good from this trial."

There were also families for whom religion played little or no role in their everyday lives, and other Christian faiths did not place the same emphasis as mid-twentieth-century American Catholics did on sanctification through suffering. But as Karen Sánchez-Eppler notes, death is always both individual and intimate, and also culturally constructed in its expression.[40] Whether a family had a particular faith tradition or not, they lived in a culture in which religion held a prominent place, and they were living the kind of loss that called forth religiously grounded explanations. They no doubt heard words from well-meaning friends, family, and community members that all things happen for a reason, that it was better their child had died than live with prolonged suffering or disability, that their child was now in a better place, that God does not give us greater burdens than we can carry.

And many lived in a sort of silence, made to feel like they should not speak their dead child's name, that talking about their child or his death meant dwelling on the past when they should be focused on the future. Or they lived a silence grounded in survival. Having lost this child or these children, their own ability to carry on with life meant not speaking their child's name, clearing a house of a child's belongings and the painful memories they held.

In the face of the unimaginable, marriages and family bonds were tested. Some were undoubtedly deepened, others strained beyond repair, and others still destroyed. Five-year-old Stanley Krzeczkowski and his seven-year-old brother, Casimir Jr., their parents' only children, were burned in late 1943; Stanley died later the same day; his older brother ultimately survived. Casimir Sr. and Stella Krzeczkowski divorced shortly thereafter.[41] Richard Szumita would ultimately survive his burns, but the accident changed his parents' marriage. Margaret Roberts Szumita had acceded to her husband's authority and beliefs in baptizing their first two living children Catholic. But at age one, Richard, who had been born in 1942, developed polio, and at age six, he was horribly burned wearing a Gene Autry cowboy suit. It seemed he would not live. Like many whose children died or hovered on the verge of death, they were likely encouraged to have another child. But when they did in 1949, Margaret refused to have him baptized Catholic, and so he remained unbaptized until the birth of a final child in 1955, another son, at which point Margaret had both boys baptized as Protestants.[42]

The loss and grief of siblings and playmates went mostly unacknowledged. The playmate that Marco Antonio DiTrapani had been playing with, who had seen his friend in a blaze of flames, was "sent away" for a while. "They sent him away while Tony was in the hospital," Mrs. DiTrapani remembered; "then he was away some two months after he was buried."[43] Children who died in the midst of a school year, like Michael Blessington Jr., Tommy McCormack, and William Augustus Strong III, were there one day and not the next. What were their classmates told? And for young children who lost siblings, few likely ever saw their sibling alive again, even where they had survived for days or months in the hospital. The relaxed visiting rules for those in critical condition applied to parents, not young children. Children who lost a sibling also lost their parents in a sense, for at least a time, in the hours they spent at the hospital and, afterward, absorbed by their own grief.

The Szumitas were not alone in having another child when it seemed their child who had been burned might die, or their child had died, or it had become clear he would never recover. The advice came from doctors and lawyers, and I expect also from relatives, friends, ministers, priests, and rabbis. As Tommy Habina lay in the hospital near death, his doctor told Mrs. Habina that she should get pregnant.[44] Maybe he thought pregnancy and a new baby would distract and occupy her, sparing her from her son's suffering in the immediate term and providing the comfort and demands of a new baby should Tommy die. Almost exactly a year after Gerald Sukinik's death, a birth announcement of a son, Richard Jeffrey Sukinik, appeared in the paper. The announcement noted that "the Sukiniks also have a daughter, Beverly, 19, and were the parents of the late Jerald [*sic*] Sukinik, who died June 12, from burns received when his cowboy suit became ignited."[45] But these children did not, could not, replace what had been lost. *The possibilities of one human soul will never be found in another.*

Documents like birth and death certificates ground a life in time. Religion makes claims to the eternal. Families who lost a child lived somewhere between these worlds: They were in time and out of time. In the final pages of David Grossman's prose poem *Falling Out of Time*,[46] Walking Man says,

> And he
> is dead
> I understand, almost,
> the meaning of
> the sounds: the boy
> is dead. I recognize
> these words
> as holding truth. He is dead,
> he is dead. But
> his death,
>
> his death
> is not
> dead.

Centaur's words close the book:

> Yet still it breaks my heart,
> my son,
> to think
> that I have—
> that one could—
> that I have found
> the words.

heavy

Dear Frances,

Today is the five-month anniversary. . . . I felt today like I was carrying around a heavy load. I felt literally weighted down. It was hard to walk. I bicycled slowly to school, just didn't have any energy and pushed my bike up the hill.

. . .

I have a funny story to tell you. On Monday—the day I sent out the announcement of the cat-bed-making project in your memory, I got a response in the afternoon from Carrie's mom and she mentioned that their copy of Animal Tracks from the Animal Humane Society had arrived and how nice the picture of you was. And I rushed to the mail and there was our copy and on the front was a picture of a happy-looking dog and then three cover stories, beginning with "Unforgettable Sweet Girl." And I think, "oh, that's the story about Frances." And I open the cover to check the table of contents to find the story about you and there it is, p. 14, title's a little strange—"A Long Way Home: Helping Unforgettable Sweet Girl on her Journey"—but I'm still thinking it's about you. I flip to p. 14 and that is a story about—a dog, of course. The story about you [as a volunteer] is in the back appropriately with other "memorials and honorariums." I had to laugh and what made it special on a day that had been very hard and emotional was that I knew you would have thought it was very funny. So, Frances, my unforgettable sweet girl . . .

. . .

Early on I felt like "I can't do this"—and I still do often enough. But I also find now that I often feel "I don't want to do this." And the fact that I don't have a choice increases the feeling.

. . .

I found myself thinking about some of those evenings when it was just you and me at home. I loved those evenings. Sometimes I'd be upstairs working and I'd hear your footsteps on the stairs and then there you'd be standing at the door with books in hand and you'd say, "I thought I'd come up here to do my reading to keep you company." And it was so wonderful to have you there and while I cleared papers from the couch, so you'd have a place to sit, you'd hug Sam on the floor. And then the two of us would work quietly together— the studying the working made better by the companionability of it.

. . .

I have so often this feeling of "haven't we proved ourselves worthy enough? Haven't we grieved hard enough? Haven't we been without her long enough? Can't we then have her back now?" It's not directed at God. I don't know where it's directed. It's just a feeling—by someone who has always worked hard, often giving that extra push to achieve some goal and yet now, no matter how hard I work, no matter that I've shown how much I love, how much we need you, how important it is that you have the opportunity to live your life, we don't get to have you back.

. . .

I've been thinking about your room. It's just as it was when you had your stroke. It hasn't been dusted or vacuumed or anything since you died. It feels less inhabited right now because of all the dust. Once or twice I've gone in there to think about beginning and I open a drawer or I look at the top of your dresser and I don't know where or how to begin, so I don't begin at all.

. . .

Dad and I drove up to the cabin tonight for the final time before it has to be closed down for the winter. I think it is almost one year exactly since you, Dad, and I were here last year. I asked Dad on the way up here if he has a hard time sometimes really realizing or understanding that you are gone. He said, "often." I feel that way now: a dull, dawning aching awfulness that leaves me wanting to scream: "Nooooo" and run from this reality, literally run, screaming until I can run no more.

. . .

I remember at the beginning of your junior year you initiating a conversation about bedtimes as though you were expecting a battle. You wanted to change your "bedtime" to whatever time it was (10:00 p.m.?) that Wilder had gone to bed his junior year and then, I remember your doing the same at the beginning of your senior year. And my replying in each case that, "yes," that was fair or right, or of course, that you should basically use your judgment about when to go to bed and just be sure to get enough sleep. And the funny thing was, that except on a rare occasion, you were in bed by 10:30 at the latest. You simply got ready for bed and came for hugs (Sam hugs and me hugs) and I love yous and off you went to bed. Except weekends, of course, when it was me who came to you for hugs, and I love yous and off I went while you stayed up.

. . .

Some days I just want the day to come to an end so I can climb into bed and have a few hours where I don't have to know that I've got to live the rest of my life without you.

. . .

Frances, I just realized this morning when I looked at the calendar that I had turned Monday to Friday into the 26th through the 30th—the week we spent in the hospital with you. But today isn't the 30th, it's the 29th. I woke up early this morning with a deep sadness filling my whole body. But I was off a day. In this strange world where nothing means what it used to mean, I find myself feeling that I have yet one more day with you before I have to let go again. I had planned to work on your room. And maybe though it's not the 30th that is what I will do anyway because I feel raw and fragile.

. . .

I finished cleaning your room. It's 9:00 p.m. It is hard for me to imagine that your room will never be messy again.

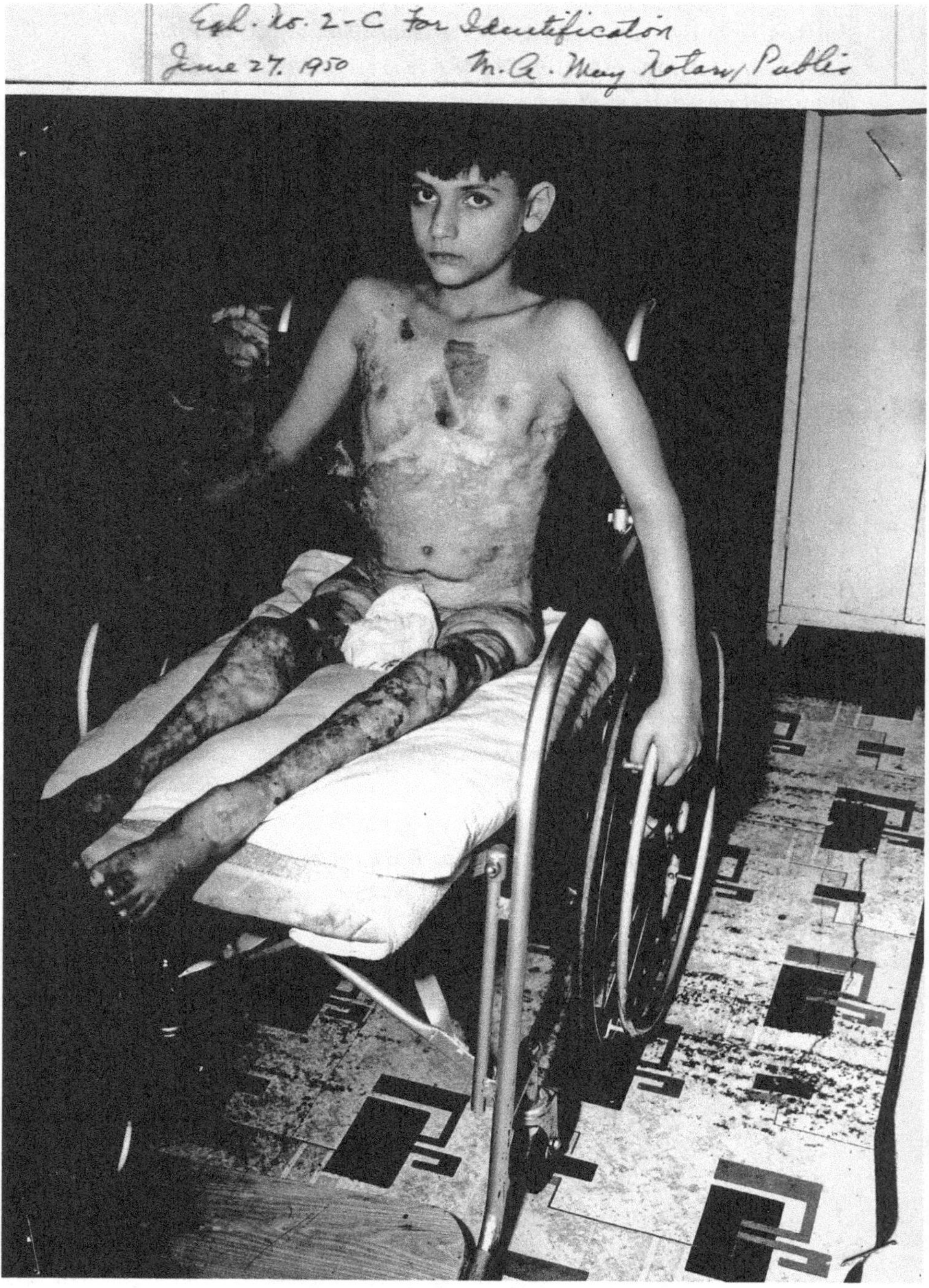
Exh. No. 2-C for Identification
June 27. 1950
M. A. May Notary Public

chapter nine · lost years

Perry Caparco was five years old when his Gene Autry cowboy suit caught fire in spring 1944 near his family's home in Providence, Rhode Island. He suffered third-degree burns encircling both legs, from his ankles to his buttocks. The doctors and nurses initially fought just to keep him alive with infusions of penicillin, plasma, and blood, the blood given by relatives, friends, "public-minded" individuals in the community, and co-workers of Perry's father, who paid from his own meager earnings for the wages that his co-workers lost in time giving blood. The first skin grafts came from Perry's father. The grafts failed. Ultimately, as was true for all the children, to have a hope of "taking," the skin had to come from their own bodies. And so, when they thought he could survive it, the doctors began to take skin from Perry's chest and back and stomach. At one point, they had him "pretty well covered." But then the skin sloughed off, and they were back to where they had started.

Photographs taken close to five years after he was burned show a slender boy with large, dark eyes in a wheelchair, his misshapen legs a mass of scars, scabs, and open sores, one leg permanently shorter than the other, his chest, stomach, and back a mass of scars; the smooth, unmarred shape and skin of his arms magnifying the distortions of his legs.[1] By the time he was twelve, Perry Caparco had spent more than half of his life in a hospital.

"But they weren't 'lost years,' were they?" a colleague said to me.

Roy Cizek was three years old when over 40 percent of his body burned in April 1946. Burned from his ankles to his waist, his face singed, his hair and eyebrows and right ear burned, he was in agony. "We could do nothing with him to start," the doctor explained, "except to put him to sleep with methyl-chloride and ether, and take the rest of his clothes off and [remove the dead skin] and clean him the best we could." Months of care passed.

"No matter what we did we had to hurt him in our treatments which made him suffer more. . . . you really couldn't give him enough medicine to stop all his suffering." The doctor searched for words to describe the pain this child endured: "It was—I don't know, except to say it was so severe that little fellow would seem to me to just about fall apart because of that."[2]

Emily Dickinson writes,

Pain has an element of blank
It cannot recollect
When it began, or if there was a time when it was not.
It has no future but itself,
Its infinite realms contain
Its past, enlightened to perceive
New periods of pain.[3]

Once, when talking with my daughter Frances about these children, she asked what I would rather have, my child die or live in such pain. She wasn't asking me how a historian would answer the question. She was asking me as a parent, a mother, her mother. That was the same day she asked me why I did this work.

Burns are defined by degree—first, second, and third—with third-degree burns being the most severe—and by the percentage of the body affected. Though some of these children escaped with a combination of second- and third-degree burns concentrated on parts of their legs, most of them suffered third-degree burns on almost the entirety of their legs, covering at least 25 percent of their body. In some cases, another article of clothing shielded other parts of their body: a leather jacket snug at the waist, wool underwear with a double layer of fabric at the crotch, wool socks, shoes. But many were burned over 30 or 40 percent of their body or more. Seven-year-old Casimir Krzeczkowski suffered third-degree burns from his feet to his stomach, including his penis and scrotum; his five-year-old brother, Stanley, had not survived the day. Six-year-old Billy Greatorex from Washington, DC, was burned on April 14, 1944, from his ankles to his waist, the burns encircling his legs and buttocks. Seven-year-old David Gagnon of Westbrook, Maine, suffered third-degree burns two years later on April 19, 1946, and like Casimir his burns included penis and scrotum.

A photograph of Richard Szumita, a year after he was burned at age five in Pawtucket, Rhode Island, on June 21, 1948, shows an emaciated child on a hospital bed, his head seeming too big for his body, his skin blackened from just below his rib cage to his ankles.[4]

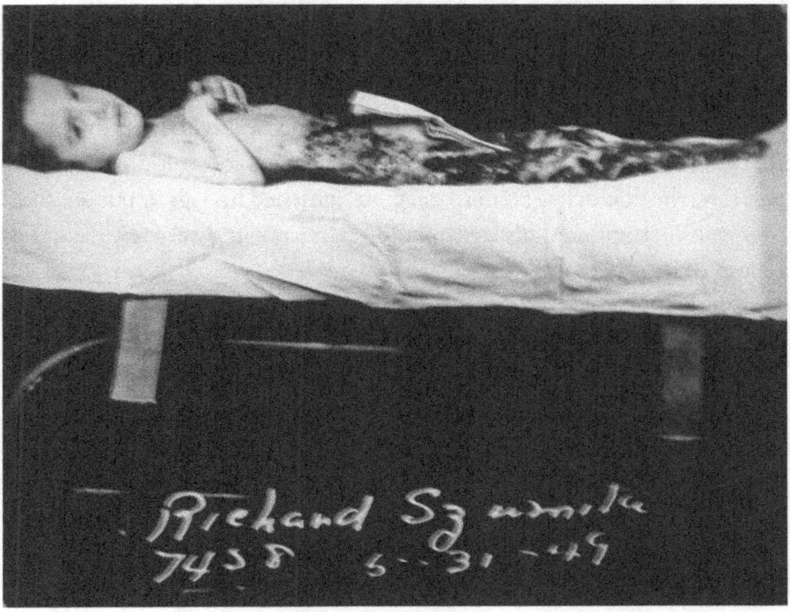

"Working against the odds"—as Eddie Bradley's doctor put it—applied to the treatment of all the children. Six-year-old Eddie Bradley arrived in the emergency room of Children's Hospital in Washington, DC, on February 27, 1945, in severe shock, with third-degree burns encircling both legs from his ankles to his groin, less severe burns on his chest, his pulse thready, his respiration shallow. The doctors thought it was more likely than not that he would die. On the fifth day his temperature rose to 105° and remained between 103° and 105° for two weeks; then, for several weeks, it hovered between 101° and 103°.[5]

At first, Eddie Bradley's doctors changed his dressings every day or every other day. But the pain and blood loss risked sending him into secondary shock, only avoided by blood transfusions. His life hung in the balance for months as he drifted between semiconsciousness and violent awakenings to pain. Toby Cumberledge was burned in Washington, DC, a month after Eddie Bradley. Some seventy years later, his voice shaking with emotion, he remembered the sound from the hospital room next to his of Eddie Bradley's screams.[6]

Toby's parents referred to the time after he was burned as his "siege." It was a siege for these children. And in the battle, doctors and nurses fought pain with everything at their disposal as intensely as they fought to save the children's lives, the two efforts intertwined. As would be true for many of the children, to reduce the pain, blood loss, and risk of secondary shock, Eddie Bradley's doctors began using pressure bandages, changing dressings less frequently and under anesthesia.[7] The slightest movement meant excruciating pain and so the children held their bodies rigid. Realizing that if Roy Cizek were ever to walk again, they could not allow the joints to stiffen and fuse, the doctors put him to sleep, straightened his legs to put on dressings, and then splinted his legs to hold them straight. Every few days, they repeated the process.[8]

Death hovered over these children. Describing the second time he changed six-year-old Billy Greatorex's dressings, his doctor explained that he thought the child would die in the process.[9] Medical terms for near death dot the children's hospital files: "cachetic," "moribund." Five-year-old Tommy Habina, burned in October 1944, was at the point of death after six months: his wounds infected, unwilling to eat, his "morale low." Moved from Philadelphia General to Temple University Hospital after six months, a doctor at Temple explained that at the time of the boy's transfer, "a simple redressing was sufficient to almost cause his death."[10] Richard Szumita hovered between life and death in Pawtucket Memorial Hospital for almost a year before he was transferred to the Shriners Hospital in Springfield, Massachusetts, a move that saved his life.[11]

Fever brought dangers of its own. Five-year-old Scott Timberlake of Kansas City, Missouri, who had suffered second- and third-degree burns of both legs from his ankles to his hips on April 3, 1948, ran a dangerously high fever in the first month after he was admitted to the hospital. At one point his fever spiked at 106 degrees and he went into convulsions lasting much of a day. His fever remained high—103° or 104°—for several weeks. Even before it subsided, the cost was clear: He had lost all speech, lost control of his limbs, and seemed to have limited comprehension.[12]

Their only chance was to get the children re-covered with skin. But many of the children could not initially survive grafts taken from their own bodies. Explaining why skin could not be taken from three-year old Roy Cizek early on, the doctor said that all that was left unburned on his tiny body was "but a little on his belly and back." Noting that most children in these circumstances would have died already, he explained that, "denuded" as the boy was, "to take more skin from him . . . might cause his death."[13] For Eddie Bradley the first skin grafts—each a foot square or more, larger than an 8½" by 11" sheet of paper—came from a policeman and fireman.

Most "heterogeneous" grafts, as they are called, though came from parents.[14] In some cases, like those of Perry Caparco or Pat Peterson, from their father who was out of work. But more often mothers—Margaret Szumita,

Florence Cizek, Kathryn Timberlake, Bessie Izzo, Euthemia Lockhart, and likely others—donated skin, some more than once. Learning only many years later why she had been there—giving skin from the inner thigh of both her legs for her son—Jack Lockhart had felt so comforted to discover his mother there on a bed beside him in the operating room.[15] Family economics alone made it more likely that mothers would give skin where needed. Even for mothers who were wage-earners, their wages lost by time away from work were less than their husbands'.

At every stage, the risk of infection loomed. Infections delayed skin grafting, compounded the initial injury in life-altering ways, left oozing ulcers, ate through apparently successful grafts, and sometimes brought death. Infection left three-year-old Roy Cizek permanently blind in both eyes, with one eye removed and deaf in one ear. It led to the amputation of both Jackie Izzo's legs and the almost total obliteration of both her hip joints, leaving her unable even to maintain an upright position. One aches to hear Jackie who, only after close to two years was sufficiently alive to comprehend that her legs had gone missing, asking her doctor to "bring her pretty long legs back." Six-year-old Chuck Baragona, burned in September 1947, lay for a month in the little clinic in Hodge, Louisiana, where the doctor who had attended his birth seemed destined to attend his death. Infection had set in with its telltale putrid smell. The doctor advised his parents that to have a chance of saving the boy they would need to amputate his legs. His father refused. If there was any chance his son might live, he wanted him to have his legs. They won that gamble, but only with the lifesaving aid of admission to the Shriners Hospital for Children in Shreveport, Louisiana, some seventy-seven miles away. Infection left Perry Caparco, six years after being burned, with open ulcers on his legs. It claimed the life of boys like Tommy McCormack.[16]

Infection did not signal a failure of care. The character of the children's injuries made it almost inevitable. The question became one of degree and consequences. In an article published in the *Journal of the American Medical Association* (*JAMA*), the doctors who treated Tommy Habina, Joseph Moore, and Eddie Klinck at Temple University Hospital in 1946 listed infection second in "the three clinical stages of third degree burns."[17] Infection was signaled by fever, odor, and appearance. Doctors came into a ward and lowered their nose to a child's bandaged legs and sniffed for the odor of infection.[18] But once it set in, the putrid smell did not require close examination. The staff in Hodge, Louisiana, moved six-year-old Chuck Baragona to the last room at the end of the Hodge clinic's long hall and put a fan in the window blowing out so that other patients would not have to smell him. Through their lives, Baragona and others found it impossible to shake the memory of that smell.[19]

For Roy Cizek, the infection began in his legs. As his doctor explained, "he was a little boy 3 years old and frail, and had a tendency to suck his thumbs and suck his fingers all the time, and under the crusting and sloughing he was burned high enough on the hips that he reached down there and he would scratch into his hips, and of course he had blood on his fingers, and he sucked those fingers and he pulled at his mouth, at his ear and pulled at his nose, and wiped his eyes, and he transferred those infections from below until he had a burned area—I mean a sore, around one side of his mouth, he had a sore around his ear, and an inflammation with an infection around his nose and his eyes." The hospital staff tried everything they could to keep his hands away from the infection on his hips and thighs: "We tied first one arm up to the bed, and that didn't work, he used the other arm, and we tied the other arm up, and finally put splints on his arms in order to keep his arms straight or away from it." But "we couldn't keep him splinted all the time. There are certain humane things to do; we couldn't keep him tied up all the time."[20]

For many children, the grafts from a parent or community member marked a critical turning point. But heterogeneous grafts were at best a temporary blanket of sorts to tide the child over. Ultimately, "to take," the grafts had to come from the child's body. And so doctors would begin the long, uncertain, painstaking process of taking skin from unburned areas of the child's body—stomach, chest, back, buttocks, upper thigh—and applying it to the areas where their flesh had been burned away. The heterogeneous grafts for Eddie Bradley held up about a month, by which time the doctors thought he could survive grafts from his own body.[21] Their age, size, critical weakened condition, and extent of burns presented special challenges. Billy Greatorex was six when he was burned, but his doctor's words echoed those of three-year-old Roy Cizek's doctor: "The child was very small . . . and I had a great deal of difficulty finding areas of his body to take skin from."[22]

Nor was there any guarantee that any particular graft from a child's body would succeed. The limited area the children had to take skin from, and their weakened, critical condition, together with the consequences if a graft failed, led doctors to proceed in a piecemeal fashion. As the doctors treating Joseph Moore, Tommy Habina, and Edward Klinck at Temple University Hospital in 1946 explained in their article in *JAMA*, "In general, we have feared massive, one stage coverage grafts where the recipient areas were so huge (30 per cent of the body surface) and the donor areas so limited, since failure would be a catastrophe."[23] The first graft Billy Greatorex's doctor tried "was unsuccessful and didn't take." The next graft succeeded partially. And so it went.[24] Jackie Izzo underwent some fifty skin grafts in the attempt to save her legs and, at the end, to cover her stumps. Over two years' time, Richard Szumita underwent fifteen operations.[25]

In the process, the children were left permanently scarred from their ankles to their necks. Their tiny torsos and legs bodyscapes of skin-grafting technique at mid-century: the square and rectangular scars of split-thickness grafts; the circular scars—a polka-dot pattern almost—of small deep grafts, sometimes referred to as "pinch grafts," involving a circular cone of skin; the telltale linear sucking-in scar across the stomach left by a flap graft. and the matching site where the tube of flesh had been spread on a child's leg.[26]

Machines like the Padgett Dermatone, designed for the sole purpose of taking skin grafts, made it possible to slice rectangular grafts of any desired and uniform thickness even from concave portions of the body, something not possible using a razor. Paper-thin grafts made it possible too to take several grafts from the same area over the course of many months.[27] But many hospitals did not have a Dermatone or doctors experienced in using one. Richard Szumita's father, Alexander, drove from their home in Pawtucket, Rhode Island, to Pennsylvania to buy a Dermatone machine for the hospital for grafting his son.[28]

Cecil Warnick, like Perry Caparco and, later, Jack Lockhart, suffered the long ordeal of multiple flap grafts. First, a strip of skin on the abdomen was sutured, making a sort of tube of flesh, and the child's hand was sutured to the end of the tube so that the blood flow to the tube of flesh would shift from the abdomen and begin to come from the hand. Once the direction of the blood flow from the hand was assured, a process that took at least three weeks, the tube of flesh was cut away from the stomach and the end of it attached to the child's leg, meaning that now the child's hand (and arm) stretched down to his leg. And he remained bound in that position for another three weeks until the blood flow again shifted, this time so that blood from the leg would nourish the tube of flesh. Finally, the child's hand and arm were cut free from the tube and the tube of flesh spread across an area on the child's leg. Each stage required at least three weeks' preparation. Cecil Warnick underwent two of these operations at Children's Hospital of Johns Hopkins Medical School, with one of the operations extending an additional six weeks because of an infection.[29]

Each stage of treatment, each operation was an ordeal. Speed mattered.

In some cases, when the child was out of immediate danger and the doctor judged the mother competent in nursing the child—including monitoring for infection and changing bandages—doctors sent the child home between skin-grafting operations, with the goal of building the child up for the next ordeal. Toby Cumberledge underwent his first skin graft operation three months into his stay at Children's Hospital in Washington, DC. Ten days later, he was sent home under his mother's care. In late June, he was readmitted for a second and third grafting operation and discharged a week later.

This schedule meant care, and with it the burden of causing pain shifted from hospital staff to mothers. "[The bandage] had to be taken off and usually it stuck in one or two places, and it was a matter of pulling the bandage off the raw flesh and it usually bled quite a bit," Toby's father explained. "Toby always had to be led up to this business slowly because he knew it was time for his bandages to be changed, and he would actually start to cry and complain before the bandages were touched." The process was slow. His mother would "take a little bit off and soak it a little bit and let him get his nerve back and soak it again and pull a little more off."[30] There were other reasons in the summer of 1945 to discharge any child they could from Children's Hospital in Washington, DC: infantile paralysis, polio. Except for polio patients, the hospital stopped admitting young children at all for fear of exposing them. In August, Toby's final skin graft was completed at a different hospital.[31]

Toby Cumberledge made his first trip home three months after being burned. He was then in and out of the hospital for three more months. There were other children who were "in" the hospital for only a few months.[32] But there were many whose time in a hospital stretched on for a year and for many others well beyond that. What did it mean to be in the hospital for months, even years, at a stage of life in which a year's time marked dramatic developmental changes? Cecil Warnick, burned on May 13, 1945, spent the next two and one-half years in the hospital. Burned when he was almost seven years old, by the time he was discharged on November 21, 1947, he was nine years old. More hospitalizations were to come. Eddie Bradley was in the hospital for a year; Tommy Habina for twenty-three months; Roy Cizek for over two years.[33] But these descriptions are themselves inaccurate. They express the time as a known period. In fact, neither the children nor their parents knew when or how it would end, and that fact shaped the experience of time itself.

Tommy McCormack's doctor had talked about taking Tommy off the "critical" list at the hospital because it offered a way to spare parents the pain of seeing their child in such suffering. General hospital practice of the time allowed only children on the critical list to be seen at all times by their parents. In the first months after Toby Cumberledge was burned, his mother arranged for a neighbor to look after Toby's brother and sister, so that she could be at the hospital in the day with him; his father went to the hospital every evening and, especially on nights when Toby was in great pain, remained late into the night until his son found sleep.[34] But once a child's life was no longer in immediate peril, hospital rules limiting time for visitors applied. Other factors too—the demands of household and family, work, distance, expense—meant that parents became visitors. Few were in the position of Eddie Bradley's mother, Laura, a trained nurse, who spent eight to twelve hours a day nursing her son in his first six months in the hospital.[35] Distance made visiting all the more difficult and expensive for families of limited means.

Though most were initially treated in local hospitals, many were later moved far from home and were away for months and years.[36] Expensive for any of these families, the time and cost of being away was harder for families with other children. Hospitals too, in some cases, limited visits even more strictly. When Charles and Teresa Baragona brought Charles Jr. to the Shriners' Hospital for Crippled Children in Shreveport a month after he was burned, he was taken into another room for an examination by the doctor and then, without opportunity for any form of goodbye, his parents were told the hospital would keep the boy and they were dismissed. Remembering the day, Chuck Baragona said, "It was better that way," making a gesture with his hands suggesting a clean break.[37]

He would not see his parents or they him for close to a month after he was admitted to the Shriners' Hospital. The week after he was admitted Elizabeth Mills, an RN and the superintendent, sent the first of many postcard updates on the boy's condition. It read simply, "Charles is improving and is perfectly contented." Perfectly contented? Could he have been? Or were these the words of a nurse and administrator, meant to soothe absent parents' hearts and minds? Two weeks later, her letter held out the possibility of their making a visit: "Charles is improving each day and it will not be very long before you can come back to see him." Superintendent Mills sent brief, typed postcards every week or two for the six months Charles was in the hospital, almost all addressed to the boy's father. Even in a context such as the Shriners' Hospital, in which the medical care was free of charge, fathers were the legal guardians of children. Visits—whether from his parents or others—were limited, their occasion and duration determined by the hospital. "Dear Therese," Sister Celeste wrote Charles's mother early in his time in the Shriners' Hospital. "Your darling Charles is doing fine! I went to see him the two past Sundays but they admitted me only last Sunday."[38]

What gives dimension to time in the life of a child? Pain and shock erased days, weeks, and, for some of the children, months and years. Newspapers stories with photos of children in the first weeks after being burned show them in hospital beds, their legs swathed in bulky bandages, supported by pillows or suspended in air.[39] The first words of the caption beneath a photo of four-year-old Joseph Intelisano were in bold print and read simply, "**HE'S IN PAIN**."[40] Toby Cumberledge's burns were far less extensive than many of the children's, and yet, describing his son in this early period, Toby's father explained, "He was out of his mind on several occasions, talking incoherently and screaming."[41]

There was anticipation of birthdays and holidays. The focus of a news story with a photo of Richard Szumita a year after being burned was his excitement for his seventh birthday the next day. So too, a news story with a photo of Bobby Flesher, nine months after being burned, described the nurses helping him celebrate his birthday with gifts of books and games.[42] Holidays order the undated letters Chuck Baragona "wrote" his parents from the Shriners' Hospital in Shreveport: Halloween, Christmas, Valentines Day, Easter.[43] Chuck Baragona was only just learning to spell his name. In one or two letters, his name appears at the bottom of the letter in his hand, the orientation of letters jumbled. Learning to write, beginning with his first name, and writing letters were part of how he passed time in the hospital. Events like birthdays, Christmas, and other holidays structured time and broke the rhythms of hospital time. But they were bittersweet. Tommy Habina's mother took any gift he received home, saying, "It will get lost here."[44]

Events like parades, fairs, and special visitors provided something to look forward to and then remember and talk about. A week after Chuck Baragona arrived at the Shriners' Hospital in Shreveport, the fair put on a show for the children.[45] Three months later Gene Autry visited the hospital.[46] I suspect that the Shreveport trip, including a show, an appearance at McCrory's Department Store, and the Shriners' Hospital visit was scheduled long before Chuck Baragona's arrival, perhaps even before the boy was burned, and I doubt that Autry knew there was a child at the hospital who had been burned wearing a Gene Autry cowboy suit.[47] Autry was long past making visits to children burned wearing the suits. But there is little Chuck Baragona, sitting up in bed, his legs under a blanket tent following a skin graft operation, a sort of a smile on his face, looking up at Autry with his big white cowboy hat, who in turn is smiling warmly down at Chuck and another boy standing beside the bed.

Newspaper coverage broke the boredom of hospital routine and held the excitement of having their picture in the paper. One leg bandaged and splinted, but sitting up in bed, Robert Viands radiates happiness in a photo taken three months after he was injured.[48] A photo of Jack Jacobs, six months after he was burned, shows him sitting up in a hospital bed, his legs and feet wrapped in bandages following a round of skin grafts, but his face alight, smiling brightly into the camera lens.[49] "Pilots Brighten David's Day with Surprise Hospital Visit," read the headline in a front-page story of the Portland, Maine *Press Herald* on June 25, 1947. A photo of David Gagnon, fourteen months after being burned, having just undergone another skin graft, shows him lying on a special brace in the hospital bed to limit the pain, smiling brightly, holding a baseball, surrounded by the players from the Portland Pilots who had come to visit after a game.[50] Eleven months later, in May 1948, the Westbrooke Memorial Day parade made a mile detour in their route to march past David's hospital window. The year after that, David Gagnon, still in the hospital, was taken to the parade in a special automobile bed.[51]

How much time could anticipation and the joy of a special moment fill? David Gagnon was still in the hospital three and one-half years after being injured. Perry Caparco, burned at age five in April 1944, had his first trip home, a month's stay, in August 1949. That Christmas was the first holiday he would spend with his family since being injured. His sixth, seventh, eighth, ninth, tenth, and eleventh birthdays were all lived in a hospital, as was every Christmas from 1944 through 1948. Discharged from the hospital on March 18, 1950, just shy of his twelfth birthday, Perry had been in the hospital for 2,031 days and was far from recovered. Burned when he was in first grade, his classmates were now in seventh grade.

Hospitals are not dwellings, not living spaces. It is easy to lapse into constructions of time that avoid references to living. We refer to time "spent" in a hospital or, more obliquely still, to someone "being" in the hospital. We resist saying that Perry Caparco or Eddie Bradley or Jackie Izzo or any other of these children lived in the hospital, some for significant portions of their childhoods. Did the structure of hospital time and authority replace for them family time and authority? In place of the freedom particular to childhood, there was hospital time, not family time. Seasons and with them the passage of time are experienced differently indoors. One of the usages of *curriculum* in classical Latin was the passage of the seasons.[52] Summer gave way to fall, fall to winter, winter to spring, spring to summer. The length of the daylight hours waxed and waned. There were moments outside. Tommy McCormack's father referred to having taken his son in a wagon to the rooftop of Mt. Sinai Hospital in New York City. Family photos too show children in wheelchairs and hospital beds moved out into the

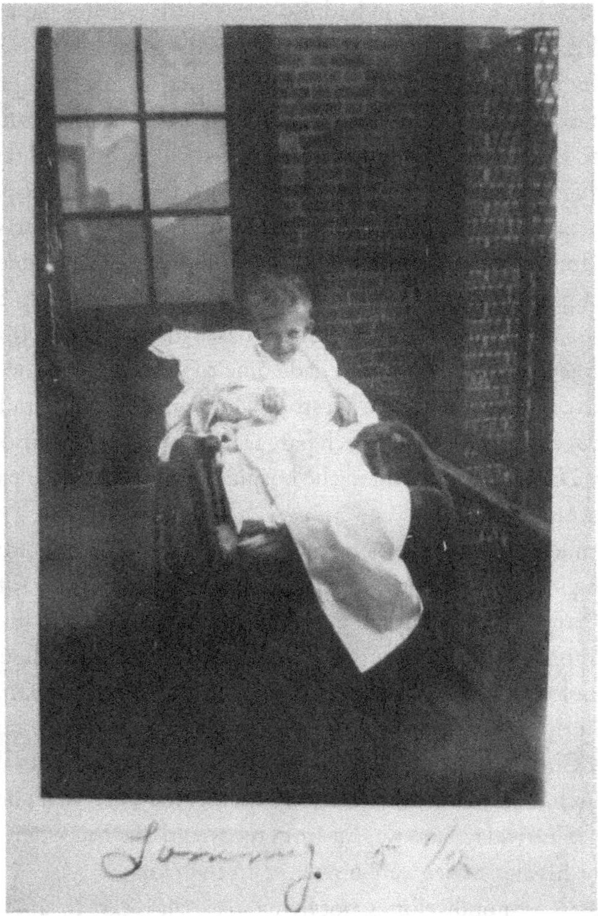

open air.[53] But these were exceptional moments against a world of artificial light and antiseptic smells.

In contrast to adults who often describe time as racing by, children often describe time as moving with infinite slowness. How much truer would that have been for these children, many of whom were not yet able to read or write, who were bedridden for months on end? There was the unbearable sound of other children crying. Loneliness. The sound of small puffs of air in the darkness of the boy's ward as the boys in the quiet time between day and sleep worked to keep tiny tufts of "fur" they had pulled from the stuffed bear they had each been given afloat. Nightmares. The comfort of a nurse gently waving a washcloth above a boy's face so that he might fall back asleep. There was fear in anticipation of the next dressing change. Fear of the ether. And there was pleading. A child begging his mother to buy the sheet on which he lay when he was set to leave the hospital because each time he was lifted the skin stuck to the sheet and ripped away.[54]

But there were also memories of world-making, of living. There was the work and excitement of relearning how to walk: "MOTHER," Charles Baragona began a letter, with big, square letters, "I HAVE BEEN UP THREE TIMES. I WALKED WITH MILLS. / LOVE / CHARLES." And in the superintendent's lovely cursive hand at the bottom, "Be sure to tell Sr. Catherine that the little boy can walk—he is not entirely well yet, but so happy to walk. E. Mills."[55] There were picture books brought by a favorite nurse. There were improvised games: a child saving the little white pills—penicillin—he was given every day to have enough to play "marbles"; wheelchair races down a hospital corridor.[56] Boredom: a child picking the little white wriggling things—maggots eating the dead flesh—on his legs beneath the blanket tent and tossing them over the balcony where he had been rolled outside in a wheelchair for a family visit. And there was radio. Jackie Izzo remembers shushing her mother when she would arrive in the midst of one of her favorite programs.[57] There was even escape: a cousin sneaking into the hospital after her school day ended, plopping Jackie, her stumps bandaged, on a hospital cart and wildly wheeling her away for an adventure. Learning how to smoke in a hospital bathroom. Laughing as she told me stories of her cousin Mary Jo, Jackie Izzo said, "She taught me everything about life."[58]

On March 8, 1948, six months after Charles Baragona was admitted to the Shriners' Hospital in Shreveport, Superintendent Elizabeth Mills wrote to his father, "Charles is ready to go home. You may come for him between nine and four o'clock."[59] Cecil Warnick's parents only learned that their son could again walk and that they could take him home when they visited on November 21, 1949.[60] Jackie Izzo's life had been despaired of for the first two years after she was burned in the summer of 1944. It was Easter over three years later that her mother walked into St. Mary's Hospital, picked her daughter up in her arms, and simply walked out of the hospital with her.[61] So many of these children, burned in the midst of a global war, returned home after war's end. The tide of the war had begun to turn in Europe but not in the Pacific when Jackie was burned. By the time she returned home, the war had been over for several years, but she did not know it.[62]

· PART III ·

Markets & Families

first snow

Dear Frances,

First snow. I'm not ready for snow without you. But like summer, like fall, like the change in time, it comes anyway.

...

Dad & I just finished eating dinner here in the family room. The green candle is still burning. Last year I thought that once you were gone to college we would have the kitchen table back, but now the only table surface that's clear to eat at is here in the family room. The dining room table is piled with your school books; the table in the living room is covered with things of yours from school or from the memorial service. . . . I need to tackle all of these spaces. The first floor is largely uninhabitable at the moment, but I don't really have the energy.

...

Somedays I go through the motions & seem okay, others I don't even bother to start. But I think this is how time passes. One day follows another and then it's been several months, and then a year and then two and somehow you're (I mean me/us) still living without having made any decision to do so.

...

I'm at the airport. It's very busy. The approach of a holiday is palpable. My heart aches. I find myself glancing up, hoping to see you heading my way, knowing also though that it's not to be. I knew we would have to do holidays, but it seems unreal that they're here. I would like to retreat.

...

It's Thanksgiving. Last May I didn't even imagine this day, but as the summer went on I knew we'd have to face the holidays. I couldn't really imagine getting there, but I knew they would come all the same. The snowstorm from yesterday has left all the trees covered in a blanket of snow. The sun is out today. It is sparkling white and still after the gray and wind of yesterday. I am heartsick not to have you here.

. . .

With Thanksgiving past many houses now have Christmas lights on. I can't imagine Christmas without you. The word even looks funny on the page.

. . .

Today is the 28th. It is Sunday. But in the calculus of your last week, it is Wednesday. I miss you. I long to have you here. "I want you where I am" you told me at age 5. Now I want you where I am because it would mean you were alive.

. . .

I question that I have to go on at all. I am caught short—almost like having your breath taken away—when I realize that you are gone. Realizing it seems to happen again and again and again. I think it would be easier if I thought that I would get to be with you again someday.

. . .

The other day it dawned on me that the one picture we have of me is when I too was a senior in high school. It's the photo of me in my cheerleading uniform leading a cheer and looking up into what is clearly the stands with a football game going on behind me. I found myself thinking that if I had died then, that year people would have thought I too was headed somewhere with my life, but I don't think anyone would have seen the path my life would take. I thought about that in relation to you. We don't know what path you would have made for yourself.

chapter ten · an academic marketplace

Professional academic norms had long cast open, individual job seeking with a taint. In the years following World War II, those norms remained strong. As a 1958 guide issued by the Teaching Division of the Columbia University Placement Bureau put it, "For the person with a doctorate, there is a certain professional prudence in not making independent inquiries to other schools unless there has been some previous contact with the appointing officer."[1] A senior scholar at the Annual Meeting of the American Historical Association in 1961 put it more bluntly: "No intelligent young historian would ever approach anybody *directly* about a job. . . . If he did, he'd automatically be finished."[2] His view was widely shared and not just in history.

But the experience of depression and war had transformed employment expectations of Americans, including those pursuing PhDs, many of whom had served in World War II or would serve in Korea. The uncertainty and academic job shortages of the early and mid-1950s, in turn, increased the pressure on professional societies to advance the employment of their members. The American Historical Association (AHA) had toyed with the idea of a placement bureau in the 1930s, only to formally consider and reject the idea in 1941. It was with the hiring of a new executive director, Boyd C. Shafer, in 1953, that the AHA finally established a "Job Register" in spring 1954.[3]

The AHA reflected a broader pattern of professional societies in the 1950s and 1960s, establishing placement services that offered registrants and hiring institutions year-round services, including making brief biographies of registrants available to hiring institutions and providing interviewing services at annual meetings.[4] They sought to distinguish their services from ordinary job seeking and did so in part through a professionalized vocabulary. The AHA dubbed its registration form the "vita form." Many other professional societies likewise used "vita" to describe the forms required of registrants.[5] Those seeking academic jobs both took for granted that they would need to complete a form and resisted the distinction societies sought to maintain.[6]

The labor intensiveness and inefficiencies of professional societies' placement systems in the 1950s and 1960s boggle the mind. At the AHA, Executive Secretary Boyd Shafer himself responded to every request from a prospective hiring institution—pulling vita forms of "likely candidates," often commenting on the availability or dearth of individuals in a given field, requesting that hiring institutions return the vita forms.[7] Though registrants completed four copies of the AHA vita form, numbers dwindled as they were mailed to institutions for consideration and often not returned.[8] Each December, the whole "register" was packed and mailed to the convention site, where hiring officials could themselves comb through vita forms for possible candidates for positions, with the consequence that for a time before and after each annual meeting, the system was completely, you might say, "offline."[9] Even institutions that happened to find a man through this system who met their needs were as likely to discover others who were uninterested in the position or no longer available.[10] And because most positions were not advertised, most candidates never knew their vita form had been sent for consideration.

The American Institute of Physics took a somewhat different approach: "Qualification Books"—giant compilations of registration forms—for purchase for a small fee by hiring institutions.[11] But it had its own absurdities. The forms were organized by registration date, not keyed by subfield of training, experience, or type of position (academic, industrial, research) in which a man was interested. And like other professional societies' systems, the actual availability of any man in the book was not clear. Though physics required registrants to re-register annually, a year is a long time in the life of a man looking for employment, and the fact that the hiring cycle in industry and research was not tied to an academic year further complicated the issue of availability.[12] All of which meant that the books, like other placement systems, were bound to be out of date.

The structure of placement services at annual meetings, moreover, was bound to produce annoyance and frustration. A report on the AHA Job Register's operation at the annual meeting in 1956 gives one a sense of things. Two separate "offices" were set up: one for employers, the other for registrants. "This is indispensable," the report noted. It mentioned confusion if registrants and hiring colleges and universities used the same or adjoining offices. But confusion seemed less the issue than assuring employers that their search would not become public and that they "saw only those whom they wished." Individuals registered for the service either in advance or at the meeting. In the employer's room, an employer filled out a form noting the requirements of their search; a staff member then selected "vitae [forms], from 5 to 30, depending on the wishes of the inquirer."[13] In any event, two white three-by-five-inch cards were completed for each registrant an employer wanted to see. One had the registrant's name only on it and was posted on a bulletin board outside the registrant's office. Registrants were directed to consult the board periodically during the meeting to see if their name was posted. "If your name appears here, take it down and present it at the desk inside, where details will be given you." The details were on the second three-by-five card held at the desk and included whom to call and where and when to arrange an interview.

The system led to disappointment on both sides. Employers discovered that many registrants were not at the meeting; registrants, excited about the service, were disappointed to not see their name posted.[14] In subsequent years, the AHA attempted refinements of the system: indexing vita forms by field, providing first one and later three typewriters for the use of those registering for the service at the meeting, having registrants at the meeting note their name and local address on a card held in the registrant's room. But other elements held firm, above all the importance of the separation of the rooms and the assurance that under no circumstances were registrants to be given access to the employer room.[15]

The AHA did not begin regularly circulating lists of advertised vacancies to registrants until 1962.[16] Though some other professional societies had begun circulating advertised vacancies to registrants multiple times a year much earlier, the advertising of positions shared two basic characteristics: larger and elite institutions resisted advertising of positions at all, and among institutions that did advertise, almost none appeared by name. Lacking any authority to force institutions to advertise jobs and eager to cultivate use of their personnel services, professional societies allowed institutions to elect whether to appear by name. None had done so in the 1930s, when the first published vacancies appeared in the *AAUP Bulletin*.[17] The passage of time did little to change institutional attitudes. Even with the protection of anonymity, larger and elite academic institutions did not advertise their vacancies. In the 1950s, vacancies appeared then not by name but by geographic location and institution type: "southern university," "Midwest university," "Midwest state college," "small New England college," "Eastern university," "large coeducational Catholic university."[18] When the AHA began listing vacancies in 1962, they, like most other professional societies, vaguely described but did not list institutions by name.[19]

Even without institution names, published listings of vacancies were a dramatic opening. They provided a somewhat public listing of at least some vacancies and enabled those seeking a job to put themselves in consideration. But the opening was circumscribed in all sorts of ways. Most vacancies would be filled without ever appearing in the pages of a published listing. The lists were shared only with those who were members of the professional society and had registered with the society's placement service. Moreover, candidates were left to guess as to the identity of the institution.

Attempts to rationalize listings nonetheless held to the value of institutional anonymity. For example, in the 1960s, the APSA adopted a new system dividing the United States into eleven geographic areas and listing vacancies accordingly. Each issue of its personnel service *Newsletter* included a map showing "area designation codes." Except for Hawaii and Alaska, each of which was the only state in its "area," "area designation codes" included multiple contiguous states. The system provided registrants with both more and less information. Knowing that a vacancy was in "designation code 10" (New York, New Jersey, or Pennsylvania), for example, obscured as much as it revealed, and no longer did a registrant necessarily know the type or size of institution—college versus university; private versus public; secular versus religious; small versus large; and so forth—that had a vacancy.[20]

Institutional anonymity had another consequence: Correspondence was directed through the professional society in which the listing appeared. As the numbers of those registering grew and staff attempted the near-impossible task of assuring that the records they sent to hiring institutions were current, the overwhelming workload on professional societies led them to direct registrants to "enclose a *curriculum vitae* for each position they wish to be considered for."[21] The American Sociological Society referred to its system "as a means of putting people in touch with each other." *As a means of putting people in touch with each other*, it was absurd. Registrants were left to wonder whether their reply had been forwarded and, assuming it had, whether they were in consideration. As a 1956 ASS *Employment Bulletin* noted, "Acknowledgements of replies, cannot, of course, be guaranteed."[22] Or, as the renamed AHA "Professional Register" put it, "The registrant who hears nothing must assume the institution was not interested in negotiation."[23]

The protection of anonymity may have led more institutions to advertise vacancies, but it did not resolve a more fundamental objection. Advertising a vacancy in effect solicited letters from strangers. Professional societies struggled to define their mediating role. The American Economic Association had been clear from the start and retained the position that it took "no responsibility for making a selection among the applicants"; the "Secretary's Office [would] merely afford a central point for clearing inquiries."[24] But as one scholar pointed out at a 1959 roundtable conference on the market for economists, "big universities do not advertise because they do not want to be flooded with applications from incompetent people and also because of prestige."[25]

Even as the number of registrants for professional societies' placement services increased over the course of the 1950s, professional societies labored under the reality that their services offered little tangible proof of success. "We need to discuss the Job Register," Boyd Shafer wrote the AHA Committee on the Register in October 1960.[26] "At present, I see the following obstacles." Among these was that "hiring is chiefly through departments and individuals—this is custom well established. Some historians think, quite wrongly, that only the incompetent register and that any register is infra dig." Translation: unseemly, demeaning, unbecoming, unbefitting, degrading, debasing, shameful, humiliating, dishonorable. Yet Shafer argued that there was both a need and demand for the Register. The longstanding practice of a man writing to friends at other institutions seeking recommendations to fill a vacancy was "hit or miss" at best; "many good men [were] overlooked. . . . The growing number of historians," he argued, made "personal knowledge" of all those available impossible. And beyond that concern, the system ignored the desires of those wishing to make a change in their appointment.[27] Everything he said about the current system of hiring and its inadequacies held true for every academic discipline.

The stigma that professional societies placement services were "infra dig" would hold so long as elite universities refused to openly advertise positions or encourage their best men to register with professional societies' placement bureaus. The same year that Boyd Shafer wrote his plea for action to the AHA Committee on the Job Register, Stan Katz, an early student of Bernard Bailyn, was finishing his dissertation in history at Harvard. Katz's personal story highlights the challenge professional societies faced.[28] Katz was not a member of the AHA; he had never heard of the AHA Job Register; he did not have a vita; he did not know that Harvard had a placement office.

Stan Katz was born in Chicago in 1934 into a cultured, upper-middle-class Jewish family. But their immigrant and ethnic roots remained close to the surface. Though Katz's parents had been born in the United States, his grandparents came from Kiev and Latvia. Stan's father was in what Stan called "the egg-breaking business" with his older half-brother, Uncle Isadore. "Imagine you're the Sara Lee Company and you have an order for ten thousand sponge cakes. And your employees set off to do this. Where do they get the eggs for ten thousand sponge cakes? Nobody ever thinks about this," Stan explained to me. "The answer is Willy Katz." The reference was to his father. Whether it was a tank car full of egg yolks, or whites, or shelled whole eggs, the place companies got them in Chicago was the SK Produce Company.

It was assumed that Stan would go to college. Katz was one of seven, as he recalls, from his high school class to go to Harvard; others went to Yale or Princeton. That was his world. By virtue of age and class he fell in that narrow generation of men who were too young to serve in World War II, and who by 1951, with the outbreak of the Korean War, were in college and draft-deferred under the Selective Service Act. As a boy, Katz had spent hours at the Art Institute; as an undergraduate at Harvard, he fell in love with seventeenth-century English history and literature. Having applied to Harvard for graduate school to study Tudor Stuart history, the buzz among graduate students about a new young faculty member named Bernard Bailyn led Katz to American history.

By the time Stan was finishing his dissertation in 1960, he was married. It was his wife, Adria, who raised the question of what they would do the next year. As he recalled, Stan responded, "I don't know." "Well, don't you think you should ask Professor Bailyn?" she asked. So, as Stan tells it, he told Bailyn that his wife thought he should be worrying about next year, to which Bailyn replied, "Don't worry." And when Adria asked about the conversation, Stan said, "He said, don't worry." "What did he mean by that?" she asked. To which Stan replied, "I don't know. But he, if he said, 'Don't worry,' I'm not worried." Later that spring Adria raised the question again. And again, Stan talked with Bailyn, who told him, "Don't worry. I think you'll hear something soon." Sure enough, the next week Stan got a call from the chair of the Harvard History Department. "'Stan, it's Bobby Wolfe,'" he said, "'I'm calling to tell you that next year you're going to be an instructor in the History Department.'" Stan shook his head in wonder remembering the moment, "He did not ask me. He told me. I mean, what a different world."

But the funnier part of the story in Katz's eyes was what happened a few weeks later. William "Bill" McNeill, chairman of the History Department at Chicago, telephoned. He said something about plans to be out East and wanting to talk with Katz. When he arrived, he offered Stan an assistant professorship at Chicago. The two men had never met. Katz had completed a mammoth dissertation, but he had not published an article, presented a paper, or even attended a professional conference. "So how would Bill McNeil have known about you?" I asked. "I don't have a clue. I don't have any idea. I never stopped to ask myself that question." When Stan told McNeill that he had already accepted an instructorship at Harvard, McNeill, after pressing Stan a bit, asked if he could use Stan's telephone. And then, as Stan listened in, McNeill dialed a number. "'Is this Jesse Lemisch? I'd like to come talk to you. I would like to offer you an assistant professorship at the University of Chicago.'" As Stan noted, "Jesse was number two on his list. And off he went." We laughed together at the story.

"So let me ask you a question," I said. "The AHA had established a Job Register. Did you know about the Job Register?" "Well, see," Stan responded, "I wasn't in that kind of game. . . . People like me were not in that game." "And when you say, 'people like me,' you mean men at Harvard?" "I mean at elite institutions. They were going to take care of us."[29] Katz's words capture the facts of life for many men completing PhDs at elite universities. What stood out in the story is that by the 1950s, the privileges of placement that had long accrued to men at Harvard and a small number of other elite universities had been opened to those like Katz who were Jewish.[30] After three years as an instructor at Harvard, Katz was promoted to assistant professor. Understanding that with Bailyn at Harvard he would not be promoted to associate professor, when Katz got a call from Wisconsin in 1965 and then an offer, he went to Wisconsin. And from there to the University of Chicago Law School in 1970, to a named chair in the History Department at Princeton in 1978, and to the presidency of the ACLS in 1986. As Stan said to me, "I've never applied for anything."[31]

But that world was changing. By 1956, the number of PhDs awarded annually by American universities had climbed to more than 8,500. By 1961, American universities were awarding more than ten thousand doctorates a year.[32] Universities like Columbia and Wisconsin that had long led in the production of PhDs were, by the late 1950s, awarding hundreds of PhDs per year; their graduate-student populations numbered in the thousands.[33] But it was not just the expansion of graduate programs at old-line PhD-granting universities that led to the exponential growth in the number of PhDs. In 1948, ninety-seven universities in the US awarded doctorates. By

1956, that number had grown to 162.[34] The increasing numbers of graduate students, coming from an ever-broadening range of institutions and within large universities—literally a sea of graduate students, searching for positions at a dramatically expanded number of colleges and universities—would of necessity have to be their own agents, requiring personal forms for their own introduction.

"Dear Dr. Birenbaum, I am about to compile my 'dossier' with Columbia Placement Service, in order to be available for a full time teaching job after completion of my Ph.D. in American history in the fall of 1966. Would you be good enough to give me a letter of reference?" The letter, dated March 29, 1965, was from Gerda Lerner. By virtue of personality perhaps, but as certainly by life experience, gender, and age, Lerner was well suited to Columbia University's culture of self-reliance. As David Hollinger reflected on his own experience at Columbia in the 1960s, students "were expected to study and survive by their own wits." The inattention extended to funding. In the humanities, for the most part, Hollinger noted, students "had to fend for themselves."[35]

Gerda Lerner had been fending for herself since escaping alone to the United States at age eighteen from Austria. She had arrived in the United States in April 1939, "after a terrible voyage of seasickness, loneliness and fearful anticipation," only to almost be turned away—an unattached female—under suspicion that her supposed fiancé was in fact a ruse to prostitution.[36] Lerner was young, life as a scholar not even part of her self-imagination, and so the non-quota visa through which some academics were able to escape Nazi Germany was not a possibility or even consideration for her. If she were turned back, she knew she would be incarcerated on her arrival in Germany because she was Jewish.[37] She was allowed into the US only on the condition that the couple return within a week's time with a marriage license. They hardly knew each other and had not seen each other for over a year, but now her life depended on their marrying. It was an unhappy, short marriage lasting little over a year.

Gerda Lerner arrived in the US—like so many other Jewish refugees in the 1930s—facing a depressed job market, with limited English skills, desperately trying to secure the escape and safety of family members. She learned that the only jobs potentially open to her were at the bottom of the wage labor force and depended on creating a new biography. She learned quickly the art of survival. "Never admit to having anything but a high school education. Don't say you're a refugee; don't say you're Jewish. Get some phony reference letters; pretend you've been here two years. Don't ask any questions; don't volunteer any information." Lerner left New York City in 1941. Close to twenty years passed before she returned. In the intervening years, she had remarried, raised two children, and begun writing fiction. She began taking classes at the New School for Social Research in 1959 in the hopes they would help her in her new craft. But then, captivated by history, she completed her BA in 1963 and went on to Columbia for an MA and PhD in History. By the time Lerner began compiling her Columbia dossier in spring 1965, she was forty-five years old and had more experience in the art of survival and self-realization than many people acquire in a lifetime.[38]

Lerner would prove as fastidious a record keeper of her own life as she was of the lives of the women whom over the course of her long career she would recover from history. Together with her correspondence with William Birenbaum and others were multiple versions of her completed registration form for the Teaching Division of the Columbia Placement Service and a May 1958 booklet advising Columbia students in securing a teaching appointment. The booklet was titled: "Columbia Assistance in Your Search for a Teaching Position." The title summed up Columbia's "philosophy of placement": Job seekers were expected to be self-reliant. "Your Search," the title read. The Teacher Placement division at Columbia was one of three university placement offices that David Brown featured as outstanding models in his 1965 study, *Placement Services for College Teachers*.[39] Columbia had been one of the first elite PhD-granting institutions to establish a placement office.[40] By the mid-1950s, the Columbia Placement office had distinct divisions, including for placing college and university teachers.[41] By the mid-1960s, a decade later, it had 2,692 active candidates.[42]

That the 1958 booklet in Lerner's files was still in use in 1965 was made clear by the fact that Brown, in his survey, written in cooperation with Columbia's placement office, quoted extensively from it. As the brochure described, a candidate's search should not end with registration with the university's placement office. A section of the booklet titled "Your Campaign" began, "The Placement Bureau is only one thoroughfare to placement. The person of initiative will doubtless want to make use of several." Included here were "the assistance of interested faculty members" and the candidate's own inquiries. "In making these unsolicited contacts to uncover possible teaching positions it is a good practice to enclose a copy of your personal resumé with a fairly brief letter."[43]

Gerda Lerner absorbed every piece of advice that booklet offered. Writing to William Birenbaum in spring 1965 to seek a letter of reference for her placement dossier, she included a resume.[44] "I am including my resume for your files and hope you will keep me in mind for any possible openings at L.I.U." William Birenbaum did not need Lerner's resume for himself. He knew her well. He had been dean of the New School for Social Research when Lerner was an undergraduate there, and she had begun her teaching career as an instructor at the New School in 1963, the final year of her BA, and had continued teaching there as she worked toward her MA and PhD at Columbia. In 1964, Birenbaum had left the New School for an appointment as vice president and provost at the Brooklyn Center, Long Island University (LIU). As Lerner understood, her resume was not for Birenbaum; it was a formal part of an inquiry for a job at a new institution where she was not known. In other job inquiries that spring, she also included her resume.[45]

Gerda Lerner and David Hollinger were both PhD students in history at Columbia in the mid-1960s. The differences in their paths to what Hollinger referred to as his "first full-time academic berth" spoke not just to differences in their age and gender but also to the multiple worlds of academic placement in the mid-1960s. Neither secured a position through Columbia's placement office. Nor had either of them been registered with the AHA Job Register.[46] But as Lerner neared completion of her degree, she had created a dossier with the Columbia University Placement Service, crafted a personal resume, and written letters seeking teaching appointments. And yet even for her a personal relationship was key to her first full-time academic appointment. Less than a month after writing to Birenbaum at the Brooklyn Center, Long Island University, Lerner received a letter from the chair of the History Department, inviting her to call to discuss a possible teaching appointment in the department.[47] In June, Lerner was formally offered and accepted a position as an assistant professor at LIU.[48] She defended her dissertation and received her PhD from Columbia that November.

While Hollinger returned multiple times in an essay he wrote in the early 1980s about becoming a historian to the self-reliance required of students at Columbia in the 1960s, when it came to securing a "full-time academic berth" he acknowledged that he was the beneficiary of "the old patronage-based, male way of placing students." Two years before completing his PhD he was hired as an instructor at Princeton. "No doubt someone at Princeton placed a call to Hofstadter, who recommended me. Within a few days of a perfunctory interview, I learned that I had passed muster and been invited to join one of the world's premier departments."[49]

Neither of the positions that Lerner or Hollinger took had been advertised. In a short piece that appeared in the *Talk of the Town* in *The New Yorker* in January 1961, Dean Albertson had described a radical move they had made in the AHA Job Register at the convention. "This year," he noted, "we're trying something revolutionary. We've put a big white sign in the lobby, where everyone can see it, which for the first time will make many of the available jobs public knowledge, instead of closely guarded secrets."[50] *Something revolutionary.*

Change came, not with AHA Job Register's revolutionary experiment or any other professional society's efforts. Rather, it was spurred by the Cold War explosive expansion in the number and size of institutions, by the tidal wave of students in the mid-1960s, and by universities and colleges that had neither an investment in nor the luxury to follow old models. "Newly organized California State College has vacancies for assistant, associate, and full professors." The ad in the *AAUP Bulletin* in December 1964 listed salary ranges at each rank and noted the attractive "three course (12 hour) teaching load. . . . Apply to California State College at San Bernardino." The ad was repeated for field after field: art–art history, biology, chemistry, drama–theater, economics, education, English, French, German, history, mathematics, music–music history, philosophy, physical education, physics, political science, psychology, sociology, Spanish. And in each an immediate need for faculty at every rank.[51] Imagine. Stocking an entire new institution with faculty in every field. Now multiply. Not just one new institution, but hundreds.

In 1940, there were 1,252 four-year colleges and 456 junior colleges in the United States. By 1960, there were two hundred more four-year colleges and another fifty junior colleges. Not all these institutions were new, of course, but they nonetheless expanded the number of faculty appointments. By 1970, the number of four-year colleges had grown to 1,639; the number of junior colleges to 886. These numbers captured only part of the transformation. Alongside the dramatic expansion in the number of colleges and universities was an explosion in the size of—especially—public universities.[52]

The number of advertised vacancies grew exponentially almost overnight. In 1960, in the field of history, there were ninety advertised vacancies. In 1964, there were 450. Speaking at the annual meeting in San Francisco in January 1966, Robert Zangrando, the new AHA executive secretary, suggested that the number of advertised positions might reach 550 that year. "One can hazard the comment that unlike in the mid-1950's we are now in something of a seller's market."[53] Flush times. Listing institutions now almost universally appeared by name. The same pattern held in other fields.[54] As a 1965 brochure on "Finding Employment in the Mathematical

Sciences" put it, "At present the new Ph.D. is not confronted with the problem of finding an academic position, but with the question of choosing one position from several offers."[55]

It seems surprising that the AHA had not always listed vacancies by field in its *Newsletter*, but that they had not said volumes about how few vacancies were advertised. That changed in 1966.[56] The wealth of positions was staggering. In American and European history, hundreds of positions, but also positions in Latin American, African, and Asian history. At many institutions, two or more positions were offered in various historical fields; a few simply said, "several." Reading through the list, one could chart the expansion of state systems. Wisconsin State, Eau Claire, Stevens Point, River Falls. Flagship public universities, like the University of Wisconsin at Madison, too, were on the list. But absences remained. Columbia University listed a position for a medievalist in the December 1965 AHA *Newsletter*.[57] But scanning listings from February 1965, when the default for listings began to include institutions by name, through 1968, there were no listings for the likes of Harvard, Princeton, or Yale.[58] It was only later, facing the mobilization of antidiscrimination law, that elite universities would join others in advertising vacancies.[59]

Bill Tuttle drafted his first vita in fall 1966.[60] Tuttle was born in 1937 in Detroit, Michigan to an upper-middle-class family. His parents were graduates of the University of Chicago; his father was a highly regarded young thoracic surgeon. As was true for hundreds of thousands of children in the United States, including the children burned in Gene Autry cowboy suits, Tuttle's world was shaped in important ways by World War II. For Tuttle, as for many, the impact came from the experience of his father's absence during and then return after the war. His father enlisted when Tuttle was four; Tuttle was almost eight when he returned. Tuttle's second monograph, *Daddy's Gone to War*, focused on the impact of the war on American children and families.[61] But that came later. In fall 1966, he was less than a year away from completing his PhD in history at the University of Wisconsin.

"The Big Red Machine." That is how Stan Katz, who had gone to Wisconsin from Harvard in 1965, referred to the department in the 1960s.[62] "Red" referred to the school's colors, "big" to its size. By the 1960s, the department was admitting as many as two hundred graduate students a year in American history alone. "Machine" referred to the department's finely tuned process for placing its PhDs. Each fall, the department chair and two faculty assigned as placement coordinators met with students to explain the departmental and university system. Students were encouraged to publish while in graduate school; were directed to develop a set of credentials, including references, with the university placement office and to complete a brief curriculum vitae for the department placement coordinators. Every member of the department assiduously collected news of vacancies. "A casual inquiry at a convention, a brief note from a former graduate student, an addendum in a cover letter accompanying a thesis chapter, an aside in a reaction to a journal article, a telephone call from a nearby acquaintance—the grapevine carried job vacancies by many routes." News of vacancies was in turn shared with the placement coordinators, who each week circulated news of openings to the graduate faculty—not students—and solicited faculty recommendations for whom the department should nominate. The placement coordinators bore the brunt of the work in this system, coordinating decisions of the two or at most three individuals the department would nominate for any position. Describing the system, David Brown noted, "Prestige is taken into full account, and a candidate who is not fully qualified for a position will not be suggested. When the department nominates a man for a job, it is recommending him, not merely referring him." The result was a consistently strong record of appointments, including at top-rated institutions across the United States.[63]

Bill Tuttle was the beneficiary of this system and this moment. "I hope that we will be able to find you a good slot," one of his faculty departmental recommenders wrote in October 1966, on notifying Tuttle that he had completed a recommendation for his Placement Bureau dossier.[64] By December, Tuttle had received invitations to meet at the AHA annual meeting with members of several departments: Stanford, Boston University, the University of Connecticut, and NYU. Though these conversations did not ultimately lead to a job offer, they nonetheless showed the system at work.[65] Had Tuttle not acted on his own, I expect the Big Red Machine would yet have found a "good slot" for him. In a sense it did. By the mid-1960s, in addition to its mighty departmental placement machine, Wisconsin encouraged graduate students to apply directly for jobs, and in doing so, even more so than Columbia, it broke ranks with the personal model of placement. It is not surprising that the break came from an institution like Wisconsin. Large public universities had long outstripped private universities in their number of undergraduates, but only in the 1950s did they do so in the number of PhDs they trained.[66] And Tuttle did seek his own opportunities.

But as was true for Gerda Lerner, more was at work than a department's or university's philosophy of placement. Stan Katz, who had gone directly from college to graduate school in the 1950s, had said "they were going to take care of us." That casual assurance represented a different time. The cohorts of graduate students in the 1960s were caught up in a maelstrom of social and political change—change that many took a direct hand in producing.[67] Many men in graduate school in the 1950s and 1960s had had their collegiate careers interrupted by military service. The interruption meant they were older, were more mature and had had broader experiences that fostered independence by the time they entered or completed graduate school. Tuttle had gone directly into the Air Force when he graduated from college in 1959. His term of service was three years. By the time he got to Madison in 1963, as Tuttle explained to me, he was ready to work. Moreover, like many other graduate students of his generation, he was married and had children to support.[68] Marriage. Children. Broader life experience in a time of radical social change. In other words, change in the material practices of academic life did not come simply from the expansion of higher education or the initiative of professional societies; it was produced as well from below.

"Mr. John Hollister suggested that I write you," Tuttle opened a letter in November 1966, to William Cartwright in the School of Education at Duke. He described his fields of training and research and noted that he would be completing his dissertation in June. "I am now looking for a teaching job for next fall. . . . The history department of the University of Wisconsin is handling my placement," he explained, "but I hope to do some searching on my own. Mr. Hollister thought that you might know of job openings which have escaped Wisconsin's attention, or that you might forward my vita to somebody who would be interested." As had been true for German émigré scholars in the 1930s, so too here: Vitae traveled. William Cartwright wrote in reply that he was sending Tuttle's vita "to friends in a couple of history departments."[69] Tuttle wrote other letters seeking a position, always enclosing his vita, and often receiving a reply that his vita had been passed along.[70] The networks through which Tuttle's vita traveled were complex. Harvey Sapolsky in the Department of Political Science at MIT had Tuttle's vita and was sending it to others, including Harvard and the Department of Humanities at MIT. The chairman in the Department of Humanities at MIT wrote to say they had no vacancy at present, but he recommended that Tuttle send his vita to the Department of Humanities at Caltech.[71] And so it went. The point is not that any of these initiatives led to a job for Tuttle—they did not—but they spoke to the fact that by the mid-1960s many PhD candidates, like Bill Tuttle, no longer felt bound by the conventions of the past. And equally, that faculty receiving his vita treated it as part of the normal course of securing a position.

At the 1966 AHA meeting too, Tuttle had his vita in hand. This time it bore fruit. It was common in the 1960s for major university presses and large universities to host convention cocktail parties. The University of Kansas was hosting a cocktail party, and Tuttle had gotten the word that Kansas was hiring. Describing the scene to me, he noted "a long line of students waiting to hand their resumes" to the chair of the History Department at the Kansas reception, "express their interest in the job, maybe talk for just a minute or two." He did not want to wait in a line, deciding he would hope to "run into" the chairman—George Anderson—later and give him his vita. And he did.[72] Or at least that is how he remembered it. Within a week after the convention, Tuttle received a letter from Anderson. They were looking for candidates "in what we have described as the Post-1945 period." It is fascinating that in the mid-1960s, history departments—or at least one department—were beginning to think of "Post-1945" as a field. He asked if Tuttle was interested and said that, if so, "we would be glad to study your credentials." Two months later, Ted Wilson, a faculty member in the History Department at Kansas, was welcoming Tuttle to the department. "You might be interested to learn—if you did not know already," Wilson wrote, "that at last count seven new people will be coming next year. That makes, I think, 38 permanent appointments in the department. I am unable to explain how this is possible in a university of 15,000. We must accept our good fortune and hope it continues."[73] Tuttle joined the History Department as an assistant professor at the University of Kansas in fall 1967.

The explosion in the number of academic appointments was an engine for the vita. Professional societies and university placement services had struggled to hold the line. In its 1958 booklet, the Teaching Division of Columbia University's Placement Office had directed candidates that "information received from a placement officer about a specific position is intended for the candidate's personal use only. If the candidate is not interested in the position, he is free to recommend to the placement officer another person who might be interested and qualified, but it is a breach of faith to share that information with another candidate."[74] *A breach of faith.* What was true enough in the 1950s was wildly out of date a decade later. Professional societies too clung to the past. Even as they began to list hiring institutions by name in newsletters and bulletins alerting candidates to positions, they resisted the idea that candidates should apply directly for positions. Professional societies struggled to remain the broker through which information passed. "A member of the Register should ask that his vita forms be sent only to vacancies for which he is obviously qualified," the AHA directed in 1965.[75] "Please select your choices for referral very carefully," the APSA May 1966 *Newsletter* noted. "The success of the service depends in part on not burdening employers with credentials of unqualified candidates."[76]

The line could not hold. The era of the vita had fully arrived.

calendars

Dear Frances,

Yesterday spiraled out of control emotionally. I suddenly felt we were in danger of not being a family anymore. I felt that I had to get busy and get a Christmas tree, that I needed to get decorations up, that we needed to remind ourselves that we were/are still a family. And all this was going through my head as I drove to the Department meeting and sat through the meeting feeling utterly disoriented.

. . .

It finally stopped snowing. We got somewhere between 14–20 inches of snow. I wish you were here to see it.

. . .

I can't really account for today. Sam had an awful night last night. I worked on recommendations letters until close to midnight then Sam went all nervous on us: panting, trying to get up on our bed, tail between his legs, shaking, pacing, and fur coming out by what seemed the handful. We tried everything: taking him outside, lying on the floor with him, petting him, leaving the bedroom door open. I slept for a couple of hours and then at around 4:30 heard a sound of frantic panting and digging only to discover him on your bed digging madly at the comforter. That was it. I got up. One could hardly expect much good to come from a day after that.

. . .

Today is the third anniversary of Grandpa Dick dying. I've been sad today and it just makes me sadder to think that someday we will be facing the third anniversary of your death. The thought fills me with despair. That's strange, isn't it? Why should one year be harder than seven months, two years harder than one. Maybe it's the idea of distance, the idea of being taken ever farther from when you were alive.

...

Tonight, I found myself thinking that we had no idea what was ahead when we spent that final afternoon together with you at the hospital. "Take as long as you need," the doctor had said. Could I have ever left that hospital if someone had said to me—remember you'll never see her again. You'll never hold her again.

...

Tonight is Christmas Eve. What an impossible day. To be followed by a greater impossibility: the first Christmas without you, past, done.

...

It is the final day of the year. Why is this so hard? I have been dreading entering a new year without you.

...

I couldn't buy a new calendar and so dates for "next year" have just been adding up with nowhere to put them. It was my way of refusing to have a calendar that didn't have you on it/in it. I remember last year when the Sierra Club calendar arrived. You immediately flipped to March and were so disappointed by your birthday month picture: a field of flowers in the Sierra Nevada mountains in California. I thought it was a beautiful picture, but you were really disappointed and started flipping to other family member's birthday months and were so bummed by the comparison.

...

This morning I was frantic. I hadn't seen my cell phone since Tuesday and I had become convinced that I had lost it. It felt like the last link I had to you alive had been lost. But then after despairing, feeling like this was the last straw and I just couldn't live, I found it on my messy desk in my office.

...

Last night was one of those wakeful, tearful nights. . . . Peace, which so many wished for us in their cards and notes, eludes me. What did they mean by peace? Did they mean acceptance? I expect that most would not be able to define, explain what they meant. It would be helpful though to know so I could look for signs or way-posts.

...

We took Wilder back to school today. When we first took him in September it had only been four months since your death. Four months seems like such a short time now. It has now been 8 months. By the time Wilder is done with the school year it will be over a year. Although I have marked each day, each month, it struck me hard to realize that in the time between our first big leave-taking of Wilder in September and this one, the time you had been gone had doubled. It left me feeling somehow that I had not been careful enough or thoughtful enough in thinking about the passage of time.

...

There is something strange in thinking that you would only be in your second trimester of college, through one trimester, but still very new at it all. In some ways, our position might seem similar—we are still novices in knowing what it means to live without you. And yet death in its absoluteness is different. In life, we are always in a state of becoming. Is there any parallel in death? Are you learning, Frances, how to do this? And though death may be absolute, a sharp line or dividing point, knowing death for the living seems anything but absolute.

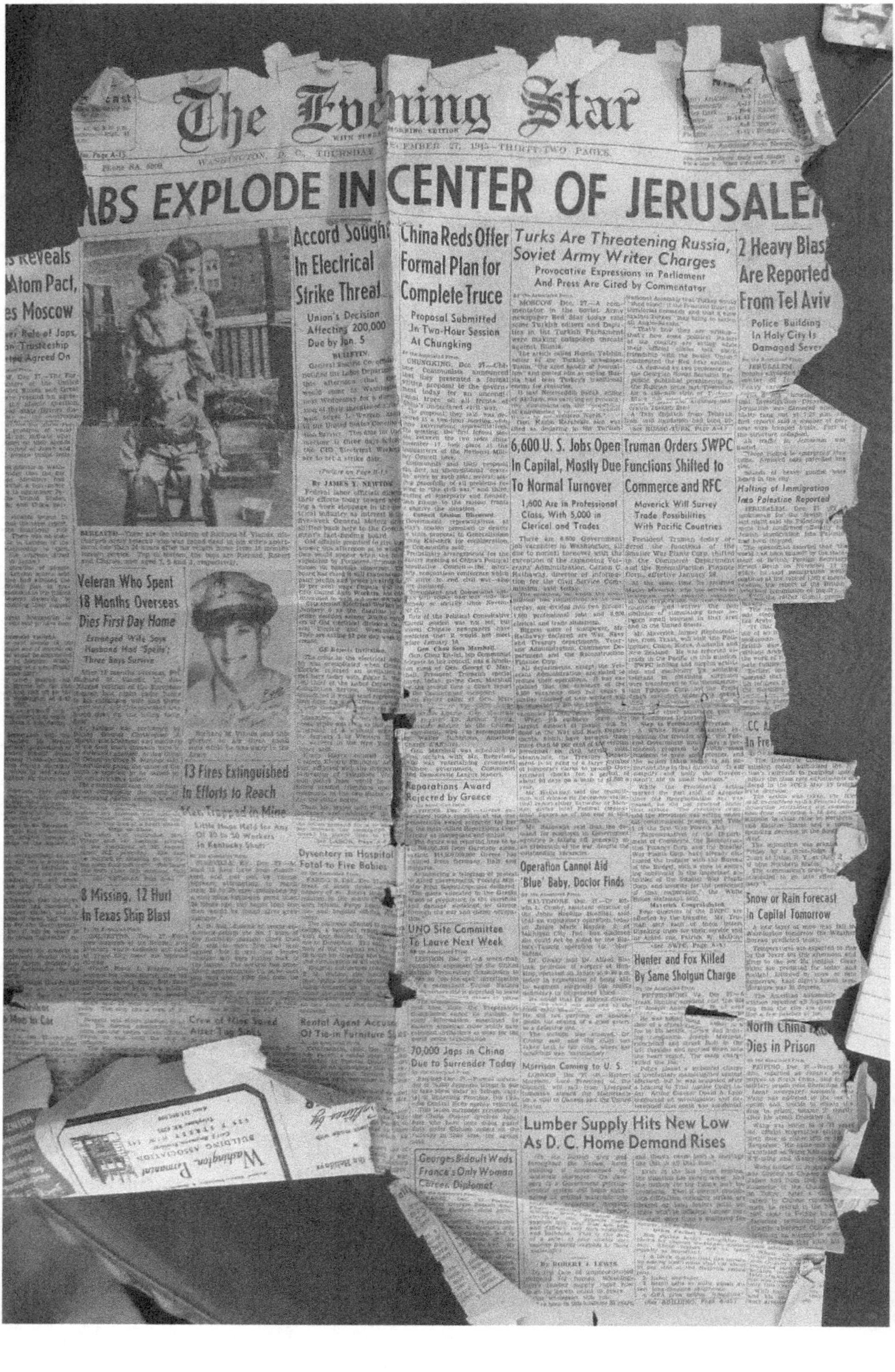

The Evening Star

WASHINGTON, D. C., THURSDAY, DECEMBER 27, 1945—THIRTY-TWO PAGES.

...BS EXPLODE IN CENTER OF JERUSALE...

...s Reveals Atom Pact, ...es Moscow

Accord Sought In Electrical Strike Threat

Union's Decision Affecting 200,000 Due by Jan. 5

China Reds Offer Formal Plan for Complete Truce

Proposal Submitted In Two-Hour Session At Chungking

Turks Are Threatening Russia, Soviet Army Writer Charges

Provocative Expressions in Parliament And Press Are Cited by Commentator

2 Heavy Blas... Are Reported From Tel Aviv

Police Building In Holy City Is Damaged Seve...

6,600 U. S. Jobs Open In Capital, Mostly Due To Normal Turnover

1,600 Are in Professional Class, With 5,000 in Clerical and Trades

Truman Orders SWPC Functions Shifted to Commerce and RFC

Maverick Will Survey Trade Possibilities With Pacific Countries

Halting of Immigration Into Palestine Reported

Veteran Who Spent 18 Months Overseas Dies First Day Home

Estranged Wife Says Husband Had 'Spells'; Three Boys Survive

13 Fires Extinguished In Efforts to Reach Man Trapped in Mine

Reparations Award Rejected by Greece

Operation Cannot Aid 'Blue' Baby, Doctor Finds

Dysentery in Hospital Fatal to Five Babies

8 Missing, 12 Hurt In Texas Ship Blast

UNO Site Committee To Leave Next Week

Hunter and Fox Killed By Same Shotgun Charge

Snow or Rain Forecast In Capital Tomorrow

North China ... Dies in Prison

70,000 Japs in China Due to Surrender Today

Morrison Coming to U. S.

Lumber Supply Hits New Low As D. C. Home Demand Rises

Georges Bidault Weds France's Only Woman Career Diplomat

By ROBERT J. LEWIS.

chapter eleven · family portraits

"I wonder if we could start by talking about your family, your parents." Somehow, I thought that asking about family might be easier, less traumatic, than beginning with the day over seventy years ago that Robert Viands was burned when he was four years old. "I don't know a lot about my father," he replied. "I think I know where he was born." "What was your father's name?" I asked. "Richard Moore Viands. He was born in Virginia, I think." "And what part of Virginia was it?" His question was directed to his wife, Cathy, not me. "Rileyville, we think," she said. And Robert added, "That's about all I really know about my dad," and then by way of explanation, "Because I was at such a young age." "Do you know when he was born, what year?" "Mmm. We could find out in just a second. We keep it wrote down." His wife got up from the kitchen table where we sat and went to check. Robert continued, "My mother was born Anne Louise Allen. And she was born in Etowah, North Carolina. And she grew up there until, I think she went to beautician school when she went to Washington, DC. And that is where she met my dad." His wife's voice came from the next room, "1913," she called out, filling in the year that Robert's father was born.[1]

We come to the lives that lie at the heart of the histories we write through particular incidents or elements of those lives, and we often write about them knowing no more than that, sometimes by necessity of sources, time, or scale, but often in the thought that their lives as a whole are not important to the history we are writing. On the kitchen table where I sat with Robert and Cathy Viands in their home in Graham, North Carolina, in November 2016, was the tattered front page of the Washington, DC *Evening Star* from December 27, 1945.[2] The page was yellowed, its edges jagged where pieces, brittle with age, had broken off. A sharp crease ran down the center of the page with other fold lines cutting across it. As we talked, Robert Viands kept picking the page up, studying the photographs and words as though answers to questions that had long troubled him might be found there.

The headline that ran across the top of the page in full caps read "Bombs Explode in Center of Jerusalem." But the headline that held Robert Viands' attention, the reason someone, probably his mother, had saved this page from the paper and that the family had kept it all these years, was to the left of the sharp crease that ran down the center of the page. It read "Veteran Who Spent 18 Months Overseas Dies First Day Home." Next to the story was a photograph of a soldier in uniform, smiling and inscribed, "To My Little Men & Ann, From Daddy." His little men were pictured in a photograph above the story: three small boys, identified as Richard, Robert, and Charles, ages seven, five, and three, dressed in soldiers' playsuits. The opening paragraph of the accompanying story read: "After 18 months overseas, Pvt. Richard M. Viands, 32, discharged veteran of the European theater last night came home to his estranged wife and three small sons and this morning was found dead on the living room floor."

The article turned to the possible cause of death, noting that an autopsy had been performed that morning with the results expected later in the day, and that "Mrs. Ann Louise Viands" expressed the belief that her husband, who had had "spells," had died of a heart attack.[3] "Dry-eyed and controlled," the story continued, "Mrs. Viands said her husband arrived at the apartment . . . yesterday. She said he insisted on sleeping on the living room floor last night. She found the body there this morning, fully clad. Mrs. Viands said they had"—the story cut off there—"(See VETERAN, Page A-4)."[4] Whoever had saved page 1 of the newspaper had not saved the page on which the story continued, and so all that Robert Viands had had through the years was that fragment of the story of his father's death, supplemented at some later point with his father's death certificate, which showed that his father had died of a heart attack due to congestive heart failure. He was thirty-two years old.

Long taped next to the photo of the three "bereaved" children had been a second news clipping: a photograph of a smiling young boy in a hospital gown, his one leg splinted and wrapped heavily in bandages, his other leg showing healed scars, with the brief caption "Robert F. Viands: Burned in Cowboy Suit."[5] The tape, yellow and brittle with age, had cracked and split, and the photograph broken loose. Whatever story had accompanied it had not been saved. There was nothing to identify the newspaper the clip-

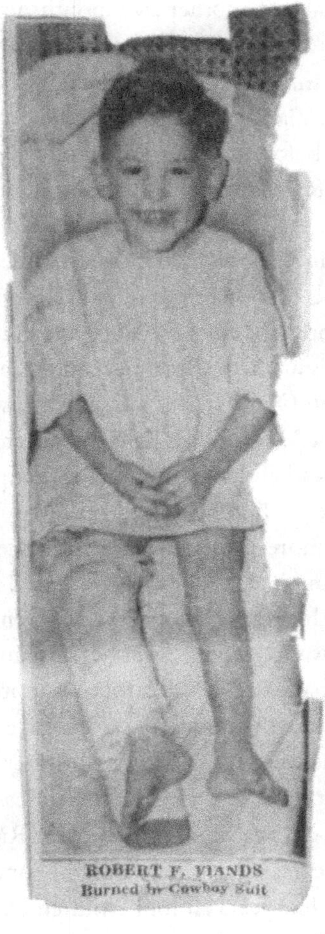

ROBERT F. VIANDS
Burned in Cowboy Suit

ping was from or the date. Robert Viands did not even remember for sure whether he had been burned before or after his father died.

Because I was at such a young age. Robert Viands was four years old when his father was inducted into the army. Seven months later, on January 15, 1945, with his father overseas, Robert's new Gene Autry cowboy suit, a Christmas present bought by his mother, caught fire as he played in the kitchen of their apartment. With his father in the service and his mother having other young children to care for, the first skin grafts came from strangers: a fire fighter, his mother told him, and some other "adult volunteer."[6] But as was true for all the children, to take, ultimately, the grafts had to come from his own body. He was away from home half a year, four months in the hospital and another two months in a convalescent center. The cost of that care, running to five thousand dollars, was well beyond the family's means, more than a middle-class man would have earned in a full year in 1945.[7] And the Viandses were not middle-class. Richard Viands had been a baker's helper before being inducted into the US Army. Whatever support came to his family from his service pay, and whatever he might have provided had he survived, he was now dead. And so, to the burdens that Anne Louise Viands shouldered was now added the financial burden of unpaid medical bills that there was no possibility of her paying.

And there was more. The *Evening Star*'s headline suggested that Richard Viands died on his first day home. But, in fact, he had been discharged two months earlier on October 31, 1945, just a few months after Robert himself returned home.[8] Maybe the night his father died was the first time he had seen his wife and children since his discharge. The missing end to the sentence in the news clipping that began "Mrs. Viands said they had" was "been separated more than two years."[9] But her statement to the reporter that her husband had had "spells" suggested that they had possibly seen each other since his return. In any event, when Richard Viands died, Anne Louise Viands was pregnant. After her husband's death, she took her three small children back to North Carolina and moved in with her parents. Eight months later, in August 1946, she gave birth to a fourth son, George. And then she went to pieces. Her brother and his wife took the two youngest boys—the baby, George, and Charles. "The welfare" put the older two boys—Robert, age six, and his brother Richard Allen, age seven or eight—into foster care, where they went from one "unfit" abusive home to another. Within a few years all four children were in an orphanage in Union Mills, North Carolina.[10]

It is hard not to put the topic one is studying at the center of another's life. But there were other hardships, other losses in these families' lives independent of and yet, as I came to understand, bound up with this childhood tragedy.[11] The Viandses were not alone in this. There were husbands, fathers, and sons lost in the war. There were fathers whose work led to disabling injuries and deaths. There were men who had lost a wife to sickness or childbirth. There were women who got pregnant in the shadow of marriage or outside it. There were miscarriages, stillbirths, and babies who lived only a few months. There were the terrors and unknowns of polio. There were separations and divorces. There was the daily strain of living from paycheck to paycheck and when there was no paycheck at all.

In the course of a life there are moments and events that become absorbed into time, more felt than specifically remembered, and others that divide time into before and after. But through memory, time moves across both kinds of moments and events, not just forward, but backward and forward, like the movement of water washing against a shoreline. Experiences distinct in time—joys, hardships, loves, losses—shape others, becoming part of the fabric of individuals' and families' lives. And so it was here. The burden of striving, hardship, and loss cumulative. And in its incident and the material resources to weather it, its weight fell more heavily on families like these, the Viandses and so many others, those with the least.

Charles Baragona Jr. was the first of six children born to Charles and Teresa May Baragona in the tiny mill town of Hodge, Louisiana. His parents were both born in small Louisiana towns, but as he described them, "My dad was Sicilian and Italian and my mother was Slavonian, Yugoslavian."[12] "How did they end up in Hodge?" I asked. "Well," he began and chuckled. "Dad was an excellent athlete. He was a small man, but he was very good at baseball, in particular. . . . Short stop, third. Good hitter too." And he explained how each paper mill had its own baseball team. "And he would play for one town, a town of Sterlington, and played against a team from Monroe, Louisiana, and they liked him, they'd give him a nickel raise if he'd transfer to that town." "So, was what he got paid for baseball separate from his . . . ?" I started to ask. And Charles Jr. interrupted, "No, they would give him another job classification that paid a nickel more." By 1940, Charles Sr. was working as a laborer in the paper mill in Hodge, with earnings in 1939 of $1,570 and playing for the Hodge Red Socks. One of his father's baseball buddies introduced his parents. The outcome seems almost predetermined. His father was, in Charles Jr.'s words, "a good-looking Italian fellow," a star baseball player, and had a car, "an old '39 Pontiac Coupe, which was a hot car back in those days." And Teresa May Turk had charms too. She taught piano and dance, and she and her sister had a dance school and traveled, and so "they would see each other." They got married in August 1940, and a year later Charles Jr. was born.[13]

Hodge was a town of about 1,000 or 1,100 people. "Everybody," Charles Jr. explained, "worked for the paper mill." And lived in mill housing. "We lived in a 1,200-square-foot house; it was a thirty-by-forty mill house." The house had indoor plumbing and electricity covered in the rent of "a dollar a day, thirty bucks a month . . . the whole neighborhood consisted of similar houses," he explained. "Same key fit every house." Well, maybe. "The Blacks lived on the other side of the railroad track," he explained. They lived in mill houses too, "but they weren't as nice as ours."

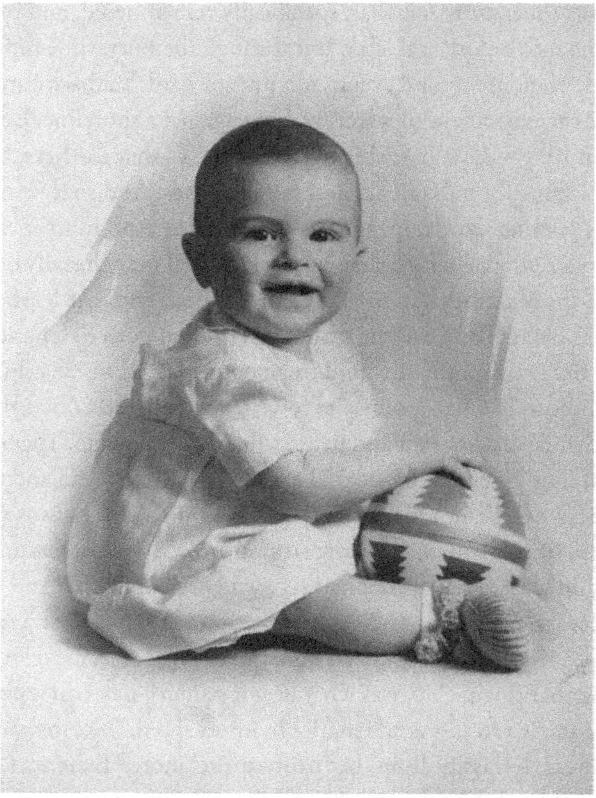

When I asked if work in the mills was dangerous, Charles Jr.'s reply was quick, "Oh, it was dangerous as heck, yeah." What made it dangerous was more complicated. "He worked in the powerhouse," Charles Jr. explained, "where they generated the steam that ran all the equipment in the mill. He died when he was seventy-nine of complications from lung cancer. . . . I'm sure that he was one of those mesothelioma guys, because he, all he did for thirty-five years was wrap pipes with asbestos." Charles Jr. remembered having asked his father once why he would not accept a promotion. His father's answer was quick, as quick as Charles Jr.'s to my question about the dangerousness of working in the mill: "Because I could get fired. . . . Who's going to take care of you six kids and mom if they promoted me, and the next day fired me? But if I'm with the union they can't fire me."[14]

That working-class families would be the primary buyers and so in turn bear the brunt of the loss from the Gene Autry cowboy suit was, in a sense, designed into the product itself. Working-class Americans were the heart of Gene Autry's fan base, and he took care to license his name to products priced accordingly. The Gene Autry cowboy suit sold in mid-line department stores, five-and-dimes, chain stores, and across the country in independent mom-and-pop stores, hardware stores, and auto supply stores. It sold in stores in coal country, steel towns, paper and textile mill towns, auto and industrial cities.[15]

Teresa May Baragona bought the Gene Autry cowboy suit for Charles's sixth birthday in August 1947 at Namie's five-and-dime store in Jonesboro, Louisiana.[16] Most cowboy suits, like most family purchasing generally, were bought by women, wives and mothers. But what it was—a cowboy playsuit—and where it was sold meant that men purchased some Gene Autry cowboy suits. That the Gene Autry cowboy suit sold at auto supply and hardware stores, sites in which men were the predominant customers and the customer base of which crossed class lines, meant that some middle-class boys would receive a Gene Autry cowboy suit. Mike Felton's maternal grandfather, who owned a Hudson dealership in Lewiston, Idaho, purchased the Gene Autry cowboy suit for his grandson from the Goodyear Store in Lewiston.[17] In some Pennsylvania cities, the Gene Autry cowboy suit sold at record stores as well. Jackie Jones's father, Elwyn, was a successful lawyer, the county solicitor in Pottsville, Pennsylvania, a town on the banks of the Schuylkill River in the heart of Pennsylvania coal country. He bought the Gene Autry cowboy suit for his son at a Speedy Record Store that opened in Allentown in 1943.[18] And some of those men were professionals; they worked in offices, not factories, mills, or mines; they earned a good living. David Lonneman's father was the manager of a wholesale toy company in Cincinnati, Ohio, and got a suit for his son in 1942, the first year that Milton Henry substituted the viscose rayon by Du Pont for the fur he originally had used on the chaps.[19]

The war too played a role as mid-level chain stores proliferated and families relocated across the country for war service and war work. With the war, Arthur Cumberledge Sr., a graduate of Annapolis and Navy commander, relocated with his family from Pasadena, California, to Washington, DC, where his wife, Mary Louise, bought their son Toby a Gene Autry cowboy suit at the same Hecht store where Robert Viands' mother had bought his cowboy suit.[20] Hecht's, an East Coast chain, was not a store the Cumberledges would have encountered in California.

Postwar shortages of consumer goods meant that some stores in smaller markets that otherwise would not have carried the Gene Autry cowboy suit did for a season because it was what they could get. As the manager and salesman at a bicycle and sporting goods store in Terre Haute, Indiana, who bought a dozen of the cowboy suits in the fall of 1945 for the holiday sea-

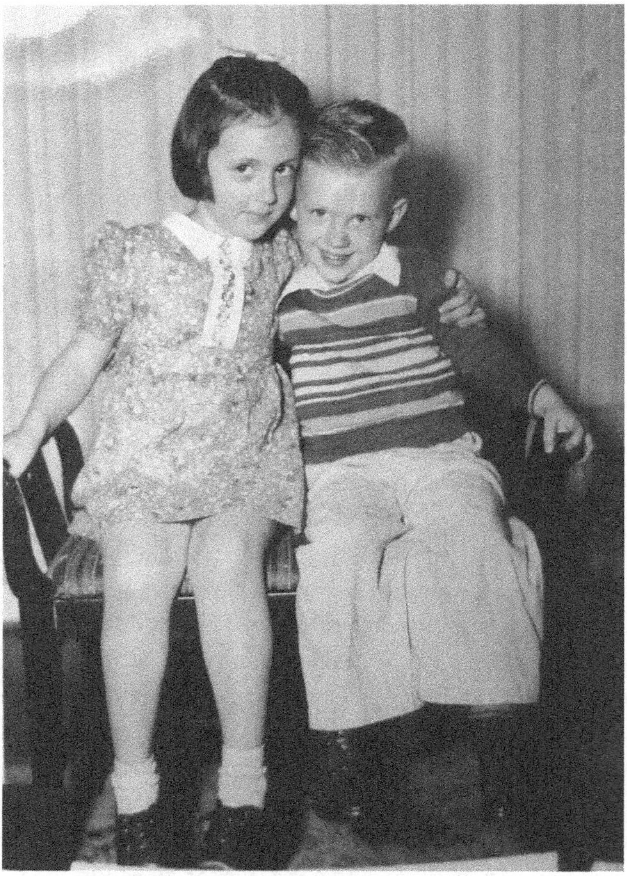

son from a "traveling man" explained, it was the first season after the end of the war and "our other lines were hard to get . . . we had to have something to sell, see."[21] That may well have been how the Gene Autry cowboy suit found its way onto the shelves of the Marks-Rothenberg Department Store in Meridian, Mississippi, where Hassie Watley Strong bought it for her grandson William Augustus Strong III, Billy, for his sixth birthday.[22]

The middle-class families among the children who were burned in Gene Autry cowboy suits were exceptional, highlighting the circumstances in which goods crossed class lines, even as in the main they reinforced them. Among the parents were not only a career Navy officer but also several managers, lawyers, and bankers, a teacher, an engineer, and a chemist.[23] They stood apart in education as well. Before the war and the GI Bill, going to college was exceptional in the American population. Fewer than 10 percent of Americans went on to college.[24] Yet many of the fathers and some of the mothers in these middle-class families had at least one or two years of college, a number had completed degrees, and the lawyers had advanced degrees.

Whereas many of the working-class families who had a Gene Autry cowboy suit lived in the largest cities in the United States, cities like New York, Philadelphia, and Baltimore, most of the middle-class families lived in significantly smaller cities and even smaller towns.[25] Edward Johnson was a teacher and coach in Wilkes-Barre, Pennsylvania, population 86,236, in the heart of coal country. Michael Felton described his family—father a lawyer and his father before him a banker—as a "First Family" in Moscow, Idaho, population 6,014. William Strong Jr. was in law practice with his father in Louisville, Mississippi, population 2,000. In this respect, they were more like the working-class families from whom they otherwise stood apart, the localized consumer markets in which they lived bringing them into this world of loss from which they might otherwise have been protected.

But most families that bought a Gene Autry cowboy suit were not middle-class. The fathers in these families were laborers, section hands, janitors, kitchen helpers, and bakers. They were grocery clerks, taxi drivers, firemen, truck wagon salesmen, and doormen. They were repairmen and utility men. They were steel layout men and body bumpers. They were dye manufacturing operators, spinners, cloth inspectors, weavers, and pressers. They were cabinet makers and painters. They were stonecutters, tracers, coal miners, machinists, machinery operators, mechanics, electric cranemen, screw machine operators, mold runners, and truck drivers. While some worked in skilled trades, others had no trade. Most had limited formal schooling.[26] Had the federal government been charting the "problem of low-income families" in 1940, fully a third of them would have fallen below the bar, and fully two-thirds of them did not make enough to support a family at what the Bureau of Labor Statistics would later call "a modest but adequate standard of living."[27]

Many of these families were first-, second-, and third-generation immigrants. Intelisano, Caparco, Porreca, Giacomarro, DiTrapani, Izzo, Furmanski, Szumita, Marszalek, Piechota, Tetla, Moore, Krau, Ulich, Gidlund, Krzeczkowski, Zibor, Gorab, Gerber, Gagnon, Lockhart, McCormack, Blessington.[28] The one African American family I found who had lost a child in a Gene Autry cowboy suit, a DC family, I was not able to find in the 1940 census.[29] That so many were white ethnics is not surprising. Immigrants had provided the labor that fueled America's dramatic industrial expansion at the turn of the twentieth century. By the 1930s and 1940s, they had young families of their own.[30] Jack Lockhart Jr.'s father was born in Edinburgh, Scotland, in 1889 and raised in Aberdeen. In 1905, at age sixteen, he borrowed money from an uncle and immigrated to the US. By 1917, when he registered for the US draft, he was living in Detroit, working for the Ford Motor Company, and was married with one child, a daughter. One year later, his wife died in the global flu pandemic. His parents would raise the child. In 1922, he remarried. His second wife, Euphemia Greer, like him, was born in Scotland. She was eighteen; he was thirty-three. Their first child, a girl, was born the next year. Over a sixteen-year span, they had five living children. When their last child, John Lockhart Jr., "Jackie," was born in 1938, his parents were still renters. Two years later, they owned their own home in Royal Oak, Michigan, valued at $2,000. John Sr., "a steel layout man" at Ford's Dearborn plant, was earning $1,500; he was the sole-wage earner for a family of seven.[31]

Daniel Marszalek, born in 1939, was the last child and only son of George Marszalek and his wife Mary Fialkiewicz. George Marszalek had immigrated to the United States in 1907 at the age of eighteen. Petitioning for naturalization in 1920, he listed his birthplace as Kroscenko, Austria, and noted that he was a subject of the Republic of Poland and Austria.[32] Later, he listed his place of birth simply as Poland. By 1920, he was married, living in the small town of Taylor, Pennsylvania, had three daughters, and worked in the mines. His wife, Mary Fialkiewicz, was born in the US, likely to immigrant parents, and like him had limited formal schooling. He had completed third grade; she had completed fourth grade. By 1940, the couple had nine children: eight daughters and one son, ranging in age from twenty-four to one. Eight of their children, plus a son-in-law, were living at home. The family had moved to Clarks Summit, a tiny town a few miles north of Scranton. George Marszalek was working as a laborer; his earnings in 1939, $640. The only other wage earner in the household was their twenty-two-year-old daughter Stella, who, with a third-grade education, worked as a clerk, earning $180 in 1939.[33] Their combined income was $820 for the support of a household of ten. In 1942, at the age of fifty-three, George Marszalek registered for the US draft. He was unemployed. In the space to note "obvious physical characteristics that will aid in identification," the registrar had written in, "No Left leg."[34] Three years later, their youngest child and only son, Daniel, would be burned in his cowboy suit, dying a day and a half later.[35]

Tommy McCormack's parents, James and Catherine, were Irish immigrants. By 1940, the couple had filed first papers for naturalization, lived on New York City's Upper East Side in an apartment that they paid $27 a month for in rent, and had four children, all boys, a child born roughly every two years between 1929 and 1937. James McCormack supported his household of six as a doorman earning, in 1939, $1,100. Michael Blessington Jr.'s parents too were born in Ireland. They had immigrated to the US with his mother's brother and his wife, settling into a shared household in Queens. Michael Blessington Sr. was a stonecutter, but work was unsteady. His earnings for 1939, to support a family of five, were a meager $720. The $20 a month they paid for rent represented one-third of his earnings. Like so many others, they made ends meet by sharing a household with relations. By 1940, the Blessingtons were naturalized US citizens and had three children under the age of four. Michael Jr., born on August 23, 1937, was their only son. Burned in a Gene Autry cowboy suit two days after Christmas in 1944, he died three months later on March 28, 1945. He was seven years old.[36]

Among the treasured narratives, an article of faith of twentieth-century American history has been that mass consumption became a fact of American life between the two world wars, and that mobilization for World War II ended not only the Depression but also precarity in American life, ushering in a long era of broadly shared prosperity. But as historians set out to trace the lived contours of these narratives, many have found something different. Call it scraping by or eking out a living, the struggle to make ends meet remained after the war, as before, a defining fact of life for millions of Americans.[37] Susan Porter Benson's words echo in my head. Referring to the working-class families at the heart of her study of consumption in the interwar years, she wrote, "People do not function in the marketplace as autonomous individuals solely in response to marketing and desire but as part of families in which consumption is an object both of struggle and of shared aspiration."[38]

Benson might have been speaking of the largely working-class families that bought Gene Autry cowboy suits for their children in the 1940s. This simple gift, a child's playsuit, reflected the shared aspiration of all these families. Fire transformed that aspiration into a nightmare. It made the Gene Autry cowboy suit an object of struggle for these families, radiating out from them to extended family members and others who had given the suit to a child, to the children a child was playing with and the communities in which they lived.

Neighbors, friends, and strangers responded to these children's and families' plight with altruism and selflessness, including by giving skin from their own bodies. Charitable and community fundraising efforts reflected the class divisions that defined American life. The first news stories of Pat Peterson being burned in Tampa, Florida, in early January 1946 appeared in the Tampa papers the day he was burned.[39] Over the next several months, stories regularly appeared charting the seriousness of his burns, his status, the progress of skin grafts, the family's mounting financial expenses, and community efforts to allay the burden.[40] Richard Peterson, Pat's father, worked at the post office, but because he was a substitute, he did not have the benefit of sick leave or disability. He received no pay when he was off for a month following more than a dozen skin donations to his son, the grafts taken from him because his blood matched, giving a chance that the skin donations would take. Only able to work part-time as he recovered from the donations, he lost more pay.[41]

The Tampa papers' coverage spurred fundraising efforts. Three months after Pat was burned, the Tampa Elks lodge announced that it was appropriating $50 to start a "Pat Peterson Fund," noting that they hoped the boy could convalesce at the Elks Harry-Anna Crippled Children's Home in Umatilla. Pledges and donations from children, mothers, couples, church groups, other fraternal organizations, and businesses followed, all reported in the press and generating more gifts, as well as visibility for the Elks civic activities and their own fundraising for the Harry-Anna home.[42] The presentation of a $1,500 check to Pat Peterson in the hospital by the chairman of the Elks Committee on Social and Community Welfare and his statement "I feel confident now, that Pat Peterson may walk and play again" were carefully staged, the press on hand to capture the moment.[43] So too, seven and a half months after Pat was burned, when Elks leaders saw the boy into a waiting ambulance for the drive to the Elks home in Umatilla, where his expenses would be covered and he would relearn how to walk.[44] Their efforts mattered materially for the Petersons and for Pat. They mattered too to the Elks goal of raising $10,000 for the home. Pat Peterson became a sort of poster child for the Elks campaign.[45]

Community fundraising efforts like that for Pat Peterson and his family, as well as for others, reflected and reinforced the narrative that this was an accident for which no one was to blame. They reflected, as well, the gendered, class-bound, and ethnic structure of the American private social-welfare system. It was Jack Lockhart's mother's lodge—the Bonnie Jean Lodge no. 221, Royal Oak Daughters of Scotia—that organized a concert to raise funds for a surgery for Jack, still unable to walk three years after being burned.[46] The woman who organized a variety show as a benefit for Jackie Izzo only knew about Jackie from having read about her in the papers.[47] "Jackie Attends Benefit with Her Proven Friends," read the headline the day after the event. Jackie had been wheeled into the crowded auditorium on a hospital bed. The story's opening sentence read, "Jacqueline

Izzo should be one of the proudest girls in Saginaw today, she has so many friends." They had raised $3,000.[48]

The money mattered. But it did not address the underlying inequalities that in part placed these children in harm's way. Nor did it come close to meeting the expenses that families faced. The Elks $1,500 fundraising goal was based on a statement by a friend of the Petersons early in the boy's treatment. But Pat was ultimately in the hospital over seven months and in 1948 faced another set of surgeries. The Elks covered his care at the Harry-Anna Home for Crippled Children after both hospital stays. But the $1,500 raised by the Elks for his hospitalization fell far short of the costs for his medical care. The hospital, nurses, medicines, and medical appliances costs (wheelchair, leg and ankle braces, crutches, and special shoes) totaled $4,352.94. The doctor's bills were another $2,150, bringing the total to $6,502.94.[49]

Social structures that created inequality decided which families bore a greater risk of tragic accident. In turn, the relative poverty of these families and the limited public social-welfare net made the burden of the tragedy that much heavier. Michael and Angela Caparco had four children, including their five-year-old son, Perry, who was burned in 1944. For four years, Perry was treated in Roger Williams General Hospital in Providence, Rhode Island. But the desperation of his situation led to a move to Massachusetts General Hospital in Boston in April 1948. By April 1950, he had been in a hospital for six years. At Roger Williams Hospital alone, Perry had had seventy-five blood transfusions, innumerable plasma transfusions, and twenty-five skin-grafting operations. Even apart from the blood, which had to be paid for or replaced, the hospital's expenses exceeded $8,000. The expenses of Perry's medical care at Massachusetts General by April 1950 were over $6,000.

Michael Caparco was a painter by trade. During the war he had been employed in the Kaiser Shipyards in Providence. But that security ended with the war's end.[50] By spring 1950, the Caparco's had long since exhausted their limited financial means. The $300 they had in the bank had gone to the hospital. Michael Caparco had reimbursed the lost wages ($12 a day) of the fifty fellow shipworkers who had donated blood for Perry. A Blue Cross hospital policy had paid just over $1,000.[51] Public welfare from the Providence Department of Public Welfare and the State of Rhode Island had paid over $7,000. Both the hospital in Providence and Massachusetts General Hospital had written off part of the expenses. But there was still an outstanding balance owed to the hospital in Providence of close to $3,000, and it was not clear how long Massachusetts General would keep the boy—especially since, as Rhode Island residents, they had no call on welfare in

Massachusetts. The family had run out of places to turn. They owned no real estate. Their only property was a 1939 Plymouth automobile valued at $150.[52] And though temporarily home, Perry was confined to a wheelchair, unable to walk; had to be taken to Massachusetts General Hospital every two weeks for bandage changes; and soon enough would be back in the hospital for more skin grafts and other surgeries. What was a family to do? The Gene Autry cowboy suit had effectively made the Caparcos wards of the state, and even that future was unsure.

Traumatic and fatal injury, especially involving a child, weighed on marriages that already bore the burden of limited income. And when those bonds failed, family livelihood was further imperiled. Chesley Franklin Johnson, Rachel and Chesley Lee Johnson's only child, survived for over seven months after he was burned, treated first at the McLeod Infirmary in Florence, South Carolina, where they lived and then moved to Duke University Hospital in Durham. His parents faced medical expenses of over $1,200 as well as travel and hotel expenses to be with their son after he was moved to Durham. In the wake of his death, they divorced.[53] Stella Krzeczkowski and her husband, Casimir Sr., divorced in the wake of the accident in November 1943 that led to the death of their son Stanley and debilitating injury to their only other child, Casimir. Casimir was in the hospital for two and a half years. Legally, Casimir's father remained responsible for his son's expenses, but realities were often far different. "Mr. Kresokowski don't pay any medical bills since I had been divorced from him," was how Stella Krzeczkowski put it. She remarried, and her second husband's support for her and her son was a critical supplement to her own wages working in a spring factory in Passaic, New Jersey. But the medical expenses for Casimir remained her burden alone.[54]

Even in families that remained together, injury of a child often meant the interruption or end of a mother's wage-work and the loss of income critical to the fragile financial balance of working-class families' lives, compounding the burden they faced from unexpected medical bills. Three years after Tommy McCormack's injury and death, his mother, Catherine, had not returned to her evening job.[55] Margaret Szumita, who like her husband worked in the Raycrest Mills in Pawtucket, Rhode Island, was out of work for two years caring for her son Richard.[56]

Like the Viands, many families brought to this hardship other losses that shaped this loss. By the 1930s, infant mortality had dropped dramatically. In 1930, the US reported infant mortality at sixty-five deaths per thousand live births.[57] But statistics distance the shadow of death from individual women's and family's lives; they obscure that the burden of infant mortality was not spread evenly in the population.[58] Alexander Szumita and Margaret Roberts had married in Pawtucket, Rhode Island, in 1935. Their first child, a boy they named James, born in 1937, was either stillborn or died within days of birth. Margaret was twenty-one years old; her husband Alexander was twenty-two. A year later, in 1938, they had a second child, a boy they named Edward, who again was either stillborn or died within days of birth.[59] What anxiety she, they, must have felt through her third pregnancy. But in 1940, their third child, another son, was born alive and survived, and less than two years later, in 1942, a fourth son, they named Richard. Four pregnancies in five years' time; two living children.

Hardly was Margaret Szumita out of the shadow of that fourth pregnancy when Richard, not even one year old, developed polio, leaving his right arm and shoulder crippled. How could these other losses and trials not shape the trial they endured when Richard at age six was burned in a Gene Autry cowboy suit?[60] It casts in a different light Margaret Szumita leaving her work at the mill for two years to care for her son Richard. What was true for the Szumitas was true for many of the families who had a child burned in a Gene Autry cowboy suit, families who had also lost children in miscarriages and stillbirths, had borne infants who died within a few months of birth. Their lives reflected the cumulative burdens and losses that shadowed the lives of these families.[61]

In the moment, none of these families knew the role the war played in the hazardous nature of the Gene Autry cowboy suit. But all the same, especially for those whose child was injured or died during the war, the two events were bound up together. When the Selective Service Act was passed in October 1940, married men with dependents, like Richard Viands, were classified as III-A and protected from induction. But beginning on October 1, 1943, the ban on inducting men with dependents was removed, and by April 1944, more than half the men inducted were fathers.[62] Robert was burned when his father was overseas. Robert survived. But there were other fathers in the service whose boys were burned in Gene Autry cowboy suits who did not survive—like Ernie Bell, Arthur Lunsford, Richard Johnson, and William Augustus Strong III. Edward Johnson got to see his son Richard only because his son had survived for five months. Other boys, some of whom died, were burned after their fathers had returned from the service.[63]

For all these families, there had been other joys, hardships, loves, and losses that were part of the fabric of their lives and that they brought to this loss. It could not have been otherwise.

memory

Dear Frances,

I found myself thinking last night or earlier today why recent pictures of you are so much more important to me than baby pictures of you. We did not lose you as a baby—that part of your life was already and for a long time had been a memory; it was good and natural that it be so; it was a signifier of the fact that you had, in fact, grown up. It is you now—or in recent pictures—that I hold fast because this you was not a memory and has now been rendered a fundamentally different memory—not a memory of you "before" but a memory, in a sense, cut short, incomplete, because there is no after.

. . .

It snowed more today. Great, big, beautiful floating flakes of snow. I so associate snow with you. I imagine you in the snow, tromping along in your boots, the snow collecting on your hat or in your hair, you tilting your head back to catch snowflakes in your wide open mouth, you collapsing into the snow and making snow angels and always, your laugh, and your smile.

. . .

Dad and I went cross-country skiing this afternoon along the river. I could feel the cold air against my face and for a moment or moments at a time felt that it was your face that the cold air was blowing gently against.

. . .

Dad pointed out to me yesterday that it's starting to stay light a little longer now each day. It's no longer dark at 5:00 in the evening.

. . .

I thought for the first time today how hard it will be to have your classmates finish their freshmen year of college. It will be one of those benchmarks that we simply assumed, took for granted, and yet no longer is.

. . .

I had planned to do the keynote lecture for the WAWH as a braided narrative about loss in our lives & the way it is hidden/masked by our CVs, about the families who lost children in the cowboy suit tragedy, and about my experience of losing you. But recently I have found myself thinking that my loss is mine, that it is private, that I don't want to share it with others. I have also found myself questioning why I ever thought talking about our sense of loss in any way mirrored the loss suffered by these families. You had gotten to celebrate your 18th birthday. You were on the verge of adulthood, independence, college. You had the inklings of who you might become, of what you might believe in, of the commitments you might make. We don't know what you knew, but we were told at least that you were not in pain. The families who lost children in the cowboy suit tragedy lost children who were only 4 or 5, 6, 7, 8, 9—children, truly. They suffered horrible pain, horror, terror. Some died almost right away, others suffered for months, others lived. My/Our loss is not theirs, theirs is not ours. And there is the differences as well of the times—the 1940s vs. 2010s.

. . .

I was thinking the other day about you and photographs. I think your having photographs all over your room—of family . . . was your way of expressing emotions of love, happiness, and belonging. Your room feels like a happy place because it is so full of love.

chapter twelve · "married, two children"

The resume that Gerda Lerner enclosed with her cover letter as she searched for a university teaching position in 1965 included only the barest hints of the life that shaped her identity and values. It did not include any reference to her family background, to how, why, or when she emigrated to the United States, to the factory and working-class jobs she held in the first years after her arrival, or her first marriage. Organized by categories, formatted as a list—academic training, teaching experience, publications—it was exactly as expected: profoundly impersonal.[1] Bill Tuttle's 1966 vita was much the same. As Lerner and Tuttle understood, in writing their vitae they were fashioning a professional life and identity.

That self-fashioning was, in important respects, formulaic. "Form, *n.*, a set, customary, or prescribed way of doing something"; "a document with blanks to be filled up." "Form, *v.t.*, give form or shape to"; "mould (a person, the mind, a faculty, etc.) by discipline, experience, or education."[2] A personal resume or vita was and is both noun and verb. It is a customary, prescribed way of doing something. It is as if the individual were responding to a series of invisible questions, filling in an unlined blank. And in so doing giving form or shape to a life, disciplining as certainly as a field of knowledge does. What stood out about the resume or curriculum vitae as it took form in the United States, what remains true today and gave shape to this book, were its limits for accounting for or representing human experience. It as much as said that lived, personal experience and background were irrelevant to teaching, research, knowledge. Its form, structure, and contents reinforced the view that knowledge was and should be impersonal, objective, and detached.

But if the vita of the 1950s and 1960s was marked in the main by its profound impersonality, there was one category of personal status that was almost uniform in its inclusion: marital and parental status. Just beneath her name and address, Lerner's resume read:

> Born April 30, 1920, Vienna, Austria
> American citizen, 1943
> Married, two children, ages 20 and 22

Tuttle's vita too began with "married, two children."[3] In this respect, as in others, their vitae were formulaic. But what those three simple words—"married, two children"—meant for a man differed radically from what they meant for a woman. They were the foundation of two distinct, gendered academic career paths. Women, and others who did not fit the academic template, might tweak the categories to distance themselves from or bring themselves closer to the gendered narrative script, but the script itself was written.

Like lawsuits for personal injury, vitae are bound up in prediction. A verdict and calculation of damages rests on a prediction about what a "natural" life would have amounted to in a way that produces a dollar value in the present. So too a potential or current employer reads a vita as a prediction of the productive course of an academic life as a teacher or scholar. And just as a verdict and damage award or legal settlement shape the life that follows, so too predictions relating to the productive course of an academic life shape the future course of that life.[4] Marital and parental status read through gender were fundamental to the prediction that the vita was bound up with.

The career-bounding significance of marital and parental status read through gender flew in the face of the claim that *merit finds its own place*. In the late nineteenth- and early twentieth- century United States, newly professionally trained PhDs had struggled against status, forming professional societies and seeking academic appointments based on their training rather than on their family background.[5] But their rebellion was incomplete. The privilege of sex assumed. (And whiteness, and ableness, and . . .) The consistent echoing refrain in letters between men filling academic appointments: *We want a man.* Logan Wilson's 1942 study of the American professoriate titled: *The Academic Man.* David Reisman's unselfconscious 1956 description of individual transformation through higher education: "A small-town boy who goes to college may be lifted by that encounter into the wild blue yonder of the mind: a discipline with its national and even international market of ideas, can free him from the ethnocentric nest of home and parish, give him a new past (the traditions of 'his' field) and a new identity."[6]

The material practices that provided grounding for the vita took for granted the relevance of sex and gender in academic life. Just as letters between men seeking to fill an academic appointment had long begun, "We want a man," so too, from their beginnings in the 1930s, the few "position available" advertisements in professional journals in every field had routinely, explicitly included sex as a qualification for a position. Most sought a man.[7] Candidates for appointments understood this. "Teachers available" notices across academic fields from the early 1930s on, had regularly included gender identifiers. From its start in 1932, each listing in the American Sociological Society's Personnel Exchange in the *American Journal of Sociology* was preceded by an "M" or "W." Perhaps someone inquired, because in the third issue the letters were explained: "The numbers are assigned in the order in which the entries are received, with the prefix M (man) or W (woman)."[8] In other disciplines, as in economics, it might as well have been a requirement—so uniform was the practice of men, at least, following the statement of their field with the word "Man."[9]

Men's and women's references to their sex were not parallel. Women understood that they would be attractive to women's colleges but that more generally their sex would exclude them from consideration even at coeducational institutions. Their listings capitulated to the realities of the professional world they had entered. For men, the calculus was different. Federal, state, and private employment policies and practices in the Depression limiting or giving priority to men likely played an important role in men beginning to note their sex as the most prominent element of their professional identity beyond field. But it meant that men were being trained to think of their sex not as incidental but as a fundamental qualification, and women were being trained to think that their sex was disqualifying.

But privilege takes its purest form when it requires no explicit claim. Such was the power of a man's name at the top of a vita. "William M. Tuttle, Jr." "Herbert Gutman." "Morton Keller." "Peter Novick." "Peter Rossi."[10] We think of a name as identifying a particular individual. And it does. But so much more information is contained in a name: ethnic heritage, possibly religion, and most certainly, sex.[11] Beginning in the late 1950s and even more so by the 1960s and 1970s, the curriculum vitae became the gateway form of academic life. Hiring, retention, promotion, merit, fellowships, and introductions at presentations all came to require a vita. Folders filled with vitae became common in individual, departmental, and administrative academic files.[12] Every element of these vitae was read in light of and through the name at the top. A personal resume or vita must, of course, identify its subject. But the name at the top of a vita did more than this: It placed one within or outside the borders of academic and intellectual belonging. In their 1958 book *The Academic Marketplace*, Theodore Caplow and Reece McGee could write without critique, "Women tend to be discriminated against in the academic profession not because they have low prestige but because they are outside the prestige system entirely and for this reason are of no use to a department in future recruitment."[13]

The screening and evaluative work done by the name at the top of a vita was in turn compounded by other personal data that was fundamental to the predictive value of vita in the 1950s, 1960s, and early 1970s. Job candidates did not have to guess at what was expected on their vita. The material practices of academic life—information, application, and employment forms; university placement service forms; vita forms; advice from professional societies—provided direction.[14] A "Note to Applicants" in the supplement to the *American Sociological Review Employment Bulletin* in February 1960 advised applicants that each listing "should include the following items of information in order: type of position preferred; two subjects with best preparation; highest degrees and awards; experience; publications; present residence; age; family status; date available." Together with the *American Sociological Review*'s identification of every applicant by sex, every applicant's disciplinary training and experience was framed by personal identity: sex, age, and family status.[15] The sciences and math were no different.[16] Professional societies were uniform in their advice to candidates: Vitae should include marital and parental status.[17]

University placement office forms reinforced this professional norm. If in the 1910s, 1920s, and 1930s a minority of PhD students registered with university placement offices, by the 1960s, establishing a dossier with the university placement office was expected of graduate students.[18] The Columbia University placement form that Gerda Lerner completed in 1965 was typical of forms in the 1950s and 1960s. The Columbia form had five sections: Academic Training; Experience; Courses Capable of Teaching; Personal Qualifications; Details of Training. Personal questions relating to smoking and alcohol use, standard in the 1910s and 1920s on such forms, were long since gone, along with the moral codes that led to them. Other questions, on subjects like religion, church membership, and church attendance, once pervasive, were now far less common, barred by law in some states, removed in others in the wake of the horrors of the Nazi regime.[19] But questions related to "Personal Qualifications," including marital and parental status, physical condition, and height and weight remained standard on university placement forms in the 1960s. Gerda Lerner filled in her height, weight, and physical condition on the form. She did not include this data on her personal resume. But she did include her marital and parental status.[20] In both regards, Lerner's resume was like hundreds, thousands of other resumes and vitae from this period.[21]

Flipping through vitae circulated to faculty in the Department of History at the University of Chicago between 1965 and 1968—vitae that included both established scholars and PhD candidates—marital and parental status were listed on all but a few.[22] So, for example,

PETER NOVICK
PERSONAL: Born Jersey City, N. J., 26 July 1934
Married, one child.

CURRICULUM VITAE – Stephan Albert Thernstrom
Date and Place
Of Birth: 1934, Port Huron, Michigan
Married, two children

Curriculum Vitae of Richard E. Ellis
Born: 7 September 1937
Married: two children (and expecting a third)

In the 1950s, 1960s, and early 1970s, listing marital and parental status on vitae and resumes was the norm in every field.[23] On most vitae, this information was the first item or category beneath the individual's name.

In one sense, the personal data at the top of a vita was just that—"personal," administratively relevant to employment, but irrelevant to one's academic credentials. And yet, in fact, all the other elements of a vita—educational training, academic appointments, other experience, honors, professional society memberships, publications—were shaped by and read through that status.

As in the power in a name, the meaning of marital status on vitae was fundamentally gendered. "Married, two children" at the top of a man's vita defined him as mature, settled, a provider. In US census terms, he was the family or household "head."[24] His obligation of support, both legal and social, provided a certain assurance of a man's stability and gave him claims to a salary greater than those without such obligations had. In the context of the Cold War, moreover, with its intense homophobia and heightened pressure for "normal" family life, "married" at the top of a man's vita could provide cover against career-ending suspicions of homosexuality.[25] But this was not all: "Married" on a man's vita weighed into the form's predictive value. This status said that because he could depend on the unpaid labor of a wife to care for home and family life, he would be able to focus on his professional career.[26]

The value of a wife to colleges and universities was not only indirect. University life had long depended on the unwaged labor of the faculty wife.[27] The many references to happy marriages and charming wives as assets to college or university social life in so many replies to letters beginning, "We want a man," reflected this reality.[28] In 1949, the dean of the faculty at Princeton wrote to department chairmen inquiring about their methods of assisting and evaluating junior personnel. Among the questions in which he was specifically interested: Was there a person or committee who provided "assistance in personal problems such as housing, office accommodations, community adjustment, family illness, or general orientation in case of new men?"[29] In 1949, only men were on the Princeton faculty. But it was the labor assumed of faculty wives that the replies to the Dean's query highlighted. The chairman of the Department of Economics replied, "In such matters as housing and family illness, it is only fair to say that the Chairman's wife has done more than her share." The chairman of the Department of English replied, "Appointment of a faculty wife, who can (and does) solve problems of housing and unexpected illness or expense." Their replies were mirrored in others'.[30] Little had changed by the point that John Gillis joined the faculty of the History Department in 1965. Describing Princeton as a junior faculty member, Gillis wrote, "With the exception of a few bachelors, we were all married, a condition that was an unstated condition of success in a place where social and intellectual life were so tightly joined. Junior and senior faculty found themselves in one another's houses almost every Saturday evening, a situation made possible by the fact that at this time faculty wives were expected to be helpmates to their husband, whatever their own educational attainments."[31]

Gillis described the sociality that underlay intellectual life as "very Princetonian." But the fact of the matter was that Princeton was not so very distinct in the importance it placed on marriage for a man, the status and labor it assumed of a faculty wife. In academic institutions of every rank in every region, the status of wife as helpmate to her husband had long extended not only to the care of children, husband, household, social gatherings, and settling new families into university life but also, in many cases, to their husband's research and teaching. A faculty wife might chauffeur her husband to and from campus, grade student papers, type and edit her husband's manuscripts, read galley proofs, and help with her husband's research, including work in his lab.[32] Marriage *an unstated condition of success* for a man. Wives, *whatever their own educational attainments, helpmates.* The word "married" on a man's vita promised quite a lot.

In a pathbreaking article on marriage and the polity in the nineteenth-century United States, the historian Nancy Cott argued, "Men's civil and political status grew . . . from being independent heads of units that included dependents."[33] And so it was here. "Married, two children" on a man's vita was the professional and intellectual corollary to the civil and political function of family headship marked by Cott. That many wives saw their work as part of a partnership with their husband, vital not only to his career and to university life but in many cases to the original creative, scientific, and other intellectual contributions that established their husband's reputation, spoke not just to the character of their personal relationships and the benefits of being part of a college or university community but as much to the straitened life expectations of women as individuals in this era.

The vita is an individuating document, lacking even a biography's or obituary's potential to color in the world around its immediate subject. In her history of women scientists in America to 1940, Margaret Rossiter relates a number of examples of married women with doctorates who collaborated in their husband's research. Noting the difficulty of even finding biographical information on many women scientists, she notes that their work can be "glimpsed indirectly in the biographies and bibliographies of the prominent scientists who employed them," as in the *Biographical Memoirs of the National Academy of Sciences.* "Most invisible of all are the wives of these high achievers, who are usually mentioned only once, with very high praise, but then ignored, while their husbands' achievements are discussed in full."[34] While many men may have viewed their wife as a partner in their careers—and universities assumed their un- or under-waged labor—a man's wife's name almost never appeared on his vita. It was his vita and his name only that appeared at the top; her identity and contribution subsumed in the word "married."[35]

Few married men included their wives' names on their vitae. Most often where they did, it was not so much naming his wife as an individual as it was as a faculty wife. For non-European international scholars in the 1950s and 1960s, as had been true for earlier generations of foreign scholars, marriage to an American woman (or for Jewish scholars, marriage to a Protestant woman) could improve their chances, evidence that they would fit into and be assets in American collegiate or university life.[36] In such instances, a wife's name was part of a search for academic belonging for the man whose name appeared at the top. The addition of her American academic credentials served as yet additional evidence that the couple would fit in in an American institution.

Instances of a man including his wife's name or credentials on his vita as an individual or scholar in her own right were rarer still. An example: one curriculum vitae in a thick file of vitae circulated by the history department chair to faculty in the department at the University of Chicago in the mid-1960s. Just below his own name: "Married (wife a candidate for a D. Phil. at Oxford in political theory)." The vita went on to offer the man's academic credentials, his area of concentration, thesis and thesis supervisor, honors, languages, fields of interest, possible fields of research, and teaching experience. The vita attracted enough interest for what appears to be follow-up on the candidate's wife. Scribbled in handwriting on his vita, not her name, but details of her credentials: her date of birth, college and graduate school credentials, thesis title; languages; fellowships and other honors; and teaching experience. The man, in what seems a calculated silence, had not mentioned children on his vita. This detail too had been part of the due diligence on his wife. Along with the other notes, scribbled in the margins was, "M [married] 3 children."[37]

"Married, __ children." How different the meaning in these words at the top of a vita bearing a woman's name. What for a man was a professional asset was for a woman a professional liability, the predictive value of "married, two children" on a woman's vita the inverse of that for a man. By definition, a married woman was understood to be dependent, not independent. By law and social norms, provided for, not a provider.[38] She did not have a wife freeing her to concentrate on her professional career, there to serve as an unwaged research assistant. Her first obligation was understood to be owed not to herself, her career, or an employer but to her husband, household, and children.

A woman might choose to not marry, focusing on her career—the vast majority of the small number of women with faculty appointments in the early twentieth century had remained unmarried—but not only did men not face a choice between career and marriage, marriage in fact boosting their careers, but also single women were marked as anomalous in a world that assumed marriage as the normal state of adulthood.[39] The words "married, two children" on a woman's vita reflected inverse gendered obligations and burdens that were socially deep-wired and reinforced daily, shaping the course of a life not only through individual choices made within their constraining frame but through choices made by others acting on their predictive value.

Whereas few men included their wives' names on their vitae, many women included their husbands'. And this practice, too, reflected the differential gendered meaning of marriage for women and men. Elizabeth Cady Stanton, the intellectual leader of the nineteenth-century women's rights movement, challenged women's loss of civic identity on marrying. "A [married] woman has no name!" she decried in an 1856 letter.[40] The not-so-distant echo of her words lay in the common practice of even professional women in the 1950s, 1960s, and early 1970s signing correspondence with both *their* married name and their own, and vitae on which a woman listed her own name with her married name immediately following or just below in parentheses.[41] Women may no longer legally have been required to take their husband's last name at marriage, but by social convention most still did. And by social convention they became known not just by their husband's last name but also his first: Mrs. Herbert B. Lewis; Mrs. J. Barkov M. Kassarjian; Mrs. E. W. Monter Jr.[42] Alison Cornish Thorne, noting the practice at Texas A&M College of listing faculty wives in the yearbook "by their husband's name as Mrs. without their own first names being given," found herself listed in the yearbook as "Mrs. D. Wynne Thorne." It did not matter that, like her husband, she had a PhD or had taught; she was a faculty wife.[43] Married professional women lived a divided, double identity. Their inclusion of their husband's name on their vitae reflected that they were known, and in some contexts defined solely, through their relationships to their husbands, even as they had identities as individuals.

Women's inclusion of their husband's name, and sometimes of his occupation, reflected the geographic constraints that marriage imposed on many women's professional lives. Though Gerda Lerner did not list her husband's name on her resume, her letters made explicit the geographic limits of her job search and the reason for those limits. "Due to my husband's business, I must stay in the New York City area."[44] A husband's name and occupation on a vita implied the same. Just below her own date of birth on Dorrian Apple Sweetser's 1964 "Personal Data Sheet" were the words, "Marriage: to Professor Frank E. Sweetser, November 23, 1960." Reading her vita, Everett Hughes, chair of the Sociology Department at Brandeis, understood. Frank Sweetser was on the faculty at Boston University, a specialist in social psychology; Dorrian's search for a position was limited to the Boston area.[45] The freedom men enjoyed—to go where merit led, whether single or married—most women lost on marriage.

"The Physics staff recommends appointment of Mrs. Dinah Rozen as a lecturer with a 3/5th teaching load for 1965–1966," read a May 1965 memorandum from the chair of the Department of Physics to the dean at Queensborough Community College. The chair went on to note and extoll "Mrs. Rozen's credentials," closing, "We are fortunate she is interested since well qualified candidates in physics are not available at the rank and salary we offer." Unlike the title "Mr.," which was the same whether or not a man was married, "Mrs." signaled that a woman was married, and—like "married" on a woman's vita—it allowed potential employers to assume, whether true in the particular case or not, that she was provided for, that her husband's career came first, and that at the very least her husband's career location defined the geographic orbit of her search for a position. And for many women, by social convention as much as by economic necessity, it did. That Mrs. Dinah Rozen was available and interested in an appointment at Queensborough Community College was most certainly a product of her marital and parental status.

Dinah Levine married I. Robert Rozen in 1955, while she was still an undergraduate at Radcliffe College. She was working toward a BA in physics; he was working toward his law degree at Harvard. After their marriage, she completed her BA, graduating magna cum laude in 1958, followed by an MA at Columbia in 1961, receiving the highest degree on the MA exam in physics that year, and then continuing coursework toward a PhD. While a student at Radcliffe, she had held a teaching assistantship in physics at NYU; and, as an MA student at Columbia, she held a teaching assistantship in physics and then a research assistantship in the Columbia Radiation Laboratory, an appointment she continued after completing her degree. In 1963, she held a one-year instructorship at Bronx Community College. Then motherhood intervened with the birth of their first child and, by 1966, a second child, both daughters. A part-time teaching appointment was the most she could manage alongside her familial obligations. Her husband's career, by contrast, flourished. With a law degree from Harvard Law School, by 1966 he was a corporate general counsel to the DCA Food Industries, Inc., a vice president of the Mayflower Doughnut Corporation, and a trustee of the Riverdale Hebrew Day School.

The predictive value of "married, two children," so different for a man than for a woman, assumed the natural course of a life. But as Dinah Levine and Robert Rozen's lives highlight, the dependency imposed on women was an unsure source for the future. When she applied to Queensborough Community College for a part-time instructorship in 1965, she was a married woman with children. A year later, she was a widow, her husband dead of a heart attack at his office desk at the age of thirty-four.[46] "Dinah L. Rozen," read the name on her vita in late 1966. "Widow, two children." She was thirty years old.

"Literary history and the present are dark with silences," began a 1965

Harper's Magazine essay titled "Silences: When Writers Don't Write," by writer Tillie Olsen.[47] "The silences I speak of here are unnatural," she wrote, "the unnatural thwarting of what struggles to come into being, but cannot." As she explained, "the very great have known such silences," but it was "unmined genius," particularly that of women, on which she focused. She drew on the words of Honoré de Balzac, Rainer Maria Rilke, Joseph Conrad, and Thomas Mann for what is required for creation: "constant toil . . . without duties, almost without external communication . . . unconfined solitude . . . the flow of daily life made easy and noiseless . . . time as needed for the work . . . totality of self."

And then, she contrasted the lives of women. As she noted, "women are traditionally trained to place others' needs first, to feel these needs as their own . . . ; their sphere, their satisfaction to be in making it possible for others to use their abilities. . . . The needs of creation," Olsen wrote, "illuminate women's silence of centuries." Searching literary history, she noted that most of those whose literary achievements endured had not married or had married only late in life and had household help. Few had children.

Having drawn on the words of great male writers for what was needed to produce original creative work, Olsen turned to the words of great women writers for expression of the burdens of married family life. "The house seems to take up so much time," the late nineteenth-century writer Katherine Mansfield Murry wrote, early in her relationship with John Middleton Murry, when, as Olsen notes, "they both dreamed of becoming great writers."

> I mean when I have to clean up twice over or wash up extra unnecessary things, I get frightfully impatient and want to be working [writing]. So often this week you and Gordon have been talking while I washed dishes. Well someone's got to wash dishes and get food. Otherwise "there's nothing in the house but eggs to eat." And after you have gone I walk about with a mind full of ghosts of saucepans and primus stoves and "will there be enough to go around?" And you calling, whatever I am doing, writing, "Tig, isn't there going to be tea? It's five o'clock."

And, Olsen asked, "if, in addition . . . to the daily responsibilities, there are children?"

> Motherhood was "almost certain death to creation."

> Not because the capacities to create no longer exist . . . but because the circumstances for sustained creation are almost impossible. The need cannot

> be first. It can have at best, only part self, part time . . . More than in any human relationship, overwhelmingly more, motherhood means being instantly interruptible, responsive, responsible. Children need one now. . . . It is distraction, not meditation, that becomes habitual; interruption, not continuity; spasmodic, not constant toil.

Little wonder was it that women whose children were grown, like Gerda Lerner, included the ages of their children on their vitae or resumes—signaling their children's adulthood and with it their own independence from the cares of motherhood. "Married, two children, ages 20 and 22," read Lerner's 1966 resume, at the start of her academic career.[48] For married women who had not had children, the words "no children" on their vitae, combined with their own date of birth to show their reproductive years were past, signaled that motherhood did not and would not compete with the demands of an academic life.[49]

"For some years, I have been playing the triple role of part-time writer, part-time teacher and part-time homemaker," wrote Maxine Kumin in her 1961 application to the Radcliffe Institute for Independent Study. The Radcliffe Institute was the brainchild of Mary Ingraham Bunting, a microbiologist by training and the sixth president of Radcliffe College. Her goal: to stem the exodus of highly trained women in the arts and sciences derailed from promising careers by marriage and the demands of raising a family. Kumin's application, like the hundreds of others Bunting's "messy experiment" produced, spoke to the challenges women faced in balancing marriage, motherhood, and career. "The rigors of a regular teaching and homemaking schedule have not permitted me to develop as intensively as I would hope in the area of creative writing," wrote Kumin.[50] In 1946, the same year she completed her AB in history and literature at Radcliffe, Kumin married Victor M. Kumin, a research chemist. After her marriage, she continued her education at Radcliffe, earning an AM in comparative literature in 1948, but that year the demands of motherhood were added to those of marriage with the birth of their first child. A year later, a second child; and in 1953, a third child. Six years passed between her master's and her return to writing, but even then, marriage and children came first. When her youngest was five and started kindergarten, Kumin finally was able to seek a teaching appointment. Part-time.

There were thousands of women like Maxine Kumin, their educations cut short, their ability to pursue an academic career circumscribed, their creative and intellectual aspirations if not silenced, then reduced, by the demands of marriage and motherhood. In the blank provided for "special talents and training" on her application for the Radcliffe Institute in 1962, Tillie Olsen wrote, "Rather than say 'none,' I list these, even if not academic: . . . 3. Jugglery of mothering, wifehood, fulltime work on a job, running a household, and somewhere writing or hope of it. (not talent for, but training)."[51]

The differential gendered impact of marriage and parenthood on vitae and in the lives they captured was seen in its clearest form in the lives of academic couples. Describing his years at Princeton in the mid-1960s, in which "a few faculty wives like Lois Banner and Jane De-Hart Matthews taught down the road at a place called Douglass College, while my own spouse took part-time jobs at the local community college while deciding whether she wanted to enter graduate school," John Gillis finished his statement by saying, "No one questioned, however, the priority of the man's career."[52] Certainly not most men, including hiring officials.

Peter H. Rossi completed his PhD in sociology at Columbia in 1951, marrying a fellow sociology doctoral student that same year. Given the date of his degree, Rossi likely did not have a vita in 1951. Nor did he need one. At Columbia he had been an instructor and research associate at the Bureau of Applied Social Research, and the illustrious faculty there—led by Paul Lazarsfeld and Robert K. Merton—were undoubtedly the source of his appointment as an assistant professor in the Department of Social Relations at Harvard. Four years later, in 1955, he accepted an appointment as a full professor at the University of Chicago. 1955 was a full year for the Rossis: the family move to Chicago with a promotion; the publication of his first book, *Why Families Move*; the birth of the Rossis' first child. In 1957, a second child. That same year a research grant from the Social Science Research Council, with a second, and then an auxiliary grant in 1958 supporting the research for his second book. In 1960, the Rossis had a third child. That same year, in addition to his position as a professor of sociology, Peter Rossi accepted the directorship of the National Opinion Research Center at Chicago (NORC). In 1961, his second book, *The Politics of Urban Renewal*, was published. A decade out from his PhD, Peter Rossi had built a vita that led him to be sought after by elite universities across the country.[53] His vita listed his education, his occupational history, and his awards, supplemented by a "select" bibliography, and at the top "Family Status: Married, three children."[54]

The fellow sociology doctoral student Peter Rossi married in 1951 was named Alice. Taking his last name, she became Alice S. Rossi. When he was appointed an instructor at Harvard, she went with him and found a position as a research associate, first on a project in the Russian Research

Center and then two years later on a project in the Graduate School of Education. When he was appointed as a professor at Chicago, she again followed. But with this move motherhood became the center of her working life. For the next four years—the years in which their children were born (1955, 1957, 1960)—she had "no regular employment." She did complete her Columbia doctorate in 1957, and in 1959, she did some teaching as a lecturer at Chicago. From 1961 to 1967 there were a succession of appointments as research associate in anthropology, sociology, NORC, and the Committee on Human Development.[55]

In the ten years of their marriage, he built a distinguished vita. Hers was a disjointed record of fits and starts, silences, a helpmate to the work of others. On a curriculum vitae from 1966 or 1967, Alice Rossi began, as so many men's and women's vitae did, with family status. The first category beneath her name read: "Family Status: Married, three children, ages 10, 9, and 6."[56] "Education" followed, and then "Professional Experience"—that long succession of positions as a "Research Associate." At the bottom of this list, she included a "Note" describing her work during the war years from 1943–1946 and then "No regular employment during 1955–1959. Children born in 1955, 1957, 1960."[57] Those children had been her work, as well as maintaining a household while finishing her long-delayed degree and facilitating the flowering of her husband's career. In listing their ages, just as Gerda Lerner and so many other women did, she signaled that she no longer had preschool-age children demanding her full attention throughout the day. A decade from her doctoral degree, itself slowed by marriage and the birth of their first child, Alice Rossi had published a few articles but had held no faculty academic appointment. Her vita was not one which led to invitations from across the country.

Responding to one of the invitations he had received in 1961—this one from James Coleman in the Department of Social Relations at Johns Hopkins—Peter Rossi spoke indirectly to the toll of marriage and motherhood on his wife's career. It was a difficult time for them to move, he explained, because Alice had begun work only a few weeks ago on a project of a professor in the Anthropology Department that offered an "extraordinary opportunity" for her. "It would be difficult for anyone to break back into a professional career after an absence of five or six years," he explained. "It is especially difficult for a woman to do so when those five or six years have been taken up with non-professional activities." What he did not say was that the work Alice had done in those years had made it possible for him to concentrate on his career. He could move across the country, move between the spheres of private and public, be husband, father, and academic star because she bore and cared for their children and their household. "From the point of view of the profession," he continued, "she is way over age in grade with very little opportunity to make up for this gap without making some substantial scholarly contribution."[58]

What in fact came out of what Peter Rossi described as an "extraordinary opportunity" was a hard professional lesson that many women and others as research associates learned. Once Alice Rossi had designed and fielded the study, the anthropology professor (male) who was principal investigator fired her. The dean's response, as Alice Rossi later noted, was to protect the professor, leaving her to find another research position to try to close the yawning gap on her vita.[59] It would be years still before she had an academic appointment of her own. That she did was in part a product of a challenge to discrimination against women in academia that she, with many others, led.

The only personal information that the feminist political theorist Susan Moller Okin included on her curriculum vitae in the 1970s and early 1980s were her date and place of birth and her citizenship. As her vita noted, she was born in July 1946 in Auckland, New Zealand; she was a New Zealand citizen with US citizenship pending. Okin completed her PhD in political theory at Harvard in fall 1975. Her advisor, Michael Walzer, opened a letter for her dossier with the Harvard University Office of Placement Services, by saying of her dissertation—"Women and Citizens: The Treatment of Women in Western Political Thought"—"It is, I think, a complete success. I must confess that I am not only delighted with her for writing it, but delighted with myself for not pressing her to write on a more conventional subject."[60] Okin was a visiting assistant professor at Vassar in the year she finished her doctorate. She began an appointment as an assistant professor in the Department of Political Science at Brandeis in fall 1976.

Though she had married in 1972 while still a graduate student, Okin did not include her marital status on her vita. In the years that followed, she revised her vita, adding new articles, her first book in 1979—*Women in Western Political Thought*—and her promotion to associate professor at Brandeis. She did not include her marital status. Nor did she include that in the years she was working toward tenure, she became a mother.[61] In July 1977, Moller Okin gave birth to the couple's first child, a girl, and in May 1979, the same year she published her first book, she gave birth to the couple's second child, a son.[62] "Married, two children" on vitae and professional-society vita forms, and as expected categories in "position-wanted" advertisements, had been as damning for women as it was advantageous for men. The absence of marital and parental status on Susan Moller

Okin's early vitae, as much as the topic of her dissertation and her Harvard degree, reflected the successes of the feminist movement of the late 1960s and early 1970s, of which women's challenge to sex inequality in academia was one piece.

In early 1985, Okin added her marital and parental status to her vita.[63] She was then working on a book she would publish four years later titled *Justice, Gender and the Family*.[64] The book focused on the failure of contemporary theories and theorists of social justice to address the gender-structured inequality of family life. "In the past," she wrote, "political theorists often used to distinguish clearly between 'private' domestic life and the 'public' life of politics and the marketplace, claiming explicitly that the two spheres operated in accordance with different principles." They did so, she argued, based on claims about the nature of women and family life. "Men, the subjects of the theories, were able to make the transition back and forth from domestic to public life with ease, largely because of the functions performed by women in the family." Strikingly, as she showed, contemporary theories of justice were little different: "In one way or another . . . almost all current theorists continue to assume that the 'individual' who is the basic subject of their theories is the male head of a fairly traditional household."[65]

In 1958, close to three decades before Okin published *Justice, Gender and the Family*, the Hungarian-born physical chemist, economist, and philosopher Michael Polanyi published what came to be regarded as his philosophical magnum opus, *Personal Knowledge: Towards a Post-Critical Philosophy*.[66] His preface began, "This is primarily an enquiry into the nature and justification of scientific knowledge. But my reconsideration of scientific knowledge leads on to a wide range of questions outside science. . . . I start by rejecting the ideal of scientific detachment." Polanyi acknowledged that the words in his title, "Personal Knowledge," "may seem to contradict each other: for true knowledge is deemed impersonal, universally established, objective. But the seeming contradiction is resolved by modifying the conception of knowledge." His project was showing that "into every act of knowing there enters a passionate contribution of the person knowing what is being known, and that this coefficient is no mere imperfection but a vital component of his knowledge."[67]

Polanyi divided his argument into four parts: The Art of Knowing, The Tacit Component, The Justification of Personal Knowledge, and, finally, Knowing and Being. In a chapter on the Justification of Personal Knowledge, Polanyi wrote, "Let me declare accordingly my true position as the author of what I have written so far, as well as of what is still to follow. I must admit now that I did not start the present reconsideration of my beliefs with a clean slate of unbelief. Far from it. I started as a person intellectually fashioned by a particular idiom, acquired through my affiliation to a civilization that prevailed in the places where I had grown up, at this particular period of history. This has been the matrix of all my intellectual efforts. Within it I was to find my problem and seek the terms for its solution."[68]

Susan Moller Okin did not begin with a clean slate of unbelief. She was trained as a political theorist. Hers was a different world from Polanyi's, but just as he was fundamentally shaped by the period of history in which he lived and was trained, so were scholars, men and women, of Okin's generation. Okin came of age in a world shaken by the American war in Southeast Asia and by movements challenging racial and sexual inequality, only to find herself living in a world that seemed to have moved on, the goals of these movements far from fully achieved. It was within this context that she found her problem and sought the terms for its solution. *Justice, Gender and the Family*, like the book I now write and that you are reading, was rooted in personal knowledge.

The personal knowledge Okin claimed was as distinct from the personal knowledge Polanyi claimed as the embodied liberty claimed by nineteenth-century abolitionists and feminists was from the political liberty claimed by the authors of the Declaration of Independence.[69] In her preface, Okin noted that "a number of concurrent factors [had] spurred" her into writing the book and writing it as she had. There was the state of academic feminism, the current political climate, and her "direct experience" as a woman, wife, and mother "of the difficulties of being a fully participating parent while being a member of the workplace as currently structured." In revising her vita to include her marital and parental status, Okin claimed her personal knowledge—and in so doing, she challenged the meaning for women that "married, two children" on vitae had for so long held.

That she could do so depended on a social movement that in 1970, when she entered graduate school at Harvard, had only just begun.

work

Dear Frances,

You are on my mind. I just finished reading an article in The New York Times about smiles: what sparks them, how they operate, how those who see them know what they mean. I read it as though reading an article about you, about what [one of your teachers] called "your thousand watt smile." I read it thinking about the connection you forged with people who knew you and people who didn't through your smile. I read it thinking about the way your smile was like a fire in a fireplace—brightening up a room, making it feel warm and inviting, offering the assurance that everything would be okay. Writing this now I feel like one way to carry you forward is to smile, to offer others the reassurance you offered with your smile . . . I'm thankful for this article today that helped me be warmed by your smile even in your absence.

. . .

Dad and I went to the movie tonight. It was my first theatre movie without you. Such an awful milestone. I sat there in the dark & wept. This is work I never dreamed I would have to do.

. . .

Tomorrow it will be 9 months since you had your stroke. 9 months. It is a phrase I associate with baby clothing & babyhood. At 9 months you were crawling, could stand holding on to a table, and had many words.

. . .

I talked with [the minister] today. I had gone to talk with her about this WAWH lecture. I made a list of my questions—should I do it, would I be able to deliver it, did it have value, did I want to, would you want me to . . .

She very much liked the idea for the lecture, but didn't want to shape my view. By the end of our conversation, I felt again that I could do this. But then 2 things happened: I left the church & collided once again with the reality that you are gone. It seems absurd to say that I re-remembered that you were gone. I knew when I sat & talked with [her] & tears ran down my face that you were gone. But there is something about that kind of talking that then leaves me momentarily suspended—I have a sort of anesthetized feeling that it will all be okay, everything is going to be okay. There's a feeling that you too are there somehow. And then I leave that space and suddenly find myself confronting the fact that it will not be okay, it will never be okay again because you are gone. But I forced myself to push on. I came home and started reading an article that Leslie Reagan wrote about her experience of a miscarriage & how the hospital staff responded & the research effort it sparked for her to consider/place treatment of miscarriage in historical perspective. The article was so unsettling & then too reading a chapter in a book about child death & commercialization in the 19th century & then about women in the historical profession. I found it all upsetting, unsettling. You are not a subject of intellectual interest to me. You are my child. Your death has not made me interested in situating the experience of childhood death in the 20th/21st century. Leslie Reagan had a note at the end of her article saying that a danger of such a personalized narrative was that an audience might not feel able to critique the views offered. I do not want to have my experience critiqued. You are not a subject. Your death is not a subject of study for me. I love you and I ache to have you back. So that is where I am.

· PART IV ·

Law

chapter thirteen · verdict

A simplistic reading of circumstance would say that chance led the McCormacks to be the first family to file a lawsuit.[1] But their filing suit was no more a matter of chance than was how they came to have the cowboy suit itself. The same class structures that segmented Americans' living, working, and shopping lives had long structured who served whom in service relationships. James McCormack had immigrated from Ireland in 1927 at the age of twenty-three with a seventh-grade education, settled in New York City where he had first arrived, and married a woman who was an Irish immigrant like himself. They had their first child in 1929, and through the years of the Depression, at two- or three-year intervals, came three more children, all boys. A family of six living on a working man's wages in a tiny, four-room railroad-style apartment in a walk-up at 98th Street on the city's Upper East Side.[2] Sometime in the mid-1930s, James McCormack became a doorman at 15 West 81st Street, a luxurious sixteen-story co-op building on New York City's Upper West Side, overlooking Central Park West.[3] Where James McCormack worked, Milton Henry lived.[4] James McCormack exchanged greetings with Mr. Henry, on occasion did small things for him. That was his job. He greeted residents, opened doors, called taxicabs, helped residents into their cars, received and carried their packages and parcels, and did other small things as they requested.[5] He was "James." They were "Sir" and "Madam," "Mr.," "Miss," "Mrs." with surname.

Class structured every element of their relationship. Building residents might give the doorman a gift for Christmas, never the other way around. And so, about a month before Christmas in 1944, Mr. Henry asked James how many children he had, how old they were, and, noting that he was in the toy business, promised that by Christmas he would have something for the two younger boys. A day or so before Christmas, he invited James up to his apartment and gave him two Gene Autry cowboy suits.[6] Two weeks later, Tommy McCormack was burned wearing the chaps of the cowboy suit as he played in the kitchen of the McCormack apartment. James McCormack was off work for four or five weeks from the burns to his hands where he tried to put out the flames; he returned to work in early February, his hands still bandaged.

Residents knew his son had been burned and James himself, too, in trying to save his son. They were, he testified, "very considerate about me."[7] He wore heavy mittens to shield and protect his hands as he carried on with his usual work, made more painful by the cold of a New York winter. Though James McCormack and Mr. Henry continued to see each other as Mr. Henry came and went from the building, James McCormack never approached Mr. Henry about what had happened, and Mr. Henry never spoke to James McCormack again. It was Mr. Henry's wife who approached James McCormack in early April—"when the news broke"—to say how sorry she was about his son. The Henrys moved out of the building a year after Tommy was burned.[8]

But the character of service relationships and the fact of proximity made other connections possible as well. At some point, another resident in the building, Bernard G. Nemeroff, a name partner in the law firm of Nemeroff, Jelline, Danzig & Paley, approached James McCormack and talked with him about what had happened. And in mid-May, three days after Tommy McCormack died, Mr. Nemeroff's firm brought suit on behalf of the McCormacks in New York state court.[9]

Over the next three years, as James and Catherine McCormack learned to live with the death of their youngest son and Tommy's three brothers learned to live with their parents' grief and their own loss, the pending lawsuit hung over their lives. In the summer and fall of 1945 and early 1946, alerted by the breaking news in Washington, DC, of the chaps' dangerous inflammability, a handful of other families, mostly DC-area families, filed suit for incidents from early 1945.[10] The lawyers learned from each other and later coordinated discovery.[11] The McCormack lawsuit initially had named as defendants only the Henry Company and E. F. Timme & Son.[12] But a lawsuit filed in January 1946 included as defendants the Woonsocket Falls Mill—the mill that had woven the fiber into a high-pile fabric—and Gene Autry.[13] And other plaintiffs moved to sue these defendants as well.

The McCormack case was particular in one regard: The cowboy suit had been a gift from Milton Henry himself. A year after initiating the lawsuit for the McCormacks, their lawyer added Milton Henry individually and the Woonsocket Falls Mill as defendants.[14] But they did not add Autry. In contrast to other families, Autry's name had not been an impetus in their acquiring the cowboy suit.

It was almost three years to the day after Tommy McCormack was burned that his father, James, took the stand on January 5, 1948, as the first witness in the McCormack case.[15] Why did the defendants let this case go to trial? Why not settle the McCormacks' claims? By early January 1948, there were at least thirty-one pending Gene Autry cowboy suit cases.[16] McCormack was the first case to come to trial. But with many other cases pending, the defendants knew that settling here would mean paying out money to other families. There was also the possibility that they—the defendants, that is—would win at trial, either on the law or the facts, and so put an end to this business. And finally, the defendants did not all have to win for any one of them to escape liability. For the plaintiffs' lawyers there was a different sort of calculus: McCormack would be a test case for all the others. And for James and Catherine McCormack, there was perhaps the hope that a trial and a finding that the defendants were liable would bring some sort of closure.[17]

It was not easy for James McCormack to be there. It had been two and a half years since their son Tommy died. The day after the trial opened would be the third anniversary of the day he was burned. Even if James McCormack could now get along from day to day, retracing out loud, in the foreign and formal space of a courtroom, under oath, before a judge and jury, the sequence of events that led to his youngest son's death opened the wound that lay just beneath the surface. Returning to the day that Mr. Henry gave him the cowboy suits was unbearable. "Mr. Henry gave me two cowboy suits," Mr. McCormack said early in his testimony. "He took them out and showed them to me. He asked me the ages of the boys, and—" Emotion overcame him. When the judge said, "We will have a short recess," James McCormack said, "It is all right. I will be all right." But the judge insisted on the recess, and with the jury excused the lawyers turned to other matters.[18]

Elliot Paley, another partner in the firm representing the McCormacks, had taken over the case. He was gentle in his questioning of Tommy's father. Responding to the emotion in James McCormack's body and voice, he offered at several points to "try to carry some of the evidence with me, so you won't have the difficulty."[19] But there was no way around it; the evidence had to be gotten before the jury. James McCormack had to describe that night and the months that followed in the hospital. And so he retraced the evening of the accident: when he arrived home; when his wife left for work; the layout of their tiny apartment, in which one could see from the front room where he sat back to the kitchen where Tommy was playing; hearing Tommy scream; seeing him "on fire"; Tommy's older brother Jackie attempting to throw a thin cotton bedspread over his brother; his own actions in grabbing his blazing son and plunging him in the bathtub; calling to neighbors to get a cab. He told of the nursing supervisor being "lenient" with him in that first week when he too was in the hospital for the burns to his hands, of getting "a look at him"—that is, at his son—"through the glass" in the little room next to the nursing supervisor's desk, of the first time he was allowed to visit Tommy.

"When you visited him what did you see?" Mr. Paley asked. And again, James McCormack broke down. And again, the judge called a recess. In law, as in intellectual inquiry, emotion is suspect, seen as a source not of knowledge but rather of potential prejudice. When James McCormack returned to the stand, the lawyer representing both Timme & Son and Woonsocket objected to his testifying to anything further that might be covered by a doctor's testimony. But as Mr. Paley explained to the court, the question of pain and suffering—the child's, not the parents—was "a vital element in the case."[20] And so, James McCormack had to retrace the four long months of his son's suffering until Tommy died. Catherine McCormack was likely there for her husband's testimony. When he spoke, he spoke not just to the jury but—maybe even more importantly—to her. How many times had they rehearsed the events of that night, trying to make the story come out differently? Or had it lain between them, a silent, devastating crevasse?

In building the McCormacks' case, Elliot Paley called only a handful of witnesses. In addition to James McCormack, there was his son John ("Jackie"), who had witnessed the event and tried to extinguish the flames; the chief chemist of the New York Testing Laboratory; the principal doctor who treated Tommy at Mt. Sinai Hospital from his injury to his death; and, finally, Tommy's mother, Catherine.[21] These witnesses were key to establishing that Tommy was wearing the chaps of the Gene Autry cowboy suit made by the Henry Company on the night he was burned, the course of events that evening, the burning properties of the fluffy fabric on the chaps, and the character of the burns and their role in the child's death. Together these facts told a story. But they were not sufficient to establish the defendants' liability. The plaintiffs bore the burden of proof, and that included establishing the chain of production: the relationship of one defendant to another, the role each played in the fluffy fabric on the chaps of the cowboy suit.

A whole series of issues complicated the proof: The Henry Company had used multiple high-pile fabrics from Woonsocket over the time it produced the cowboy suit; there were no records identifying which Woonsocket fabric was on the chaps of any given cowboy suit; when the chaps Tommy was wearing were manufactured was not clear; and, finally, the chaps—the key evidence in the case—had been completely consumed by fire. The plaintiffs had to show that the Henry Company had used only fabrics from Woonsocket on the chaps of the cowboy suit from early 1942 to March 1945, that each of those fabrics had the same basic characteristics, that differences among the fabrics—things like color and a bright or dull finish—were immaterial to the facts. And so, as is true in many cases of products that cause injury, only a small fraction of the plaintiffs' evidence focused on the event and its aftermath.[22]

Interleaved with that testimony, Mr. Paley read from the pre-trial testimony of first one and then another of the key officers and employees of the defendants.[23] What was a commonplace of courtroom trial practice for the judge and lawyers must have seemed strange to the jurors. But that testimony was critical to establishing the legal foundation for introducing into evidence as exhibits samples of the fabrics that Henry had purchased from Woonsocket and used on the chaps and the cowboy suit, and whose burning properties Marvin Kramer, chief chemist of the New York Testing Laboratories, had tested.[24]

On the stand, Marvin Kramer testified that the fabric on the chaps was "composed of viscose rayon and in a very fine, fluffy form." He described taking a one-by-seven-inch strip of the fabric, holding it upright, in a draft-free space, and touching a match to it. "The material burned so rapidly I was unable to work a stop watch quickly enough to get any record of that time."[25] The fabric would not spontaneously combust, but once it made contact with a flame, however small, it would burn in its entirety in a flash. As he explained, its burning properties were very different from those of animal fur, which tends to naturally put itself out. It was like kindling.[26] Listening to his description, the jurors would have thought back to the testimony of James McCormack. He had been close at hand; there had been a tub of water in the kitchen for Saturday evening baths; he had plunged his burning son into the water that was right there; and still the child had been horribly burned over most of his body.

The burning properties of the fabric established, Mr. Paley returned to the pre-trial testimony to establish what the various defendants had known, possibly known, or should have known, about the fabric's properties, about who was using it, and for what. Mr. Henry had testified that he first used a Chinese goat fur on the chaps of the cowboy suit, that circumstances—no one mentioned the war by name—led him, in late 1941, to begin looking for an alternative fabric for the chaps. When had Mr. Henry switched from fur to the fabric purchased from Timme? Early 1942. Over what time period had he used the fabric? From early 1942 to March 29, 1945. Had he told anyone from Timme what he planned to use the fabric for? "I told them that we were going to use them to make cowboy suits." Who specifically had he told? A Timme salesman named Henry Bullwinkel. When? "When he originally came into our showroom and I showed him the cowboy suits and told him exactly what we wanted it for."

Back to William E. Roschen's pre-trial testimony. Roschen's testimony established that Timme was the "sole agent and factor" for Woonsocket. Paley introduced into evidence the contract setting out the terms of their relationship. All the fiber Woonsocket wove into fabric was viscose rayon from Du Pont, purchased for Woonsocket by Mr. Roschen of Timme. Where was Timme's first contact with the Henry Company? Here the stories diverged. "As I understand it," Mr. Roschen had said, "the first contact was made when Mr. Henry came into our office and selected certain merchandise." Referring to the fabric, he said, "many of our customers use it" for stuffed children's toys, teddy bears and the like. "And you sell to these customers knowing they are going to use it for that purpose?" He dodged: "I really don't know what everybody uses merchandise for." "Did you know at the time that these were sold to Henry what Henry was intending to use them for?" "No, I did not." Back to Arthur Robertshaw Jr.'s pre-trial testimony. What was Woonsocket's business? "The manufacture of pile fabrics." Who purchased the fiber Woonsocket wove from Du Pont? Mr. Roschen of Timme. What firm handled all the billing for fabric shipped by Woonsocket? Timme.

With this, Mr. Paley turned to his next witness: the doctor who had had direct charge of Tommy McCormack at Mt. Sinai Hospital, Dr. Ernest E. Arnheim. His testimony was brief. Tommy McCormack was brought to Mt. Sinai Hospital around 7:30 p.m., the evening of January 6, 1945; he died four months later on May 12, 1945, never having left the hospital. In a trial transcript that ran over a thousand pages, Dr. Arnheim's testimony took up a mere fourteen. There was no cross-examination. "Thomas McCormack" had arrived at the hospital in severe shock, with third-degree burns over the greater part of his body: legs, thighs, buttocks and lower back, lower abdomen, and hands, all burned.[27] He described their giving the child blood transfusions, plasma, and large doses of penicillin, and efforts they made beyond medication to allay his pain and suffering. "Most severe burns of this type are fatal," the doctor explained. "That is, they result in death very quickly. This boy lived for some time." An autopsy after the child's death revealed that the veins in his legs were filled with blood clots and organisms causing blood poisoning—both were results of the burns and both reinforced how hopeless his case had been.

If the jurors felt a sense of emotional relief when the doctor left the witness stand, it was short-lived. Elliot Paley returned to William E. Roschen's and Arthur A. Robertshaw Jr.'s pre-trial testimonies to establish that E. F. Timme & Son and its partners owned a controlling share of the stock in Woonsocket and that both firms knew the hazardous character of the fabric and sold it to the trade anyway. In one answer after another, Arthur A. Robertshaw Jr. admitted that they knew the fabric burned, that they had run tests in their attempt to find a finish that would retard the fabric's burning properties on which they might get a patent, that everything they tried "spoiled the fabric," and that they shared the results of their tests with Timme & Son. He admitted that raising the nap or fluffing it made the fabric more inflammable and then described the processes they used to raise the nap further and the special creels they shipped the fabric on to avoid crushing it. Reading from Mr. Roschen's pre-trial testimony, the jurors heard him admit that he too knew the fabric was inflammable, that the burning increases as the rayon is fluffed, that having failed to find a flameproofing solution, they sold the fabric anyway.

A final point related to the fabric had to be made. Had they known what Mr. Henry intended to use the fabric for? Had they told him it was inflammable? Had they told him it could not be used for clothing? The second Timme salesman to work with Mr. Henry, a man named Henry Bobsin who no longer worked at Timme by the time of the trial, testified that Mr. Roschen had told him the fabric was never to be sold to the clothing trade because it was inflammable. He had taken over the account when the first salesman, Henry Bullwinkel, went into the US Navy.

Bullwinkel had returned to Timme as an employee after the war and been promoted. His testimony was riddled with inconsistencies. Mr. Paley had asked if he had ever said to Mr. Henry "in words or substance, these materials are inflammable and not to be wrapped around the body in any way." Mr. Bullwinkel said, "Never did." But then he also claimed to have visited Henry's Passaic, New Jersey, plant on March 6, 1942, and told Mr. Henry himself that day that the fabric was only for stuffed animals and not to be used in wearing apparel because it was inflammable. He claimed that Mr. Henry had asked in response, "Can you find out about having it flameproofed for me?" On the day that Mr. Bullwinkel claimed to have visited with Mr. Henry at his Passaic plant, Woonsocket sent a large shipment of fabric to the M. A. Henry Company. The shipments—altogether more than seven thousand yards of fabric—continued for the next three years.

The final witness in the McCormacks' case was Tommy's mother, Catherine. Her testimony consumed less than five pages in the trial record, but it returned the jurors to Tommy and the events of the evening of January 6, 1945.[28] Catherine McCormack affirmed that she had left for work at 6:30 p.m., that she learned of the accident when she got off around 9:00 p.m., that when she got home from the hospital that night she had thrown away the unworn top of the cowboy suit that Tommy had been wearing the chaps of, as well as the second cowboy suit that had never been worn. But the center of her brief testimony was on whether she had had a conversation with her son about what had happened that night.

James McCormack had testified that just minutes before the accident, Tommy had asked if he could come into the front room where his father was sitting and he had told him no; it was cold in there, even James was wearing his coat, and Tommy had just had his bath. So, Tommy had gone back to the kitchen where he was playing Crokinoles, a game where you shoot one piece against another. James could hear him from the front room, see him from where he sat.[29] The stove was not going; the pilot light was not lit; the matches were kept in a can on a shelf in the kitchen over the stove, about six feet from the floor.[30] When Mr. Paley asked James McCormack, "Did you have occasion to ask him how the accident happened?" Mr. McCormack replied, "No. I never could get around to asking him that." On the defendant's motion, everything but the word "No," was stricken from the record.[31] Catherine had asked her son and shared whatever he told her with someone at the hospital.[32] That was all the jurors would hear. The rule of hearsay, part of the law of evidence, prevented Catherine McCormack from repeating what he had said to her. As the judge would direct the jurors at the end of the case, there was no evidence on how the cowboy suit caught fire, and they were not to speculate.[33]

At the heart of this case lay the wrongful death of a child, but the jurors heard almost nothing about that child. Mr. Paley had asked James McCormack a handful of questions about his son. Tommy had been seven, almost eight, years old; his birthday was in February; he was in his second or third year at the parish school paid for by the parish; he was a healthy, playful child.[34] No photographs of Tommy McCormack were introduced. But in the lower right-hand corner of a photograph of the McCormack apartment—introduced as evidence to establish the view from the living room—was a photograph of a boy. Perhaps it was of Tommy.[35]

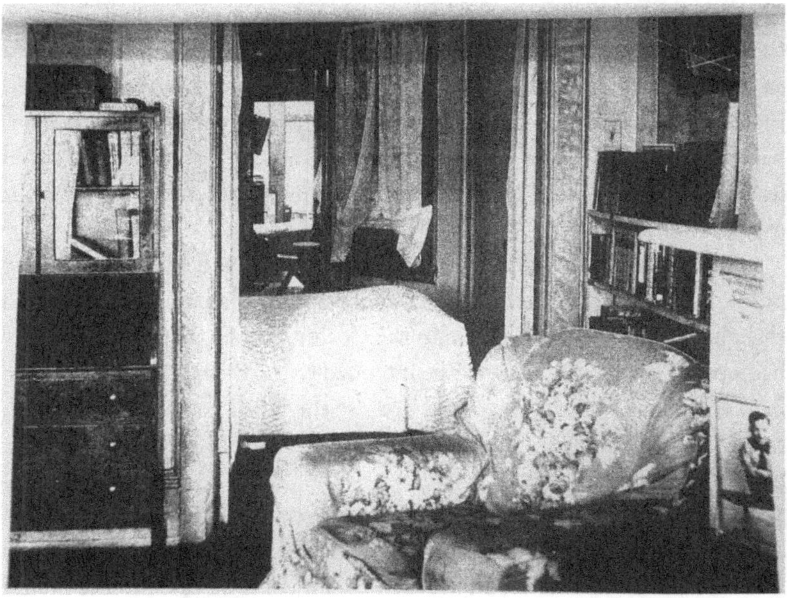

One small, but important detail remained: introducing mortality tables into evidence. The judge said he would take judicial notice of the tables. And with that, the plaintiffs rested their case.

Now it was the defendants' turn to make their cases. For three years, the Henry Company had done business with Timme & Son and, through it, Woonsocket. The events of late March and early April 1945 brought that business relationship to an end. What followed was a demonstration of what happens when a product with components involving multiple enterprises leads to injury and death. The defendants fought against not only the plaintiffs but, as importantly, against each other. There was, as well, the lingering potential of criminal charges for their actions.[36] The defendants were engaged in their own multifront war. It was a war of truths, half-truths, and lies. The trial stretched on for over two weeks. In the Record on Appeal, the plaintiffs' case took up 177 pages; the defendants', 799.

The jury had heard the words of Milton Henry, William E. Roschen, Arthur Robertshaw Jr., and Timme salesmen Henry Bullwinkel and Henry Bobsin. Now they would see, hear, and be asked to judge the credibility of these men themselves. Henry was intent on convincing the jury of four points: first, that he, individually, did not know when he gave the Gene Autry cowboy suits to James McCormack for his youngest sons that the fabric on the chaps of the suit was dangerously inflammable; second, that Timme and Woonsocket had known the fabric was inflammable and known that there no effective permanent flame-retardant treatment and had sold it to the trade anyway; third, that Timme's salesmen knew what he intended to use the fabric for and not only sold it to him but in fact recommended it; and finally, that the M. A. Henry Company, of which he was president, had reasonably relied on Timme's expertise and did not know and could not have been expected to know the dangerous character of the fabric it used on the suits.

Timme and Woonsocket's case directly challenged Henry's on every point. They admitted to knowing the fabric was inflammable but insisted that they did not sell this fabric to the clothing trade, that Milton Henry had not told them initially what he intended to use the fabric for, and when he had, he was told that he could not use the fabric for wearing apparel, that it was inflammable, and that Henry told them to ship it anyway, that he had another use for it.

At the heart of the defendants' case, Milton Henry's word was pitted against that of the young Timme salesman Henry Bullwinkel. Mr. Henry said that his first contact with a Timme salesman took place in the Henry Company showroom on Broadway. Mr. Bullwinkel said that first contact took place in Timme's showroom. Mr. Henry said that in that first meeting he showed Mr. Bullwinkel one of the Gene Autry cowboy suits and asked for a recommendation for a substitute for the fur on the chaps of the suit, and that Mr. Bullwinkel sent him a set of samples. Mr. Bullwinkel said Mr. Henry came into the Timme showroom and picked out several fabrics without saying what he intended to use them for, later asking for another fabric with an even higher pile. Mr. Henry said Mr. Bullwinkel knew from the start what he intended to use the fabric for, that after he had made up several sample cowboy suits with the fabric on them, he showed them to Mr. Bullwinkel in the Henry Company's Broadway showroom and asked Mr. Bullwinkel's opinion on which fabric looked best, the men agreeing that the higher-pile fabric was better. Mr. Bullwinkel said it was only on Friday, March 6, 1942 that he learned of Mr. Henry's intended use of the fabric, that Mr. Henry showed him one of the cowboy suits for the first time, that he told Mr. Henry the fabric could not be used for wearing apparel, that it was inflammable, and Mr. Henry asked if it could be flameproofed, and then told Mr. Bullwinkel to ship the material anyway, that he had another use for it. Mr. Henry denied that any such exchange had taken place, said Mr. Bullwinkel had never visited him at the Passaic factory, that he never went there on Fridays and most certainly knew he was not there that day.

Henry challenged Timme's claim that it had not known from the start what he intended to do with the fabric, but he also pressed the point of

Timme's broader business practices in the sale of this fabric. Henry introduced a letter on the company's letterhead he had sent to Mr. Bullwinkel at Timme in February 1942, at the top of which was an image of a cowboy on horseback and beneath it the words "play suits" and "fur chaps"—clearly references to products the Henry Company made.[37] In his pre-trial testimony, Mr. Roschen had tried to dodge the question of the fabric's inflammability, insisting that the fabric was not made for the clothing trade and was not sold to that trade because it would not "wear." He was pushed on that point at trial. Question: "Let me ask you this: Wasn't there a reason, namely, not only because they wouldn't wear well, but also because it was inflammable?" Answer: "First, because they wouldn't wear well, and secondly, we would not recommend them to the clothing trade because they were inflammable."[38] Adding to the tangle of words and documents, Henry introduced all Timme's invoices. The fabric was identified only as "plush" or "peach" or "peachfox fluffy." The word "inflammable" was not stamped on Timme's invoices.

Timme had its own testamentary and documentary retort. Milton Henry had been in the business for fifteen years. Was the jury really to believe that as the person who purchased all the fabric for his business he knew nothing about the fabrics he used, including on the chaps of the Gene Autry cowboy suit? To suggest Henry's knowledge of fabrics, the availability of alternatives, and that he had not settled on a fabric before March, Timme introduced a letter Henry sent to Bullwinkel in mid-February, with a fabric sample enclosed, asking if Timme had "anything similar." The sample was a mohair, goat fur. A fabric that would not burn.[39] Bullwinkel had replied the next day saying that they had been making a fabric like it, but that the scarcity and the high cost of mohair yarn forced them to discontinue it. He suggested as an alternative a fabric "made of 50% Wool, 50% Rayon Pile and 100% Cotton Back" that was available, enclosing a sample.[40] Henry insisted he had not known what the fabric in the mohair sample was when he sent it. The cost of the wool blend was $4.00 per yard. The cost of the high-pile plush fabric Henry had from Timme in January was just $2.10 per yard.

There were lines of testimony cut off or left unpursued, physical evidence that the jury never saw, excluded by the court on its own or on a defendant's motion as immaterial or prejudicial, sometimes following heated exchanges between counsel and judge out of the hearing of the jury. Any reader of this book comes to this trial knowing many things that were carefully kept from the jury as irrelevant or prejudicial to this case. You know, for instance, that Du Pont worked closely with Timme and Woonsocket and other manufacturers to develop viscose rayon threads with properties that met their needs, that Du Pont had made the rayon fiber it supplied to Woonsocket to be woven into a high-pile fabric, that it knew the fiber and fabric were inflammable. But Du Pont was not named as a defendant in McCormack; its liability was not even before the court.

And you know that Tommy McCormack was far from the only or even the first child burned in one of these cowboy suits. The jury heard opaque references to "when the news broke" and references to exchanges that Mr. Henry had with someone in Washington, DC. But they were there only to establish time in reference to the McCormacks' case, not the substance to which they referred.[41] The jury never saw the letters, never knew their content. The incidents they described had taken place after Milton Henry gave the cowboy suits to the McCormacks, after Tommy McCormack was burned. The judge excluded their contents as irrelevant and prejudicial to this action.

Even the line of questioning as to when Mr. Henry learned that Tommy McCormack had been injured was cut short. In his pre-trial testimony, Mr. Henry had said that he first learned that the cowboy suits were inflammable in March or April 1945. Mr. Paley sought to show that Mr. Henry knew earlier, that he knew about Tommy McCormack. But the judge, sustaining Henry's lawyer's objection, would not let Paley pursue this line of inquiry. "It is liable to be prejudicial," the judged explained, "giving the appearance that this man, after learning of the child's serious injuries, deliberately ignored the father." Paley admitted, "That is the purpose of it actually."[42]

There was nonetheless no shortage of damning testimony and physical evidence against each of the defendants. The most damning piece of physical evidence against Milton Henry and the Henry Company was the carbon copy of a letter dated March 6, 1942, with the names and addresses of four flameproofing companies, sent—as Mr. Bullwinkel of Timme noted in the letter—at Mr. Henry's request.[43] The letter reinforced Timme's argument that they had told Mr. Henry that the fabric was inflammable and not to be used on wearing apparel; it gave meaning to Mr. Roschen having written on an order that same day, "Stamp bills Sold For Use in Toys Only."[44] Mr. Henry insisted that he never received such a letter. Each side swore in secretaries to buttress their claims. For Timme, the secretary whose initials appeared at the bottom of the letter. For Henry, his longtime secretary at the Passaic factory. She insisted that she opened and read all the mail, had never seen the original of this letter, and would remember if she had. Moreover, she insisted that she had never seen the man in the courtroom identified as Mr. Bullwinkel. When Timme's lawyer pressed her on the sureness of her memory as to Friday, March 6, 1942, she responded, "Mr. Henry was getting married." A question that might have been asked, but was not, was—given that Timme and Woonsocket knew there was no way of flameproofing the fabric, why send a list of flameproofers to a customer?

But whereas the flameproofer letter hung over Mr. Henry's general credibility, the New York City fire marshal's investigation in early April 1945 of the hazard posed by the Gene Autry cowboy suit hung over Mr. Roschen's. Arthur Robertshaw Jr. and William E. Roschen had both admitted that they had long known the high-pile viscose rayon fabric was inflammable, that it could not be flameproofed, and they had continued, nonetheless, to sell it. But that was not, apparently, what William E. Roschen told the men from the New York City fire marshal when they called on him in early April 1945. The interview had taken place at the offices of E. F. Timme & Son on April 11, 1945. Assistant Fire Marshal Cassidy told the judge and jury that he spoke with a man who identified himself as Mr. Roschen, a partner in the firm, that he had said that E. F. Timme & Son had sold four thousand to five thousand pounds of rayon pile made by Woonsocket to the Henry Company. Question: "Did he tell you what he knew about that material concerning inflammability?" Answer: "He told me that he did not know this material was very inflammable, until he tested same by burning a small quantity in the presence of myself and Fire Marshal Shaughnessy." Question: "And you made a report of that?" Answer: "The following day," from notes he had written at the time. On the witness stand, Mr. Roschen admitted to having been interviewed by individuals from the fire marshal's office in April 1945 but flatly denied that he had said he did not know the fabric was inflammable until the tests that day.

What did this jury make of these two men—William E. Roschen and Milton A. Henry—who were so cagey about the facts? In submitting the case to the jury, Judge Corcoran told the jurors that while he was "the judge of the law," they were "the judges of the facts."[45] It was for them "to determine from the evidence in the case where the truth is." He directed the jurors to use their "intelligence as practical people" to judge each witness's credibility. What would that intelligence have revealed? Henry was in his early forties at the time of the trial; Roshen was in his early fifties. Both men were successful New York businessmen, but they no more shared the same class or status than Milton Henry did with James McCormack. Milton Henry may have been the president of his company, but it was small fry compared to Timme and Woonsocket. Henry's company had a short history and sold cheap goods: novelties, leather goods, pistol and holster sets, children's cowboy suits. Timme and Woonsocket had been in business for half a century; their lines included trademarks like "Timme Tufts" that the jurors might have known, even worn. And then there was a fact that was both more subtle and pointed. Milton Henry dealt with Timme salesmen. As William E. Roschen said, "I never met Mr. Henry until Monday morning here"—referring to the start of trial. And just in case his meaning was not clear, "I didn't meet him then; I never saw him before."[46]

The trial had taken over two weeks. The burden of proof—that is, proving the case by a preponderance of the credible evidence—rested on the plaintiffs. While a unanimous verdict was desirable, it would be enough if ten of the twelve jurors agreed on a verdict. A separate verdict was required for each cause of action. "When you took your oaths as jurors in this case," the judge directed, "you undertook to decide the issues fairly and impartially, without being influenced by sympathy or bias or prejudice one way or the other."[47]

The plaintiffs' case depended on the defendants having failed in a duty they owed the plaintiff. The duty that manufacturers of goods like Milton Henry, the Henry Company, E. F. Timme & Son, and Woonsocket owed consumers like James and Catherine McCormack and their son had been spelled out over thirty years before in the case of *MacPherson v. Buick*. "If the nature of a thing is such that it is reasonably certain to place life and limb in peril when negligently made, it is then a thing of danger," and the manufacturer was under a duty to the ultimate consumer to make it carefully. If it failed to do so, liability would follow.[48] Just three years before the McCormack trial, the New York courts reiterated the rule from *MacPherson* in a case very much on point: A woman had suffered severe burns when the netting on her evening gown brushed across a lit cigarette on the floor and exploded into flames. As the appellate court wrote, "Underlying the manufacturer's liability is the danger reasonably to be foreseen from the intended use of the article. Clothing is worn to cover, adorn and protect the human body."[49]

One could hear these precedents in the judge's instructions to the jury in McCormack. The first question for them to determine, he directed, was whether the Gene Autry cowboy suit was "a thing of danger."[50] He reminded them that they were not to speculate as to what ignited the suit. But it was for them to determine whether the manner, intensity, and time in which the suit burned, the possibility of it being extinguished when aid was close at hand, made it inherently dangerous if worn by young children like Tommy McCormack.[51] If the jury found that the rayon chaps were highly inflammable and dangerous, that the defendants knew that and did not warn of the danger, they should find them liable.[52]

But what was the jury to do if they found that a defendant had not had actual knowledge? First, Mr. Henry individually. That the Henry Company might be liable would not by itself mean that Mr. Henry individually would be liable. The jury must determine whether he individually knew that the cowboy suit presented a danger when worn by young children. The Henry Company would not be liable if it did not know the fabric was inflammable and could not have ascertained its inflammability "by the exercise of reasonable care." But it was not absolved from its own duty to use reasonable care by virtue of having purchased the material from someone else.[53]

As to Timme and Woonsocket, the judged the instructed the jury, "there appears to be no dispute" that both "knew that the high pile fabric delivered to the Henry Company was inflammable." Their contention was that they did not know that the Henry Company was going to use the fabric in wearing apparel or cowboy suits. If the jury found that they did know, it was for the jury to decide whether they had exercised reasonable care to give warning of the danger.[54] Their duty was not necessarily met by notifying Mr. Henry or the Henry Company that the fabric was inflammable. The question was whether they had taken steps "that an ordinary, reasonably prudent person would take to see to it that these fabrics were not used in a way to create a danger to the ultimate user."[55]

To recover for negligence, the individual injured must have been free from contributory negligence. As the judged explained, a person, like James McCormack, who endangers himself attempting to rescue someone "imperiled by the wrong of third persons" is not contributorily negligent unless his action would be deemed reckless.[56] Moreover, as to Tommy, the judge explained that "the law does not expect from a child of that age the degree of care that is expected of an adult." It was for the jury to decide whether he exercised "the standard of care that you would ordinarily expect of a boy of that age, experience and background."[57] But whereas, he directed, the plaintiffs bore the burden of proof as to whether James McCormack had been contributorily negligent, because the child had died, the burden of proof relating to Tommy's contributory negligence rested on the defendants.

To this point, the law was not complicated. But Henry's and the Henry Company's cross-claim against Timme and Woonsocket involved the complicated law of agency and joint ventures. The claim was basically this: that Milton Henry and his company had been at most passive wrongdoers, whereas Timme and Woonsocket had been active wrongdoers and as such would have to reimburse Henry and his company for any judgment they faced in the case. But the jury did not have to get to these questions if it found that Milton Henry individually or the Henry Company knew the fabric was inflammable.[58] The burden of proof, moreover, on the cross-claim was on the Henry Company and Milton Henry individually.

The jury only got to the question of damages if they determined that the defendants were negligent, that their negligence "directly produced the accident," and that there was no contributory negligence. The jurors would have to place a dollar figure on the death of Tommy McCormack, his pain and suffering before his death, and James McCormack's pecuniary losses and pain and suffering for his own injuries.

The law offered hard lessons on the worth of a life. "You are not to allow any damages," the judge directed, "to the parents for their grief or for the loss of the love and companionship of their child." The parents could recover only "their pecuniary"—that is, monetary—losses: medical expenses, funeral and burial expenses, and the sum of money that the jury determined "the parents would have realized from that child."[59] A brief tutorial on the history of "wrongful death" statutes might have softened the apparent harshness of the law. Under the common law, an action for negligence died with the individual. Responding to the terrible human toll of industrial accidents in the nineteenth century, state legislatures across the United States had passed statutes that made a cause of action survive death of the individual, enabling next of kin to bring a claim for damages.[60] Public outcry and lawsuits for the accidental injury and death of children came later, at the turn of the twentieth century, driven by the rising toll of accidents to children in workplaces and industrialized urban streets.[61]

The judge acknowledged the challenge in arriving at an amount for damages. Determining what these parents might have realized in a monetary way from this child was "indefinite." His parents would have had a legal right to any wages Tommy earned before he reached the age of twenty-one, and as an adult he might have given money to his parents. "All you can do as honest jurors is this: You have seen boys, you have seen them grow up. You have seen what parents have or have not realized in the way of money from those boys. Judge as nearly and honestly as you can what sum of money these parents would have realized from this boy, taking into account his and their life circumstances."[62] In the cause of action for the child's injuries before his death, only damages for pain and suffering, not death itself, were allowed. There are "no guides that I can give you," the judge explained, in calculating these damages. For James McCormack, the jury's award should compensate him for his injuries, including consideration of whether they were permanent, and, just as for Tommy, pain and suffering.[63]

Each cause of action required a separate verdict.[64] The jury was not "to attempt to punish any of the defendants."[65] Nor were they to apportion blame and damages among the defendants. As the judge explained, "A defendant is either liable to the plaintiff on a given cause of action for the full amount, or not liable at all."[66] The plaintiffs could only recover the damages awarded once, but if others were insolvent or more difficult to collect from, any given defendant might find themselves carrying the full burden.

It was late morning when the judge released the two alternate jurors, and the jury of eleven men and one woman retired to deliberate. It was evening before they reached a verdict.[67]

"How do you find?" Judge Corcoran asked the foreman. "We find for the plaintiff against M. A. Henry Co., Inc., E. F. Timme & Sons, Woonsocket Falls Mill." They assigned damages of $3,500 for Tommy McCormack's wrongful death, $60,000 for his pain and suffering, and $1,000 for James McCormack's injuries.[68] The jury ruled against Milton Henry and the Henry Company on their cross-claims against Timme and Woonsocket. There was only one final claim: that of the McCormacks against Milton Henry, individually. The jurors had been unanimous on the cause of action for Tommy McCormack's death and his father's injuries. But in calculating damages for Tommy McCormack's pain and suffering, only ten of the twelve had agreed. And on the final claim—that against Milton Henry individually—the jurors could not agree. Four believed that Milton Henry had known that the fabric was inflammable; eight were not convinced of this or at least not willing to hold him individually liable—and so, Milton Henry himself was found not liable.[69]

I don't know whether James and Catherine McCormack were there to hear the verdict. If not, they would have learned from their lawyer, Mr. Paley. And with it, the news that the case was not over. The defendants' response to the verdict had been immediate and emphatic. They moved for the court to set aside the verdict as against the law, against the evidence, and against the weight of the evidence. They moved for a verdict in their favor. They moved that the damage award on pain and suffering be set aside as "grossly excessive." And when Judge Corcoran denied their motions, they gave notice that they would appeal the verdict and the damage award for Tommy McCormack's pain and suffering.[70]

Tommy McCormack's death had not made the news. The verdict did. The *New York Post*, *New York World-Telegram*, and *The Sun* all got the news out on Wednesday, January 21, 1948, the evening of the verdict. The headline in the *Post* read, "$64,500 for Death of Boy, Father Wins Suit over Fatal Burns." The *World-Telegram*'s front-page story was headlined simply, "Award $64,500 in Boy's Death."[71] The next day, the story was in the other New York City dailies.[72] News of the verdict fanned out across the nation.[73]

While the level of detail varied, the headlines made two points clear: A jury had awarded a verdict in a case involving the death of a child, and the damages were substantial. With one striking exception—Gene Autry's hometown paper, the *Los Angeles Times*—the dollar figure "$64,500" screamed from every headline.[74]

But even as the news fanned out across the country, there were far more towns and cities in which the verdict was not reported, in which news of the hazard had never broken.

your backpack

Dear Frances,

This summer [a friend] said that I would keep learning about you. [The minister] echoed that today. I wish I could remember her exact words, it was something about me coming to know you in new ways, so that although you would not be getting older, our relationship would nonetheless keep growing. She said it so much better than that. It was affirming. It is probably part of the reason I left there & then like a tsunami the fact that you were gone shocked me, stopped me in my tracks.

. . .

Walking from the parking lot into school today, I saw a girl with jeans on and knee-high brown boots. And for a split second I felt a whole different kind of sad. I think it was what fits the term bittersweet. For just a moment, I could see us heading out, light, laughing, for a shopping adventure. And then as fast as that light sadness came, it went. And I knew I'd never get to shop with you again. And when I left school, it was close to 5:30 and beginning to get dark. And I realized in what again felt new that it was Friday evening. That I was going home to a home without you and I wanted simply to sit down, cry, and melt away.

. . .

Sam is here asleep right beside my bed. His presence is comforting. He now sleeps every night snuggled up right against my side of the bed. Do you think he knows I'm fragile? Or, is he thinking that by keeping very close tabs on me he won't lose another person he loves?

. . .

After that night when Sam was so upset and digging on your bed, I've started closing your bedroom door every night as I go to bed. It's hard to do emotionally. It's even harder to open it in the morning because each time I do, I go back to the morning of April 26th.

. . .

I need to empty your backpack, but like the box of things from your locker which is still in the living room, I don't know what to do with the things. And so the box sits in the living room & your backpack sits at the end of your bed.

. . .

Dad and I skied yesterday. We didn't talk at all. I've told him that skiing together is like canoeing was this summer: something he and I can do together where I feel at one with you. But yesterday that spell was largely broken—the binding on one of his skis wasn't working and he got angry and upset about it. To me it seemed like such a small, insignificant thing—here it was the 30th, the day of the month where each month I walk those final hours with you. It is a day which for me the only thing that matters is you and here he was upset about a ski binding. In fairness to him, he was likely upset about the ski binding because we lost you. His frustration, his helplessness came out there on a piece of malfunctioning equipment. But the point is that I didn't feel together with him then. It was a sort of not quite hostile silence, but not shared either because he knew that I thought that a ski binding, all the ski bindings in the world, just didn't matter.

. . .

I'm not sure I fully understand the meaning of surreal, but conversations and conversational moments like one I had today feel surreal to me. You died nine months ago and I'm sitting, having tea, talking with a group of people who know but we are all talking as though things are normal. In fact, I don't think surreal is the right word. It's absurd—it is, as the dictionary says, "out of harmony with reason or propriety; incongruous; inappropriate; unreasonable; ridiculous; inharmonious. That which is absurd, especially human existence in a purposeless, chaotic universe." That is how life feels to me now: chaotic, purposeless. I work to steer a course, to go through the motions, but even doing so is part of or is what makes up the absurdity.

. . .

When I left school this evening, I was stunned by how warm it was, and then I was hit with the realization that spring is coming and it will be the first time we face leaving winter behind without you. Each season has felt this way. But spring, well spring will be especially hard: your birthday, the 1st anniversary of your stroke and your death; the end of the school year with no end to the school year for you. Can it be spring without you? We still have two feet of snow and much winter ahead, but the sunshiny warmth of the day told me we cannot stay in winter.

chapter fourteen · finding their way to law

By the time of the McCormack verdict, it had been three and a half years since Jackie Izzo was burned in July 1944 in Saginaw, Michigan, leading to the amputation of both her legs at the hip. Like other families whose children were burned in Gene Autry cowboy suits, Jackie's parents in the intervening years had shouldered the financial and emotional burdens of their child's injuries as best they could with the support of family, friends, and community. But on January 22, 1948, a friend of Jackie's father saw the headline in the *Detroit Free Press*, "Award $64,500 in Boy's Death." The story was brief. A jury had awarded a verdict for the death of an eight-year-old boy who died from burns after the chaps on the "Gene Autry" cowboy suit he was wearing caught fire. The rayon used in the chaps was "highly inflammable." There were "35 similar actions" pending.[1] Hadn't Jackie been wearing a Gene Autry cowboy suit?

One might think that in a national market of goods, there would be federal rules for determining how long one had to bring a legal action. But in fact, how long one had to bring suit was determined by the law of the state in which the injury happened. Gene Autry cowboy suits were sold in at least twenty-four states between 1942 and 1945. They continued to be sold and worn and cause injury and death well past that time in yet more states. And every state had its own laws—and within states different laws—limiting how long one had to bring suit for negligence, for wrongful death in cases where the child died, and for breach of warranty for actions against a retailer. "Statutes of limitations," as they are called, are intended to ensure that claims are made in a timely fashion when evidence for their pursuit and defense can be readily obtained. Availability of evidence, fairness of defense, and finality are weighed against other variables including the public welfare.

For many violent crimes such as murder, there is no statute of limitations. But civil actions for monetary damages are always subject to time limits.

It did not matter for purposes of statutes of limitations whether a family knew they had a cause of action. Nor did it matter if they had gone to a lawyer and been told they had no legal claim. The statutes of limitations continued to run. The dramatic variations, both among and within states, for different causes of action suggest the role of power and politics in their determination. They demonstrate as well the fractures federalism produced in a national consumer market. But most importantly here, the laws limiting the time to bring a lawsuit, together with vagaries beyond any of these families' control that impacted when and whether they learned they had a cause of action, became yet another structure profoundly shaping these children's and families' life chances.

The myth of America as a litigious society, the hazard in what we know by the term "flammable fabrics," the special outrage of injury to children, make the resort to law seem so obvious to us today that it requires work to enter the world of Americans at mid-century. Likely most families who had a child burned in a Gene Autry cowboy suit never found their way to law.[2] Beyond the all-absorbing anxiety and grief of having a child whose life was hanging in the balance or had been extinguished, a whole array of social, cultural, and geopolitical factors worked against families making legal claims in the early years of this tragedy. There was most immediately that the tragedy unfolded in the midst of World War II. The same newspapers that carried stories of individual children burned when their cowboy suit caught fire also carried stories of "boys" whose lives had been lost or bodies maimed in service of their country.[3] Papers too carried news of polio outbreaks claiming the lives and health of children and adults alike.[4] The context cut against making legal and monetary claims out of one's suffering. For many, religious belief confirmed that suffering and loss was a part of life.

The known world, moreover, and the rhythms of everyday life, predisposed not just parents but also police, fire officials, doctors, and newspapers to interpret the facts before them in terms of accident; sadly, this was what happened when children played with fire or matches. Long accustomed to clothing made from natural fibers like wool that did not easily or readily burn, families had no basis for suspecting the cowboy suits the children had been wearing. The concept and term "flammable fabrics" did not yet exist. It was brought into being in part through the cowboy suit tragedy and the legislative battle for protective regulation that followed it. Confronted with a particular incident, the cultural narrative trumped other facts before them. Its depth and tenacity haunted the lives of the burned children and their families. And still the clock ran.

Had more families known the cause of their child's injury, more would have brought suit. When and where there were investigations that specifically identified the hazardous character of the fluffy fiber on the chaps of the Gene Autry cowboy suit and identified local victims, lawsuits followed. Tommy McCormack's father, James, had described early April 1945 as the moment when news "broke in the newspapers."[5] But the difference between New York City and Washington, DC, highlights the importance of the character and scope of the investigations and reporting. None of the short articles in New York City dailies in April 1945 identified any victims in New York City or across the river in New Jersey where the Gene Autry cowboy suit was manufactured, although there had been many. The New York City fire marshal insisted there had been no local victims.[6] That the McCormacks were the only New York City or New Jersey family to bring suit in spring 1945 suggests that it was the lawyer who lived in the building where James McCormack worked, and who knew that his son Tommy had been burned, who told James McCormack about that news.[7]

The New York City fire marshal's investigation had been triggered by the investigation in Washington, DC.[8] Unlike the coverage in New York, the *Times-Herald*'s reporting and the DC fire marshal's investigation specifically named the hazard and identified burned children and their families by name and address.[9] Its warnings of the hazard were specific and repeated. At least ten of the fourteen families named in the coverage filed suit against the retailer and manufacturers. That at least six were represented by the same Washington, DC lawyer, Robert E. Lynch, suggests he may have approached them.[10] If the McCormacks had not brought suit, one of these lawsuits would have been the first to go to trial and, assuming they won, played the role that the *McCormack* case ultimately played for families like Jackie Izzo's.

The importance, for families finding their way to law in time, of news coverage that specifically identified the hazard and identified victims by name played out equally in other cities. Just over a month after the *Times-Herald* coverage, the *Cumberland Evening Times*, in a story with the headline "Booby Traps: Child Burned When Cowboy Pants Ignite," reported on the injury of two boys in the Cumberland area.[11] In subsequent coverage they identified two more boys by name who had been burned in Gene Autry cowboy suits.[12] All four of the boys' families brought suit before the verdict in *McCormack*. In contrast, *The Philadelphia Inquirer* ran a single story on the DC investigation. Had reporters searched Philadelphia-area hospitals that day, they would have discovered three boys burned wearing Gene Autry cowboy suits being treated at Temple University Hospital.[13] None of the boys or their parents were identified in the article, and there is nothing to suggest that these families whose attention and energies were focused on their children's survival even saw the news. But the doctors treating the boys either saw the article or learned of it and referred to it in an article about their course of treatment for the boys that they published in the *Journal of the American Medical Association* (*JAMA*) in April 1946.[14] Two of the boys, Thomas Habina and Edward Klinck, were still in the hospital when the article was published; the doctors gave their parents a copy.[15] Both boys' families retained lawyers that fall.[16]

The importance of the breaking news was reinforced by the experience of families who had sought out a lawyer earlier. John Lockhart Jr. was burned on January 3, 1944, in Royal Oak, Michigan, a suburb of Detroit. Shortly thereafter, his father went to a lawyer to ask about possible legal remedies.[17] "Jackie" Lockhart, playing with another boy, had found lighter fluid and lit a fire in an empty garage down the alley. No adult was present. When Jackie's chaps exploded into flame, the other boy, out of fear or sensing they would be in trouble, ran. What made Jackie's father nonetheless see what happened as potentially having a legal remedy? Did it matter that as a sheet-metal man at the Ford Motor Company he likely knew something about clothing and fire, or that he was a union man, or was it that he was older, fifty when Jackie was born, that led him on his own or with the encouragement of co-workers to seek out a lawyer?

Whatever led John Lockhart Sr. to a lawyer, the lawyer told him he "had no remedy."[18] Personal-injury lawsuits are generally brought on a contingent-fee basis, meaning that the lawyer takes the financial risk in bringing suit in exchange for a percentage of any verdict or settlement.[19] A contingent-fee agreement was, in any event, the only basis on which most of these families could afford to bring suit. For lawyers in places where the news had not broken, taking such a case seemed a bad gamble.[20] The pernicious hold of the assumption that "this is what happens when children play with fire" not only weighed on families emotionally but also in effect blocked them from legal recourse.[21]

Other families too in areas where the news had not broken sought a lawyer before the verdict in *McCormack* and were rebuffed. So, for example, Andrew Javinsky's father tried to find a lawyer shortly after his son was burned in Muskegon, Michigan, in September 1944, but could find no one willing to bring the case on a contingent-fee basis.[22] Soon after their son was burned on September 9, 1947, in Hodge, Louisiana, Charles

Baragona Jr.'s parents went to a lawyer without success. They were advised by "others"—who? Family members? His father's co-workers at the mill? The parish priest?—"that they would be unable to recover anything for the injuries" their son had suffered.[23] How many families never pursued a lawsuit or were delayed in bringing suit because they could not find a lawyer to represent them? And still the clock ran.

Three years passed before John Lockhart Sr. again went to a lawyer. Perhaps that his son Jackie still could not walk, his knees drawn up in a fixed flexed position, another surgery the only hope for straightening his legs, a surgery the Lockharts could not afford, drove him once again to seek out a lawyer. In March 1947, by which point many suits were pending, John Sr. found his way to a Detroit lawyer, Elmer Groefsema, who specialized in personal-injury litigation and was already representing two other families in Gene Autry cowboy suit injury lawsuits. Groefsema took the case.[24]

The path to law was more difficult still for mothers on their own. Stella and Casimir Krzeczkowski Sr. divorced in the wake of their two sons being burned in November 1943, the incident claiming the life of their youngest son, Stanley, and leaving their only other child, Casimir Jr., two years later, still in and out of the hospital. Local coverage in the Passaic *Herald-News* had laid the blame squarely on the boys' playing with matches and their mother's absence.[25] It was almost three years later, in June 1946, in light of new incidents in Passaic, that reporters at the *Herald-News* reconsidered the longer history of injuries and fatalities to area children wearing Gene Autry cowboy suits.[26] Casimir Sr. remained legally liable for his son's support following the couple's divorce, but that he did not meet that obligation simply added to the burdens the children's mother bore.[27] Casimir Sr. was opposed to and wanted to have nothing to do with a lawsuit.[28] The burden of tragedy, divorce, supporting herself and her surviving son, the hostility of the boy's father toward a lawsuit, the pursuit of treatment to spare her son a life of disability, any of these things alone but certainly all of them collectively must have absorbed her energies and attention.

For Stella Krzeczkowski, as for the Izzos and many others, the first truly "breaking news" was the AP story announcing the verdict in *McCormack* in January 1948. For families who had been shouldering an economic burden well beyond their means, the verdict held out the possibility that through a lawsuit they might pay their mounting medical bills as well as the medical expenses yet to come. Following news of the *McCormack* verdict, the number of lawsuits multiplied dramatically. Many of those lawsuits involved incidents that occurred well before Tommy McCormack had been burned or died. The lawsuits came from across the United States: New York, New

Jersey, Maine, Rhode Island, Pennsylvania, Ohio, Indiana, Michigan, Mississippi, South Carolina, Florida, Idaho, California.[29] And in the years that followed, more lawsuits in more states.

The *McCormack* verdict changed the calculus for lawyers who might represent these families. Assuming the judgment in *McCormack* held on appeal, the case established the liability of the principal defendants. All a lawyer now had to do was prove that the particular child had been wearing a Gene Autry cowboy suit and that the lawsuit was brought on a timely basis. Within a week or two of the article in the *Detroit Free Press*, Jackie Izzo's parents had taken the news clipping to a lawyer in Saginaw, Michigan, and signed a contingent-fee agreement with him. The Izzos' lawsuit was formally filed in New York in June 1948.[30] Other families, like the Baragonas and Javinskys, who had unsuccessfully sought out a lawyer before, now found lawyers willing to take their case.[31]

Regardless of where a child had been injured, reaching the principal defendants required that suit be filed in either state or federal court in New York, and filing suit there required New York counsel. For the lawyers, early connections mattered. All but one family identified in the DC coverage who brought suit were represented by the same New York City lawyer, Edmond Borgio Butler, of the firm O'Connell & Butler.[32] News of the *McCormack* verdict, including that the family had been represented by Elliot Paley of the firm Nemeroff, Jelline, Danzig, & Paley, led other families to them. Butler and Paley came to represent dozens of families in Gene Autry cowboy suit cases.[33]

But how did families in other cities find their way to a lawyer in an era before it was legal for lawyers to advertise their services? Several boys—including "Jackie" Elwyn Jones, William Augustus Strong III, and Michael Felton—had fathers who were lawyers and themselves hired local counsel in New York to file suit. But they were exceptional in terms of their professional status and class. Two of the three were from small towns.[34] There is less mystery generally in how families found their way to a lawyer in small towns where the name of the local lawyer or lawyers would have been more widely known than in large metropolitan areas. Especially where there was no evidence that families would have known of each other or encountered each other in hospitals where their children were treated, one is left wondering exactly how multiple families came to be represented by the same local counsel. Elmer Groefsema signed his first retainer with a Michigan family in May 1945; he went on to represent at least five Michigan families, families living in different cities, each of whom had a child burned wearing a Gene Autry cowboy suit.[35] As was true more generally in the litigation, in every subsequent case the lawyer returned to the same New York City firm that they had worked with in their first case.[36]

For many families, their lawsuits came too late. Jackie Izzo had been burned on July 21, 1944, in Saginaw, Michigan. One month later that same year, Joseph Moore was burned in Philadelphia, Pennsylvania. Jackie's parents filed suit on June 24, 1948. Joseph's parents filed suit six months later, on January 17, 1949. Both families filed suit in federal court in the Southern District of New York. The statute of limitations in Michigan for actions based on personal injury was three years, but for minors (those under twenty-one), the statute tolled during the child's minority and did not run until three years after they reached the age of twenty-one. By the time Jackie's parents knew they had a cause of action, the statute had already run, barring any action for their losses and expenses, but the tolling of the Michigan statute in cases of minority meant that Jackie Izzo's case would proceed.[37]

The law of Pennsylvania was harsher. Actions for personal injury had to be brought within two years of injury.[38] There was no tolling provision for injury to children. Applying the Pennsylvania statute in Joseph Moore's action, the court granted the defendants' motions for summary judgment.[39] Given the timing of Joseph Moore's injury (August 26, 1944), Pennsylvania's two-year statute of limitations meant that his parents would have had to file suit for their losses and their son's before August 26, 1946, close to two years before the *McCormack* verdict and the AP story that alerted many families they had a cause of action. Moore's family challenged the harshness of Pennsylvania law, arguing that having sued in New York—the only place they could reach all the defendants—the New York statute of limitations should apply. The court rejected their claim. As the court explained, the New York Civil Practice Act was explicit in providing that the statute of limitations that controlled a suit was the statute of the state where the cause of action arose. In other words, where the injury occurred.[40]

The burden of lack of awareness of a cause of action, coupled with the uneven toll of death from Gene Autry cowboy suits, was compounded by statutes of limitations that almost uniformly set a shorter time limit for wrongful death actions than for actions where the injured individual survived.[41] Richard LaVerne Dorsey was injured in Buffalo, New York, on Christmas Day 1943. Two weeks later, on January 12, 1944, Dennis Duffy Jr. was burned in Brooklyn. Later that year, Michael Blessington Jr. was injured in Queens on December 27, 1944. All three boys were horribly burned. Dennis Duffy and Michael Blessington both died, Dennis two weeks after being burned, Michael three months after he was burned. Richard Dorsey survived. None of these families had any idea that they had a cause of action. The Duffys and Blessingtons learned when the *McCormack* verdict hit the papers; both families filed suit within a few months of the verdict. Richard's parents learned even later, not filing suit until June 14, 1950.[42]

New York's statute of limitations for actions in negligence was generally three years. But in cases involving injury to a minor, the child had until the year after he reached the age of majority to pursue a legal claim. Unless he died from his injuries. And in that event, the administrator for the child's estate had three years from the date of accident or one year from the date of death, whichever was longer, to bring suit.[43] Dennis Duffy Jr.'s and Michael Blessington Jr.'s families met neither standard. One by one, the defendants in the Duffys' suit filed motions to dismiss on the ground that the action was barred by the statute of limitations. One by one, the court granted those motions. The Duffys' lawyer tried to make the case that the suit was not for wrongful death but only for the pain and suffering that the boy had suffered in the two weeks he survived. The court rejected that it made any difference.[44]

The Blessingtons' lawyer was even more determined, adding new causes of action for nuisance and punitive damages and a supporting long recitation of the facts. He highlighted the defendants' knowing use of a highly inflammable fabric on the chaps of a playsuit for children, making the suits "fire traps" without warning to consumers, and the number of children injured or killed, including many before Michael Jr.[45] The court rejected it all. The defendants had moved for dismissal on the ground that the action in negligence was barred by the statute of limitations and that the other claims were just attempts to get around the statute. The court agreed. Citing *McCormack*, the court noted that actions had been permitted in "other incidents . . . when such actions were timely brought. . . . We cannot," the court continued, "allow sympathy and the exigencies of a particular case to give the Statute of Limitations any effect other than that which the Legislature intended it should have." The court noted that the statute of limitations was "'a declaration of public policy governing the right to litigate'" established by the legislature. "'At times, it may bar the assertion of a just claim. Then its application causes hardship. The Legislature has found that such occasional hardship is outweighed by the advantage of outlawing stale claims.'"[46] The Duffys had missed the statute of limitations by over a year; the Blessingtons by less than three months. Joseph Moore had been injured before either of these boys; his parents brought suit later—six and one-half years after their son was burned—but that he had survived meant that under New York law his action too survived. In fact, because he was still a minor, the statute had not even begun to run.[47]

There were a few exceptional states with longer statutes of limitations for wrongful death actions, and there the harshness of barring a just claim was not added to the burden of death. William Augustus Strong III was burned in Louisville, Mississippi, on November 3, 1945; he died the next day. The Mississippi statute of limitations for personal injury actions was six years, significantly longer than most states, and six years as well for cases of wrongful death, with an additional year added for bringing suit where death occurred in the final year of the statutory period for personal injury actions more generally.[48] Billy Strong's father, a lawyer, might well have known all this or at least would have known to check the statute. His firm brought suit just within six years after Billy's death, meaning that both the son's and parents' claims for loss could proceed.[49]

Wrongful death statutes extended the ability to bring suit for actions that otherwise would have been extinguished by death, but the insistence that the public-policy objective of "outlawing stale claims" outweighed the harshness of barring "just claims" rang hollow in these cases.[50] Edmond B. Butler had filed suit on April 2, 1946, for the death of Marco Antonio DiTrapani, "Tony" as he was known to his family. In the complaint, Butler noted that "by reason of the burns sustained by the said infant decedent on March 13, 1945 . . . the said infant died in Alexandria, Virginia, on April 2, 1945." But as the facts would emerge, there was a question of whether Tony had died on April 1 or April 2. In a deposition, Mrs. DiTrapani had replied "19 days" when asked "how long did your son linger in the hospital before he died?" The hospital record and autopsy that Butler had been provided cited April 2 as the child's date of death. But hearing Mrs. DiTrapani's testimony raised another possibility. If one counted the date Tony was burned, March 13, 1945, 19 days would mean that the child had died on April 1. No one asked that follow-up question in the deposition. But there was other evidence: The child's death certificate said he had died on April 1, 1945. The Henry Company had not raised the one-year statute of limitations as a bar to the action in its initial answer; it did so in an amended answer filed in October 1946. Whatever Butler said in court—"I make no representations as to the time of the death of the boy, as I am not a doctor and was not there"—he most certainly understood that the death certificate crippled the DiTrapanis' claim.[51]

All these children were wearing the same make of cowboy suit, and their lawsuits involved the same principal defendants. The distinctions in the time to bring an action for personal injury versus one for wrongful death were felt most acutely by families who confronted both. Casimir Krzeczkowski Jr. and his little brother, Stanley, were burned on November 1, 1943.

Stanley died that day; Casimir survived with horrible injuries. On March 18, 1948, less than two months after news of the verdict in *McCormack* appeared in the Passaic *Herald-News*, Stella Krzeczkowski brought suit for her son Casimir Jr.'s injuries. Six months later, she brought suit for the November 1, 1943, death of her son Stanley.[52] The New Jersey statute of limitations for actions for personal injury was two years. But as in New York, in cases of injury to minors, the statute tolled during the child's disability so that a child had until one year after turning twenty-one to bring suit. And as in New York, death ended the "disability" of being a minor. New Jersey provided that wrongful death actions had to be filed within two years of the date of death.[53] Applying these rules, Casimir Jr.'s case would proceed; Stanley's was dismissed. Even had his mother acted on it, the Passaic *Herald-News*'s June 1946 investigative story came too late for a lawsuit for her son Stanley's death.

Some families whose actions for negligence and wrongful death were barred by statutes of limitations nonetheless obtained some measure of justice through a claim for breach of warranty against a retailer. Barred from pursuing an action against the manufacturers, the families of both Michael Blessington Jr. and Dennis Duffy Jr., for example, pursued claims against the retailer they had bought the cowboy suit from, benefiting from the six-year New York statute of limitations for actions in warranty. But that too only came with a fight that itself took years. By 1953, close to a decade after both boys had died and five years after their families brought suit, the companies that had actually placed this fiber, fabric, and cowboy suit on the market were off the hook, the families left with but a rump of their original claims—a breach-of-warranty claim against the retailer—their suits still unresolved.[54]

Even this measure of financial justice was not available to many families. Breach of warranty was a claim in contract and was limited to instances where an immediate family member had bought the cowboy suit for a child. In the many instances where the cowboy suit was a gift from or purchased by a relative or family friend, or was a hand-me-down from one family to another, there was no claim for breach of warranty, because the original purchaser themselves had not been injured, and the legal fiction that applied within families that enabled recovery to a child based on a purchase made by a parent did not apply. The Blessingtons and Duffys too were fortunate, if that term can be used at all, in that the retailers were major department store chains, McCrory's and the Hecht Company—businesses, in other words, that had insurance and whose corporate form made suing them different from suing the owner of the neighborhood five-and-dime.

Many families' suits came only days before the statute would run. The burden was heaviest for families whose children were burned early and lived in states with short statutes of limitations lacking tolling provisions for injury to minors. Thomas Habina was burned on October 16, 1944, in Philadelphia. His family only learned of the role of the Gene Autry cowboy suit in his injuries two years later, in midsummer. They filed suit on October 15, 1946, one day before the Pennsylvania two-year statute of limitations for negligence actions would have run. Having twice been counseled against legal action, the Baragonas' lawsuit came only a week before the one-year statute of limitations for negligence actions in Louisiana ran.[55] Had the *McCormack* case not been decided in that interval, it seems likely that the Baragonas would not have found a lawyer to bring their case.

Legal incompetence too cost some families dearly. Five-year-old William Touhill was burned in Philadelphia two days after Christmas 1944. Sometime thereafter, his father, John, went to a Philadelphia lawyer who he understood was beginning an investigation. But inquiring later, he "was informed that nothing had been done." He turned to another Philadelphia lawyer, who referred the matter to a New York firm. By this point it was late December 1946. Under Pennsylvania law, the Touhills had only two years to bring suit. Hurriedly, the firm filed suit just days before the statute would have run. But they named as a defendant only the M. A. Henry Company.[56]

It was another two years, after the decision in *McCormack*, before the firm turned the case over to Elliot Paley, who had represented the McCormacks.[57] Paley succeeded in getting the court to allow the plaintiffs to add four additional defendants: E. F. Timme & Son, Woonsocket Falls Mill, Du Pont, and Gene Autry.[58] But one after another these defendants raised the Pennsylvania statute of limitations as a bar. Paley challenged their motions, arguing that only the Henry Company's name appeared on the box of the Gene Autry cowboy suit so that in 1946 there was nothing to alert counsel of the role these other defendants had played in the manufacture and sale of the fiber and fabric. He argued that not to allow this action to proceed against these defendants would bar the action before "the infant plaintiff had knowledge of the fact that he had such a cause of action."[59]

But one by one, the court granted summary judgment in the defendants' favor.[60] "While [plaintiffs] urge understandably liberal construction of the limitation statutes," the court noted, "yet the law of Pennsylvania clearly and inexorably bars the action." And of the plaintiffs' claim that time of discovery of the existence of the cause mattered to the statute of limitations, the court said only, "Wholly without merit." The court closed, "The plaintiffs have presented their contentions with considerable vigor, ingenuity and earnestness (and I have unhurriedly sought to study and analyze them) but unfortunately the action is barred, and the motion must be granted."[61] Paley appealed the orders only to have them affirmed. New York's highest court, in turn, refused to accept the case.[62] By 1954, a decade after William Touhill was burned and eight years after the Touhills began legal action, only the original claim against the Henry Company survived—a company whose insurance had been exhausted years earlier and that had "discontinued its business." It was more than many families managed but far less than what they deserved, given what Paley described as the "murderously inflammable" instrument the defendants had introduced into commerce.[63]

Many, in fact likely most, of those whose children were burned in Gene Autry cowboy suits never found their way to law. There were a number of news reports where a burned child was explicitly identified as having been wearing a Gene Autry cowboy suit in which no lawsuit seems to have followed. Some of those instances involved children who died.[64] It is not hard to imagine that such a family, consumed by grief, would see nothing to be gained through a lawsuit. In many other reported instances of children burned in what seem likely to have been Gene Autry cowboy suits, there is no evidence of their family bringing suit.[65] By spring 1945, the Henry Company claimed to have sold two hundred thousand Gene Autry cowboy suits distributed across the United States.[66] Every one of those suits presented the same hazard. Borrowing the phrase Ralph Nader would use some twenty years later, the hazard was "designed in."[67] And that fact meant that every child wearing one of these suits was at risk. "There are just two things to remember," DC Deputy Fire Marshal Warfield had warned in April 1945: "The suits are highly inflammable, and regardless of what anyone can do, kids at one time or another are going to get around a fire."[68] How many children were burned? How does one argue from absence?

The only thorough investigation of children burned in Gene Autry cowboy suits was that of the DC fire marshal and the *Times-Herald* in spring 1945. Their investigation identified twelve DC-area children burned in Gene Autry cowboy suits between April 1944 and March 1945. Eleven of those incidents were concentrated in a six-month period (October 1944–March 1945); at least seven (possibly as many as nine) were concentrated in a three-month period (January–March 1945). The one injury that predated October 1944 was from the preceding April, a child brought to the newspaper's and fire marshal's attention by his return trips to Children's Hospital for treatment where four other children were in the hospital in spring 1945 for burns from a Gene Autry cowboy suit. The focus on one year only, and likely not capturing even the toll in that year fully, suggests that even in the DC metropolitan area the toll was higher. But focusing solely on those identified in the coverage, fully one-third, four out of twelve, did not bring a lawsuit even though the hazard had been named, something that was not true in most of the country.

Other factors too suggest something of the potential magnitude of the number of children injured or killed. I have identified ninety-eight lawsuits by families against the Henry Company and other related defendants. One might use the percentage of DC-area families identified in the *Times-Herald* coverage who did not bring suit to argue that the number who brought suit represented only two-thirds of those injured or killed. That would suggest that at least 147 children were injured or killed from burns wearing Gene Autry cowboy suits.[69] But that number, resting as it does on a percentage of families bringing suit for whom the hazard had been identified, is likely far too low. Consider again the DC investigation and that at least eleven DC-area children were injured in a six-month time frame from October 1944 through March 1945. It seems inconceivable that the total incidence of injury from Gene Autry cowboy suits was ninety-eight and that fully 11 percent of the victims lived in a single metropolitan area and were hurt in a single six-month time frame.

The evidence related to retailers in the DC investigation also suggests that most families whose children were injured or burned in Gene Autry cowboy suits never brought suit. At least eight of the twelve families identified by the *Times-Herald* had purchased the cowboy suit from the same department store in Washington, DC. Hecht's was a major retail chain in the 1940s, with stores in New York City; Washington, DC; Baltimore; and Maryland more generally. Yet of all the other lawsuits that I am aware of against the principal defendants, only three other cases involved a purchase from a Hecht's store: John Zibor burned on October 29, 1944; Dennis Duffy burned on January 12, 1944; and Dennis McCarthy burned on November 1, 1945. All three were burned in Gene Autry cowboy suits purchased from the Hecht's store in New York City. Dennis Duffy's mother had purchased the cowboy suit that led to her son's death in December 1943. The case files do not say when the cowboy suits worn by the other two boys were purchased. It defies probability that eight of the Gene Autry cowboy suits sold by a single Hecht's store (the DC store) in a single month (December 1944) led to injury in a three-month period and that only three other Gene Autry cowboy suit sold at any other of the chain's stores left a child injured.

In 1942, another major department store chain, McCrory's, purchased 498 Gene Autry cowboy suits distributed among stores in forty-six towns and cities in sixteen states plus the District of Columbia. In 1943, the retailer purchased 1,170 Gene Autry cowboy suits distributed among sixty-seven towns and cities in twenty-one states plus the District of Columbia.[70] McCrory's continued to sell the suits in 1944. Of the ninety-eight lawsuits against the Henry Company and others in the manufacturing chain, only five involved a purchase from a McCrory's store, one in each of the following cities: Toledo, Ohio; Cumberland, Maryland; Washington, DC; Queens, New York; and Philadelphia, Pennsylvania. None involved the purchase of a Gene Autry cowboy suit from a McCrory's store in 1942; only one from a purchase in 1943; four from a purchase from a McCrory's store in 1944. Drawing on the experience of sales by Hecht's Washington, DC, store in December 1944, can it really be that not a single child was injured by a cowboy suit sold by McCrory's in 1942, and that only one child, from McCrory's 1943 sales of as many as 1,170 Gene Autry cowboy suits, was burned?

Or, to take another approach: Social-scientific studies of the percentage of individuals who suffer consumer-product-related personal injury suggest that 93 percent of those injured do not bring claims.[71] So, what if we assume that the ninety-eight lawsuits I have found represent 7 percent of those injured? This tack would suggest that possibly as many as 1,400 children were injured in Gene Autry cowboy suits.

Or we might take yet another approach. I do not know the number of Gene Autry cowboy suits Hecht's DC store sold in December 1944. But I do know that those sales led to at least seven children being burned. In 1943, McCrory's Pittsburgh store purchased forty-eight Gene Autry cowboy suits. It is not unreasonable to assume that Hecht's DC store sold forty-eight cowboy suits in December 1944. That would suggest an injury rate of 14.6 percent. Multiplying this percentage times the number of cowboy suits that the Henry Company sold between 1942 and 1945 (two hundred thousand) would mean that as many as twenty-nine thousand children were injured or killed by Gene Autry cowboy suits. That number seems staggering and so improbable. But is it? A statistician would reject the calculation for any number of reasons. But remember the DC fire marshal's warning that children at one time or another would get around fire and that if they did, the dangerously inflammable character of the fire on the chaps made it certain what would follow. The defendants' explicit worry about stirring up claims suggests that they believed the number of lawsuits brought fell far short of the number they might have faced.

States with short statutes of limitation in which many Gene Autry cowboy suits were sold further mask the scale of injury. The statute of limitations for personal injuries in the state of Pennsylvania, for example, a state where hundreds of Gene Autry cowboy suits were sold, was two years. In 1942, McCrory's sold Gene Autry cowboy suits in fourteen cities in Pennsylvania; in 1943, the company sold the cowboy suits in eighteen cities in the state. Collectively, these McCrory's Pennsylvania stores purchased 117 cowboy suits in 1942 and 276 in 1943, and likely more in 1944.[72] Yet only one of the lawsuits brought for injuries in Pennsylvania involved, as far as I can determine, a Gene Autry cowboy suit sold by McCrory's: a sale by McCrory's Philadelphia store in December 1943. Sales of the cowboy suit across the United States were concentrated in the years from 1942 to 1945, with injuries following often within days, weeks, or a few months of receiving a cowboy suit. What seems likely is that the incidence of injury in Pennsylvania was masked by the lack of knowledge of the hazard, coupled with the harsh two-year Pennsylvania statute of limitations for actions for personal injury and one year for wrongful death. Taking the *McCormack* verdict in January 1948 as a baseline for when many families found that they had a cause of action, any family whose child was injured in Pennsylvania before January 1946 who did not otherwise find their way to law before the *McCormack* verdict would have had their action barred by the Pennsylvania statutes of limitations.

Though there is no way of knowing how many children exactly were injured or killed in Gene Autry cowboy suits at mid-century, what seems undeniable is that many, perhaps even most, families never found their way to law. These families were left to rely on their own limited resources, the generosity of family, friends, and community, of doctors and hospitals who treated the children as charity cases, of state welfare offices that paid some portion of their medical expenses or kept a family afloat. For the burned children, there were additional needed treatments that never happened and pain and suffering and the loss of future earnings uncompensated. Siblings in families that never found their way to law bore the financial burden of these injuries in changes to their material lives. Caretakers, primarily mothers, carried the burden of caring for a horribly burned child in the months and years after they were released from the hospital, without additional support. And for the children, their siblings, and their extended families there was the guilt in thinking that what had happened to them was their fault.

The defendants intended that this would be so. A key part of their calculus was working to limit the number of families who found their way to law. From the start, in words and actions, the defendants made a priority of not stirring up cases.[73] Their actions contributed to both more children being injured and fewer of those children and their families finding their way to law. When Milton Henry was asked by the *Times-Herald* reporter in April 1945 what actions he planned to take, given the number of cowboy suits the company had sold across the country, he replied, "Why wave a red flag and scare everyone to death when we aren't sure what the trouble is?"[74] Silence and delay served the defendants because statutes of limitations continued to run. And so, with each lawsuit filed, the defendants requested a jury trial not because they wanted a jury but as part of the strategy of delay.

The McCormacks had filed suit in spring 1945. The case did not reach a jury until January 1948. The verdict was damning, the AP story broadcasting the verdict equally so. But the delay in reaching it held a silver lining: By January 1948, many potential lawsuits were barred by statutes of limitations. For pending cases, settlement would become the defendants' new strategy—in part because settlements, unlike verdicts, could be kept quiet.

an unbridgeable gulf

Dear Frances,

Dad and I are both on the road today. Dad had a flight to Chicago and I had a flight to Vermont. There was a family behind me on the flight—mom, dad, and three little kids, maybe 18 months to 5 or 6. For most of the flight all three of the kids sat on the side with their dad behind me. They were going to visit grandparents. I loved listening to their excitement over things that adults overlook ("Dad, are we backing up? Yeah, we're moving, we're backing up.") or tolerate ("Whoa, Whoa, Whoa . . ." as the plane was tipping & bumping like a rollercoaster ride coming in) & along the way the joys, trials & tribulations—tears, laughter, big brother telling little brother what to do & so on & parents working all the while to have the kids keep their voices soft. Listening to them brought back memories of you & Wilder when you were little & our flights. When I heard they were coming to visit grandparents, I felt & still feel a deep sadness. Down the road you would've been coming home with your children. I had assumed that and looked forward to it however unconsciously.

. . .

The end of a trip like this is hard. It's the moment when I should be coming home to you or to 'my' 'our' world. It's one of those moments when I come face to face with the realization that you are gone and I start down that path of remembering, knowing, realizing all over again.

. . .

I have found myself thinking more about your room. When I finally faced it and cleaned it with love this fall, I hadn't imagined that there would be more stages, that your room would become a site of my imagining you chang-

ing. Looking at it now, already, there are elements that I wonder how you would feel about . . . Would you have taken the posters down? Would you want me to take them down?

. . .

I'm having a hard time getting started today. I still find the sound of an alarm clock in the morning hard because it reminds me of your alarm beeping and beeping on the morning of April 26th and your not hearing, understanding, or being able to turn it off. But then I also found myself thinking about how you and I had settled into a pattern your senior year of you hearing my alarm go off and coming in to sit on the edge of the bed and talk until you had to go to school. I loved that time. Sometimes you needed to turn on the light so I could help you decide about earrings or help you get a necklace on. But mostly, we just talked, with light streaming in from the hallway, and beginning to creep around the blinds, about your day ahead. I always groaned when you had to leave both because it meant this most wonderful, companionable way of waking up was at an end and because I really had to get out of bed and into the shower.

. . .

There were two articles in the paper this morning I wanted to tell you about . . . the second was about the practice—very common—of people sleeping with their pets. It made me laugh out loud several times, especially relating to the pay-back (urinating on the clothing of an unwelcome new romantic interest of their master seemed the most common) animals have when a potential new romantic interest comes into the household. You would have loved the story and heartily approved of all these pet owners whose mates (human) are the ones who have to adapt to/be accepted by the animals who are already in bed. You, no doubt, Frances, would have become one of those people who shared not just your house, but your bed with many creatures, and bed-hogging, sharp nails aside, I think would have felt so loved & so happy with your animal companions.

. . .

The scholar presenting at the noon workshop today had met me before. Being reminded of when and where powerfully reinforced the invisibility of our personal lives within our professional identities. Fall 2009, he was at our house as part of a large group. When I went up to him today to shake his hand and said who I was, he reminded me of that occasion. But all I was thinking about was that our "meetings" "our crossings" his and mine had leapt over a crucial defining fact: when we first met, you were a [high school] senior; meeting again now, you are gone. And yet he doesn't know about this transformation. There is to him continuity, where there is to me an unbridgeable gulf.

chapter fifteen · to be "judged on our capabilities alone"

In early 1969, a year before Susan Moller Okin started graduate school at Harvard, students at the University of Chicago seized administration offices to protest the university's decision not to renew the contract of Assistant Professor Marlene Dixon in the Department of Sociology. Jo Freeman, a graduate student in political science, responded to the administration's decision by conducting a "simple sex census." Using university catalogs as a source, she began with the Sociology Department for the preceding ten years. She then expanded her search to the history of women faculty over the whole history of the university in the six major social-science departments: anthropology, economics, history, political science, psychology, and sociology. What her census revealed surprised even her: In the employment of women as faculty, the "normal" university career was not there at all. Although the University of Chicago had been coeducational since it opened its doors in 1892, over the entire course of the university's history, not a single woman in the graduate division of any of these six social-science departments began her career as a junior faculty member and rose in that department to become a full professor.[1]

But if no women had had a "normal" university faculty career at the University of Chicago, there was nonetheless a pattern to women's employment as faculty. It was simply this: Few women were hired at all; initial appointments of women were generally at the rank of instructor or lecturer; the few women whose appointments were renewed remained untenured for an abnormally long time; and the tiny number of women who had become full professors had for the most part risen through "women's departments." Freeman had suspected and had hoped to show that the turnover rate of women was considerably higher than that of men. But as she said, "I could find no such pattern because I could not find any women." Marlene

Dixon, appointed in 1966, had been the first woman to hold a faculty appointment in the Department of Sociology in nineteen years. In the entire history of the six departments, Dixon was only the fifth woman to hold a first appointment as assistant professor. "Where are the women Ph.D.s?" Freeman asked, and answered, "Look to the 'temporary' position of Research Associate. Some women stay in it for years." In fact, more women had been employed as research associates in the six departments Freeman surveyed than as faculty members.

Presenting her sex survey at the minority groups workshop at the American Political Science Association (APSA) annual meeting in winter 1970, Freeman noted that "the patterns of discrimination are clear": "Women can get their training in the major departments, but they cannot rise up through the academic ranks in the faculty." Nor was Chicago an anomaly, she noted; the pattern held at all comparable institutions of higher education. She closed on a personal note. "As I plied the catalogs and catalogued the plight of the female faculty, I could not help but feel a serious concern for those women currently in graduate school who, like myself, believed the myth that we would be judged on our capabilities alone and that the opportunities open to us were no different than those open to men. . . . I felt a concern and I felt an urgency that we should not complacently wait for the men who control the departments to decide how many token women they might allow on their faculties. If we do so, the situation will change no more in the next 77 years than it has in the last 77." Going through the catalogs, she said, her mind continually returned to the example of early Black civil rights protesters picketing stores where they were not hired with signs reading, "Don't buy where you can't work." "Women can buy at the University of Chicago," Freeman explained. "But once they have their Ph.D., their status changes. Women can buy here, but they cannot work."[2]

Between 1968 and 1971, the question of women's status in academia exploded across the United States—in universities, colleges, and disciplinary professional associations, and for individual women. The ground was laid by the dramatic expansion and democratization of access to higher education in the years since World War II, the exponential growth in the number and size of PhD programs and the professoriate, the dramatic growth in the number of women in college and college-educated women pursuing and holding advanced degrees, and the explosion in federal dollars for research and student aid to institutions of higher education.[3] Rights movements and the anti-war movement crashed across this landscape, turning college and university campuses and professional society meetings by the late 1960s into tinderboxes.[4] This was the combustible environment in which women's challenge to sex inequality in academia emerged. Individually, for some women it was a dawning consciousness, for others a movement that met their deeply grooved experience of discrimination. Their challenge would transform the vita even as it reinforced and deepened, in unexpected ways, the vita's centrality to academic life.[5]

In 1930, women had made up over a quarter of faculty at colleges and universities in the United States. By 1966 that percentage had declined from 27.1 percent to 22 percent. The percentage of those receiving doctorates who were women had also declined: Women accounted for 15.4 percent of doctorates in 1920 and 1930; by 1950, only 9.6 percent.[6] Moreover, women were largely excluded from tenure-track faculty appointments at the most prestigious colleges and universities. Where were the women? Relegated to positions outside the tenure system at elite universities and to teachers' colleges and junior colleges.[7]

And yet despite the decline in terms of percentages, the growth in the professoriate and the size and number of graduate programs, especially in the 1960s, meant that in absolute terms the number of women in academia had grown significantly. And this growth too mattered.[8] There were women at institutions of every rank, large and small, public and private, single-sex and coed, across the United States. And in many disciplines by the late 1960s, even at the most elite universities, women made up close to a quarter of graduate students.[9] In other words, there was a force that once mobilized might produce change.

The data on women's status in academia was stark. In 1969, Harvard's Faculty of Arts and Sciences had 411 tenured professors. Not one was a woman.[10] Women made up 22.6 percent of current students in the graduate arts and sciences at Harvard and 19 percent of the PhDs Harvard awarded in 1969. But of Harvard's 194 assistant professors, only nine were women.[11] To the extent that there were positions for women with advanced degrees at Harvard, as Jo Freeman had found at Chicago, they were largely outside the tenure system.[12] And this, in turn, meant that most women with advanced degrees at the university were not eligible to apply for research funds or sabbaticals, could not be principal investigators on grants, and could not formally advise graduate students. These restrictions mattered not only for the individual women affected but for knowledge itself.

Columbia, like Harvard and Chicago, had long been a major producer of PhDs, including women. In the 1960s, the percentage of doctorates awarded to women at Columbia grew from 13 percent to over 24 percent.[13] Yet the tiny percentage of women with tenure in the graduate faculties (2 percent) did not budge. Nor was the difference simply a matter of faculty appointments for women catching up with doctorates awarded to women. Men who had received their doctorates between 1960 and 1970 held positions at every rank of Columbia's graduate faculty: ninety-one assistant professors, seventy-four associate professors, thirty full professors. The picture for women who had earned their doctorates between 1960 and 1970 was different: twenty-four assistant professors, one associate professor, no full professors. And at Columbia, as was true at Chicago, Harvard, and other elite universities, women with advanced degrees were largely relegated to non–tenure ladder positions, with all the consequences that followed in terms of heavy teaching loads at introductory levels and lack of access to research funds and sabbaticals. The one category in which women constituted a majority was outside the tenure system in part-time employment.[14]

The employment of women on faculties at major public land-grant universities differed little from their employment at elite private universities despite their difference in size, longtime coeducational character, and production of huge numbers of PhDs. In 1969–1970, at Berkeley women made up only 5 percent of assistant professors—sixteen of 296—and only 3 percent of associate and full professors—twenty-nine of 899.[15] In many departments, including large departments like history, mathematics, and physics, there was not a single woman on the faculty. Some had never had a woman faculty member; others had not had a woman faculty member for decades.[16] At Berkeley, as elsewhere, given the low proportion of women on the faculty, most graduate students were trained by men. And as was true elsewhere, the only place that women were represented in significant numbers was in appointments outside the tenure system.[17] The record was no different at other large public, major PhD-producing universities. In 1969, Michigan's huge College of Literature, Science, and the Arts had nine hundred faculty members of professorial rank; thirty-four were women.[18] The picture for women in the sciences was even bleaker. At the University of Minnesota, for example, the eleven departments of the Institute of Technology had only two tenure-track women out of some four hundred faculty members.[19] Nor was Minnesota an anomaly.[20] The patterns held as one moved down the ranks of PhD-granting institutions.[21] Wherever one turned, the basic facts were staggering in their consistency.[22]

Statistics and the *N*s they are based on capture one kind of truth, the experience of individual women another. Suzanne Gossett was one of the thousands of women who pursued a PhD in the 1960s. She was in the first cohort of women PhD students (thirteen in total) admitted to Princeton in 1963.[23] She had been admitted to the PhD programs at Columbia and Yale but had gone to Princeton because her husband Philip was starting a PhD there in music history. Philip was given a fellowship his first year; Suzanne, despite her distinguished record, was not. The faculty member who would become her advisor in the Department of English was away her first year in the program. On his return he informed her that he had voted against her admission, and when she was completing her degree in fall 1967 he took no steps—no mentoring, no letters, no phone calls—to help her find a position. By the time of the MLA annual meeting, all the other members of her PhD cohort in English on the job market, all men, had positions. She did not. Suzanne's husband Philip was on the job market the same year and received an offer from the University of Chicago—next to Princeton, the top program in music history in the US.[24]

Left to "place" herself, Suzanne wrote widely seeking a faculty appointment. Many of the replies came addressed to "Mrs. Philip Gossett."[25] None offered even an interview. As Suzanne Gossett explained to me, "Everyone said, 'Have a baby. Go to Chicago. Something will turn up.'" She got pregnant but had a miscarriage.[26] And so she found herself without a job, without a baby, angry, and deeply depressed. That April she received a phone call from the interim chairman of the English Department at Loyola—one of the local universities that had initially sent her a rejection addressed to Mrs. Philip Gossett—asking if she was still available. She flew out, gave a lecture, and was offered a position as an assistant professor. This was how the Gossetts began their academic careers: Philip at one of the nation's elite research universities; Suzanne at a teaching institution where many faculty had only MAs and where she was the only faculty member with an Ivy League degree.[27] They arrived in Chicago in fall 1968 as the city erupted in protests and violence.

That same year, Bernice Sandler began her search for an academic position. When she had first applied to the PhD program in counseling at the University of Maryland in the mid-1960s, she was rejected on grounds of age. She was married, thirty-six years old, and had two children. But she persisted, was admitted, and as she was finishing her degree, she began looking for a faculty position. There were six openings in her department. Though she had an excellent record, including teaching in the department, she was not considered. When she asked a faculty friend why, he responded, "Let's face it, you come on too strong for a woman." Sandler's initial response was to go home and cry. She blamed herself. "I bemoaned the fact that I had spoken out at staff meetings with suggestions for improving procedures. I lamented the times that I had discussed teaching and professional issues with faculty members. I regretted my participation in classes as a graduate student." It was her husband who said this was "sex discrimination." Shortly thereafter, she received two similar rejections, in one of which an employment agency counselor looking at her resume said that she was "not really a professional" but "just a housewife who went back to school." The rejections set her to thinking. Sex discrimination was "immoral"; surely it was also "illegal."[28]

Four years earlier, in spring 1964, as the Civil Rights Bill was debated, an amendment adding "sex" to Title VII of the bill was proposed on the House floor. Opponents of the amendment feared it was an attempt to and would sabotage passage of the law; proponents saw it as necessary to protect women, especially Black women, who without the amendment would continue to face pervasive discrimination in employment. The Civil Rights Act became law that summer, with "sex" listed in Title VII—along with race, color, religion, and national origin—as prohibited grounds for discrimination in employment.[29] But as Bernice Sandler discovered, neither Title VII, nor any other law passed by Congress in the 1960s prohibiting discrimination against women, applied to women in education. Title VII expressly exempted educational institutions.[30] Nor, as Sandler discovered, could women in education look to other federal laws passed by Congress in the 1960s. The Equal Pay Act, the first law prohibiting sex discrimination, passed by Congress in 1963, did not apply to professional and administrative employees. Moreover, sex discrimination was not among the categories of discrimination prohibited in federally assisted programs under Title VI of the Civil Rights Act.[31] Nor, as of 1969, was the US Constitution any help.[32]

But as Sandler discovered, there was a legal route to challenging sex discrimination in colleges and universities. She found it reading a footnote in a report of the US Commission on Civil Rights. In fall 1965, President Lyndon Johnson had issued Executive Order 11246, setting out the requirements for nondiscriminatory practices in hiring and employment by federal contractors. The original order applied only to discrimination in employment on the basis of race, color, religion, and national origin. But in October 1967, President Johnson issued a second order, Executive Order 11375, amending Executive Order 11246, so that it applied as well to discrimination in employment on the basis of sex. Allowing a year for the development of new regulations, Executive Order 11246, as revised, went into effect on October 13, 1968.

The order was broad in its application. It applied to every federal contractor with more than fifty employees and holding federal contracts totaling $50,000 or more. It prohibited discrimination on the basis of race, color, religion, sex, or national origin. And it required federal contractors "to take affirmative action" to remedy past discrimination and have a "written plan of affirmative action" with "specific goals and timetables." Enforcement fell to the Office of Federal Contract Compliance (OFCC) within the Department of Health, Education, and Welfare (HEW). A compliance review could be triggered by a complaint or, in the case of contracts over one million dollars, was to be completed before the award of the contract. Failure to meet the terms of the executive order could be penalized by the withholding or withdrawal of all federal contracts.[33] By 1968, universities and colleges were receiving billions of dollars annually in federal contracts.[34] And though there were dramatic differences in which institutions benefited most generously from federal largesse, well over 80 percent of universities and colleges held federal contracts in excess of $50,000, making them subject to the terms of Executive Order 11246.[35]

When Bernice Sandler discovered Executive Order 11246 in late 1969, the Department of Labor had not yet developed or issued guidelines, and HEW's Office of Federal Contract Compliance had not conducted a single compliance review or pre-contract compliance review including sex. The silence surrounding the order's application to sex, its application in higher education, led even Sandler to question her research. Yet on contacting the Department of Labor she learned that her research was correct—and, what was more, that at least one federal official, an attorney named Vince Macalouso, assistant director of the Labor Department's contract compliance division, was anxious to see it enforced.[36] On January 31, 1970, Bernice Sandler, in her new position as director of the Women's Equity Action League's Office of Federal Contract Compliance, filed the first official complaint alleging an industry-wide pattern of sex discrimination in academia and demanding a class action and compliance review of all universities and colleges holding federal contracts. That same day, Sandler filed a complaint against the University of Maryland.[37]

Bernice Sandler was a trailblazer in discovering the legal path for challenging sex discrimination in academia. But it was critical that there was a larger social movement to take up and act on her discovery. Between 1968 and 1971, women in academia—graduate students, research associates, faculty—organized in departments and across university and college campuses. They formed caucuses in dozens of professional societies, and they joined feminist organizations like the Women's Equity Action League (WEAL) and the National Organization for Women (NOW).[38] Their actions were bound up with the larger social ferment and yet also responses to distinct catalysts, as for example, the denial of tenure to Marlene Dixon at Chicago or the consolidation of Radcliffe College into Harvard University. Individually, as members of committees, and through feminist organizations, using the skills of their advanced training, women lent thousands of hours of uncompensated labor to gather the data that documented discrimination against women in academia.

It was an awakening. Sitting in the audience in a packed ballroom at the annual convention of the American Historical Association in 1970 as Willie Lee Rose shared the shocking pattern of discrimination against women in the historical profession, Linda Kerber—two years beyond her Columbia PhD and still unemployed—understood her situation in a new light. "We were unemployed because a profession that prided itself on its commitment to the life of the mind measured its colleagues by nonintellectual criteria."[39] "Higher education." That lofty term. Academia was a workplace. And sex discrimination, as the data showed, was an industry-wide pattern. University committees on the status of women and women's local and national organizations joined Sandler in filing complaints against universities.[40] By October 1970, formal complaints of sex discrimination under EO 11246 had been filed against over two hundred colleges and universities. More were to come. And with each complaint came press releases, letters to the state governor and to US senators and representatives.[41]

The evidence of sex discrimination in academia that had for so long gone unexamined now provoked a fiery political response. On March 9, 1970, Martha Griffiths (D-MI), longtime advocate of women's rights, excoriated both universities and federal agencies in a speech on the House floor, demanding immediate action: "It is shocking and outrageous that universities and colleges, using Federal moneys, are allowed to continue treating women as second-class citizens, while the Government hypocritically closes its eyes."[42] Shortly thereafter, Representative Edith Green (D-OR), chairman of the Special Subcommittee on Education in the House Committee on Education and Labor, introduced legislation to close the gaps in Title VI and Title VII of the Civil Rights Act of 1964 that had left women in academia with no legal protection against discrimination on the basis of sex. In June 1970, she held the first hearings on sex discrimination in academia, ultimately leading to the Education Amendments Act of 1972, passed on June 23, 1973, which extended the protections of Title VII to women employed in education.[43]

Women's challenge to sex discrimination in academia was not explicitly about the vita. But like so much else in this story, women's challenge and universities' response to it were fundamental to the transformation of the vita in its substance and its centrality to academic life. With universities and colleges facing legal sanctions, women eagerly organized, the urgency of their pursuit heightened by a collapsing job market. As was true in the women's movement more generally, young women were at the heart of the challenge.[44] By the late 1960s, the vita was an integral part of the job search. In every discipline, jobs were a first concern and so the vita became bound up in their effort.

Committees on the status of women in professional societies and new women's professional organizations scrambled to connect women and their vitae with news of positions.[45] In its first newsletter in October 1970, the ASA Women's Caucus Steering Committee urged women seeking an appointment for the next year to send a curriculum vitae and letter, "so that if any of us are asked for recommendations, we can refer potential employers to you."[46] By spring there was a formal organization—Sociologists for Women in Society (SWS)—and among its newly established committees was the Committee on the Job Market. In its March 1971 newsletter, the committee announced itself and its task: "to act as a clearing house for jobs for women and for academic teams. . . . Therefore: Those of you who are seeking employment should fill out the form marked 'SWS Employment Form.' Be sure to attach a current vita to the form. If your spouse is also looking for a new job, be sure he attaches a current vita to the form he completes."[47] In turn, those who knew of jobs were asked to fill out the "Job Opportunities Form": "We are especially interested in the assistance of people who know of job openings, and would be willing to personally forward the vitae of qualified applicants."

Professional disciplinary societies had been running job registries for at least a decade and a half. Newly formed women's organizations learned as they went. In the May 1971 SWS newsletter, the report from the Job Market Committee was emphatic: "Please send FOUR (!!4!!) vitae with the Employment Form."[48] They began their jobs file drawing on news passed through the grapevine, but they were preparing to send letters to a thousand four-year colleges on jobs for the 1971–1972 academic year, "so our files should start to grow." In an addendum to their report, Job Market Chair Rita Seiden Miller wrote, "PLEASE: We need women who want jobs—we can't believe the response we've gotten (already) to our job questionnaire." The character and location of those positions though was made clearer by the next sentence: "Especially looking for women who would be interested in jobs in small colleges in the South and Midwest (also have a few in New York state, Conn., and R.I.). . . . HELP!! Who would believe??"[49] The sense of possibility in that moment was palpable.

In every discipline, women organized. In its March 1971 newsletter, the Coordinating Committee on Women in the Historical Profession, for example, eagerly announced that the AHA had agreed to their request to "maintain a special job file for women historians."[50] Whereas women in sociology initially collected women's vitae to send directly to schools with positions and later listed jobs in their newsletter for women to forward their vita independently, the AHA Committee on Women Historians followed the example of the AHA Job Registry, drafting a vita form for women to complete.[51] The work of building rosters of women scholars in a discipline was immense and unending. They distributed the form to all women who registered at the annual meeting and published the form in the *AHA Newsletter*, collecting and retyping completed vita forms onto "McBee" sort cards, drafting and mailing a form letter to 1,200 history department chairmen announcing the service. And that was only the beginning. When a letter with notice of a position arrived at the AHA, it was xeroxed and mailed to all the women registered to whom it might apply, and the cards of these women in turn xeroxed and sent to the department.[52] And with each notice of a position, the process was repeated.

At the same time, women worked to dismantle the pervasive institutional structures that closed academic jobs to women—including disciplinary-society placement services that included sex-specific job ads and required candidates for positions to include their sex.[53] Among Bernice Sandler's earliest official complaints under Executive Order 11246, as well as Title VII, were two in April 1970 against professional societies in her field, the American Personnel and Guidance Association (APGA) and the American Psychological Association (APA), for advertising positions in which sex ("man") was listed as a qualification for the position.[54]

It might not be accurate to say that every professional society was vulnerable to the same charge, but the vast majority were.[55] In the same month that Sandler filed formal complaints against the APA and APGA, Linda Kerber—in a letter to Willie Lee Rose, the chair of the newly established AHA ad hoc Committee on the Status of Women in the Historical Profession—wrote, "If I may add a personal note, may I suggest that the Committee on the Status of Women undertake the relatively simple move of convincing the AHA to omit sex identification (and perhaps age) in the candidate availability notices in the Professional Register? Volume II No. 4 has 16 such entries."[56] A new AHA policy for listings in the Professional Register—now excluding sex and number of children—went into effect shortly before the December 1970 association annual meeting, at which the ad hoc Committee on the Status of Women presented its report on the status of women in the historical profession.[57] Quietly in the early 1970s, professional societies eliminated sex as a qualification from ads placed by hiring institutions, and sex, marital, and parental status from listings by candidates for positions.

Eliminating sex as an explicit qualification for academic positions was an important step in opening positions to applications from women. But the break was neither simple nor complete. In 1970, the final line of the American Institute of Physics (AIP) Placement Service registration form read: "Married _____ Children ______ Health ______ U. S. citizen? _____ Age _____." With their signature (required at the bottom), registrants agreed, "The AIP has my permission to show this sheet to any employer."[58] When exactly the AIP placement service revised its form is unclear, but by 1974, a new form was in use.[59] A cover letter noted, "Check the following items if you want us to provide such information to prospective employers—otherwise omit." The items? Age, sex, and current employment. In a stack of completed forms and vitae that stood some six inches thick, only one registrant left the questions blank.[60] Men had everything to gain, nothing to lose, by revealing their sex. Only a tiny number of registrants for the AIP Employment Referral Service in 1974 were women. It was one of these who left the three questions blank. She could only hope a college, university, or industrial employer looking at her full resume detailing her training, skills, experience, and publications would see something more than her age, sex, and present employment.[61]

That hope flew in the face of deeply ingrained assumptions about women's nature, place, and commitments that women now openly challenged. The Committee on the Status of Women at Harvard in 1970, for example, interviewed women lecturers and junior faculty and held open hearings. Again and again in those interviews and hearings, women voiced their anger, frustration, and humiliation at the assumptions and questions they faced from men about their marriage and family plans, their "commitment" to teaching or research, as though for a woman marriage and children were inconsistent with a career and intellectual life.[62] Single women were asked if they planned to marry. Married women without children were asked their family plans. Women who could not have children were asked if they planned to adopt. The message was not lost on them. So, in one of the committee's interviews with an unmarried assistant professor came this question and answer: "What if you were married, with children? Would this make a difference?" "Oh God, yes!" (laughs) "They don't believe in academic women with children."[63]

As Caroline Bynum and Janet Martin, assistant professors with Harvard PhDs and co-founders of the Women's Faculty Group at Harvard, wrote in the *Radcliffe Quarterly* in June 1970, "Nobody asks a man, do you want to choose between [being] a husband and a father or have a career. And yet conditions are such that women are constantly being forced to choose between one or the other."[64] But it was more even than an expectation that women make a choice; men made the choice for them.[65] As one of the many women in the hearings at Harvard who spoke put it, "what you have to prove is that you're not a woman."[66]

As her testimony highlighted, there was a deeply ingrained misogyny in academia, a dismissal of women as a sex as intellectual equals. When Caroline Bynum and Michael Walzer, co-chairs of the Committee on the Status of Women at Harvard, sent a letter to department and program chairmen asking them to respond to a series of questions related to women in their field and women graduate students and faculty in their department, close to one-third did not bother to reply at all.[67] Several others penciled in cursory responses in an exercise that could not have taken them more than five minutes.[68] But it was the question about women's success in a given discipline that was most revealing of underlying attitudes about women. Some chairmen simply responded, "Yes," to the question of whether women were as successful as men in their discipline, treating this question with the same vague annoyance as they did the rest of this unwanted exercise. Other chairmen gave voice to their views of women's intellectual inferiority. The Math Department chairman scribbled in, "They are not as successful in creative research." The chairman of the Statistics Department wrote, "It is very difficult to find women who have proven outstanding ability." The Music Department chairman wrote, "In composition women are not as successful as men, they seem always to lack the very highly creative instinct of men. The record throughout history confirms this." The chairman of the Sociology Department replied, "All I can say is that of the persons generally recognized as prominent sociologists in America today, none are women." In a letter written to a colleague with a "cc" to the committee, historian Oscar Handlin impugned not women's lesser intellectual capacity across time but the "puzzle" that contemporary women seemed less capable than an earlier generation without fault of the university.[69]

The deeply ingrained assumptions, beliefs, practices, and rationalizations about women as a sex, and about women and family life, gave the vita a particular importance to women. It offered a tool by which a woman could present herself as an individual. Education, honors and awards, professional-society memberships and service, fellowships and grants, publications, students trained. Each of these categories on vitae, so essential to building professional and scholarly identities and reputations, held a greater weight for women and other minorities long excluded from or limited to subordinate positions and institutions in academic life.[70]

Moreover, discrimination in any of its elements—and women and other minorities faced discrimination in all of them—mattered not only in an immediate sense but cumulatively for the credentials that they could present in a vita.[71] And in that regard, a critical starting point for women to be seen as individuals was the erasure from vitae of marital and parental status. In an exchange in June 1970 with a young sociologist whose husband was also in sociology, the two of them struggling to find positions where both they and their careers could thrive, Alice Rossi wrote, "From a long-range point of view . . . marital status must become totally private and no business of employers."[72]

Initially though, the importance of marital and parental status on vitae was reinforced by the elimination of that data from professional-society registries. The instruction sheet for registrants of the American Institute of Physics Placement Service in 1974 directed registrants to provide an "informative and concise . . . personal resume" which should include "information which does not appear on the standard form."[73] In physics as elsewhere, marital and parental status no longer appeared on standard registration forms. Most AIP registrants included that data on the personal resumes and vitae they submitted. Nor were they alone. But gradually over the decade, personal data, especially marital and parental status, disappeared from vitae, first from women's vitae and more gradually from men's.[74] There were differences by field and a scholar's age, and personal data did not disappear entirely, but increasingly its presence on vitae more than its absence was what stood out.

The heady excitement of the first discipline-specific job market committees for women did not last.[75] In her December 1972 report to the AHA council on behalf of the Committee on Women Historians (CWH), Linda Kerber noted that "despite euphoric predictions women are not monopolizing new openings"—far from it—"and the imbalance perceived two years ago persists."[76] As Kerber noted, 1,400 women were registered in their women's roster. The committee received 108 notices of positions from universities and sent over six hundred letters to women notifying them of the positions. Inquiring of those institutions, the committee received only eighteen replies. Ten reported that they had hired a woman from the CWH's lists.[77] In an effort perhaps to put a better light on those returns, the committee's update noted that "many institutions wrote that the roster had helped them take affirmative action in response to the government's Executive Order banning discrimination in institutions under federal contract."[78] What they—that is, the AHA Committee on Women Historians and their equivalents in other professional associations—did not know was that simply asking for a list of women seeking positions was at many institutions part of the theater of compliance.

Needing in any event to keep up the pressure in the hope that the number of inquiries and placements would grow, they took every possible opportunity to encourage the listing of positions and women's registration in the roster. One can hear the echo of the early boosterism of the AHA Job Registry in their call, "We are updating the roster and have enclosed on the last page of this Newsletter a tear-out form to be filled in and returned to us. . . . **Please Return this Form Quickly**." A year later, they had a revised vita form and reported that they had shifted "to computer." More urgent calls for women to complete new vita forms, more retyping of those forms into a system the returns of which were slim.[79] But as Charlotte Quinn, special assistant to the Committee on Women Historians, wrote in May 1973, "The clear danger is that as pressure slackens, those in sympathy with women's aspirations will feel that the need has passed."[80] If the returns for the work of job registers for women were slim, it nonetheless and perhaps all the more deepened women's need for and dependence on the vita.

There are unexpected parallels between women's experience of sexism in academia and the cowboy suit tragedy. Disaggregated experience and narratives of the known world or the common sense of the matter had been as important in obscuring sexism in academia as the character of the hazard that led to the injury and death of children wearing Gene Autry cowboy suits. Like families in the cowboy suit tragedy, women pursuing advanced degrees and academic positions in the post–World War II era knew only their own individual experience and read that experience through broader cultural assumptions. Data on women's status in academia had largely existed only in disaggregated form, scattered across thousands of colleges and universities in staff and faculty catalogues, department and administration files, and chairmen's memories.[81] Collecting that scattered data provided the foundation for a different narrative, a different kind of knowing, just as breaking news of the hazard and the *McCormack* verdict had in the cowboy suit tragedy.

But as was true in the cowboy suit tragedy, so too for sex discrimination in academia. Law was central not only in producing a new way of knowing but equally in defining its limits. For even as women turned to the vita as a tool in their pursuit to be "judged on their capabilities alone," universities with very different intent discovered that the vita served their needs.

can I have a body when you cannot?

Dear Frances,

I woke up this morning feeling like crying. Still feel that way now two hours later. I just sat there cleaning out my cell phone mailbox. Dad said when you get more than 100 messages, the oldest ones start dropping off without you even knowing it. The idea of losing your last messages had me in a panic. . . . But I did something wrong and it deleted all the sent messages, so now the sent mailbox is empty. I feel dizzy and sick. Now, I don't have my last texts to you.

. . .

I have now done a Yoga class. It was hard. Like going to the doctor or dentist, neither of which I've managed, going to yoga feels like a decision to force myself to re-inhabit my body, to take care of myself. It feels like one more step in joining the living. How can I have a body when you cannot? Can I have a body, be in my body and not lose touch with you?

. . .

For the first time since you died I listened to NPR on the way to school this morning. The radio was on—as it often has been when someone else was the last to drive—but this morning it didn't sound just like noise that I had to get off right away and so I listened. I suppose it's a sort of mental well-being sign-post, but it brings a sort of sadness along with it. I still can't imagine reading a book for pleasure, having dinner with friends, anything that is about leisure or relaxation. There's a feeling that if I have you out of my mind for an instant I risk losing you.

. . .

It's the first of March. You would have been turning 19 this month. Wilder and I have each had to have a birthday without you. Dad hasn't yet . . . But this month we face the hardest birthday—yours.

. . .

I'm trying to remember if it was only beginning in your senior year or as early as your junior year that you announced that you would be looking for a man who was like Dad to marry. You had such good judgment, Frances. A guy like Dad would have been perfect for you. It's good there are guys like that in the world for women like us. I think Wilder's that kind of guy too.

. . .

Do you think dogs look at photographs? Does Sam see all the pictures of you and recognize you, remember you through them?

. . .

I had a dream last night that [two of your friends from high school] came over and I was surprised to see that already they looked different from last year and it left me feeling such a deep sadness to realize that the change that I thought of in the future was already happening, that you already would look different than the pictures we have of you from last spring.

. . .

Dad mentioned on the way home from dinner that he was thinking about you. He spent much of the day doing the not particularly satisfying, but unfortunately necessary work of tax returns. And he had realized that this would be the last tax return he would ever do for you . . . He said he felt like it was kind of a silly thing to be thinking about. But it doesn't seem that way to me. He has worked hard over his whole adult life and most of that work has been directed to being a good provider for his family, especially his children. You didn't really know this yet and wouldn't have appreciated it for years to come. What makes the moment sad is that however good a job he did at providing he could not save you. And so, I imagine it's especially hard to do this last return not only because he won't get to do another, but also because it wasn't, couldn't be enough.

. . .

I have been feeling recently like it's harder to feel what it was like to hug you. Losing that feeling is so awful, it's like a parent holding on to a child's hand through some disaster and then simply it not being there anymore.

. . .

After committing myself to start today out positive and working hard, I am in shambles. I'm shaking and in tears. Whatever else would go wrong in life before you died we always had each other. Now the public (teaching) becomes a prop for the private and when it fails as it has this morning, there is nothing.

· PART V ·

Power

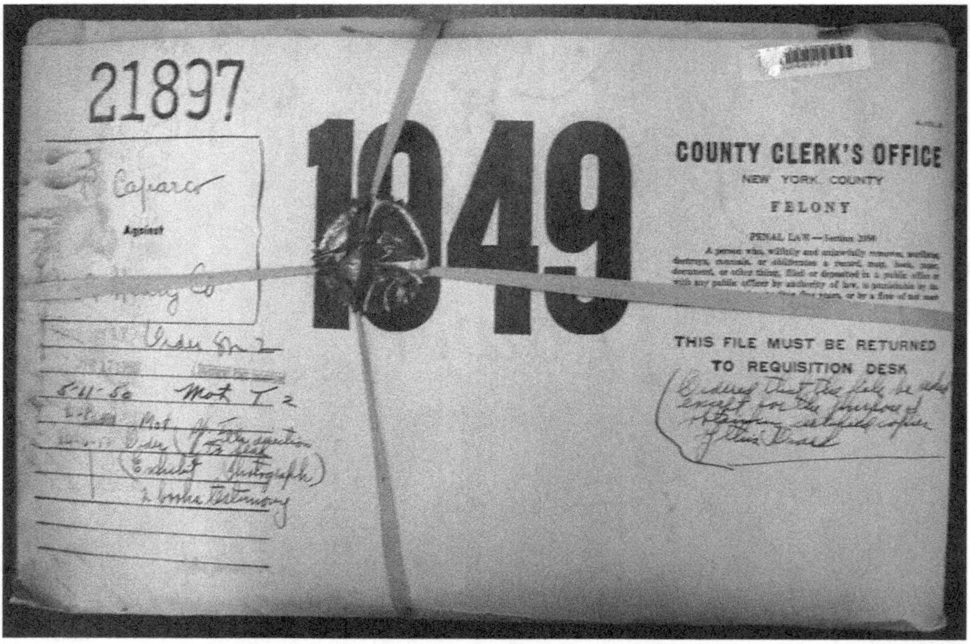
21897
Against
1949
COUNTY CLERK'S OFFICE
NEW YORK COUNTY
FELONY
THIS FILE MUST BE RETURNED
TO REQUISITION DESK

chapter sixteen · the price of settlement

For two and a half years after news of the dangerous character of the Gene Autry cowboy suit was first published in April 1945, the defendants dug in their heels, resisting every legal claim that followed. Then came the *McCormack* jury verdict in January 1948.[1] With the exception of Milton Henry personally, the jury's verdict had been against all the named defendants: the M. A. Henry Company, Woonsocket Falls Mill, and E. F. Timme & Son. The only prospective defendants whose liability remained untested were those not named in the case: Du Pont and Gene Autry. When Judge Corcoran denied the defendants' post-verdict motions, they filed an appeal.[2]

That appeal was still pending on the morning of March 25, 1949, when the trial in the case of *Jackie Izzo v. M. A. Henry Co., Inc., et al.* was scheduled to begin in the US District Court for the Southern District of New York, the Hon. Vincent L. Leibell presiding. When he called the case, the lawyers informed him it had settled for $97,500.[3] He asked about the child's injuries. The lawyers noted they were terrific; her suffering had been awful. Burned in July 1944, when she was six years old, both her legs had been amputated at the hips. She had been in the hospital and "practically at death's door for a period of two or three years." But she had, as one of the lawyers for Jackie noted, "made a remarkable recovery, so to speak." She would never be able to be fitted with prosthetics, but he assured the court, "there is no suffering at the present time" and "the prospects of life to the child is good." "She has become quite happy in her predicament."[4]

Judge Leibell asked if he was "to pass on the sufficiency of the settlement." Lawyers on both sides of the case quickly responded, no. They explained that the Michigan probate court where the family was from would do that as well as approving attorney's fees. But one of the defendants' lawyers suggested it would be good to have the judge's approval of the settlement: "I mean I would not like anything to be left open so that there was any question about it being a valid and final settlement," he said.[5] When the judge noted that if the case went before a jury, the award would likely be higher than this settlement, the Izzos' Michigan lawyer quickly responded, "That is, if we recovered."[6] The defendants' lawyers joined him. As one noted, "it would lie on my conscience if I did not accept the settlement that has been offered here," thereby subjecting the child to the uncertainty of a jury trial.[7] Gene Autry's lawyer, William Martin, added, "I think we all have more or less the same feeling, as we have tried to look at this just as though it were one of our own youngsters, so that I think this child is being dealt with as well or better than a number of these unfortunate children."[8] As they talked, Jackie Izzo and her parents waited in a hotel room a short distance from the courthouse. Prepared to come to court, they were not called. Accepting the lawyers' assurances, Judge Leibell approved the settlement. Only later would he learn how much of that settlement had gone to the lawyers.

While many families, like the Izzos, learned they might have a legal claim through the AP story reporting the McCormack verdict, others had learned earlier, and by January 1948 there were dozens of lawsuits involving children burned in Gene Autry cowboy suits from across the United States pending in state and federal court in New York, with dates on jury trial calendars looming. Before the *McCormack* verdict, the defendants had refused to settle. The verdict changed the calculus. Joint and several liability meant a plaintiff could collect a damage award in its entirety from any one of the defendants that had been found liable. If one defendant was insolvent or harder to collect from, the plaintiff could collect the award in full from any of the others.[9]

By settling, the defendants could bargain among themselves as to who would pay what and avoid the uncertainties and sympathies of juries. The defendants also understood that the parents, desperately in need of money to pay for their children's past and ongoing medical care, would accept the trade-off of less in settlement now rather than risk the delay and uncertainty of a trial and appeal. After all, the McCormacks might end up with nothing. And so long as the *McCormack* appeal was pending, the defendants argued that their liability remained undecided as a matter of law. The cowboy suit litigation would continue for another six years, but in that time no other case involving the principal defendants and any of the injured or dead children would go to trial. The only additional case tried was one brought by a Maryland retailer to recover against the principal defendants the amounts it had paid in judgments to three families who had brought suit against the retailer in state court.[10]

Settlement became the order of the day. But the defendants were not in a rush. Time was money. In every case, both plaintiffs and defendants demanded a jury trial.[11] Plaintiffs hoped for a jury of their peers or at least a bargaining tool for settlement. Defendants bought time: cases that languished, children who died in the wait for their case to come up for trial, liability determinations postponed or avoided altogether, settlements delayed, plaintiffs pressed by need, worried that the money would run out, settling for less. Whether in state or federal court, the wait for a bench trial was long, the wait for a jury trial longer. The defendants settled, as in *Izzo*, only when a trial date was imminent. The defendants' lawyers were skilled at their craft. Every case had a price. And as they understood, "pricing the priceless child" would cost them in aggregate in settlements a small fraction of the cost of going to trial, as families competed for what was treated as a limited pool of money.[12] This was the price of settlement.

The first settlements came within months of the *McCormack* verdict, before the Izzos had even filed suit. Billy Greatorex, burned from his shoes to his waist at age six in April 1944, the third-degree burns fully encircling both legs and his buttocks, was among the boys included in the Washington, DC, papers' coverage in April 1945.[13] With Edmond Butler and Robert Lynch representing them, his parents filed suit in October 1946. Their case became the first to settle after the *McCormack* verdict. The settlement: $28,000.[14] Three more settlements came in quick succession. The family of John Wrobbel, burned at age seven in Lancaster, New York, settled for $7,500. Three days later, Billy Weatherell Jr.'s family settled for $39,000.[15] Tommy Habina's parents settled on April 16, 1948, for $33,000. Tommy was now eight years old. Thick scar tissue limited the range of motion in his knees so that he walked with difficulty, had scars from burns and grafts from his ankles to his neck, and close to four years after being burned had unhealed "deep ulcerations" remaining on both of his knees and ankles.[16]

Because these cases involved children, settlements had to be approved by a court to be legally valid. Judge John C. Knox, chief judge in the US District Court for the Southern District of New York, oversaw more settlements in the cowboy suit litigation than any other judge. The month after the *McCormack* verdict, Judge Knox called a collective pre-trial hearing in the cases pending in the federal court. Two weeks later, he asked the parties to waive their demand for a jury trial—all but two did—and then he consolidated the twenty-one cases before him with a "trial" date of May 17 and ordered each plaintiff's counsel to provide a statement of the child's injuries and the related medical expenses.

When Judge Knox opened what was in effect not a trial but a consolidated settlement proceeding on May 17, 1948, his courtroom was crowded with men.[17] There were lawyers for the twenty-one plaintiffs.[18] And though there were far fewer defendants, there may have been even more men in the courtroom representing them: their own and their insurers' lawyers, as well as insurance adjustors. The cases before the court involved children injured in 1944, 1945, and 1946. Timme and Woonsocket had both been insured by Traveler's for all three years, but the Henry Company had different coverage for each year, and so the number of men in the room multiplied. It made for a strange trial. No witnesses sworn, no evidence introduced. Only lawyers, insurance adjustors, capsule summaries of the boys' injuries and related expenses prepared by their lawyers, a few photographs, a court reporter, and the judge. His goal was not to try these cases but to create the conditions that fostered settlements. And he was proud of the work he did. Pre-trial hearings were his stopgap solution to what he referred to as "the dreadful congestion" in the federal district courts.[19] Several years later, at a meeting of the Superior Courts Committee of the Association of the Bar, he noted with pride his work in the pre-trial settlement of a number of the cowboy suit cases. That his assessment was defendant-focused was made clear by his explanation that the settlements had saved the litigants time, a great deal of money, and adverse publicity.[20]

Within the first few minutes of the consolidated settlement proceedings before Judge Knox in May 1948, four settlements were announced. A lawyer would call out the plaintiff's last name—as in "The Wilks case is settled"—and then the lawyers would note the total settlement, what portion would go to the parents for medical expenses, what portion to the child, who among the defendants was paying how much, and the amount from the settlement for the plaintiffs' lawyers' contingent fee.[21] In lulls in the announcement of settlements, Judge Knox would ask whether any other cases had settled, grant a recess or take a late start to a day to give the lawyers time to settle additional cases, ask lawyers to split the difference where they were close to agreement, or agree to talk in chambers where the parties were at an impasse. There were moments when Judge Knox suggested that he thought the "asking price" for a case was reasonable, and a case in which he knocked $10,000 off the plaintiff's asking price, but not once in the proceedings did he suggest, much less demand, that a settlement be higher. By the end of four days of hearings all but one of the consolidated cases had settled. It was one of two cases in which the plaintiff had not waived their demand for a jury trial. The family's lawyer asked if they might try the case right then. Judge Knox's response was immediate: "Not before a jury . . . [I]f you want to go before a jury there is not the slightest hope of getting a disposition soon."[22]

The consolidated proceedings before Judge Knox in May 1948 made clear any number of things that otherwise would have remained in shadow. In the opening minutes of the proceedings, the Henry Company's lawyer said, "We have, as your Honor knows, a certain amount of money available." He was referring to the Henry Company, but the view governed the entire cowboy suit litigation. There is nothing in the law that limits a defendant's liability to its insurance coverage, but in these cases everyone, judges included, in effect adopted that coverage as a limit as far as the money could be stretched. And so, insurance adjustors speaking on behalf of one of these defendants could say in the discussion of a case, "This is not an endless chain as far as the money is concerned. We have a number of suits in this policy period and there is just so much money."[23] And announcing the settlement of a 1945 case, the plaintiff's lawyer noted that they had been informed that the Henry Company's insurance was exhausted for that year, and so Timme's and Woonsocket's insurer would be paying the full amount.[24] Even where a given defendant did not contribute to a settlement, they were included in the general release the plaintiffs signed, barring any further legal claims.[25] Nor was the issue of insurance limits related to the Henry Company alone. Other defendants too disputed the division of particular settlements, arguing that "our money isn't going to hold out for these other cases."[26]

Our money—meaning, in fact, the limits of their insurance coverage. And so, insurance became part of the facts of a case. "What are the facts in this case?" Judge Knox asked the group assembled in one of their many conversations in chambers. The family's lawyer, Edmond Butler, explained, "This is a different insurance coverage. It was in 1946 that the accident happened." Debates over insurance and the money left in a policy ran through the proceedings before Judge Knox; ran through, in fact, the cowboy suit litigation as a whole.[27] Settlements became negotiations with insurance company lawyers and adjustors who knew, as they put it, what they could get from the home office and what they could not and about how much they wanted to spend on each of these cases.[28] Each settlement reflected negotiations in the shadow of the law between the lawyers and, often, insurance adjustors, representing the parties to a case.[29]

Insurance limits meant that the year in which a child had been injured took on new weight. It made competitors of families. It pushed them to take the money offered in fear that holding out for more risked their getting nothing. As Edmond Butler noted at one point in the consolidated proceedings, "The father said to me he was not wealthy enough to gamble when he was offered $58,000."[30] But for most families the offer was far lower, and they took it. "It was necessary to seriously consider the settlement and adjustment of this case," one family's lawyer noted, "before the insurance coverage was exhausted by other judgments or payments in settlement therefor."[31] Some such statement was a recurring refrain in parents' and plaintiffs' lawyer's affidavits seeking approval of a settlement in these cases.[32]

The defendants understood that fear of the money running out drove these families to accept less. They used it against the families. I suspect too that some plaintiffs' lawyers used this fear to get their clients to accept what had been offered. Guaranteed a percentage by way of a contingent fee of whatever settlement was reached, they too had an interest in taking the money on the table.[33] The families' and lawyers' fears had grounding in fact. By the time of the consolidated hearing before Judge Knox, the Henry Company's insurance for some years was already exhausted. Timme was left carrying the weight of settlements. By 1949, Timme's insurance coverage for children burned in 1944 was exhausted, and by 1950, their coverage for 1945 cases was exhausted. Woonsocket, which had escaped from some settlements, was close behind. By the time some families brought suit, the defendants' insurance coverage for the year their child was injured was already exhausted.[34] And for children burned in 1948 and after, none of the principal defendants had any insurance at all.

Insurance coverage mattered for another reason: The M. A. Henry Company was barely solvent by spring 1948. When Judge Knox asked why the Henry Company was not contributing to the settlement of a 1945 case announced in the third day of the consolidated proceedings, the family's lawyer told the judge, "He has got no money."[35] In a case settled on the final day of the hearing, the lawyer for the Henry Company's wholly owned subsidiary in Newark, New Jersey, noted that with the company's insurance for 1945 exhausted, other cases from the year still pending, and its assets limited, it could only afford to make a nominal contribution of $250.[36] He would repeat this litany for each of the final three cases settled in the proceedings.[37] Solvency is a tricky business in companies where the principal assets are often intangibles including a founder's name, reputation, and contact list. And so it was here. Milton Henry continued in the business of children's novelty goods under new corporate names, but the M. A. Henry Company became an empty shell.

With the fear of the Henry Company's insolvency and of the money running out, plaintiffs' lawyers might threaten to take their chances at trial, but everyone in every one of these negotiations knew that they could not, would not, take the risk.[38] Waiting for a jury trial meant more time would pass, and any verdict for the plaintiff would be appealed, and so more time would pass. Any family going to trial, moreover, risked the possibility of a verdict against the Henry Company alone and so the possibility of recovering nothing at all. That fear benefited Timme and Woonsocket as much as it did the Henry Company. The risk of ending up empty-handed was too high. Parents and lawyers in their affidavits in support of settlement said all these things. And so, plaintiffs' lawyers pressed for what they could get and convinced their clients to take what was offered.[39]

What they could get, or from the defendants' perspective what they would pay, depended not just on the child's injuries or other important facts in the case but on what might be called the money in the case. And the money in the case depended on not only the year in which the child had been injured and how much remained in the principal defendants' insurance coverage for that year, but also on whether a major national retailer was named as a defendant. Many of the cowboy suits had been bought from small, local businesses that only a separate lawsuit by the plaintiffs in the local jurisdiction could reach. And at least some families brought lawsuits against such retailers.[40] But these small, local concerns were often also the kinds of individually owned businesses that had short lives. By the time many families discovered they had a legal claim, the retailer was no longer in business, the owner retired, impossible to locate, even dead.[41]

Even larger, national chains with stores in New York could sometimes wriggle out of a case. One of the legal claims that families had against retailers was for breach of warranty, but that required a direct contract relationship—"privity of contract"—between the injured person and the retailer. Though retailers sometimes argued that there was no privity where a mother had purchased the cowboy suit for her child, most courts treated the nuclear family as a single unit for purposes of privity.[42] But where the cowboy suit had been purchased by a grandparent, an aunt or uncle, or a family friend, or where it had been a hand-me-down from a neighbor, the lack of privity gave the retailer an out from contributing to any settlement.[43]

Making the most of the money that was not in other cases became a principle in settling. Discussing the case of Charles Stultz Jr. in Judge

Knox's chambers in the May 1948 consolidated hearing, Edmond Butler explained that "there [wa]sn't any money in Henry's policy" and that there was only a "small amount available from Gene Autry." That meant it again came down to the retailer, H. L. Green, and Timme and Woonsocket.[44] Butler's price for the case was $18,000. When the lawyer for the retailer H. L. Green said, "We have a top of $3,000 and that is all there is," Butler responded that he would show it was negligence for the retailer to have sold the suit and then collect the full judgment from them: "It is only because I want to save the money from the others and not because I have anything against you or H. L. Green, but the proper way for us to handle it is to take the money that isn't in any other case."[45]

This argument worked until spring 1949, when the money in the case, in this sense, went down. In early March, *Lutz v. Henry, et al.* went to trial in the Southern District of New York. The question at stake was whether a retailer who had sold one of these cowboy suits and had to pay a judgment to a family had a right to what was called a "claim over" against the principal defendants—that is, the right to be reimbursed by them. When first sued by the families of Cecil Warnick, James Detrick, and Robert Flesher in 1946 and 1947, Louis P. and Ida K. Lutz, who owned and operated Lou's Auto Stores in Cumberland, Maryland, had notified the Henry Company, Timme, and Woonsocket. None of the three had bothered to respond. Louis and Ida Lutz were held liable to the families in all three cases. The Lutzes then brought suit in the US District Court for the Southern District of New York against the principal defendants to recover their losses. The money at stake—the amount of the state court judgments in Warnick, Detrick, and Flesher, plus interest ($24,931.69)—was less important than what the result would mean for the litigation as a whole. To that point, retailers, especially large national chains, had been pressed to and had contributed to a number of settlements. The jury in *Lutz* held that the Henry Company, Timme, and Woonsocket were liable to retailers in these cases.[46]

While only a trial court decision, *Lutz* gave retailers new grounds for resisting pressure to contribute to settlements, and they took advantage of it. "Is the Hecht Company a defendant here?" Judge Knox asked in a 1950 settlement hearing of a boy burned in 1944. Timme's lawyer replied that although they were, "they are not present because they will not pay." The cowboy suit had been purchased from the Hecht store on 14th Street in New York City. But John Zibor Jr.'s mother, with no reason to know or anticipate the legal consequences of asking this simple favor, had asked her sister, who worked for the telephone company on 14th Street, if she would buy the cowboy suit for her. As Timme's lawyer explained to the court, Hecht's insurer took the position that they were not liable on warranty because there was no privity, and if held liable in negligence, they had a right to recover from the principal defendants—and so they refused to contribute to the settlement at all.[47] "Realizing these things," Timme's lawyer explained, "we discussed it frankly with Mr. Zibor and agreed that $17,500 would be a fair settlement." "Well," said Judge Knox, "I would like to see this boy get more money, but I don't know that it devolves upon me to interfere if you feel that that is the best you can do." With the family's lawyer confirming that they couldn't get more without going to trial, Judge Knox approved the settlement.[48] "How much money is this boy getting?" he asked. The answer was $8,369.02.[49]

The decision in *Lutz* was important for a second reason relating to the money in the case. Between 1940 and 1945, Du Pont had sold to Woonsocket, through Timme, over three million pounds of viscose rayon thread. The mill had woven that thread into the fluffy fabric that the Henry Company used on the chaps of the Gene Autry cowboy suit.[50] But Du Pont was not named as a defendant in the McCormack case. It was first named as a defendant in a suit filed in October 1947.[51] It became a party more generally in many cases in the litigation through the Henry Company impleading it as a third-party defendant in pending cases beginning in April and May 1948 and in cases filed in later years.[52] Du Pont's legal counsel, Harold Medina, from the white-shoe New York firm of Cravath, Swaine & Moore, was among the lawyers in the consolidated proceedings before Judge Knox in May and early June 1948.[53] But though covered by the general releases signed in those cases, Du Pont did not contribute to any of the settlements.[54]

At the end of the evidence in the Lutz case, on Du Pont's motion, the judge dismissed Du Pont from the action on the merits from all claims in the case.[55] Du Pont's defense was simple, brilliant, and wrong. As Harold Medina would describe Du Pont's position the following week to Judge Leibell in the Izzo settlement hearing, explaining why Du Pont was not contributing to the Izzo settlement, "We are in the same position as the cotton grower. We made rayon thread, and that is the only connection with the case."[56] The company whose corporate tagline was "Better Things for Better Living Through Chemistry" erased here the chemistry, the years of research and testing, the long-term relationships with manufacturers that went into transforming cellulose fibers into a rich array of rayon threads, each carefully designed to be woven into fabrics with particular properties, including the plush fabric purchased by the Henry Company used in the Gene Autry cowboy suits. Du Pont's argument took a twentieth-century fiber produced with twentieth-century chemical processes and rebranded it as akin to a cotton boll and Du Pont as akin to the cotton farmer. But as importantly, though Du Pont had produced a fiber that it knew was inflammable and that was produced to be woven into just the kind of high-pile fabric manufactured by the Woonsocket Falls Mill, Du Pont could argue that it was not liable for a second reason: Timme and Woonsocket knew the yarn was inflammable, as was the pile fabric woven from it. As Harold Medina told Judge Liebell, "There can be no liability as against Du Pont."[57] That Timme's and Woonsocket's lawyer backed Du Pont up in this case, and never filed a cross-claim against Du Pont, is puzzling only if one does not consider their relationship.[58] Timme and Woonsocket needed Du Pont: Woonsocket's only business was making pile fabrics. They understood that they would be doing business with Du Pont long after the last of these cases settled. That Du Pont was not held to account highlights yet another injustice in the narrative of the money for settlements being exhausted.[59]

In a settlement context in which the plaintiffs competed for a limited pool of money, children who died were compared to children who had survived. Robert Flesher was burned in 1945 when he was eight years old. He died a year and a half later, never having left the hospital. Edmond Butler represented the Fleshers. Using the amount awarded by the jury for the pain and suffering of Tommy McCormack, who had died five months after being burned, Butler argued that his "price" of $25,000 for the Flesher case was actually low. "Well, I don't know," Judge Knox said, "I have no doubt that the boy suffered the torments of the damned, but each of these other boys suffered a lot of pain and suffering, too." He commented that the boy's father had recovered the medical expenses in an independent suit against the retailer in Maryland and there were other families who had not gotten anything yet. "The rest are alive with the possibility of a breakdown," the judge noted, adding, "There is nothing in the world that can benefit the kid and I don't know whether his father, in view of the entire situation, ought to get that recovery for his pain and suffering or not. I am inclined to doubt it." The defendants quickly joined the judge.[60] "What is the least that you think you can with propriety accept?" Judge Knox asked Butler. When Butler suggested possibly $20,000, the judge said, "Ask them if they will take fifteen thousand dollars.... This money that is paid here," he explained, "might go to the benefit of other children." When Butler informed the judge the next day that the family would, on his recommendation, take $15,000, but that "they were somewhat reluctant," Judge Knox said, "I do not want to force them to take it." But the choice was clear: Take $15,000 in settlement or go to trial. Taking what was offered in settlement or going to trial took most of the volition out of "it is voluntary on their part."[61]

Families who had a child who died in one of these incidents may well have accepted lower settlements rather than go to trial in hopes of putting some element of the nightmare behind them. For families whose burned child had survived, immediate financial need drove them to take what was offered. The defendants understood this need too. It had been part of their calculus from the start. For the vast majority of families, years passed before they knew they had a legal claim—an ignorance the defendants had contributed to—years in which families shouldered the financial and emotional cost of these injuries themselves, sinking more deeply into debt as they spent any limited savings they had, took on second jobs, or in the case of mothers, quit jobs to care for their injured child, took out loans, borrowed money, and depended on the generosity of relatives, friends, neighbors, and strangers.

Filing suit brought no immediate relief. It had taken two and one-half years to reach a jury trial in *McCormack*. Following the *McCormack* verdict, the defendants, in one case after another, challenged plaintiffs' motions in both state and federal court to move cases up on the trial calendar.[62] They argued that families who were not New York residents were not entitled to consideration for a "preference," that families were not truly at risk of becoming public charges, that it was unfair to other cases on the court's docket, that it was inequitable "merely because this boy has been seriously injured" to give a case preference on the calendar over other cowboy suit cases, when "in the normal course of events" the case would not come up for trial for two years.[63]

In the normal course of events none of these children would have been burned; they and their parents would not have been before the court. Responding to the defendants' challenge to a preference in the Caparco case, Edmond Butler argued that the family was not at risk of becoming public charges, that they had already been rendered public charges by the defendants' wrongful acts. Moreover, the defendants well knew that a preference was not about this case—or any of these cases—taking a court's trial time or being set ahead of other pending cowboy suit cases. Every cowboy suit case that had come up for trial since the McCormack verdict had settled, "and there is not the slightest doubt in our minds," Butler assured the court in *Caparco*, that if a preference were granted here, the boy's and father's suit too would settle. A preference was needed to force the defendants to the settlement table to meet this family's desperate financial need in their effort to save their child's life. "This plaintiff," Edmond Butler argued of Perry Caparco, "is in such a precarious physical condition that delay is desired by the defendants, apparently because they feel he may die before this case could be tried in the normal course of events."[64]

The court in *Caparco* approved the motion for a preference, as did the courts in every case following the *McCormack* verdict where a preference was sought. Still, there is something appalling about defendants that have caused a child's suffering resisting a motion to move a case up on the trial calendar. The contrast with the response of others who had had no hand in the wrong is striking: hospitals and doctors treated the child regardless of the family's ability to pay; community members and fraternal organizations scraped together funds to cover necessary surgeries, hospitalization, and rehabilitation; parents, relatives, and strangers prayed for, and gave the blood and skin from their own bodies to save, a child's life. How different the valuing of the worth of a life.

When the defendants talked about cases out of the hearing of judges and the plaintiffs and their lawyers, what they described as bad, heavy, or dangerous cases were not ones in which a child had died of his injuries but cases in which a grievously injured child had survived, including children seriously burned after all the defendants incontestably knew of the hazard.[65] What made the case of an injured child who survived heavier than the child who died was in part the expense of future medical and life support that a child who survived might require. But it was more than this. A dead child could not be brought into court; a child who had survived could. As Edmond Butler said to the defendants in one of the cases consolidated before Judge Knox, "I can assure you of this: We bring this kid into court, we show the burns, and if we get a verdict it is not going to be $15,000."[66] As trial dates loomed, the defendants worked in settlement negotiations not just to settle heavy cases to avoid a jury trial but also to ensure that a child be kept away from a settlement hearing, if there was one, or even from the judge's chambers or the court building itself. So, for example, in the Izzo case, one of the specific points of negotiation for the defendants was an assurance that Jackie Izzo would be kept at the hotel, as they feared the adverse attention and publicity her appearance in court would produce.[67]

As the defendants' efforts to keep these children out of court suggests, settlements were important to the defendants for another reason: They were a means of keeping news of a case out of the press. Verdicts produced AP stories; settlements could be kept quiet and sealed. In the opening minutes and again at the end of the Izzo settlement hearing before Judge

Leibell, the defendants asked that the settlement proceedings and case file be sealed. When news of the settlement was announced in the Michigan papers, it was under the headline "Damage Suit Ends in Sealed Pact." The terms of the settlement, the article noted, "were not disclosed." The file had been sealed, it explained, at the request of the manufacturers of the cloth "to prevent publicity which might bring 'unfounded claims' against them."[68]

Maybe the defendants in fact worried about "unfounded claims," but they used this pretext, and judges' concern with their own overcrowded dockets, to protect themselves against their real fear: adverse publicity and legitimate claims that had yet to be filed.[69] The Izzos were a powerful example for the defendants of the perils of publicity and the benefits of secrecy. The Izzos had only learned they had a claim through the AP story of the *McCormack* verdict. But even here the delay benefited the defendants because the statute of limitations had run on any claim by Jackie's parents. Dozens of cowboy suit case settlements were sealed at the defendants' request. All with the plaintiff's approval.[70] In every case in which the defendants requested a file be sealed, whether state or federal, the court approved the request without question.[71] The plaintiffs' lawyers' interest in securing a settlement for their client bought their agreement.

Three weeks after the settlement in *Izzo*, the appeal in *McCormack* was decided. As Autry's lawyer, William Martin, explained in a letter to Autry's agent, the verdict had been upheld against all the defendants.[72] The decision meant that the argument the defendants had successfully used as leverage in so many settlements—that is, that their liability had not been decided as a matter of law—was no longer a viable argument.[73] But he suggested that the appellate judge's order to reduce damages for pain and suffering by half, to $30,000, offered some solace.[74] I think of solace in this tragedy in terms of the children who survived despite grievous injury. There was no solace for the families, like the McCormacks, who lost a child. Faced with accepting the court's order or a new trial on the question of damages, the McCormack family surely felt no solace. But like all the other families here, they accepted the money on the table, as the court and defendants no doubt expected they would.

Every case in this litigation involved burns from a Gene Autry cowboy suit with the fuzzy, highly combustible fabric on the chaps. But it was only in spring 1945 that the defendants were put on notice that children had been injured and some had died. In this sense, although children burned after April 1945 were wearing the same cowboy suit as those burned earlier, their injury was not the same. There were children burned all through the year 1945, and though the numbers of children burned in succeeding years grew smaller with significantly diminished sales of the suit with the hazardous fabric, children were burned in 1946, 1947, 1948, 1949, and as late even as 1951 and 1952.

"Late cases" was the moniker the defendants gave to cases of children burned especially in 1947 and after. Even before the *McCormack* appeal was decided, the defendants shifted their approach to late cases: Investigate quickly and quietly. If possible, settle before the family takes the question to a lawyer. Where a local lawyer is already involved, work with him. Hope he can be interested in a quick settlement. If possible, keep the case out of New York by submitting to a local court's jurisdiction for approval of a settlement. A local judge won't know the whole picture. All these things will reduce the price of a settlement. And so, for example, on November 30, 1948, the Henry Company, Timme, Woonsocket, and Gene Autry submitted to the jurisdiction of the Court of Common Pleas in Lehigh, Pennsylvania, for one purpose: to open and close the legal claim of William E. Pritchard Jr., a boy burned in spring 1947 from his ankles to his waist, with the burns on his right hip so deep that they exposed the bone.[75]

One dramatic difference between a trial and settlement is that of the absence of confrontation and witness. Settlement meant that the principals never had to explain their actions and subsequent failure to act in front of the families who bore the consequences. Apart from the McCormack case, the defendants in these cases never saw or heard firsthand what their actions and inaction had done to these children and their families' lives.

The pre-trial depositions of mothers and fathers, neighbors and strangers, doctors and nurses, those who had witnessed the child ablaze, smothered the flames, worked to save a child's life, or tried to soothe their torment, were heard only by the defendants' lawyers, who listened with an ear for facts that would limit their clients' liability. Helen DiTrapani was deposed before a notary public in the offices of the lawyer for the retailer the Hecht Company on July 11, 1946, two months after the first anniversary of the death of her five-year-old son Marco Antonio, "Tony." "Mrs. Ditrapani, do you understand the purpose of this hearing?" the attorney for Hecht began. "In order to make sure you do," and then he explained their right to interrogate her about anything related to the case. She described hearing her child calling her, discovering him in flames, running across the yard, and lying on him to smother the flames. The questioning continued about when and by whom the cowboy suit was bought, what were its elements, when exactly her son had been burned, how long he had "lingered in the hospital before he died." And in her answers to these questions, the lawyer for Hecht heard that there was no privity of contract, and hence no claim against the retailer for breach of warranty, because the cowboy suit had been purchased by her sister-in-law. And the defendants' lawyers collectively started calculating whether in fact the lawsuit was barred entirely by the statute of limitations because it had not been brought within a year of the child's death.[76] The case settled on the first day of the consolidated proceedings before Judge Knox for $5,000, garnering something in settlement only because of a dispute as to the boy's date of death between the hospital records and the death certificate.[77]

The defendants' lawyers listened to pre-trial depositions calculating the risks or plusses parents or others posed as a witness in a potential trial. After attending the deposition of one boy's mother in September 1950, Gene Autry's Los Angeles counsel sent a report to William Martin. The Ulick boy had been burned five years earlier, and in the years since, his mother had worked tirelessly to save her child's life and return him to health. She described carrying him to three hospitals before finding one that could treat him, desperately calling friends to give blood plasma for her son, a year of washing out sheets filthy with pus. He did not quite say that she milked the story for all its drama, but his words came close to that. He described her testimony as emotional and convincing. And whether in fact she had washed out a dozen sheets a day for more than a couple of days, he noted that she clearly believed now that it had been for a year. What he heard in this mother's story of her effort to save her son's life was that if the case went to trial, she would be an excellent witness for the plaintiff and a dangerous witness for the defendants. They should try to find a way to not have her testify, or better still, to settle the case.[78]

Whether the parents had anticipated it or not, in the course of these cases, their children themselves became exhibits. Photographs have been used in legal proceedings in the United States and England since the mid-nineteenth century, but the first major treatise on photography as evidence in courts of law was not published until 1942, the same year the first children were burned in Gene Autry cowboy suits.[79] The first telethons produced by national disability-related charities made children the center of their televised fundraising spectacles, "the suffering of innocent children" especially powerful as a fundraising tool.[80] But charity was not the point of these photographs passed among lawyers, insurance adjustors, and judges. They were proof. But proof of what? Injury, disability, the permanence of scars, the need for continuing and future medical care. Past, present, and future written on these children's bodies—or so the photographs suggested.

Photographs that I have shared in chapters focused on the injuries them-

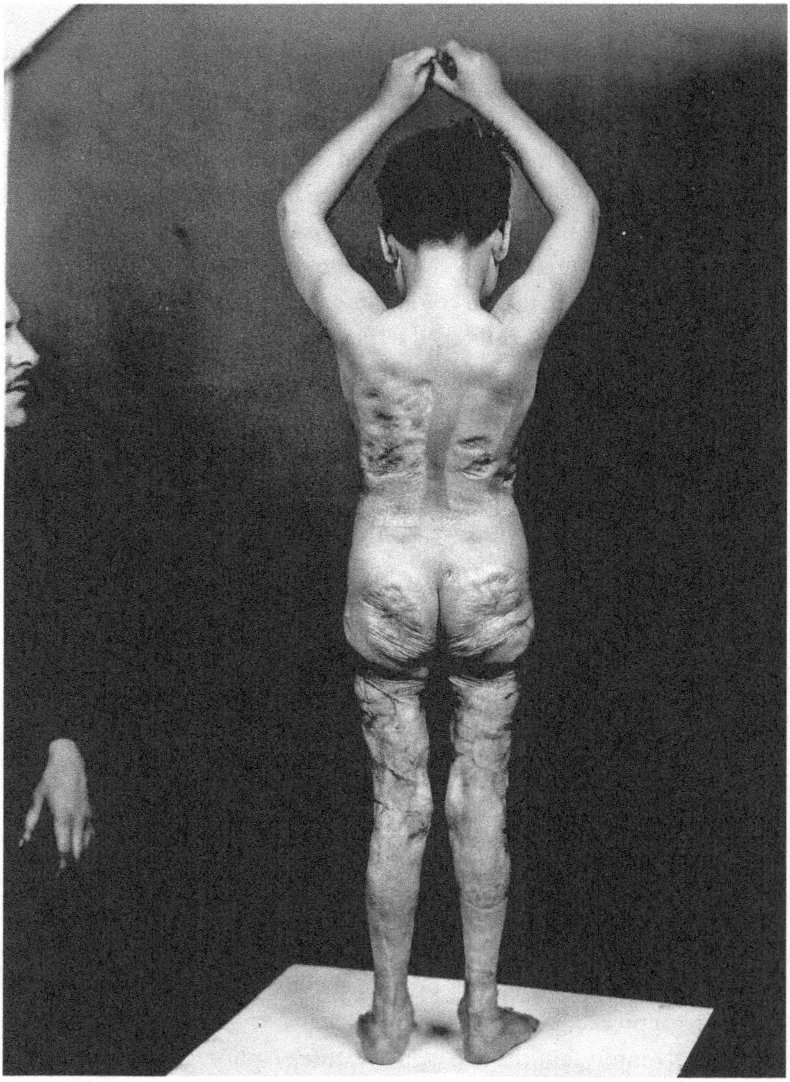

selves and their impact on families' lives—photographs like those of Perry Caparco, naked in a wheelchair, only a small cloth covering his crotch, or Richard Szumita, lying naked on a hospital bed—began as evidence. Who was the man captured at the edge of the frame of photographs of Roy Cizek? The child standing naked, his arms raised high over his head.[81] Had there been more trials in this litigation, the photos and the children themselves would have been more exposed, more public.

There were cases where the photographs showed only the portion of a child's body that had been burned. But most included the child's full body and face.[82] Many children's burns extended to their buttocks and sometimes penis and scrotum. For almost all the children, their torsos were the sites where skin was harvested to re-cover their legs, and so their torsos too were important evidence of the injuries the children had suffered. But including a child's face in these photographs was about more than establishing identity. It called on emotions: sympathy, anger, outrage. It attested that this was a person, and that, if he survived, he would carry these injuries and scars through life.

In many cases the photos were not filed with the court, and so one is left to imagine what the parties and judges saw. The answer to the judge's question, "How badly hurt was this boy?" might be that the insurance company had "the pictures"—suggesting that the settlement reflected the extent of the injuries and that the judge did not need to further concern himself with its adequacy.[83] In others, the judge had the photos in hand. "A kid that is scarred up something like that," Judge Knox said as he held a photograph of one boy, "he is going to get married some day and the effect of those scars on his wife is something to take into account, and his own humiliation from it." Contemplating the photograph, the judge voiced his support for Butler's asking price of $25,000. When the defendants began to bicker, Judge Knox responded bluntly, "I don't know anything about your liability, but I should say that you would do well to settle the case in view of what is here."[84]

In the same hearing, Butler's co-counsel handed the judge photographs "taken last week" of another boy, Cecil D'Wayne Warnick, who had been burned at age six on May 13, 1945. He was now almost ten. Butler insisted that he himself had not seen the photos before this. "I say to your Honor that I put a price on the case of $55,000 and I don't know whether in conscience I can recommend it." Looking at the photos of the boy, Judge Knox asked, "Do these doctors think that this boy will get back a fairly natural contour to his legs?" "No, I think not," was Butler's reply. "That was a horrible thing," Judge Knox said, adding, "I don't think your asking price on this is out of the way at all." When pressed by the defendants, Butler noted, "I don't think in conscience that I can come down a nickel." In fact, he added, "if I had seen these pictures the price, the minimum price for the boy, would have been $75,000, and then I would be saying to you that I wouldn't take a cent less."[85]

What did it say when a boy's lawyer could hesitate on the "price" he had asked for a case because until that moment, he had "never seen the pictures, and reading the doctor's testimony I would never have envisioned him as he is"?[86] He was, perhaps, working the defendants, making the case for his "price" of $55,000 by saying now it should be $75,000. But there is something more in his statement: Most of these cases were decided on paper records, a doctor's affidavit as to the character of the child's injuries and what they likely meant for his future. No judge, much less a jury, ever saw most of these children, not even a photograph.

No one questioned what having these photos taken felt like to the children who were made to appear in their underwear or naked in the presence of men in suits they did not know. Or what it felt like to the few children who were "produced" in court. Jack Lockhart, over sixty years later, remembered driving to New York with Elmer Groefsema, the Lockharts' Michigan lawyer, and another boy and both their fathers to appear before Judge Knox. He remembered the glossy wood in the courtroom and being taken into chambers with his father and the lawyers and asked to "drop my pants." We "weren't in there long, just a few minutes." "Do you remember how you felt about that?" I asked. He had gone through life showing his legs to no one. "Well, I never liked to show my legs to anybody, you know, but because it's adults telling me to do it, I did it, you know."[87]

Other boys, now old men, echoed Jack Lockhart's memory of being a child having to obey adults because they were adults, forced to expose what they voluntarily showed no one. "Talk about embarrassed," Gaither Bates recalled, as the memory washed over him. It had been so painful that it remained buried in his memory until my questions about whether he had appeared in court dislodged it some sixty-eight years after the fact. "I completely forgot about that." "Do you remember the judge being kind in that moment? Or recognizing that you might feel embarrassed?" I asked. "No, I mean, I was so embarrassed. I mean, you kind of draw in. And wonder when it's going to be over."[88]

Judges had the final responsibility in these cases; their approval of the settlements was required by law. But few of the children ever appeared even in a judge's chambers. Most settlements were approved on the basis of pretrial hearings, with only the lawyers for the parties present or, more commonly still, simply on the basis of affidavits of the plaintiffs' lawyer noting the settlement agreed to by the parties, and supported by an affidavit of the child's guardian, generally a parent, and a doctor. Early in the final order in many cases was some version of the following: "It appearing from the record before me and the testimony of the doctors and the photographs of the infant herein which are submitted with this application that it would be extremely detrimental to the health and welfare of said infant to require that he be transported from . . . to appear before me" or, more simply, "the Court having waived the production of the infant plaintiff and his father . . ."[89] Judges, keen to lessen the pressure on their dockets, comforting themselves that families were getting something, simply accepted plaintiffs' lawyers' descriptions and doctors' affidavits of a child's injuries, current condition, and likely future.

By the mid-1950s, the defendants had settled at least a hundred cases involving children burned in Gene Autry cowboy suits. There were late cases, unsettled cases from earlier years, and lawsuits for incidents from earlier years that would only be brought in the 1950s. The patterns held, now well-worn. The defendants capitalized on every weakness in a plaintiff's case; fought among themselves as to who would pay how much; settled pending cases only when trial loomed; worried that courts might, on learning the whole story, demand more from them; and, celebrated when they got out of a case with a cheap settlement.[90]

Having asked parents to do the impossible work of valuing their children's lives and futures, turning their children into exhibits, the parents' calculations were crudely discounted in ways that had nothing to do with the families and children's losses.[91] Law paved the way for differences. Wrongful death laws meant that a cause of action in these cases survived death, but it was still cheaper for a wrongdoer when a child died than survived. The jury that awarded $60,000 for Tommy McCormack's pain and suffering awarded only $3,500 for the child's wrongful death. The average settlement in death cases was $10,000 less than the average in cases of children who survived.[92] Short statutes of limitation for wrongful death cases meant the statute had run and the action was barred before many of these families, especially those of children burned in the early years, even knew they had a legal claim. And, finally, it was cheaper for the defendants when a child died, because many of these families did not pursue a legal claim at all.

Most families who learned in time that they had a legal claim and found their way to lawyers who pursued their claim received something in settlement. A handful led to large settlements: the case of Scott Timberlake, with a settlement of $88,000; of Jackie Izzo, which settled for $97,500; of Perry Caparco, which settled for $100,000; and of Roy Cizek, with a settlement of $180,000.[93] Settlements in most cases, though, were much lower. The average was just over $26,500.[94] But families did not receive averages. In the twenty settlements announced in the four-day proceedings before Judge Knox in spring 1948, the settlements ranged from $58,000 down to $3,600.[95] The "average" settlement would be lower still if one added in all the instances of families who received nothing—their lawsuits barred by statutes of limitations—and the families who never brought lawsuits at all.

Even among children who survived, the settlements were never only or even primarily about the severity of a child's injuries. The defendants had consistently worked to get out of cases for as little as they could, and that amount depended as much and sometimes more on factors other than the severity of a child's burns. There was when the child had been burned; when the case was brought; the defendants making the case both to judges and plaintiffs that there was only a limited pool of money with many claims to be paid from it; the urgency of the plaintiffs' need, which could be worked to allow defendants to get out of a case for less; the skill and commitment plaintiffs' lawyers brought to the case; and the leverage the law gave the defendants.

Averages mislead for another reason. Every single one of these cases, like personal-injury actions more generally, was brought on a contingent-fee basis. Families had little choice. They took the terms their lawyers offered, ranging from one-third to one-half of any settlement or verdict. As the lawyers explained, they shouldered the risk of getting nothing. No award, no settlement, no compensation for their labor. But how much risk was there for a lawyer in a case involving a highly inflammable playsuit for children that had resulted in disfiguring, disabling burns and even death? The first lawsuits were filed, moreover, only after the DC fire marshal had tested the suits, found the fuzzy fabric on the chaps to be extremely hazardous, and identified the M. A. Henry Company as the manufacturer of the cowboy suit. Still, until the verdict in McCormack, it was not clear what a jury would do. And the principal defendants' appeal of that verdict meant that their liability was not definitely decided until April 1949. Even after that, the defendants continued to make work for families' lawyers. How much was the risk lawyers took worth?

When Jackie Izzo's parents had asked Frederick Heilman of the law firm Heilman and Purcell how could they afford to bring suit when they had no money to hire a lawyer, Heilman had assured Jackie's father that they would owe nothing unless there was a verdict or settlement for Jackie. And if there was, the contingent fee—50 percent; the standard rate in Michigan, he told them, for litigation that had to be brought out of state, plus expenses—would come out of the settlement.

Presiding over the settlement of Jackie Izzo's case, Judge Leibell accepted the lawyers' statement that the Michigan Probate Court would handle approval of attorneys' fees. He did not ask what percentage those fees were. The Michigan Probate Court subsequently approved the settlement of $97,500 and awarded one-half the settlement plus expenses to the Izzos' attorneys. That sum: $48,877.50. Jackie Izzo received slightly less than half:

$48,622.50. Learning later of the Michigan Probate Court decision, Judge Leibell, as well as Judge Knox, were outraged, but they had no power to change the award. The Izzos would subsequently but unsuccessfully challenge the award. The result left them embittered, their anger directed not at the defendants but at their own lawyers.

In the only other cowboy suit case that came before him—that of another child from Saginaw, Michigan, represented by the same firm that had represented the Izzos and whose family similarly had signed a 50 percent contingent-fee agreement—Judge Leibell insisted that the fees be capped at 35 percent of the $15,000 settlement. Leaving nothing to chance, he further specified the exact dollar figure—$5,250—and added an initialed, handwritten note further stipulating "that they receive no other sum therefor from any other source."[96]

In the cases before him, Judge Knox had not allowed attorneys' fees exceeding 40 percent, even if the terms of the original contract provided for a higher percentage.[97] But the variation among contingent-fee awards represented yet another way in which families similarly situated in terms of a wrong done found themselves in wildly dissimilar positions in terms of recovery. Perhaps because the portion of the settlements to parents was largely for medical costs already incurred, contingent fees were generally taken fully from the portion of the settlement designated for the child. And so awards to the children shrank. The settlement in the case of Tommy Habina was $33,000. $6,365 went to his father for medical expenses, and $11,082.65 to the lawyers, leaving $15,552.35 for Tommy Habina. Many were left with far less—$6,900, $5,000, $4,800, $3,300—to see them through this injury for the rest of their natural lives.[98]

spring

Dear Frances,

The first walk of the spring without a hat or gloves. It is windy, sunny, bright. The river is open (ice gone), not quite white caps, but long deep ripples on the water from the force of the wind blowing against the current. Streams of water run rapidly along the sidewalk and alley from melting snow. We can once again see patches of grass in places. How I wish we could swap places right now. You would find a way to go on, losing a mother more natural, more in the normal course than losing a daughter. I keep pushing this rock up the hill, but I really don't want to now, anymore.

. . .

It feels unreal that it can be spring. Our last first time for a season without you. We were deep into spring when you had your stroke and then we were numb with shock and grief for the remainder of it. I don't remember the weather at all in the weeks after you died. This spring doesn't feel like other springs—I don't feel excitement or anticipation in the longer days, the warmth of the sun, the coming of the end of the school year. I kind of just find myself in it and feel a certain surprise that it is here. And also sadness. I loved sharing spring with you. It was the sharing that made for anticipation and excitement.

. . .

Your birthday is now past. Why was the day harder than many other days? Each of the days through April 30 is a day you were alive the year before. But now we have recognized the first birthday without you. We had thought hard about how to structure the day to remember you and be positive. But what I really needed to do, what I really wanted to do was to talk about how hard it was not to have you here, how hard it was for me to believe that last year, at the very same time the four of us were together having a wonderful, fun evening together. Imagining, without giving voice to it, that next year would be the same. We celebrate birthdays with presents, special dinners, a silly song, but behind each celebration is recognizing another year—it marks both an ending—for you what would have been the end of your 18th year—and a beginning—for you the start of your 19th year. And so yesterday all those who loved you had to acknowledge in yet another concrete way that you never got to finish being 18, in fact, hardly got started. Instead of gifts and celebration, we have a day that will forever be marked as your birthday, but that we now face without you. . . . I would so loved to have been able to give you a big hug yesterday and to have said, "Happy Birthday, sweetheart. I love you."

. . .

It's as though a higher power has given us a reprieve from having to leave winter and enter spring without you. We have at least three inches of fresh snow on the ground and expect one to three more inches today. The limbs of the trees are all blanketed once again—this time in a wet snow and the flakes of snow come floating down except when the wind catches them and blow them about in little eddies.

chapter seventeen · "on our traditional basis of quality alone"

Those with power do not easily surrender their authority. The knowledge industry was little different in this regard than the world of commerce. Facing organized challenges by women on their campuses, federal contract compliance reviews, and individual and class action lawsuits, university administrators calculated the costs of resistance, the measure of compliance necessary to keep regulators at bay, and mechanisms for preserving their autonomy. Just as the principals facing claims from families of children burned in Gene Autry cowboy suits used every tool at their disposal to limit the number and cost of claims, so too here universities resisted women's demands and federal authority.[1]

The first federal contract compliance reviews including or focused on discrimination on the basis of sex took place at Harvard and Michigan in 1970.[2] Both university administrations responded by refusing to turn over faculty employment records, arguing that to do so would violate employee privacy rights, only giving in when pending government contracts were put on hold and federal officials highlighted the provision in every federal contract that gave the federal government access to records necessary to complete its compliance reviews.[3] Reading administrators' polished responses, one can feel an underlying deep well of resentment and anger at women's and the federal government's presumption in challenging their authority. But only very occasionally did that anger boil over publicly. As for example, in February 1971, when a senior administrator tasked with addressing sex discrimination at the University of Michigan told a reporter for the *Michigan Daily*, "We just want to get those bastards at HEW off our backs" and "I don't know why I have anything to do with sex." In the same story, the university's human relations director was quoted as saying, "Once you let women know they've got you over a barrel, they'll take everything they can get from you. . . . Women just make life difficult."[4]

Universities sought refuge in arguments of institutional complexity, decentralization, and departmental autonomy. As Harvard administrators told an HEW review team, "every tub sits on its own bottom."[5] Harvard President Nathan Pusey's description of the university's structure was less colloquial but expressed the same point: He was doing all he could within his authority. He had sent Harvard's nondiscrimination policy to all department heads. It was they who held responsibility "for the elimination of any discriminatory practices, either intentional or unintentional."[6] Department heads had long held great authority within the structure of most universities. But that authority had never been unlimited and had changed with the growing size and administrative complexity of universities, until now it proved convenient to fall back on.[7]

Another strategy was to challenge the appropriate institutional unit of measurement or the relevant statistics against which a university's progress was measured. Universities argued that schools or divisions rather than individual departments were the appropriate unit of measurement on progress in hiring women.[8] Women and HEW argued that using this metric would allow universities to continue longstanding practices of hiring women only in "women's fields," sheltering departments that had long had no or only token women from having to hire women. Similarly, elite institutions resisted the metric of doctorates awarded to women in a given discipline. So, for example, the University of Chicago insisted that national statistics of PhDs in a given field were inapplicable because it did not require a PhD as a condition of employment, recruited from an international market, and, most importantly, because many who received PhDs did not meet the standards of excellence that were the hallmark of the university.[9]

A final strategy of resistance, a trump card of sorts, pervaded universities' response. In every exchange relating to discrimination, administrators took pains to explain the distinctive character of universities as workplaces, their high standards, their responsibility as sites of knowledge production, and their corresponding prerogative in assessing candidates' qualifications. Responding to the findings of the Office of Civil Rights in its contract compliance review in February 1972, Princeton President Robert F. Goheen explained, "The difference between the available supply for positions on a faculty such as this one and for factory work, or even for upper-level management positions in an industrial corporation, is immense. . . . Sometimes there are only one or two strong candidates, and occasionally we are unable to fill a position at all."[10] Forwarding Princeton's Affirmative Action Plan to the Office of Civil Rights in March 1972, he reasserted institutional autonomy. Princeton was committed to hiring and promoting minorities and women "to the fullest extent that their abilities merit and that appropriate openings exist. . . . Under its policies, rules, and procedures," the university would "continue to employ and advance people strictly according to their qualifications and achievements."[11]

But universities could not afford to simply deny or ignore federal authority. They wanted and were dependent on the continued flow of federal dollars. They resisted federal demands, dragged their feet, denied discrimination, made much of the qualifications required for an appointment, and all the while trumpeted their commitment to equal employment opportunity.[12] Within a few short years, they mastered the requisite vocabulary. Their required annual reports became sleek productions touting universities' "good faith effort," their "continuing program of positive action in the field of equal employment opportunity."[13] The measures they adopted to prove their good-faith efforts more deeply embedded the vita in university life. Central were changes in the processes of faculty hiring and promotion.

One can chart the shift in elite universities' behavior over time. At Princeton, the pressure to hire more women faculty began with the shift to coeducation in 1969. Writing to department chairmen, Dean of the Faculty Richard Lester noted that the shift made it important to "increase the number of qualified women in the regular ranks of the faculty."[14] Slightly over a year later, the stakes had grown. In late 1970, an official complaint against Princeton under Executive Order 11246 had been filed, and a contract compliance review loomed. In a memo to department chairmen in April 1971, Lester noted that the need to increase the ratio of "qualified female faculty" was not only a matter of providing "career models for our women students" but also a matter of law. His tone remained conciliatory. "It would be helpful if you could indicate," he wrote, the "supply of qualified women"; the quantity and quality of inquiries and applications from women in the last two years; difficulties in recruiting women; and what the department might expect in terms of increasing the proportion of women faculty in the next three to five years.[15] Seven months later, his tone shifted again. All inquiries to other institutions for possible candidates for positions must include "an explicit statement" encouraging the nomination of "women, blacks, Puerto Ricans, Mexican-Americans, American Indians, and persons from other minority groups." And every appointment request submitted to the administration now required "a written statement on the department's efforts to obtain qualified female, black and other minority group candidates," and "a written statement of the grounds for ranking and recommending another candidate or candidates above the highest rated female, black or other minority group candidate. . . . Obviously," he closed, "it is desirable to maintain records that will provide support for such written statements."[16]

By early 1972, the climate at Princeton and elsewhere had changed further still. The Office of Civil Rights had submitted the findings and recommendations from its compliance review to Princeton in January. Princeton President Robert F. Goheen replied within a week, and in early March 1972 Princeton submitted an Affirmative Action Plan. That plan immediately drew fire from NOW's Central New Jersey Task Force on Equal Academic Opportunities, which had filed the original official complaint against Princeton. Among the task force's objections to Princeton's plan were its vagueness on how the university would ensure that recruiting, hiring, and promoting "will meet affirmative action requirements" and its failure to require the advertising of all faculty and administrative positions.[17] The task force critique coincided with another memo from Princeton's dean of the faculty to department chairmen. His memo directed departments on the importance of evidence of compliance, record-keeping, and consistent processes. The memo included a draft form that department chairmen would be required to submit to central administration for every recommendation for an appointment, including the approximate number of letters, phone calls or other communications with other institutions seeking names of candidates, and the "use of public announcements" or other means of obtaining candidates.[18] If a department did not openly advertise, its failure would now mean a blank space on a form required for requesting administration approval of an appointment.[19]

The changed climate by 1972 was apparent everywhere. At the University of Chicago, between January and April 1972, the assistant vice president and affirmative-action officer, Cedric L. Chernick, joined by the associate provost and the vice president for programs and projects, conducted individual EEO Review interviews with every department chairman, the minutes of which went also to the provost.[20] He clearly read the reviews, which showed just how few departments had changed established hiring practices. In a memo to all academic deans, the provost highlighted the university's particular vulnerability in relation to "search procedures for candidates for faculty appointment. . . . If we are to avoid the kind of imbroglio with HEW that has characterized the experience of Columbia, Harvard and Yale (for example), our practices in this regard will have to be modified in the direction of broadening them, making them more systematic, and especially documenting evidence to support the rationale underlying any given search procedure."[21] Failure to do so, Vice President for Programs and Projects William B. Cannon wrote to all academic deans, might necessitate establishing "special procedures and approval regarding appointment and promotions," in units "which do not supply appropriate documentation."[22] Deans communicated the new imperative to department chairmen: "I do not need to tell you that this University has never been in the business of employing double standards or setting quotas as an approach to the problem," Dean Robert McCormick Adams wrote in June 1972 to department chairmen in the Division of Social Sciences at the University of Chicago. "But if we are not to be forced in that direction against our will, 'affirmative action' can only mean that we deliberately set out to broaden the pool of candidates from which we seek to make new appointments on our traditional basis of quality alone."[23]

The stakes were huge at Chicago, as elsewhere. As of April 1, 1969, the annual level of federal grants and contracts for research and training to the University of Chicago was over forty-four million dollars. And that figure did not take into account funds for capital expenditures. As was true for Michigan, Harvard, and others, federal commitments represented about one-third of the combined operating expenditures at the University of Chicago. Nor were these institutions exceptions. In the over three billion dollars the federal government committed annually to higher educational institutions, Chicago ranked about twelfth.[24]

One engine of the vita as a professional form had been the dramatic expansion of academia and the explosion in the numbers of PhDs. Here was another: law and equal employment opportunity. Advertising of appointments, with its accompanying flow of vitae, was for universities a means to fend off federal contract suspensions and the imposition of quotas. In 1972, the record related to elite universities advertising faculty positions was still mixed. By 1974, universities and colleges were uniformly openly advertising positions in every field at every rank. Chicago, Princeton, Harvard, Yale, Cornell, Columbia, Penn, Michigan, Berkeley, Stanford, and on down the list.[25] Ads like that by the University of Michigan in November 1974 for several positions in history reflected the new environment: "The department encourages applications from qualified Blacks, other minority groups, and women. The University of Michigan is a non-discriminatory Affirmative Action employer."[26] Openly advertised searches meant vitae, in some instances hundreds of them.

Vitae and resumes, in turn, became part of the documentary apparatus of compliance. The second question on the draft form that Princeton's dean of the faculty sent to department chairmen in May 1972 was, "Numbers of candidates for whom resumes were received as a result of such recruitment efforts and extent to which women and minority candidates were obtained for this position."[27] At the University of Chicago, the chairman of the Department of Chemistry, in a June 1972 memo to Vice President Cedric L. Chernick, offered a detailed description of the process the department intended to use for all future searches, including a letter "to every Ph.D. granting institution in the United States, to the national laboratories, and to a few selected foreign universities." In the letter, the department noted that individuals should "submit a curriculum vita, a brief statement of research interests, a list of publications, and a list of three or four individuals who may be contacted and who will serve as references." And in its memo, the department noted that it would collect these materials, including vitae, and contact at least one reference for each candidate, with applications being reviewed by the New Appointments Committee.[28]

Whereas the vita was a critical tool in women's efforts to be acknowledged as individuals, it proved an equally critical tool for universities in preserving their autonomy, and not only as proof of having searched broadly. Long able to ignore women's credentials, now, where necessary to defend their hiring, reappointment, tenure and promotion decisions, universities explicitly denigrated women's qualifications. *On our traditional basis of quality alone.* As in the world of women's access to credit following passage of the Equal Credit Opportunity Act in 1973—where banks, credit card companies, and other lenders used "creditworthiness" to deny women the access to credit the law was intended to ensure—so here "qualified" enabled universities and colleges to defer and deny women's and other minorities' opportunity for equal employment in academia.[29]

There had been from the start more than an element of theater to the broadening of searches and the collection of vitae. In that June 1972 memo, in which the Department of Chemistry at Chicago laid out its open search procedures, it went on to describe how unlikely it was that a woman or member of a minority group would be hired. "The graduate schools from which high quality chemists have come . . . have not turned out any significant number of high quality black chemists, nor have they turned out a significant number of high quality women chemists." The chair noted that from 1967 to 1971, no woman candidate had met their standards.[30] Department after department in those June 1972 exchanges at the University of Chicago explained why, despite their best efforts and intentions, it was very unlikely that they would appoint a woman in the immediate future. There was the fact of the small number of women trained in, say, physics or mathematics; or, as in economics, in the subfields in which the department was hiring. But the point that departments uniformly spoke to, beyond the financial constraints limiting their number of appointments, was the matter of qualifications. "We are always searching for the very best individuals," explained the chairman of statistics, "best in terms of imaginative research, stimulating teaching, and similar professional aspects. Color, sex, religion, nationality, and so on have nothing—repeat, nothing—to do with our decisions about scholarship and other professional abilities."[31]

Where it was necessary to explain the departure of a particular woman, department chairmen were ready with the (un)qualified card. "Mrs. Gray, whom you term 'the only female' in the Department," explained the chairman in history in a memo in June 1972 to a senior university administrator, "decided to accept the deanship of the College of Arts and Sciences, at Northwestern." The position was a good fit for her, he explained, given her "gift for administrative work" and "excellent background in the humanities." He might have stopped there, but he did not. He described her publication record as "not imposing." Her likelihood of advancing at the University of Chicago as "unpromising." He concluded, "The deanship therefore offered a dignified and constructive alternative."[32]

His memo referred to Hanna Holborn Gray, whose *curriculum vitae*—that is, the lived course of her life—says something about discrimination and being qualified. Two years after she left Chicago, she was appointed provost at Yale, the first woman to hold that position, and in 1978 she returned to Chicago as its tenth president, the first woman president there or at any major research university. The women's movement and law opened the possibility of those opportunities, but her preparation for them was grounded in discrimination. Born in 1930 in Heidelberg, Germany, Hanna Holborn came from a distinguished family of academics. Like so many others, her family fled Germany with Hitler's rise—her father considered "politically unreliable," her mother Jewish—securing a non-quota visa with the appointment of Hanna's father, Hajo Holborn, to a position in history at Yale.[33] Hanna Holborn grew up in New Haven, earned a BA at Bryn Mawr, and in 1951 began work on a PhD in history at Radcliffe, where, as she notes in her memoir, the unequal status of women was evident in everything from Radcliffe's lack of a faculty of its own to lower fellowship awards, women's only-recent access to the main reading room at Widener Library, and Harvard President James B. Conant's hostile views on the education of women.[34]

What is most striking in Gray's memoir are not the specifics in her experience of sex discrimination, which were like those of so many others, but how she narrates that history in her own life. At Harvard, she met and married fellow history graduate student Charles Gray, "warned by some that this would likely mark the end of any chance of an academic career."[35] She completed her PhD and was appointed instructor and then assistant professor at Harvard. But, when Charles, who was at MIT, was offered a tenured appointment in the Department of History at Chicago, she joined him. "Out of the blue," she writes, she was offered a year's research fellowship at the Newberry Library. In the next sentence, she notes that its president was a longtime family friend from Yale. "I had also started—newly appointed at the last minute when additional bodies were needed, and at the lowest level and pay of part-time lecturer"—teaching Western Civ in the college at the University of Chicago.[36] When summoned to the Dean's office and offered an assistant professorship to begin in fall 1961, she says, "I was astonished. It had not occurred to me that a regular appointment at the university would ever be within reach." She accepted as a fact of academic life nepotism policies that in intent and practice closed off positions for women.

"I was so grateful," she says, "that I was ready to do anything I was ever asked, including taking on some extra courses I was only minimally qualified to teach and taking on innumerable committee assignments as well."[37] Hanna Gray developed a "gift for administrative work." But if her own scholarly agenda was less developed, her skill in administrative work more developed, it was because of unequal burdens, and her acceptance of them because she was "so grateful." And she was asked to take on innumerable committee assignments. And again and again she said yes, including in winter 1969, when student protests against the denial of reappointment of Marlene Dixon led the University of Chicago to appoint a committee to review the decision. Hanna Gray was named chair.

Marlene Dixon had joined the University of Chicago faculty as an assistant professor in fall 1966.[38] An appointment in the Committee on Human Development had not been in the original budget, but they had been looking for a sociologist for some time who would meet their needs and also be satisfactory to the Sociology Department.[39] The faculty of the Committee on Human Development were excited about Dixon. They had reviewed her vita and a letter of recommendation from the UCLA sociology chairman, read two pieces of work from her dissertation research, and talked with two other professors in the University of California system about her. She had made two visits to campus. In a memo to the dean of the Division of Social Sciences, attaching Dixon's vita and the materials they had reviewed, the chairman of the Committee on Human Development noted that the appointment had strong faculty support. They had been "most impressed by her competence, spontaneous enthusiasm, and both theoretical and research acumen." Her research demonstrated "both theoretical structural skill and highly sophisticated empirical methods." She had offers in sociology from both the University of Wisconsin and the University of Rochester.[40] He suggested that she might welcome a joint or courtesy appointment in sociology, but that the Committee on Human Development's recommendation for the appointment "was in no way conditional upon such action."[41] The dean of the division supported the appointment. In a memo to Provost Edward H. Levi, he noted her "very substantial potential. She seems to be very able, well motivated and committed to an academic career. I doubt if her training is as good as it would have been in a better department, but I do feel that she will overcome this deficiency." As he noted, although the Sociology Department had not yet met to consider a joint appointment, "a poll of some of the major professors indicates that affirmative action will probably be taken." (And it later was.) Provost Levi approved the appointment.[42]

At the University of Chicago, entry-level appointments at the rank of assistant professor were for a three-year term. In the fall of the third year, the faculty member was formally reviewed and either reappointed to a second (final) three-year term as assistant professor or not reappointed. Marlene Dixon's review was in fall 1968. The Committee on Human Development supported her reappointment; the Department of Sociology voted against it. Noting that reappointments in the division required "a reasonable probability that the individual would earn tenure by the end of the second term," the division dean recommended that Dixon not be reappointed. "Based on the evidence that I have . . . I am convinced that her chance of achieving a quality and quantity of research output sufficient to warrant tenure at this University is significantly less than 50 percent." He admitted that if the budget were less tight, he might have modified his decision on the grounds that "she needed somewhat more time to demonstrate her potential," but noted that "her most recent efforts at research and her statement of her next efforts are rather less convincing than the work that was based upon her dissertation." The provost accepted the dean's recommendation.[43]

The denial of reappointment to Marlene Dixon—an activist professor supportive of the student movement; the first woman, as Jo Freeman's "simple sex census" showed, appointed in the Department of Sociology for nineteen years; and one of very few women faculty at the University of Chicago overall—sparked student protests that led the administration to appoint a faculty committee to review the decision with Hanna Gray as chair, which in turn led to the appointment of a committee on the status of women at the University of Chicago. The Gray Committee, after a comprehensive review, unanimously concluded that there had been "no deviation from normal procedures."[44] "We have found in this case," they concluded, "no conscious discrimination, no sign that anti-feminism was in any sense an issue."[45]

Theirs was not the only assessment of Dixon's qualifications. In response to the student protests, the Department of Sociology had issued a statement that the "intellectual quality" of Dixon's work "did not meet the standards required for reappointment" in sociology. Department faculty were asked to sign the statement. One, an assistant professor, refused.[46] He wrote a three-page, single-spaced response disputing that Dixon's sex and political activities had played no role in the decision and that her scholarly record was insufficient.[47] The point is not to say that he was correct and the voting faculty in sociology, the dean, the provost, or the "Gray Committee" wrong. Rather, it is to highlight how process, documentation, the vita, and the power to define and assess "qualified" offered tools as important to universities in making and defending their decisions as they were to women and other minorities in potentially opening pathways.

Marlene Dixon's case offered a preview of coming attractions.[48] There were legal challenges against colleges and universities of every rank in the academic hierarchy for sex discrimination in the 1970s. No discipline had clean hands. Most of those challenges, as in Dixon's case, were unsuccessful. Provided that universities could demonstrate that they had followed established rules and policies, their evaluation of candidates' qualifications was almost insurmountable. There were women who won legal challenges in these years. But their victories highlight how decidedly unequal were faculty versus university officers and administrators, the lengths to which universities and colleges would go to denigrate women's qualifications in defending their decisions and their right to make them, and the costs—material, temporal, psychological—of fighting for rights.[49]

Consider Dinah Levine (Rozen) Moché.[50] Recall, she had joined the physics faculty at Queensborough Community College (QCC) in 1965 as a part-time lecturer. The department chairman nearly crowed at their good fortune in getting a person of her training (BS magna cum laude from Radcliffe in physics, MA in physics from Columbia, and substantial coursework toward a PhD at Columbia) "willing" to accept the rank and salary QCC offered. The following year, 1966, she was appointed an instructor. A year later her husband died unexpectedly, leaving her with two small children to support.[51] She remarried at some point, becoming Mrs. Dinah Moché, and now had a blended household of four children. In 1971, she was promoted to assistant professor, her promotion coinciding with legal challenges to sex discrimination in academia. But she had been teaching physics for eight years and remained without tenure, the only woman in the physics department at QCC, the only woman hired in physics since the program's beginning.

In March 1973, members of the Physics Department at QCC received a memo that the departmental P&B (promotion and benefits) committee was beginning its annual promotion review of faculty. Interested faculty members were invited to send the committee a memo noting "new items on their vitae or any other information which they feel would aid in a fair, objective and comprehensive evaluation." Moché submitted a memo to the committee of new items on her vita. Juggling family life and teaching, she had not completed her Columbia PhD, but she had built a national and even international reputation as a teacher of physics, gaining professional recognitions and numerous NSF teaching and study grants, regularly presenting papers at the college physics teacher association meetings, and publishing. The departmental committee took no action on her memo.

The next year, in April 1974, Moché wrote the committee a memo titled "Professional Qualifications for Promotion to Associate Professor." She included her updated vita, current bibliography, publications, letters of commendation, and among other things "a packet of letters" regarding her paper "Why Don't Girls Choose Physics." The chairman notified her a few weeks later that the committee had decided not to recommend her for promotion. "I am incredulous," she responded. "By any objective standard my professional qualifications and accomplishments are outstanding for a community college teacher." She asked for a meeting with the chairman or an explanation in writing of the decision, to which the chairman replied that the Board of Education "does not permit chairpersons to give reasons for negative personnel actions."

Moché then wrote a letter to the college president, detailing her reputation, publications, grants, a position on the editorial board of the journal *The Physics Teacher*, and active research agenda. "Every man who came at the same time or after me is now in a higher position, despite my outstanding professional credentials and continuing achievements." President Schmeller acknowledged the "keen disappointment" she must feel but insisted that he could not act. "My intervention would be justified only if I had evidence of your competencies which was not available to the Committee, and I must say in all honesty that I have no such evidence." Filing a formal grievance, to which she added yet more evidence of her qualifications, Moché found no more success. In September 1975, President Schmeller denied her grievance. Her record did not matter. "You do not meet the bylaw requirements for associate professor as you do not possess the doctorate." Onward turned the wheels. In October 1975, the union notified Moché that it would not submit her grievance for arbitration.

In spring 1976, the departmental P&B committee again voted against nominating Moché for promotion to associate professor. Again, she wrote to President Schmeller challenging the decision. Surely her academic and professional credentials demonstrate "much more ability and understanding of physics than is required for the Ph.D. from less prestigious institutions." Moreover, soon enough she would have the formal credentials required in the bylaws. In September 1975, she had returned to Columbia to complete her dissertation; she had as well another physics teaching book scheduled for publication and also new articles. In June 1976, she notified President Schmeller that she had completed all the requirements for the PhD at Columbia and successfully passed her final defense. "Will you exercise your academic judgment and recommend my promotion to Associate Professor in the Physics Department at this time?"

President Schmeller asked the departmental P&B committee to reconsider Moché's nomination for promotion request. The committee voted against it. And Moché again found herself filing a formal grievance. President Schmeller, who noted that he was "not necessarily convinced that any . . . bylaw, contractual or statutory policies were in fact violated," nonetheless, exercising his "academic judgment" found her "qualifications merit[ed] consideration" by the collegiate P&B committee. It seems incomprehensible to have to write that the college committee again voted against Moché's promotion to associate professor. But they did.

The final document in the file is a letter dated December 8, 1976, from Moché to President Schmeller—formal notice of her appeal of the collegiate P&B committee vote. "I would be grateful for an opportunity to review my professional qualifications with you personally before you decide this appeal." In 1976, Moché filed a sex discrimination suit against Queensborough Community College and City University of New York. The New York State Division of Human Rights found "probable cause" supporting her complaint. In 1977, four years after her battle for promotion began, she was promoted to associate professor and two years later to professor. In the course of her career, she published over twenty books.

Moché's story was a case in point of the seriousness and intensity of women's commitment to intellectual life. It underscores the hollowness, as Helen Astin showed in her 1968 dissertation, of the claim that women dropped out of professional life when they married.[52] Moché's life spoke too to the importance of the vita for women in demonstrating and making claims for their professional qualifications. But her story also showed how powerful men in departments and administrations used formal rules, policy, and process to judge women's "qualifications," find them wanting, and make those decisions so hard to overturn. I thought of the hours, the emotional energy, that their decisions cost this woman and so many others like her in their quest to prove their commitment and their qualifications.

If Moché's story left me angry, it was another woman's story that broke my heart. And this one too, I read in the beautiful reading room at the Schlesinger Library, the collections of which have been so fundamental in building the field of women's history. I found Natalie Allon's story in a file labeled "Discrimination-Affirmative Action" in the papers of SWS, Sociologists for Women in Society.[53] Allon, a sociologist trained at Brandeis, was hired as an assistant professor at Hofstra University in 1972. She came up for tenure and promotion in 1977, the year that Dinah Moché was finally promoted to associate professor. But unlike Moché's experience, Allon's department, the dean, and the college ad hoc tenure committee all strongly supported her promotion. The provost, Harold E. Yukor, did not.[54] He summarized his assessment of Allon by saying, "She is a good professional, but not an outstanding one." Assessing her qualifications, he found her teaching "above average," the documentation of professional activities in her field—the sociology of obesity—"massive," but some of it not "substantively academic," nor the number of publications "extensive," although, he admitted, her level of research and writing stood out in a "department not notable for its publications." Given the department's numbers (declining enrollments, a highly tenured faculty with distant retirements), "I can only recommend tenure for persons with excellent qualifications.... Under these circumstances, I am unable to recommend tenure for Dr. Natalie Allon."

With the support of the Department of Sociology, Allon appealed the provost's decision, and the University Appeals Board unanimously supported her promotion. But in August 1977, Hofstra President James M. Shuart rejected the appeals board recommendation. "As President I have the responsibility to insure both the academic quality and fiscal integrity of the University now and into the future." Sidestepping Allon's qualifications, he rested his decision on grounds even more difficult to challenge—the "fiscal needs" of the Sociology Department and the university. Noting his support of the provost's assessment and exercising his own "best judgment of departmental and University needs, I must recommend to the Board that Dr. Allon not be granted tenure." Natalie Allon received notice of the decision by certified mail a few days later. "Accordingly, the academic year 1977–78 will be your terminal year at Hofstra University." Hofstra was not an elite university, but the position that Allon found as an assistant professor at the College of Textiles and Science in Philadelphia, as she pursued a lawsuit alleging sex discrimination against the university, was several more steps down the academic ladder—with the consequent differences in teaching load and support for research.

The file had not said what had happened to Allon, where she had gone from Hofstra, or what had become of her claim against the university. I wondered and began to search. I found a scholarship in her name at Hofstra University and a special journal issue originally planned by her but of necessity carried out by others and dedicated to her. And then I found that in fall 1980, two years after being dismissed from Hofstra, her legal action pending, Allon was in a devastating car accident on her way to a professional meeting. The accident left her unable to breathe or move on her own or communicate; it marked the end of her career and independent life. She would spend the remainder of her life in a nursing facility. She died in 2001 in an anesthetic accident during minor surgery.

Who can say whether Hofstra's dismissal of Allon played a role in her devastating accident. That question haunts me, as does another. Time in the course of a life does not have a uniform weight. The weight of any given period of time in a life is shaped not only by the moment or events themselves, but also by what comes before and after. Had Allon gone on to live a full life, had she been able to continue her intellectual work; the injustice of the denial of tenure would weigh less heavily than it does given that she did not. Hofstra agreed to a settlement in Allon's legal case in 1982—two years after the devastating car accident—endowing the "Natalie Ina Allon Scholarship," which awards $3,000 annually to sociology students at Hofstra. The special issue of the journal *Marriage and Family Review* she had planned was published in 1984 and dedicated to her pioneering research on the sociology of obesity and dieting. It opened with an article summarizing her career and the major conceptual and theoretical advances she made to the understanding of obesity. In their dedication, David Kallen and Marvin B. Sussman noted the importance of her intellectual work. But as they also noted, "the accident which ended her professional work also took from us the persona of a warm energetic and loving friend whose inability to interact leaves a void in our lives."[55]

Even before Natalie Allon was denied tenure, the high tide of affirmative action had passed. The shift was marked by a book titled *Antibias Regulation of Universities: Faculty Problems and Their Solutions*, published in 1974, by Richard Lester, professor of economics and the former dean of the faculty at Princeton who had been so deeply involved in Princeton's response to affirmative action. Lester assailed HEW and affirmative action as threats to higher education. He asserted that women taught lower-level courses and researched and published less because they were less meritorious. He argued that if women were promoted more slowly than men it was a product of their own commitments to household and family. He idealized the democratic process and merit-based values of university hiring and promotion decisions.[56] The history traced here shows the lie in Lester's claims. But his book and the positive response to it spoke to the times.

The social movements of the 1960s and early 1970s were one of those moments that change the course of lives. Many in academia found their life's intellectual work from within and through those movements. Their curriculum vitae speak to the fields they built and the transformations they brought to fields long established. But we see at most in their vitae a shadow of the force of this moment on their lives. Those movements also made universities far more open both in terms of education and as workplaces. In defense of their autonomy, universities changed: openly advertising faculty positions, adopting uniform procedures and record-keeping in hiring, promotion, and tenure. Those changes embedded the vita in university life. They did not bring substantive equality.[57] They did not assure women and other minorities faculty appointments. But they did mean that women and other minorities knew of positions, had the opportunity to submit their vitae for consideration, and—when hired—to have their qualifications considered rather than simply dismissed by virtue of sex, race, religion, national origin, and—later—age, disability, and sexual orientation. And as university and college faculties came to include increasing numbers of women and other minorities, they sustained the pressure from within. Looking at names of references on vitae even as early as the late 1970s, change is there. Where once those names had been all men, and largely white men, there were increasing numbers of women and other minorities.

And yet in fundamental ways universities were not changed. Women's fight to be judged on their capabilities alone came at the sacrifice of a more fundamental restructuring of work. The erasure of personal data from vitae was partly a product of law's prohibition of discrimination in employment on the basis of race, sex, religion, and national origin, and partly a product of women's effort to be seen and judged as individuals, not as a sex or as wives or mothers. But that erasure contributed to the privatization of marital and parental status and made it easier for universities to ignore women's differences from men, though the structure of women's lives had not changed.[58]

Universities and colleges resisted the assertion that higher education was a workplace to which standards that had been developed for industry, intended to measure progress there on the "under-inclusion of women" and other minorities, applied. But higher education turned out to be remarkably like industry in a broader sense. In her thought-provoking history of Title VII, *Equality on Trial*, and a related article, historian Katherine Turk argues persuasively, if depressingly, that "the law of workplace sex equality had come to view the state's main role as protecting women's right to be treated like breadwinning men." What that meant was that women's rights at work became reduced to "a choice between opting out or buying into systems that had long been designed around men."[59] The story for women in academic life fit this larger picture. As Turk argued in a 2014 article, "feminist pressure opened more faculty positions to women and established their study as a respected intellectual pursuit. But amidst efforts to redefine women's place in academia, domestic responsibilities became cemented as wholly a private sphere concern."[60] The erasure of personal data from vitae contributed to the removal of the structures of family life from institutional consideration.[61] This was the context for Susan Moller Okin's challenge: adding marital and parental status to her vita in 1985 when she had not included it in her vita in 1975.

The erasure of personal data from vitae had consequences as well for knowledge and the ends of knowledge. In this sense, there was a deep irony to the erasure of the personal from vitae. Knowledge growing out of life experience—personal knowledge—was fundamental to the women's and other rights movements of the 1960s, 1970s, and since. And those movements brought into being or into the mainstream important, new fields of knowledge and ways of acquiring knowledge. But the fight for inclusion, the tyranny of the vita, constrained the scope of their challenge to disciplinary ways of knowing. The erasure of personal data from vitae reinforced the claim to and expectation of knowledge as objective, the product of higher education, distanced from emotion and from lived experience. So that, even as the vita became the document through which academics were known, knew themselves, and produced knowledge, a document of "I," the "I" in a fuller sense was erased from it. And in that erasure, something was lost—not just for individual lives or the structure of work but for ways and the ends of knowing.

knowing

Dear Frances,

You feel so far away to me these days. This morning I found myself thinking "Can you have a fight with a dead child? Can you feel rejected, unloved by a dead child?" How unfair are such feelings, because you're not even here to defend yourself. I brood and feel down because I fear you didn't love me. If I admitted this to Dad he would tell me I'm crazy.

. . .

Today is the 29th—Thursday. I ache all the more so because I am having a harder and harder time feeling you here in the way I did and could in the first eight months. If this is healing, I don't like it. I'd rather have the searing, wrenching pain and tears than this feeling that this is just my life now.

. . .

Here I am at the end of the day hating everything because I manage . . . This past summer I wanted nothing more than to die because I wanted to be with you, because I couldn't bear living without you. But it's like someone turned the treadmill back on and so I'm in motion. I want to be true to you. I want to be with you. I would willingly die. But I'm told that I can't because it would dishonor you. You wanted to live and didn't get the chance, so I have to. And then there is Wilder. If I died how could I expect him to live? And so I'm in this position of having to live, but not wanting to, and then hating myself when I discover that I'm in motion. I feel like I'm forgetting, forgetting that you are gone, not just away. I love you, sweetheart. I know I do.

. . .

I put in words today for the first time something that has been on my mind since—I'm not sure when. Last year I assumed that this year you would be in college, that both you and Wilder would be away in school and I realized that Dad and I were on the verge of the next stage in our life—the beginning of what would be a transition to you and Wilder developing your own, independent, adult lives. . . . But now you don't get to do that. I can't imagine either going on as though the transition that I had imagined as beginning happened or that death took its place. Because you aren't getting to live your life and so I don't know how to live mine.

. . .

Dad's birthday is next Friday. He'll be 53. It will be his first birthday without you. I'm at the airport. As soon as I walk into an airport a feeling of sadness comes over me. I so associate airports with you—leaving you, the joy of returning. . . . It's funny that a space of leaving, of absence, of return is so marked by feelings about you. But it is. Seeing mothers and daughters together, hearing mothers talking to their children on cell phones—airports are full of these emotional landmines. . . . It's watching/seeing/hearing a girl say "mom" or "mommy," hearing a child crying . . . these are the little impossibilities of the everyday.

. . .

I'm really exhausted today—the cumulative result of an intense, demanding week: busy, stressful, emotional, lots of putting on a good face. I have now been at a conference where many people didn't know about our lives. It's an alienating experience. Of course, most people who've seen me, interacted with me in the past—before this last year—didn't know anything about my personal life either. But then it did not seem strange. My personal life was always part of my professional life—in casual conversations you mention kids, your dog, your spouse. But now the follow-up questions, even the conversation is different. Death, loss are not casual subjects. At dinner on Friday night, another woman in the group of people at my end of the table started talking about her kids. I asked questions, said things, hoping questions to me about kids would not come next. But then a sweet, female student—someone who had already told me how important my work had been to her and how glad she was to meet me—looked across at me and asked, "Do you have kids?" The woman who had been talking about her children knew about you. I looked at her, almost pleading, and then tried to start. "I have two children: a son who'll be 21 this summer" (still thinking desperately—how do I say what comes next in a gathering that is all about sociability, where people are talking and laughing and having a good time getting to know each other), but I forged on, "he transferred from the University of Oregon to St. Olaf this fall," steeling myself even as my voice tightened and the tears began to run down my face, "my daughter died unexpectedly last April from a stroke. . . ." And there we all sat, me with tears running down my face, the poor young woman who had asked, saying, "Oh, I am so sorry." And then we gradually began to try to pick up a conversation, but we were a new small group now in this room filled with the voices of others who did not know, who had been chatting along even as the whole room seemed in my mind to have gone completely silent for a few minutes. And so it goes.

. . .

How can it be that Friday night I was crying trying to tell someone that you had died and last night hours of wrenching conversation, tears streaming down my face—was that not knowing? And yet this afternoon, I feel all over again, as if I have just become aware, just really understood for the first time that you are gone. I have known and known anew, so many times this year. And each time I wonder if there will come a time when the knowing no longer sweeps over me anew and leaves me feeling drained, defeated.

. . .

I am disoriented, trying to grasp what happened, how it is that we are still here—seeing the new growth of spring poking up through the dirt, feeling the warmth of the sunshine on our bodies—and you are not. Can you hear me Frances? Can you feel my love? Are you okay? Is there an "okay" in death?

. . .

I have hives again all under my arms from the stress and upset like I did after you died.

. . .

I have not fully acknowledged that you are gone. I find myself still, although we are approaching a year, shocked and resistant. . . . I think those who didn't know you, those to whom you are an abstraction—a name, a category (daughter)—it is easier to place this new label ("died"—"her daughter died") and have it stick. Whereas, it is different for me. Is it because I don't want to believe, can't accept, or is it also a matter that you will never be dead to me. You will always be part of who I am, always alive to me. I keep wrestling with this because I can't fathom the gap between other people's understanding of what has happened and my incomprehension.

. . .

I'm not sure where today went. I am continuing to observe student's classes, get them prepared for prelims, write recommendation letters, and so on. But even as I do, I think "What am I doing? Frances is gone." I would like to simply curl up in a ball and let the world go on without me. And yet, feeling like I have an obligation to all these students, I keep showing up, keeping reading things for them. It remains incomprehensible to me that you are gone, that this time last year you were alive and happy and working away to finish up projects, your thoughts focused on getting the pants you needed for your internship, on discussions of a new dress for prom, but that in a couple/few short weeks it will be a year. How can a person both so fully know and not know at the same time, not just serially or in alternating fashion, but simultaneously. I miss you, Frances.

chapter eighteen · "public cowboy no. 1"

It was late November 1949. Autry had forwarded a letter from William Martin, his New York lawyer for the cowboy suit cases, to his agent, Mitchell Hamilburg, who in turn replied directly to Martin. Their exchanges often traveled in this circuit: Martin to Autry, Autry to Hamilburg, Hamilburg to Martin. Martin had noted a case in which Autry's contribution to the settlement was to be $3,000. Hamilburg wanted to know both what this case was and why it was it was costing Autry this much. The plan, he reminded Martin, had been to cap Autry's payments at $1,000 and then only if and when they had to. He also asked how this business stood, saying that he thought things should now be pretty much wrapped up.[1]

Just a few days later, in a letter with a very different tone, to a potential new licensee of Gene Autry merchandise, Hamilburg spelled out the terms of a licensing contract with Autry and made his pitch for the benefits of the Autry brand. The letter was long. It described Autry's vast empire of motion pictures—six new films coming out in 1950, shown in ten thousand theatres across the US, with each one seen by approximately five million people—as well as a highly rated weekly radio show, the Melody Ranch Hour; dozens of other Autry licensed products; and personal appearances, including rodeos across the country, capped each year by the Gene Autry World Championship Rodeo at Madison Square Garden in New York City, where Autry was the star attraction. The point was simple: Autry's celebrity drove sales of products bearing his name.[2] Toggling back and forth in Autry's records between resistance to contributing toward settlements of claims for the burned children's injuries and deaths and keeping payments to a minimum where made at all, and the pursuit of new licensees and increased sales of products bearing Autry's name, exposes an uncomfortable truth: Each was as much about business as the other.

Autry was not exceptional in this regard. The same was true for all those involved in the manufacture or sale of component elements of the Gene Autry cowboy suit. Their resistance to acknowledging responsibility or shouldering the financial burden was more telling for how inconsequential this product was to the bottom line for any of them. E. F. Timme & Son had bought over 3.3 million pounds of viscose rayon thread from Du Pont between 1940 and 1945. Over those same years, Du Pont's annual worldwide shipments of rayon increased from eighty million pounds per year in 1940 to 150 million pounds in 1945. What Du Pont sold to Timme in any year between 1940 and 1945 amounted to less than 1 percent of Du Pont's annual viscose rayon sales.[3] Timme's sales to the Henry Company between 1942 and 1945—7,681 yards of fabric—were a minuscule fraction of its sales; the Henry Company's sales of the Gene Autry cowboy suit a small fraction of its business; Gene Autry's licensing revenues from those sales a tiny fraction of his income in these years.

Autry had hired "Mitch" Hamilburg in 1938 to handle product licensing and endorsements. He was good at his craft. What began with three licenses in 1938 had grown in just over a decade's time to forty across the United States and seven more in Canada. The companies themselves were not household names. The products they made, like many consumer products, were hardly necessities of life, things like horseshoe-nail rings, flags, buttons, lunch boxes, bicycle horns, billfolds and watches, pencil cases, toothbrushes and tooth powder, comics, gloves and mittens, rubber boots and cowboy boots, cowboy hats, pistols, holsters, and cowboy suits.[4] What differentiated them in the market, generating sales, was the name they bore. Gene Autry had made himself into his own brand.

Autry was not a defendant in the McCormack case because of the unusual facts in that case: the cowboy suit a gift directly from Milton Henry to James McCormack for his sons. But he was named in many cases that came after it. While the exact language varied from one case to the next, the point the families' lawyers made was the same: Autry was a public figure whom parents and children idolized and trusted. And he had breached that trust. A child had been seriously injured and was "maimed for life, by reason of the sale and distribution of this cowboy suit by this defendant, for without Gene Autry there could have been no 'Gene Autry' cowboy suit, and without Gene Autry children would not have bought nor desired a 'Gene Autry' cowboy suit."[5]

Neither Autry nor Hamilburg had concerned themselves with the character of the fabric used in the "Official Gene Autry Ranch Outfit." Their focus had been on looks and style; their point of comparison cowboy suits endorsed by other personalities.[6] Whereas, the liability of the Henry Company, Woonsocket Falls Mill, and E. F. Timme & Son were all decided in *McCormack* in 1948, Autry's liability as a licensor of an article of clothing for children that was in fact dangerously inflammable was unresolved because he was not a party in the *McCormack* case. In the years that followed, Autry assiduously avoided a legal resolution of that question, one of many strategies for minimizing his contributions to settlements. As Autry's lawyer, William Martin, explained in a letter to Mitch Hamilburg in April 1949, there might be a point when Autry's liability would have to be tested in court, but all the more reason to get as many cases resolved before that as possible.[7]

The question of Autry's liability was complicated by a vital fact. Before March 29, 1945, some of the defendants had known the fuzzy fabric on the chaps was inflammable, others had or possibly should have known. Many children had been injured, others had died, in accidents before that date. But in late March 1945, all the principal defendants had been notified that there were children who had been seriously burned and that some had died. Autry was still in the service when he got the news from Mitch Hamilburg, who had gotten the news from Milton Henry, who had gotten the news from a buyer at the Hecht department store in Washington, DC, who had gotten the news from the DC deputy fire marshal.[8]

The question was—what had Autry and the others done next, and what should they have done? Legally? Morally? The Hecht Company immediately sent back to the Henry Company forty-eight dozen Gene Autry suits that it had in stock. Autry would later swear in a deposition that when he got the news about the danger the suits posed, he had directed Mr. Henry to take the cowboy suits off the market, and that Mr. Henry had told him both that he had done so and that he had asked the retail store to withdraw them from the counters.[9] But Autry's and Hamilburg's claimed conversations with Henry were not in writing, and so what was said and when remained open to question. Neither Autry nor Hamilburg ever followed up with Henry. More damning, Autry continued to accept royalties on the very suits that he now knew were the cause of injury and death. But perhaps most damning of all for Autry was that he did not use his exceptional celebrity or public appearances to warn of the hazard and prevent further injury.[10]

I wish I knew what Autry and Hamilburg said to each other in the spring of 1945 and in the months that followed, as the number of lawsuits relating to injuries and deaths from the Gene Autry cowboy suit grew and Autry hired William F. Martin of Martin & Clearwater to defend against the suits. But correspondence from the years before 1949 between Autry, Hamilburg, and Martin is gone, burned in a 1962 fire at Melody Ranch.[11] We do know that Autry's weekly radio program remained a staple of radio, that he returned to making motion pictures, became the star attraction of rodeos across the country, and kept up a packed schedule of public appearances. All without publicly warning of the hazard that he now knew the cowboy suit bearing his name posed. The pace was relentless, the opportunity to warn communities large and small across the nation unparalleled.[12]

From the start Autry had an advantage for avoiding being served in cases that the other defendants did not have, and he capitalized on it. All those involved in the production of the Gene Autry cowboy suit, with the exception of the mom-and-pop sorts of retailers, had bases in the state of New York, making them subject to lawsuits there. Autry, in contrast, was based in California.[13] Even though Autry's name was on every suit that left the Henry Company's factory, he was not subject to suit in New York until a plaintiff could catch him there. Autry came to weigh the benefits of appearing in the rodeo against the risk it posed of being served in more cases.[14] The risk was real: Clumps of new cases came with each appearance. So, for example, during the 1948 Madison Square Garden rodeo, Autry was served in sixteen new cases.[15] The next spring, Martin warned Hamilburg that with the filing of several new cases, Autry should avoid New York for the near future.[16] Martin was also quick to point out the importance of getting any case settled that was set to go to trial in New York while the rodeo was on.[17] In many cases, Autry escaped any contribution to a settlement on the grounds that he was not in the case.[18] Martin was clear about just how much heavier the financial burden would be for Autry if he were a defendant in all the cases. As Martin wrote to Hamilburg in April 1949, whereas Autry was currently in fifteen cases, Henry faced more than thirty.[19] And in August 1951, in a letter to Autry, Martin reported that whereas he had ten open cases for Autry, E. F. Timme & Son's lawyer had at least a dozen more.[20] Writing to Hamilburg in October 1951, Martin reported that he thought the end was in sight, adding that with Autry not coming to New York for the rodeo that year, most of the cases he was not in would be disposed of before his next appearance.[21]

For every exchange in which Autry, Hamilburg, and Martin strategized about avoiding service and minimizing payments to the burned children and their families, there was other correspondence in pursuit of profit. There were Hamilburg-planned gatherings of Autry licensees in New York City and Hamilburg's regular bulletin announcing and welcoming new licensees, congratulating and describing the promotions of the most entrepreneurial among them, announcing Autry's tours and film releases, drumming up advertising, and more. Hamilburg pressed licensees to place ads in trade magazines to complement ads Autry was placing. Writing to licensees in March 1949, for example, Hamilburg noted that he and Autry were placing an ad in the June issue of the magazine the *Boys Outfitter* that would list Autry's scheduled activities for the year and include the names of all licensees. The plan was to send a reprint of the ad to department stores across the United States.[22] Hamilburg kept licensees apprised of Autry's schedule so that they could coordinate local promotions and tie-ins, and in so doing, he reminded them of the work Autry put in to boost their sales.[23] Every appearance, every new movie offered the occasion for a promotion, a tie-in that brought sales making money for retailers and licensees and, in turn, for Autry.[24] There were Autry and Hamilburg meetings with buyers at department stores that were considering putting in the Gene Autry line and a steady flow of letters from Hamilburg to O'Melveny & Myers, Autry's Los Angeles lawyers who handled licensing contracts, with the names of new licensees and the terms of contracts to be prepared and sent.[25]

Autry was their star, and licensees were his family. Writing to licensees in October 1950, on letterhead with a large image of Autry waving his hat on his rearing horse Champion in the background, Hamilburg thanked both new and longtime licensees for making a recent gathering a success. Words could hardly convey, he wrote, his pride in greeting them and even better having them meet in person, their star, Gene Autry. They were Gene's business family and, as Hamilburg told them again and again, Gene took as much pride in them as in his own family.[26]

In a career built on publicity, much of it aimed at children and families, the cowboy suit cases meant the wrong kind of attention. And so, on occasion, with Autry's approval, Martin accepted service in a case or joined a settlement to avoid Autry being publicly served at the rodeo.[27] Martin cut deals with lawyers representing multiple burned children and their families—settling Autry's contribution to fifteen families represented by Elliot Paley, for example, for $15,000, at a thousand dollars apiece—saving Autry the "embarrassment" of being served in new cases while appearing in the rodeo at Madison Square Garden.[28] And they resisted with every tool at their disposal, including Autry's celebrity, having Autry make sworn statements in the cases. "The defendant Autry is . . . a public performer with a heavy schedule of engagements and the head of a large film enterprise which requires his constant attention. It is respectfully suggested that to order his examination before trial under the circumstances in this case would work a considerable hardship."[29] It was a strategy with its own risks. "The plaintiffs purchased their suit almost a year after the occurrence in the McCormack action," one lawyer responded, pressing his case to examine Autry, "and Gene Autry, by reason of his neglect and failure to do anything, permitted these sales to continue. This surely is not the picture of a man who is entitled to the consideration of this Court, nor is it the picture of a man who is entitled to say 'I do not wish to be examined and they only seek to examine me to harass and annoy me.'"[30]

Throughout, the main goal was to keep payments to a minimum. Autry's team sought to avoid his being named in cases, so escaping altogether any contribution to settlements. Where he was named, the goal was to avoid his paying more than $1,000. In such a calculus, the *Izzo* settlement in March 1949, which cost Autry $5,500, rankled.[31] Autry and Hamilburg repeatedly impressed on Martin the importance of minimizing the number and cost of the cases to Autry, saying that he was about to run out of money on paying off these cases.[32] In a letter to Autry and his accountants, Martin reassured them that the character of the girl's injuries had made Izzo an exceptional case, noting that he did not expect Autry to have to make as large a payment in any other pending case and that there were several in which he thought Autry would not have to pay anything at all.[33]

In this calculus, burned children became expenses on a balance sheet. Literally. Columns of names, followed by the disposition of the case, and Autry's contribution. Greatorex, settled, contributed –$1,000; Wetherell, settled, contributed –$1,000; Tetla, settled, contributed –0 0 0; McCarthy, settled, contributed –0 0 0; Baer, settled, contributed –$500. And so it went. There was the occasional case where Autry's contribution exceeded $1,000, as in Izzo, but they were the exception. By April 26, 1950, the Autry accounting was $38,750 paid in settlement of twenty-nine cases, $2,328.31 in disbursements, and $17,700 in legal fees.[34]

Legal fees were as contentious as settlement payments. Martin and Hamilburg sparred repeatedly over the legal fees incurred in defending Autry in the cowboy suit cases. In an exchange in April 1949, Hamilburg challenged a recent bill from Martin; Martin in reply reminded him of the extensive work the cases required and closed his letter noting that he had enjoyed representing Gene in these cases and looked forward to continuing to do so. But if Hamilburg or Autry felt someone else could do so more satisfactorily, they should let him know.[35] Other tussles over legal fees followed. In November 1951, Martin wrote Autry that he felt bad about the treatment he had received relating to his bills. He had sent the most recent bill for legal services three months earlier, with no reply. Autry was not returning his phone calls; Hamilburg's promises that a check was forthcoming brought no check. Martin continued to work on pending cases. But he had reached his limit. Unless his most recent bill was paid, he suggested that Autry make other arrangements for his legal representation in these cases.[36] In this instance, Autry had replied just the day before noting that he was expecting some money in the next few days and would pay Martin's legal fees. But here too, he returned to the refrain of not being as rich as people said. In fact, given tax rates, he insisted that he was lucky to keep his head above water.[37]

I wonder if Autry believed his own words. A feature story in *Life Magazine* in June 1948 detailed Autry's multimillion-dollar empire including radio stations, newspapers, ranches, oil-rich land, his own movie company, rodeos, movie houses, a song publishing company, a publishing house that turned out more than a million Gene Autry comic books a year, hundreds of thousands of dollars in earnings a year from personal appearances, and, of course, licensing profits from dozens of Gene Autry products.[38] A map of the United States with a handy key offered a visual portrayal of "Gene Autry's U. S. A.," a business empire that extended "from coast to coast." He had come a long way from the sentiment expressed in his 1932 recording "Money Ain't No Use, Anyway." Having grown up poor, would he have never felt economically secure no matter how much money he made? Or was this how money was made? Was spending money to buy another radio station different from contributing to settlements for children burned wearing a cowboy suit bearing his name, or paying the lawyer who had kept his contributions to a minimum? The summer 1948 *Life* feature story reported Autry's "empire" as somewhere between "$4 million and $7 million in paying properties," with a net income to Autry of "well over $600,000" per year, including $100,000 per year in royalties from Gene Autry licensed products.[39]

Autry's licensing royalties continued to climb. In 1949, he earned $190,078.13 in advances and royalties on product licenses. In 1950, the sum was $222,120.94.[40] Royalties on the Gene Autry cowboy suit contributed to those numbers. Autry's first licensing contracts had provided for a royalty of 3 percent on every sale, but in later contracts that royalty was set at 5 percent. Volume was key. Royalties adding up to hundreds of thousands of dollars a year began product by product as pennies on the dollar. The record of Autry's royalties on sales of the Gene Autry cowboy suit from 1941 to 1945 was, unfortunately, lost in the same fire as the early correspondence among Autry, Martin, and Hamilburg.[41] But perhaps what says more is that Autry did not end his relationship with Milton Henry in 1945. And so, the royalties kept accumulating. In 1949, a collection of Henry companies now selling an array of Gene Autry products, including a redesigned cowboy suit without the dangerous fabric on the chaps, paid Autry royalties of over eleven thousand dollars. In 1950, the Henry companies paid Autry royalties of close to thirty-three thousand dollars.[42] Between 1949 and 1957, royalties of the various Henry companies to Autry were well over one hundred thousand dollars.[43]

Autry's continued relationship with Milton Henry was all the more surprising, or maybe revealing is the right word, because Milton Henry and the Henry Company had not, as it turned out, halted all sales of the Gene Autry cowboy suit with the flammable fabric on the chaps when they learned of injuries and deaths from the suits in March 1945. Rather than destroying the suits they had on hand and facing a loss, the Henry Company offloaded the suits to unsuspecting retailers. In February 1945, the Henry Company had signed a contract with Goodyear for the purchase of Gene Autry Official Ranch Outfits. It was March of that year when the DC fire marshal notified Henry of the incidents in the Washington, DC, metropolitan area. Henry pushed on, shipping in April at least five thousand of the cowboy suits, including it seems the suits returned by the Hecht department store, to Goodyear. Goodyear in turn placed some of the suits in its own retail outlets and sold others to small retailers across the country. At least five other boys were burned in suits where Goodyear was the retailer or wholesaler.[44] But those accidents happened alongside dozens of others in late 1945, 1946, and 1947. Henry's actions might never have come to light had Scott Timberlake been burned earlier.

The cowboy suit in the Timberlake case was purchased at a Goodyear store in Parsons, Kansas, in October 1945 and given to the Timberlakes in June 1947 for their son Scott by a close family friend whose own son had outgrown the suit.[45] Nine months passed before Scott Timberlake was burned in the suit on April 3, 1948, in Kansas City, Missouri. It was the timing of the incident that first raised red flags, as well as the fact that none of the principals had liability insurance covering incidents from 1948—which led E. F. Timme & Son's lawyers to suspect Henry of making late sales. Dozens of depositions of friends and family of the Timberlakes, Goodyear employees, Milton Henry, his brother, and other Henry Company employees confirmed Timme's hunches. As Martin reported to Autry in August 1951, there seemed no doubt that the cowboy suit that burned the Timberlake boy had gone out from Henry's factory after he knew children had been burned in Washington, DC. It was an ugly mess.[46] One month later, Martin detailed for Autry just how much of a mess. Most of the M. A. Henry Company records had gone missing, and Mr. Henry, clearly worried about a possible perjury indictment and carefully coached, had become extremely vague in his statements.[47]

Whatever Autry and his agent Mitch Hamilburg had said to Milton Henry in spring 1945 when they first got notice that children had been burned in the suits and some had died, they had done it orally, not in writing. And so, Milton Henry's memory could be vague about the fact and content of the calls. As Martin reported to Autry, while Milton Henry admitted that there may have been calls, he could not now recall whether Autry or Hamilburg had said anything about recalling cowboy suits that the Henry Company had already sold. Milton Henry's brother worked in the Passaic plant and was supposed to have ordered the actual destruction of the suits. His memory too had become vague: He did not remember how many cowboy suits the company had still had on hand in spring 1945 or how many had been destroyed. He insisted that he had told an employee to destroy the suits and trusted that it would be done. Nor was his memory any better on the number of returns they had received from retailers or even the number of retailers.[48]

Milton Henry and his brother had good reason to be vague. Contradicting their prior sworn statements, there was now clear evidence that they had continued to sell the suits well after being warned that they were inflammable. As Martin noted in his letter to Autry, if a perjury indictment were to be brought against the employee who swore the suits had been destroyed, it was clear that he would not take the blame without calling out Henry and others. But the danger the case posed was not solely for Milton Henry. As Martin noted, the only thing keeping Timme & Son's and Woonsocket's lawyer, or any of the defendant's lawyers, from bringing a suit against Henry was their fear of stirring up more cases of children who had been burned and not yet brought a lawsuit. Moreover, if the Timberlake case went to trial, Martin warned, the presiding judge might notify the district attorney and then there would be real trouble.[49]

Autry had much to lose. Martin noted that Goodyear was concerned to keep their name out of court, but they were clear that Autry should be even more anxious since his name was on the cowboy suit. And whatever he or Hamilburg had directed Henry about not selling more of the cowboy suits, the embarrassing thing, as Martin noted, was that Autry had continued for months thereafter to accept royalties on sales of the cowboy suit. Worse still, perhaps, was that Autry was on record in a sworn deposition as having done nothing himself to contact retailers or alert the public to the danger. And then there was the character of the Timberlake child's injuries rendering him a custodial case for life and the number of other children who had been burned. If the case went to a jury, Martin warned, and they learned just how many children had been burned before this boy, he did not feel that they would let anyone off.[50]

In early October 1951, Martin called Hamilburg with the news that the Timberlake case had settled for $88,000. Elliot Paley, the lawyer who had represented the McCormacks, represented the Timberlakes. His settlement demand had been $105,000. In a letter a few days later, Martin explained to Hamilburg that the judge had played a key role in getting Paley to take less, but the judge had done so only on the condition that the defendants contribute to the settlement on specific terms. Timme and Woonsocket's contribution was $36,500; Goodyear's $21,000; Henry's $17,500; and Autry's $12,500, more than Autry had contributed to any case by a significant margin. As Martin noted, the judge focused on Autry's status as a public figure receiving royalties from every cowboy suit sold. In the judge's view, once Autry knew the hazardous character of the playsuit, he had a duty to publicly warn families. It did not matter that there was no case law in which a licensor had been held liable in a situation like this. Where there was no law, he noted, law must reflect the morals of a case. As far as the judge was concerned, a public personality had a strong duty.[51]

In one of the many instances of judges and lawyers showing courtesies to the defendants that were not extended to the burned children and their families, the judge, whom Martin had known for many years, had been good enough to share his views of Autry's liability privately. As the judge had also told Martin, he thought there was a strong chance that, given the late sale, liability would fall on Henry and Autry—and since a judgment likely could not be collected from Henry, that would leave just Autry. The settlement spared the defendants dangerous publicity and a great deal of money. The lawyers and judge agreed that had the case gone to trial there might have been a verdict for as much as $200,000. Explaining all this in a letter to Autry, Martin added that while the boy might live a full life span, he would be institutionalized for life, the cost of which now was $3,000 a year. Martin closed the letter by noting the three worst cases they had faced. Children long reduced in their correspondence to a last name—Cizek, Izzo, Timberlake—were reduced further here, described simply by the condition the burns had left them in: blind, legless, an animal. Because of when it happened and the condition it left the child in, it was the last of these, the case of the Timberlake boy, that, in Martin's opinion, was the most dangerous of all to Autry.[52]

Reading the exchanges between Autry and his lawyer and agent relating to the Timberlake case, it is hard to continue. But there is more, because other children had been burned. Earlier that summer, for example, with the Timberlake case still pending, Autry's secretary called him on location to share a letter that had just arrived. She read it to him over the phone. The letter was from a Mrs. Grosch in Mount Vernon, New York, whose six-and-a-half-year-old son, Bobby, had been severely burned that April when a spark from a fire caused the chaps of the Gene Autry cowboy suit he was wearing to explode into flame. She described her son as an avid Autry fan, asking if maybe Autry could send a picture of himself to cheer up the boy who had recently undergone skin grafts. Her tone was warm. There was nothing in her letter to suggest that she held Autry responsible for what had happened. The purpose of her letter, as she wrote, was to let Autry know because she knew he would not want something like this to happen to some other boy.[53] What would she have thought had she known that by the time her son was burned in 1951, Autry had known about the danger the suits posed for six years?

Autry instructed his secretary to send the letter to William Martin with a query of whether he should respond.[54] Martin wrote back, noting the friendly tone of the letter, but reminding Autry that they had learned of many other instances in just this way and the families had usually ended up filing suit. He suggested that Autry write the boy and his mother; he even included draft letters for mother and son.[55] Autry did not change a word. The two-sentence letter to the boy said simply that he was sorry to hear he had been burned, hoped he was recovering, and wished him health and happiness.[56] In writing the boy's mother, Autry also followed the script Martin provided. This letter was slightly longer, noting that his secretary had called him on location when the letter arrived and read it to him. Autry said that he was very sad about the news, wanted to learn all the details, and with that in mind had arranged for a Mr. Riley, who worked for him in New York, to come see the family. He enclosed the letter for her son Bobby with an autographed picture, noting that he hoped for the best for the boy, and that he would be looking for the report from Mr. Riley.[57]

Mr. Riley was a detective hired by William Martin. His report came back the same day Autry's letters to Bobby and Mrs. Grosch went out. It detailed how the family had acquired the cowboy suit: as a hand-me-down bought several years earlier by Mrs. Grosch's sister, who lived in the Bronx, and brought down from the Grosches' attic when a neighbor child got a cowboy suit. And it described the child's injuries and treatment: second- and third-degree burns on both legs, for which he had just had skin grafts. It described the family's modest economic circumstances, an important variable in calculating a family's financial desperation and how cheaply a case might be resolved. And most important of all, it described Mrs. Grosch's feelings about who was responsible. She did not, Mr. Riley reported, hold Autry responsible, but she did think the manufacturer should be alerted for the protection of other children.[58] She would surely have felt differently had she known of Autry's silence.

Over the next several months, Martin followed the now-well-worn path in these cases, working to limit the damage to Autry and keep the case out of court. Following up on the detective's report, he arranged a physical examination of the boy by a doctor and secured photographs of the child's burned legs. He was also able to report that the Grosches' lawyer was cooperative; his asking price, $25,000. While Martin noted that that amount might be reduced somewhat, he expected that $15,000 was the very least that a judge in the county where the family lived would approve in settlement. But he thought it was possible, if Autry were willing to contribute $2,000 to a settlement joined by the other defendants, that the claim could be settled without the family actually filing suit at all.[59]

The timing of the case raised a real hazard. As Martin warned Autry, the claim could be made that someone should have notified the public that many of these playsuits were still on the market or in use. He noted, once again, his concern relating to late burns for the possible duty they suggested of Autry as a public figure to act with extraordinary care to prevent more children from suffering harm. They had seen just that from the judge in the Timberlake case. And as Martin reminded Autry: In late cases, all the previous burns could be introduced into evidence, the cumulative force of which would be shocking. In these circumstances, he warned Autry that Hamilburg's continued resistance to contributing anything more than a paltry amount to settlements was generating ill will, and not only with codefendants. If Martin were to tell a judge in this case that Autry was not willing to pay anything or only hundreds, he expected that the judge would encourage the family to test Autry's liability by bringing suit against him in California.[60] Autry's response too followed a well-worn pattern: Martin should get the case settled as quickly as possible paying as little as possible. It might help in doing so, he suggested, if the family knew that he was not rich—Martin could tell them that—and that most other families had accepted a settlement with only a contribution of $1,000 from him.[61]

Whatever the principals involved thought when they first learned of children being horribly burned, some of them dying, their outward actions across the years were focused on denying responsibility and preserving their businesses and reputations. Autry's initial visits to some of the children identified in the breaking news in Washington, DC, in April 1945, his pledge to join the investigation, had quickly turned into a calculated distance and stony silence as it became clear that these were not just accidents. "That was a terrible thing," Gene Autry's longtime secretary, Virginia MacPhail, would later recall of the incidents. Referring to Autry, she said, "He was upset, but he didn't talk too much about that kind of thing. He was not a down person—of course, that was partly Ina's [his wife's] doing, too. Christian Scientists believe in keeping everything positive."[62]

The most durable mark of the tragedy on these enterprises were business restructurings to protect themselves from liability. By 1948, when the first settlements were reached, Milton Henry had effectively drained the M. A. Henry Company of assets, leaving it insolvent, taking his name and contact list to a new company—the Leslie Henry Company—he established in the same line of business.[63] Autry's subsequent licensing agreements included a clause specifying that he was not liable for defects, requiring companies to indemnify him in the event of liability, and requiring licensees to carry product liability insurance.[64] E. F. Timme & Son incorporated the limited partnership, thereby exchanging the risk of personal liability that came with the business form of a partnership for the limited liability of a corporation.[65]

With these changes in place, the principals moved on. How little impact the cowboy suit tragedy had on them was evidenced in their business relationships remaining intact, individuals' careers flourishing, business horizons expanding, and their personal and corporate wealth multiplying many times over. The McCormacks' apartment was one and a half miles, a thirty-minute walk, from William E. Roschen's co-op on Fifth Avenue looking out over Central Park. They had always lived in different worlds. But in the wake of these incidents the difference had a new register. As the McCormacks and families like them learned to live with death, and as others learned to live with the lifelong consequences of traumatic injury, William E. Roschen, the sole general partner of E. F. Timme & Son, oversaw the corporate reorganization and expansion of Timme's pile fabric empire. The firm's importance was reflected in extensive coverage in *Women's Wear Daily*, the fashion industry's most influential trade magazine, and often in *The New York Times* as well. It was Roschen who oversaw, in 1950, the relocation of what had been the Woonsocket Falls Mill from Woonsocket, Rhode Island, to a new 344,000 square foot plant in Wilmington, North Carolina.[66] The Roschens' prominence in New York City's social circles meant regular coverage on the society pages of *The New York Times*. There were debutante balls and cotillions, well-made matches and weddings for their children, charity balls and fetes, weekends in Connecticut.[67] When

William E. Roschen died in 1963, at the age of sixty-seven, obituaries in *Women's Wear Daily*, the *Asbury (NJ) Park Press*, and *The New York Times* heralded him "as a leader in the pile fabric field."[68]

The cowboy suit tragedy no more unsettled the careers of non-executives at Woonsocket and Timme than it did those of their executives. Charles Bergamini, who had been named chief chemist at Woonsocket in 1942, one of those who had overseen the inflammability tests of and unsuccessful attempts to flameproof the fabric Timme sold to the Henry Company, rose in the ranks in the years after, a sign of the centrality of chemistry in an increasingly synthetic fabrics world. By 1967, he was president of E. F. Timme & Son, Inc.[69] The young Timme salesman, Henry J. Bullwinkel, who had sworn under oath that he had told Milton Henry that the fabric was inflammable and should not be used in clothing, also rose in the ranks; by the mid-1960s, he was the company's general sales manager for the Standard Fabric Division.[70]

A Timme advertising campaign for its fake furs in 1970 and 1971 spoke to just how little had changed in the company's ways of doing business. A representative ad from the campaign, a two-page spread in the *New York Times Magazine* in August 1971, featured five Hollywood actresses wearing Timme fake furs.[71] "Five women who can easily afford any fur coat in the world tell why they're proudly wearing fakes," the ad copy read. The ad described Timme as "one of the world's leading suppliers of plush and flat fabrics" and that though "Timme-Tation fake fur" was only a small part of its business, its advertising focused on this product for two reasons:

1. We believe that the slaughter of wildlife in the name of fashion is cruel and, eventually suicidal. We want to do something about it. As we gain acceptance for fake fur through advertising, the demand for the real thing goes down. So fewer animals die. And that's the big thing.
2. As more and more people start turning to fake fur, we want them to know that E. F. Timme & Son makes the best fake fur money can buy. 45 different kinds. With heavy emphasis, we don't mind adding, on the Endangered Species.

E. F. Timme & Son was playing fast and loose with words in marketing its fabrics.[72] Then again, Timme always had. Timme had made the high-pile rayon fabric that took the skin and lives of many children in the 1940s and early 1950s and left those who survived scarred for life. Did anyone seeing Timme's fake fur ads know that?

Timme's longtime source for synthetic fibers, the Du Pont Company, played a starring role in transforming public attitudes toward synthetic fabrics. In doing so, Du Pont was serving its own strong financial interests. What had begun at Du Pont in the early twentieth century as a diversification strategy for its excess nitro-cellulose capacity had become by mid-century one of the company's most important sources of revenue. By the end of the 1960s, fibers accounted for a third of the Du Pont Company's sales and fully 40 percent of its $356 million in profits.[73] Rayon was not part of this future. Though in 1950, US consumption of rayon was second only to cotton, with sales reaching a high of 1,500 million pounds a year, rayon had never reached the levels of profitability that Du Pont expected of its ventures.[74] The fabrics future Du Pont forecast lay not in cellulosic fibers like rayon but in fully synthetic fibers. Over the course of the 1950s, Du Pont wound down its production of rayon, shifting facilities and employees to expansions in its synthetic fibers, a field that Du Pont dominated.[75]

Among Du Pont senior chemists involved in rayon's development who had worked closely with Roschen and Timme were a number of men who died prematurely, including W. Hale Church, head of the Pioneering Research Division.[76] But as the careers of others suggest, had they not died prematurely they would most likely have continued to rise in Du Pont's ranks. Lester S. Sinness had joined Du Pont in 1935 as a research chemist having earned his PhD in chemistry that year from the University of Wisconsin. His career is an example of the path into industry that, beginning in the late 1920s, companies like Du Pont offered PhD chemists from large public universities. By 1939, Sinness was research supervisor and, in the early 1940s, director of the Viscose Rayon Research Section. By the time Sinness gave his deposition in the Lutz case, in which he admitted that Du Pont had been aware of the inflammability of viscose yarn since the late 1930s, he had been with the company for fourteen years.[77] Du Pont's lawyers nonetheless successfully gained Du Pont's dismissal from the lawsuit. Sinness and others most certainly knew the outcome of the case. Still, the corporate veil protected employees and shareholders not just from financial liability, but as importantly, together with corporate culture, from the weight of moral responsibility for the hazards in the products they were part of making. So Sinness prospered. In subsequent years, he continued his rise through Du Pont's executive ranks. By 1963 he was a director, vice president, and member of Du Pont's Executive Committee. By 1969, he was one of the most highly paid corporate executives in the United States.[78]

That the cowboy suit tragedy had no impact on Timme's long-term relationship with Du Pont, or on individual employees and executives at either firm, is less surprising than that Gene Autry did not terminate his business relationship with Milton Henry, a relationship that began with making the Gene Autry cowboy suit. By 1947, Milton Henry's new company, the Leslie Henry Company—based in Mount Vernon, New York, with a showroom on Fifth Avenue—had a new Gene Autry cowboy suit on the market. In the years that followed, Milton Henry and Autry expanded their licensing agreement with Henry's companies, producing not only cowboy suits but a broad range of licensed Autry products. A full-page ad in the 1954 *Playthings Directory* directed buyers to the Leslie Henry Company for "*Sure-Fire* Gene Autry" pistols, cowboy suits, holster sets, and spurs.[79] No doubt the reference to "sure-fire" was intended to be read alongside "pistols," the first item on the list. It is chilling all the same in light of the Gene Autry cowboy suit's history.

In 1961, with great fanfare, the Greater Wilkes-Barre Chamber of Commerce announced the relocation of the Leslie Henry Company to Wilkes-Barre, Pennsylvania. Focused on the few hundred jobs the company would bring to Wilkes-Barre, those negotiating the move likely did not even know that Milton Henry had manufactured the cowboy suits that claimed the lives of many children and left others with lifelong injuries across the country, including in Wilkes-Barre and surrounding towns. Some of those incidents had been reported in the *Wilkes-Barre Record*, the same newspaper grandly announcing the move of Henry's companies and the jobs they promised.[80] But other elements of Henry's business biography suggest that the cowboy suit tragedy was not an anomaly. His businesses presented a long trail of scandals, lawsuits, shoddy business management, and shady business practices.[81] Though enterprises bearing his name outlived him, so did questions of shoddy merchandise.[82]

That Gene Autry continued his business relationship with Milton Henry suggested that however "upset" he had been by children being burned in cowboy suits bearing his name and manufactured by the M. A. Henry Company, business came first. The tragedy did not touch Autry's stardom or wealth. His investments had looked toward the time that, as he put it, "like a baseball player. . . . I'll have to hang up my spikes." Autry expanded his business empire with far-flung investments, buying—among other things—more radio and televisions stations, music publishing companies, and shares in oil wells, and in 1960 establishing a new baseball team in the American League, the California Angels. Alcohol abuse sullied his final performing years, but not his fame or bottom line. Between 1983 and 1994, Autry's name appeared ten times on the Forbes 400, the magazine's list of the four hundred Americans with the highest net worth.[83] Despite extramarital relationships and more casual affairs—long widely known within his circuit—he and his wife Ina remained married to her death in May 1980. Autry remarried just over a year later. On October 2, 1998, he died of cardiopulmonary arrest and respiratory failure stemming from lymphoma. He was ninety-one. His wife Jackie told Autry's biographer that he "used to say, 'I'm going to live forever, but if I go, I'm going to take all my money with me.'" Before he was buried, she said, "I put a check in his pocket for 320 million dollars—what Forbes thought he was worth on the date of his death."[84]

The last settlements in the cowboy suit cases had come decades earlier. The Legal Department at Du Pont submitted the last annual report to the Executive Committee that included any reference to the cowboy suit cases on February 11, 1955. Two short sentences were all it took: "Three cases pending from the last report alleging burns while wearing 'Official Gene Autry Cowboy Suits' were settled. This is the last of these cases and makes a total of sixty-nine cases disposed of with no contribution by du Pont."[85]

Just the week before, on February 7, 1955, one of William Martin's partners at what was now Martin, Clearwater & Bell wrote the last—or at least one of the last—letters to Autry attending to the cowboy suit matter. The "Re:" line listed three cases: Verbonitz, Touhill, and Blessington. It had been a decade since Martin had begun representing Gene Autry in the cowboy suit litigation. The letter began by reminding Autry of the firm's telegram from eleven months earlier (March 12, 1954), in which they had informed him that they had disposed of the Blessington matter with a contribution from Autry of $1,850. They now had the compromise order and general release in Blessington to finally dispose of the case. They next reminded Autry of their correspondence from five months earlier (September 1954), in which they had notified Autry and secured his approval of a settlement in Verbonitz for $2,500 on Autry's part. And finally, they reminded Autry that William Martin, in his negotiations with Paley—who represented both the Touhill and Verbonitz families—had managed to get a general release in the Touhill case with no payment from Autry.[86]

It had been over a decade since Michael Blessington Jr. and William Touhill were burned at play on the same day, the one in New York City, the other in Philadelphia, two days after Christmas 1944. Michael Blessington Jr. had died three months later from his burns; his family had been living that loss for ten years. William Touhill, burned at age five, now fifteen, still could not completely straighten his legs or touch his heels to the floor. The doctor's bill remained unpaid. More surgeries lay ahead. The third boy, Joseph Verbonitz, had been horribly burned on Halloween 1952, close to eight years after the Blessington and Touhill boys, seven years after the defendants had been put on notice of the danger the Gene Autry cowboy suit posed. But as the letter from the firm of Martin, Clearwater & Bell noted, a check from Autry for $4,350 was all that was needed to finally close these last remaining cases. A handwritten notation with the check number and amount at the bottom of the letter suggested that Autry had finally done just that.[87]

anniversaries

Dear Frances,

April has felt unreal. It is as though I had not understood until now that we would reach this month, these days in which the before and after are so clearly marked because we now are in what we know to be our final days with you alive last year. And after the 30th we will no longer be able to look back one year to a day, a world with you alive. We will enter instead into a different set of anniversaries. I do not want the 26th to come Frances. How can it be more final than it already is? And yet the inability to look back one year to a world with you in it is another kind of year—there are calendar years, and academic years, and fiscal years. What label is there for this year?

. . .

I miss so much the comfort and relaxation of Friday nights at home with you—the question about what to pick up for dinner or where to go, the question of what movie to watch and the simple satisfaction of us all cuddled up on couches and chairs together in the family room. I miss relaxing with you. I no longer can relax because it is a site and space filled by your absence.

. . .

What I wanted to tell you about was going through papers. The papers in the study were from last April and early May. Print-outs of emails from my colleagues at school on April 27th, 28th, and 30th—responses to the message [the department chair] had circulated to the Department sharing the awful news that you had had a stroke. His message brought back how little we knew or understood or could allow ourselves to believe or share with others. Our need to believe that maybe yet it would all be okay, that you would recover. And yet I also wonder whether his words were shaped by garbled transmission, by the hope at the other end of the line that everything would be okay. His message to the Department said you had had a stroke, that you were in the ICU at Children's, that they were running tests and "you would be there for a few more days." Where did that last bit come from? Reading through his message and the responses that I only read much later—after you had died—I remembered how our "knowing," coming to know, understand what had happened was both gradual and abrupt. I still cannot fully grasp how differently we on the one side and the nurses and doctors on the other understood what had happened to you and the meaning for our lives.

. . .

I asked Dad last night what the weather was the week you had your stroke. All I remember was seeing the gradual dawning light from your hospital room each morning between 4 and 5 in the morning and both the relief of having made it through the night and dreading the day for you. I also asked Dad what time your death certificate said you had died. When was it that the doctor said, "take all the time you need." Would they have made me leave at some point if I'd shown no inclination or refused? I wonder now about how reasonable a person remains even in times that are without reason.

. . .

Cold, gray day with temperatures in the 30s and several inches of snow expected tonight and tomorrow. The cold and gray have felt less unbearable this year perhaps because they are congruent with my spirits. It's the warmth, sunshine, and fresh growth of spring that I find startling and disorienting.

. . .

It is supposed to be 61 degrees by Sunday—Easter. I'm sure it's a sacrilege to think this, but writing the word Easter made me think of the resurrection. Oh, how I would love to see you again. But then I could not bear to let you go again. Because this time I know what is on the other side of good-bye for the living.

. . .

The second thing I wanted to tell you was that in the little card shop next to Longfellow Grill, I found a pair of "cheaters" that you would have loved: no color on the front, but temples at least 1/2 inch thick of exactly your shade of bright amazing green. I was so tempted to buy them for you. Would that have been crazy? If you were here, I would have told you about them, and I suspect they would have been yours. I remember last March when Wilder took you for your eye exam and you were initially so unhappy that the Dr.

said you didn't need a prescription, but the whole thing was so screwy and garbled that I called the Dr. to see what was up and learned that you did need a little help seeing, but cheaters would do it. I had no idea what cheaters were, but when they explained, you and I went off on a wonderful afternoon's search for cheaters. And you discovered that the delightful thing about only needing cheaters was that you could get many pairs. I suspect that in time cheaters would have taken their place beside sunglasses and purses and lip-gloss as things you had many, but never enough, of.

. . .

How do parents work through the transition of having a different kind of relationship with their children as they become adults and move away and how are we to make that transition with you since you will not get to grow up? Will we always have a child who remains 18 even as new birthdays pass?

. . .

I realized this morning that it was Saturday. That a week from today is the one year anniversary of the day you died. Dad and I spent much of the day trying to find the right color of T-shirts, the right shade of green, to have made for the [Walk for Animals] walk next Saturday. There's something absurd about our spending the day trying to find t-shirts, testing iron-ons, all of which ended up not looking great so at last we ordered buttons with your picture on them. I hate it. I hate it all. What I really want to do is curl up in bed and simply not get up for the next week. But instead, in this effort to put on a good face, to be positive, I am searching for t-shirts, deciding on words and font style. And all the while I just want to scream: can we talk about what's really going on? Can we talk about the fact that in one week it will be a year since Frances died? Can we talk about what we are even doing here? I feel lost and desperate tonight. If I could get in a canoe and just start paddling and not stop until I fell asleep, I would, because there's no where I can turn.

chapter nineteen · "the road to preferment"

Research had been an important value of elite universities in the United States from the late nineteenth century. The curriculum vitae as a form, rather than the lived course of life, began as a PhD requirement in Germany in the early nineteenth century and was adopted by American universities at the end of the nineteenth century attempting to replicate the research ideal. But it is important to remember that the number of PhDs granted in the US climbed slowly, as did the number of institutions requiring this credential of their faculty, much less the expectation of continued research. It was only in the decades after World War II, driven by the demands of the Cold War state for a skilled Cold War workforce and research, that research became the defining value, the production of new knowledge and graduate training the central purpose of even elite universities, displacing undergraduate teaching as the foundation of professional academic identity and life. This revaluation filtered far down the academic hierarchy. As Leonard Levy, dean of the faculty at Brandeis, told the president there in 1963, "Like it or not, teaching and related activities . . . are almost impediments toward advancement in the profession. The road to preferment, position and profit only passes through, and sometimes by, the classroom . . . The scholar who crystalizes DNA or wins a Bancroft prize receives all the publicity, advancement and take-home pay, regardless of how much or how well he teaches."[1]

That this was the era in which the vita became central to American academic life was not then incidental. Nor was it only a product of war and displacement or a growing academic marketplace, or a tool in the defense of institutional autonomy. It was emblematic of the broader shift in academic life. The vita was more than a functional tool; it was a key technology in the creation of a new kind of identity. The lack of a need for something like the vita in the early twentieth century was not then simply a product of informal methods of placement; fundamentally, the identity it was key to elaborating—research scholar—had barely existed. That the vita, or the CV as it was colloquially known by the 1970s, became central to every aspect of academic life—hiring, salary, tenure and promotion, departmental self-surveys, the establishment of graduate programs, fellowship and conference panel applications, introductions of guest speakers—reflected the transformed character and new values of the academic economy. And at the twentieth century's end, with the creation of the World Wide Web, this public-facing, entrepreneurial vita reached its full flowering.

The postwar transformation in the role and substance of the vita was bound up with the relationship forged between science, universities, and the state in World War II.[2] But it was not a foregone conclusion that that relationship would continue after the war, much less that it would expand and so transform universities, the character of academic life, and the pursuit of knowledge. "Before World War II," as Richard Lewontin writes, "there was no model of centralized government support for a broad array of scientific projects, or for a leading role for universities in providing research and development for national objectives. The atomic bomb changed all that."[3] As Lewontin's observation suggests, the flow of federal dollars for research during and then continuing after the war was a product of both planning and the course of international events. Close to a full year before the war's end, President Roosevelt had turned to Vannevar Bush, director of the Office of Scientific Research and Development (OSRD), to suggest how the wartime relationship between the state and science might be continued in peacetime.[4] Bush's report, *Science: The Endless Frontier*, would become as formative to the character and structure of the postwar relationship between the state and universities as was the OSRD to the wartime relationship.[5]

It is impossible to know what would have come of Bush's vision had the course of international events been different; but as it was, the Cold War drove the dramatic expansion of federal research support to universities. In the two decades after the war, the flow of dollars—millions, billions of dollars annually—from the federal government for research transformed American universities.[6] As former Harvard University President Nathan Pusey noted, "prior to 1940, all the colleges and universities in the United States together never had more than $27 million available in a single year to support research, and . . . virtually all of this came from private sources."[7] By the mid-1960s, American universities collectively were spending $1.8 billion a year for research, 83 percent of which, $1.5 billion, came from agencies of the federal government.[8] Delivering the prestigious Godkin Lectures at Harvard University in 1960, Clark Kerr, chancellor of the University of California, Berkeley, and subsequently president of the UC system, argued that "American universities have been changed almost as much by the federal research grant as by the land grant idea." He dubbed the new evolution "the federal grant university."[9]

State land-grant universities owed their creation to federal funding, but elite private universities had long been wary of applied research or federal support—seeing both as a threat to their independence and to the disinterested pursuit of pure knowledge. The post–World War II relationship between elite universities and the federal government offered then what Clark Kerr referred to as "a paradox": "The better and more individual the university, the greater its chances of succumbing to the federal embrace." Kerr's gendered and sexualized language to describe that relationship was telling. "The federal embrace." A "common-law marriage, unblessed by predetermined policies." And a "classic" bawdy limerick:

> There was a young lady from Kent
> Who said that she knew what it meant
> When men took her to dine,
> Gave her cocktails and wine;
> She knew what it meant—but she went.

Reciting the limerick, Kerr noted, "I am not so sure that the universities and their presidents always knew what it meant, but one thing is certain—they went."[10]

But that universities welcomed, aggressively courted even, the postwar flood of federal dollars was not a paradox at all. That money was as important to institutions as it was to the faculty whose research federal contracts supported. Elite universities' reputations had long rested on the quality of their faculty. "A university is built of men," began the report of a committee at Columbia tasked in 1953 with assessing "Columbia's Academic Eminence."[11] In the post–World War II world, as scholars and university administrators well understood, academic reputations would be built or maintained through pioneering research. The pursuit of "unquestioned excellence," the defense of "academic eminence," required support for research—and that meant time, facilities, and money. Moreover, federal contracts did not support only faculty or research centers; they were equally critical to the expansion of graduate programs and increasingly to university budgets.[12] By 1969, federal funds made up anywhere from one-third to 40 percent or more of the operating expenditures of major research universities.[13]

How those dollars came to universities was crucial not only for the course of research and the structure of universities but also for the structure of knowledge, the identity of research scholars, and the history of the vita. Rather than flowing to universities at their request to divide as they chose, federal dollars flowed to individual scholars and scholars in university-affiliated research centers under contracts with federal agencies for research that met their needs.[14] "One of the quickest ways to lose a faculty member," Kerr noted in *The Uses of the University*, "is by refusing to accept the grant he has just negotiated with his counterpart in Washington."[15] That federal dollars flowed to individual faculty transformed the relationship between faculty and the universities that employed them. It gave academics a new kind and level of independence and power. It transformed them into what sociologist Robert Nisbet dubbed "professorial entrepreneurs" responsible for securing the funds to make their research possible. The vita was a key technology in the transaction, as essential for the elaboration of faculty identities as research scholars and the assertion of intellectual independence, as it was in the pursuit of reputational recognition and the flow of funding.

Kerr's judgment that the relationship between the federal government and universities was "a productive union" was ratified by others. By 1963, when *The Uses of the University* was published, the Carnegie Foundation, the Brookings Institution, the President's Science Advisory Committee, the American Council on Education, the American Assembly, Harvard, and Princeton had affirmed their commitment to that relationship.[16]

But not everyone shared in that judgment. From the start, federal research support was highly concentrated in the federal agencies from which it flowed and in the universities and disciplines that were its principal beneficiaries.[17] Within institutions, the flow of federal funds created growing disparities among disciplines. A 1969 faculty committee report at Harvard reflected a broader, and what would remain a more sustained, reality: "The sciences were rich, the social sciences less so, and the humanities least affluent of all."[18]

The privileging power of money was not just about the imbalances it created—the institutional, disciplinary, and individual haves and have-nots. Money was both liberating and corrosive. It raised directly the question of the pursuit of knowledge for its own sake, the purposes to which knowledge was put, the commitment to teaching, and the character of university communities. In the twelfth annual John Dewey Lecture, delivered in 1970, published by Basic Books the next year under the title *The Degradation of the Academic Dogma: The University in America, 1945–1970*, sociologist Robert Nisbet argued that money had eroded the bonds of institutional loyalty, degraded the pursuit of knowledge, and left teaching largely to those who failed to earn their own keep as research scholars.[19] He bitingly described centers, institutes, and laboratories as the epicenter of the new "academic capitalism" and their directors and other faculty recipients of federal grants the "new men of power," "the professorial entrepreneur," an "academic bourgeoisie."[20] One did not have to accept his idealized vision of the university or fully agree with his critique to recognize the truth in his descriptions. Federal money had transformed universities and the professoriate. The dean of faculty at Brandeis was right; *the road to preferment, position, and profit* lay through research.[21]

The relationship between academics, universities, and the state in World War II changed both universities and individual scholars' attitudes toward sponsored research and the relationship between education and society in unanticipated and enduring ways. It offered an example of what Robert K. Merton, in an article published in the *American Sociological Review* decades earlier had called "the unanticipated consequences of purposive social action."[22] Observers have long debated whether the consequences of federal funding for the structure of knowledge and pursuit of knowledge for its own sake were, or at least whether they should have been, unanticipated.[23] But no one seems to have anticipated that the revaluation of research and the legal mechanism of the research contract would transform academics into entrepreneurs, much less how the vita—the form that is so fundamental to academic life, knowledge, and identity—was bound up in that transformation. Merton's scholarly work in the sociology of science is critical to understanding the emergence of the research scholar, the entrepreneurial professor, and its impact on the structure of knowledge in the post–World War II era. But equally important are his own life and career, which were bound up in and reflect that transformation.

The first vita labeled as such in Merton's papers at Columbia is dated August 1968, the same moment in which vitae proliferated among those just starting their careers and hungrily searching for an academic appointment.[24] A curriculum vitae is an autobiography of sorts, a selective fashioning and presentation of the self for particular ends. The name at the top of Merton's vita, Robert K. Merton, reflected a self-fashioning that began as an adolescent. He was born Meyer R. Schkolnick, on July 4, 1910, in "the slums of South Philadelphia to working-class Jewish immigrants from

Eastern Europe."[25] At the age of fourteen, he adopted the name Robert K. (King) Merton. As described in a 1961 profile in *The New Yorker Magazine* (and more than thirty years later by Merton in the 1994 ACLS Haskins Lecture), his name change was a product of his teenage career in magic. "Robert K. Merton / *Enchanting Mysteries* / 414 Wilder Street, Philadelphia," read his business card, with the image of a black top hat and magician's wand.[26] There is something especially evocative in the appearance of magic—the science of making things appear and disappear, of making things appear as other than they are—in this story. The broader context of Merton's change of name deepens that significance. As Craig Calhoun notes, "Merton's name change was not simply whimsical. . . . Nor was it idiosyncratically individual. It was part of the generational experience of Jewish immigrants and their children in the mid-twentieth-century United States."[27] As Merton would say later, "it seemed more American back then in the 20s."[28]

By 1968, Merton hardly needed a vita as an introduction. He had been at Columbia for over twenty-five years. He was the Giddings Professor of Sociology. As that distinction suggested, he was a leading figure in his field. He had served as president of the now-named American Sociological Association a decade earlier.[29] He was the author of dozens of field-defining articles and author or co-author of at least eight books.[30] He had trained dozens of PhDs. He had received eight honorary doctorates, and he was a fellow of the American Academy of Arts and Sciences, of the American Philosophical Society, and of the World Academy of Art and Science. All this was on his vita.[31] On and on went his list of honors, distinguished lectureships, and the journal editorial boards and commissions on which he had served. His vita reflected his academic distinction.

But Merton was not born to distinction. As his early biography suggests, he was by class, religion, and ethnicity a complete outsider to academia. His path to distinction, to belonging, and ultimately to the road to preferment was paved by a series of key relationships at each stage of his collegiate, graduate, and then early scholarly career. At Temple College (now Temple University), George E. Simpson, a PhD candidate at Penn who was teaching to support himself as he finished his own degree, introduced Merton to sociological research, to the American Sociological Society, and to Pitirin Alexandrovich Sorokin, a Russian exile who, by the time Merton completed college, had moved to Harvard, where he established the sociology department. Students from Temple did not generally go to Harvard. But Sorokin welcomed Merton and made him his research and teaching assistant and, soon, his co-author—as well as publishing in his new journal Merton's scholarly work and arranging for the publication of Merton's dissertation.

That Merton was not offered a permanent faculty appointment at Harvard—having been an instructor for three years after completing his PhD in 1936—was at least in part because of antisemitism, but that instance of discrimination ultimately led to the third and maybe the most important formative relationship for Merton's career. In 1941, Merton was hired as an assistant professor of sociology at Columbia. There he met Paul Lazarsfeld, a brilliant Jewish émigré empiricist, trained in applied mathematics and social and economic psychology at the University of Vienna, with over a decade of experience securing external funds for applied social research and running university-affiliated centers. Lazarsfeld, who had only arrived at Columbia two years before Merton, was the director of what would later be renamed the Bureau of Applied Social Research. In 1942, Merton became associate director. Together the two men would make the Department of Sociology and Bureau of Applied Social Research the dynamic heart of the field and of graduate training in the postwar years.[32]

Robert Merton and Paul Lazarsfeld and the broader academic world they were part of creating exemplified the new identity of professor as entrepreneur: research scholars who found financial support for their work, intellectual sociality, and the training of graduate students in professional associations and university-affiliated research centers supported by external funding.

Before 1950, the lion's share of the bureau's support came from grants and contracts from business, foundations, non-profit organizations, and government. But beginning in 1950, the size of the bureau's annual budget and the proportion coming from government contracts mushroomed, rising by 1965 to over a million dollars a year. That funding supported the research and salaries of faculty, multiple generations of graduate students seeding their careers as research scholars, and PhD-trained research staff. It underwrote thousands of studies, books, articles, reports, masters' theses, and PhD dissertations.[33]

The vita was a critical component of this world. "What is the distinctive nature of the coin of the realm and of intellectual property in science?" asked Robert K. Merton in a 1988 article.[34] He had begun addressing that question thirty years earlier in his 1957 American Sociological Society presidential address: "Priorities in Scientific Discovery: A Chapter in the Sociology of Science."[35] As he argued there, disputes over priority in scientific discovery were so "frequent, harsh, and ugly" because science assigned its largest rewards for originality.[36] Recognition of priority depended, as Merton noted, on a scientist having made "his contributions to knowledge known to other scientists" and on their acknowledgment of "his rights to his intellectual property." But all were not equal in this contest. In a 1968 article, based on a paper delivered the preceding year at the ASA, Merton began from the claim that the "coin of the realm" in science was "recognition." As he argued, because the "class structure" of science provided "a stratified distribution of chances," those who were already recognized were more likely to be recognized in the future even when the credit rightfully belonged to another. Drawing on the Gospel of Matthew, Merton dubbed this phenomenon the "Matthew Effect": "For unto every one that hath shall be given, and he shall have abundance; but from him that hath not shall be taken away even that which he hath."[37] Put more plainly, the rich get richer, the poor get poorer. Materially *and* intellectually.

Merton's article offered an example of an all too common phenomenon in academic life that compounded "the stratified distribution of chances." He drew his data for the article from research on Nobel laureates by one of his female graduate students, Harriet Zuckerman. Though he cited and acknowledged Zuckerman, he did not make her a co-author. Five years later, in 1973, when the article was republished in a collection of Merton's work, he added a footnote: "It is now belatedly evident to me that I drew upon the interview and other materials of the Zuckerman study to such an extent that, clearly, the paper should have appeared under joint authorship."[38] Zuckerman's interviews with Nobel laureates suggest that even had her name appeared as co-author on the original paper and article, listeners and readers might well have credited Merton for the ideas. As Merton noted in his 1968 article, drawing on Zuckerman's interviews, "in papers coauthored by men of decidedly unequal reputation, another laureate in physics reports, 'the man who's best known gets more credit, an inordinate amount of credit.'"[39] Indeed.

Merton's focus was on science. But many elements of the value system of science were shared in other disciplines. Moreover, the transformation in the relationship between the state and universities and the revaluation of research in the postwar years was driven by science. So even had disciplines outside science sought to operate by a different value structure, they were caught up in science's orbit—which increasingly defined the value structure of academia more generally. And so, science's forms of recognition and reputation became the coin of the academic realm.

But even as they did, the dramatic expansion and specialization of research, and the related proliferation of books and journals, meant that finding recognition became more challenging.[40] In a 1963 book, Derek de Solla Price, plotting the growth in the number of scientific journals since the seventeenth century, projected that by the year 2000 there would be nearly a million journal titles.[41] His numbers were wildly off, but not the basic point: Beginning in the late 1940s, the number of scholarly journals, most pronouncedly in but not limited to science, had grown exponentially. That proliferation had implications for recognition. As Merton noted, the "exponential increase in the volume of scientific publications," the corresponding difficulty of locating pertinent research and the impossibility of reading everything in one's field, magnified the Matthew Effect. Readers responded by reading the work of authors whose names they already knew, marginalizing the un- or lesser known.[42]

The point again was not limited to science. The context almost demanded that scholars be entrepreneurial in claiming recognition. The vita offered them a critical tool. One's vita gathered all the evidence—educational credentials; academic appointments; honors, prizes, and awards; fellowships, grants, and contracts received; every publication; every paper delivered—under one's name. The vita became the measure of the man. As a senior sociologist at the University of Chicago noted in 1986 in consideration of a scholar for a named professorship, "There is really very little that need be said on his behalf since his curriculum vitae speaks so eloquently for him."[43]

But how it was that a scholar's vita came to "speak so eloquently for him" was about so much more than publications. Merton's August 1968 vita included eight honorary doctorates. By 1994, he had received twenty. As Craig Calhoun notes, that "Merton, and also immigrants like Paul Lazarsfeld had reason to feel insecure about their status in the university even as their prestige grew" suggests the work that a vita did for even those who seemed to need no introduction.[44] The point was far truer for others, less famous. Before World War II, there had been few prizes and awards for research. The Nobel Prizes, limited to six fields, four in the sciences, first awarded in 1901, were and would remain in a class by themselves.[45] The first generation of American academics with PhDs at the turn of the twentieth century had established professional societies and scholarly journals for the dissemination of work in their fields, and universities had likewise established university presses. But they had not, for the most part, established prizes. The American Chemical Society (ACS), founded in 1876, was unusual in having seven prizes before 1945. Even the American Historical Association (AHA), with four prizes before 1945, stood out compared to fields like sociology, political science, economics, and English—which offered none. In the years after World War II, and especially beginning in the 1960s and after, the number of prizes, honors, and awards offered by professional academic associations exploded. This explosion too fed the vita. The American Sociological Association awarded its first annual book award in 1965. By 2006, in the field of sociology in the US, there were fifty book prizes.[46] The number of prizes in the sciences spoke both to the dominant place of science in the postwar era and to the broader proliferation of prizes. As Harriet Zuckerman notes, by 1991, the sciences alone in North America offered some three thousand prizes, five times as many as in 1969.[47]

In 1969, Gale Research published the first edition of *Awards, Honors and Prizes: A Directory and Source Book*. It spoke to and of the times.[48] Academic prizes and awards rubbed elbows in Gale's volumes with those relating to every field of endeavor imaginable. Badminton, bowling, ceramics, concrete . . . on and on the list went. The first edition, one volume limited to the US and Canada, listed 2,228 prizes and awards. By 1982, Gale's *Awards, Honors and Prizes* was in its fifth edition and listed more than 6,200 prizes and awards.[49] By 1997, the thirteenth edition listed approximately 17,000 prizes, honors, and awards.[50] The proliferation of prizes reflected what historian James English refers to as an "economy of prestige" and sociologist Joel Best describes as an American "congratulatory culture."[51]

The prize proliferation was bound up with post–World War II American economic prosperity. But it was more than simply a mirror of the broader society. It went hand-in-hand with and reinforced the revaluation of research in academic life. It reflected the struggle for recognition in a world in which the emergence of new fields, increasing specialization, and dramatic expansion in size made most academics, beyond a small circle, strangers to one another.

The career and vita of Steve Ruggles offer a glimpse into the proliferation of prizes. A historical demographer, Ruggles completed his PhD at the University of Pennsylvania in May 1984 and began an appointment in the Department of History at the University of Minnesota that fall. The vita he submitted in applying to the University of Minnesota had a category titled "Fellowships and Honors." There was not much there.[52] Five years later Ruggles had received three prominent honors, none of which had existed when he began college in 1973.[53] The first of those honors—the Allan Sharlin Memorial Award for best publication in the field of social history—was established in 1985, the same year Ruggles completed his PhD. The professional association that awarded that honor, the Social Science History Association (SSHA), was established in 1974, the year after Ruggles began college. A second honor—the William J. Goode Distinguished Book Award, Family Section, American Sociological Association (ASA)—was established in 1984, the year Ruggles completed his PhD. The third major award Ruggles received in the first five years after completing his PhD was a McKnight Professorship from the University of Minnesota, an award established in 1987, part of an effort to keep promising young research scholars at Minnesota.

There is a complex dynamic in the creation, bestowing, and receipt of prizes. Within academia, as was true in American society at large, the vast majority of prizes were awarded by professional societies. In academia, the proliferation of awards was bound up with the proliferation of fields of research and related professional societies. So, for example, there were no separate sections of the American Sociological Society in 1945. By 1970, there were eight sections; by 2004, there were forty-three. Under ASA's rules, each section could make three annual awards, at least one of which had to be to a student. Not surprisingly, sections eagerly established awards, part of what Joel Best explains as the search for legitimation.[54] Focusing on the proliferation of prizes in the sciences, Harriet Zuckerman notes that prizes made work in a field "more visible" and "conferred an aura of social importance and prestige" not only on the scholar receiving the prize but also on the field.[55] Academic prizes became a vehicle for writing a field's history and assuring that those scholars for whom prizes were named were written into that history. As Ruggles' vita suggests, this was as true in the social sciences and the humanities as in the sciences.[56] Prizes, moreover, reinforced the reorientation of academic life around professional societies.[57]

But unlike the Nobel, the recipients of which were widely known and thereafter recognized and remembered as laureates, the vast majority of American academic prizes had little, if any, recognition beyond the field they represented. Vitae gathered these recognitions, assured they would not be forgotten, linked them to one's name, and linked them to one's publications. The vita was the closest thing academics had to a uniform on which might be pinned or sewn honors.[58] But the vita was better than a uniform because it so often preceded or stood in for the individual, including in consideration for other recognitions, awards, fellowships, grants, and contracts. And so, one recognition garnered others.

The proliferation of journals and of professional societies and their prizes was only one element in this later-twentieth-century transformation of the vita. By August 2022, Ruggles's vita was thirty-six pages long with thirty-three separate headings.[59] His vita, like those of others in contemporary academic life, was a far cry from the brief vita of a paragraph or two appended to dissertations, a prerequisite for the PhD in the early twentieth century that garnered recognition for the author, his dissertation, and his university through acknowledgment of his academic mentors. It bore little resemblance to the one- to two-page curriculum vitae of German and other European scholars escaping Nazi-dominated Europe in the 1930s. Part of the added length of vita in the decades since the 1960s was the incorporation of publications into the vita rather than as a separate bibliography. But that shift itself was linked to the dawning of the entrepreneurial era in academia. And the added length is not only or even mostly a product of including publications on one's vita. Ruggles's publications account for only eight of the thirty-six pages.[60] Rather, Ruggles's vita reflects the pursuit of recognition and the proliferation of opportunities for its expression.

One sees in Ruggles's vita the reorientation of academic life around research, research centers, and professional societies. We might think of the first page of a vita as being like the stories above the fold in the era of print newspapers. The first page of Ruggles's 2022 vita highlights honors and recognitions that frame his status as a national, even international figure. A Regents Professor at the University of Minnesota. The long-term director of an internationally renowned research center. Past president of two major professional societies. National Science Foundation (NSF), US Census Bureau, and National Research Council advisory committees. All beneath his name and institutional address, which is not the Department of History but rather the Institute for Social Research and Data Innovation. There is an important element of service in many of these recognitions, but the honors are listed on the first page of Ruggles's vita for what they say about his professional standing. Lesser professional-service commitments are left to the end of the vita. But as telling as any element of his vita for the reorientation of academic life, the outward-facing character of the vita, is that in those thirty-six pages, "PhD Advisees Completed" and "Postdoctoral Advisees" are included, themselves a statement of Ruggles's scholarly standing—but there is no reference to undergraduate teaching.

As the substance and organization of his vita make clear, at the heart of Ruggles's intellectual work and identity has been the creation of huge public-use databases of census data, created with the support of federal funding. Five pages of Ruggles's vita are taken up by what he calls "Extramural Funding." As Ruggles remembers it, he first included a heading on his vita for "Federal Grants and Contracts" around 1992, "when I got up to three of them." When I asked why, he replied, "I probably saw it on someone else's."[61] In the years that followed, a continuing stream of external funding, overwhelmingly from the federal government, supported the founding and work of a research center which as of 2023 had 183 employees—the size, in other words, of multiple departments. All told (and the calculator is running), between 1982 and 2021, Ruggles as PI or co-PI had brought in over $171 million to the University of Minnesota. Fellowships appear on vitae because they represent an external affirmation of the merits of one's research. The larger the award, the more prestigious the grantor, the more credit the scholar accumulates. Federal grants and contracts, though, do more than this. They not only fund research that might itself bring recognition to a university, they also were and remain an essential component of the host universities' budgets.[62]

The growing length and detail of vitae was not only a product of academic entrepreneurship or the individual search for recognition. The curriculum vitae began its life as a form as a creature of universities. It should not be surprising, then, that though their interests lay in uneasy tension, universities, as much as individuals, professional societies, and the state would play a central role in this third life stage of the vita. In 1949, Columbia University—one of the first American universities to have made the vita appended to the dissertation a degree requirement—dropped the vita requirement.[63] The timing of Columbia's action was more than incidental or symbolic. For lesser universities, including those just establishing graduate programs, the vita appended to the dissertation as degree requirement still had work to do. But for elite universities, the vita in its first purpose had run its course. It had, though, a new purpose. Universities understood that in a research age, more than ever, their rankings rested on the productivity—meaning research—and reputation of their faculty. Assuring or striving for "academic eminence," as the 1954 Columbia report by that title put it, required constant vigilance. In that pursuit, the vita became universities' multi-tool.

The heated competition among universities for rank, recognition, and external funding, combined with the adoption of up-or-out tenure, led universities to be intensely focused on weeding out mediocrity. Reflecting broader trends, the University of Minnesota had adopted its first comprehensive set of regulations establishing a system of up-or-out tenure in 1945.[64] Two years later, in a 1947 message to all department chairs and deans, requesting data on their "methods, practices, and experience," William Anderson, chair of a subcommittee on tenure, warned of the threat facing the university: "During the wartime and postwar rush of things the University has added to its faculty a considerable number of men and women without having been able to pick and choose as carefully as would have been desirable." But, as he noted, with the new tenure regulations in effect, those with the rank of assistant professor were "on the high road toward tenure," and those who were instructors "must either be dropped in due time or promoted to the next higher rank." Assuring a faculty of "unquestioned excellence" meant that "many critical decisions [would] have to be made in the next few years." Failure to do so would mean that the university would become "obligated to carry on to retirement age . . . faculty members of undistinguished qualities." This "danger," as he referred to it, "could easily become a reality through easy going and careless practices of promotion and the acquisition of indefinite tenure."[65]

The anxiety was widespread. Reporting to the Harvard overseers in his annual report in 1943–1944, Harvard President James B. Conant invoked the words of his predecessor A. Lawrence Lowell: "The surest way to ruin a university faculty is to fill it with good men." As Conant noted, "nine times out of ten the normal forces working within any special segment of the University made for a good appointment, but against an excellent appointment." Harvard did not want good men; it wanted the best men. The "new invention" at Harvard, adopted in 1942–1943, of the ad hoc committee staffed with men outside the appointing department, including faculty from other universities—was intended as a check, a way of assuring that permanent appointments went to the best qualified candidates.[66]

A 1953 committee *Report on Appointment and Promotion Procedures at Columbia University*, chaired by economics professor George J. Stigler, voiced similar concerns and adopted a similar approach. As the committee noted, "The individual departments are subjected to pressures which they cannot resist completely and continuously, and yet which should be so resisted. The personal likeability of a junior man may obscure—or even outweigh—his essential mediocrity to his immediate colleagues."[67] The Stigler Committee rejected the argument that there was a long-term place for those "unworthy of promotion" who performed important "routine duties," insisting that "even simple tasks are done better by better men, and in education there are hardly any simple tasks. More important, the junior ranks should be filled with young men who now contribute to the intellectual vitality of the university and who, we hope, will one day be ornaments of the faculty." Uniformity across the university of rules and procedures in appointments and promotions, including maximum terms for nontenured appointments and the use of ad hoc committees for all tenured appointments, were essential: "We believe this systematization should take place at once."[68]

The systematization of the measurement, evaluation, and valuing of faculty in hiring, tenure, promotion, and annual reviews went hand-in-hand with the revaluation of research in the decades following World War II. Together they were powerful administrative engines for the vita. Columbia's

Stigler Committee had not used the terms vita or curriculum vitae in its description of the materials to accompany all nominations for appointments at the rank of assistant professor and above. But its recommendation that all nominations include at least "a full professional history of the candidate" and "a full list of publications of the candidate" in effect described the vita in the form it had begun to take by the 1950s. And in 1959, Columbia University's first faculty handbook explained that "the nomination of an associate or full professor . . . goes to the Dean of Faculties with a *vita* and with letters of recommendation testifying to the nominee's career and qualifications" and that it was the department chairman's responsibility to provide the ad hoc committee, in advance of its meeting, "materials relevant to the proposed appointment," including "a condensed *vita* of the candidate."[69] Elite universities were the first to systematize tenure and promotion, but in the 1960s and 1970s, systematization of tenure, the use of ad hoc or standing college-level and university-level tenure committees, and requirements for external written evaluations of candidates for tenure and promotion became the norm.[70]

The evaluation of faculty by men beyond their department required a shared foundation. The vita provided that foundation. It offered a common form. That form was all the more important for external review of candidates for tenure and promotion. In the first half of the twentieth century, leading men in a field received scores of "we want a man" letters seeking their assistance in identifying a "first rate man" for an appointment. From the 1960s on, leading men faced a new set of requests: for their expert evaluation of candidates for tenure and promotion at other universities. And these requests included the candidate's vita.[71]

But it was not only for purposes of promotion and tenure that the vita became an essential tool of universities. The vita came to pervade every element of academic life: departmental self-surveys, annual faculty reviews, approval of new graduate programs, university information services. And in those processes, universities sometimes made clear what they wanted to see on faculty vitae. In a 1975 self-survey of the Psychology Department at the University of Minnesota, for example, faculty were given a numbered list—twenty-one categories—to be addressed in their vitae in a prescribed order.[72] The list was not a printed form with blanks to be filled in, but it was, nonetheless, a form.[73] My first clue that the faculty had been given a form to follow was that a third of the vitae were numbered. Most of these included headings, but a few were simply a numbered list with "Vita" at the top, leaving the reader to discern the questions to which they were responding.[74] Without the consistently numbered vitae, it would have taken me a while to realize that all the faculty vitae responded, in the exact same order, to a fixed set of questions. Over half the faculty—including all but one of those hired since 1970—addressed the questions on the form in the order in which they had been asked but drafted their vitae as though the structure and categories were their own.

As this self-survey highlighted, departments increasingly came to know themselves through the vitae of their faculty. That they did so was a product of the centering of research in academic life, the growth of distinct fields within disciplines, the increasingly specialized character of fields of research, and the related reorientation of the intellectual lives of research scholars outward to others in their specialized fields. One can see here how categories on vitae multiplied. The specialization of research was reflected in a proliferation of journals, which produced a proliferation of editorial boards and the need for expert outside reviewers. All of which became categories on vitae.[75] Prize committees, other professional association committees, scientific advisory boards—the list went on and on. Like the branches in a tree that divide into increasingly finer stems, so it was with possibilities for recognition.

Just as departments increasingly depended on their members' vitae to know themselves, university administrators knew and measured departments and their members through vitae. From the University of Minnesota Psychology Department's opening assessment of itself as "highly productive," the text returned repeatedly to the attached vitae that were included in a second volume. It counted: grants and contracts received; articles and books published; prizes and honors received; invited appearances; conference papers delivered; editorial board memberships; prize, fellowship, and advisory committees served on; MA and PhD students graduated. And on it went: Productivity and professional status deeply intertwined with outward-facing metrics, their disciplining force deeply internalized. Reinforced within institutions not only through self-surveys but more routinely—through hiring, salary, annual reviews, rank, named professorships, and other awards. Reinforced externally through prizes, awards, and honors; fellowships, grants, and contracts; professional association, fellowship, and grant committees; lecture invitations, and introductions. All three domains—individual, departmental/university, professional—were accessed through the vita. And so, items that without the individual professional and institutional pursuit of recognition would never have appeared on vitae, became standard. Hence, the length of Steve Ruggles's 2022 vita. The growing length of vitae generally—becomes more understandable.

In 1995, Steve Ruggles was profiled in *Wired* magazine in an article titled

"The King of Quant." The subtitle read, "Can professor-cum-revolutionary Steve Ruggles armed with the first new scholastic discipline of the information age, historical demography, topple the edifice of history . . . and everything else?" Public stardom was not something associated with academics before World War II. Big science funded by the federal government, beginning with the atomic bomb, had changed that, not only bringing some academics international eminence in their fields but also transforming them into public figures. Robert Oppenheimer, Hans Bethe, and others were featured on the cover of magazines like *Time* and *Life*. Leading figures in medicine followed. In 1960, rather than a "Man of the Year," *Time* magazine declared fifteen US scientists "Men of the Year."[76] In 1961, Robert Merton was the subject of a long profile in *The New Yorker Magazine*.[77] The article in *Wired* magazine on Ruggles brought academic stardom into the information age.

The transformations that take place in our own lifetime can be the hardest to grasp. The emergence of historical demography, Ruggles's field of research, depended on the revolution in computing. But that revolution, and especially the advent of the personal computer and the creation of the World Wide Web, had broader implications for academia and the vita.[78] It is difficult to unknow the world of textual connectivity that has become so completely naturalized—and that is, for a growing number of those in academia, the only world they have ever known. Some academics, attuned to the possibilities the web offered for connection and a global public audience, were quick in creating personal websites. Ruggles offers one such example. His early personal website was rudimentary: name, university address, email, and phone, followed by a short list of links: "Research Assistantships Available for Fall 1998"; "Overview of Research"; "Curriculum Vitae"; "Integrated Public Use Microdata Series (IPUMS)"; "Demographic Event"; "'The King of Quant' *Wired Magazine*, 3 (1995), 86–90"; "History 1301 Web Page"; "History 5011 Web Page."[79] But even the simple list of links suggested something of the character of the transformation the World Wide Web would produce. Anyone with a computer and access to the internet anywhere in the world could now access Ruggles's full curriculum vitae and read his narrative "overview of research." When I asked Ruggles why he had posted his vita, he said, "I don't know . . . Advertising, I guess."[80]

The vita that had in important respects been a product of the postwar revaluation of research took on a new kind of existence, even meaning, with the World Wide Web. Before the web, vitae had circulated in largely closed circles, each with a defined and known audience. The vita was, in this sense, a transactional document. This world continued. But with the web a new world opened in which the vita was a public document that circulated or at least was publicly accessible, the audience no longer clear, fixed, or limited to academia. Many posted their vitae as a link, as Ruggles had. Others pasted in full or abbreviated vitae featuring key categories like education, prizes and other honors, and publications. But what most defined the new medium was a return to narrative. Stripped of much of the cumbersome baggage the vita as list had acquired, narrative vitae, "Bios," were a sort of credential sandwich—education, prizes and honors, fellowships, grants and contracts—for the description of research past, present, and future, and listing of major publications. Many bios were no more than a paragraph—written perhaps with an eye to fitting on a single screen—but others were long intellectual biographies.[81] These narratives might have incorporated teaching. Some did. Ruggles's early personal website linked to two courses. But the focus overwhelmingly, like that of the vita, was on research. And befitting the nature of introduction of oneself to an audience one did not know, most websites soon included a photograph of the scholar.

The web emerged in the midst of what critics disdainfully described as a "confessional culture" but what historian Sarah Igo more thoughtfully describes as a redefinition of privacy in terms of a right to "public self-definition."[82] Academics were part of this broader culture. And equally important was the changing face of academia that began with the challenge to race and sex discrimination in the 1960s and 1970s. A growing number of scholars, especially those who were members of groups that had been excluded from or marginalized within academia by virtue of race, gender, sexuality, disability, nationality, and other elements of identity, challenged disciplinary paradigms of distance, objectivity, and abstraction.[83] They acknowledged and claimed personal knowledge, embedding their life stories in their scholarly work.

Among these scholars is the Princeton-trained cultural anthropologist Ruth Behar, born in Havana, Cuba, to Jewish parents who had escaped Nazi-dominated Europe, her family moving from Cuba to New York City in 1962. In the final chapter of her first book, a feminist ethnography of a Mexican street peddler, titled *Translated Woman: Crossing the Border with Esperanza's Story*, published in 1993, Behar shared her own border-crossing story, what she called "the biography in the shadow."[84] The book, especially the closing chapter, brought her condemnation but also acclaim.[85] In the closing chapter, Behar retraced for readers her path from outsider to "a member of the professional managerial class." For her as for other outsiders, higher education was critical to that transformation. In a mix of her own words and those of two other scholars, she wrote that higher education is "'a process'" by which "'we learn to avow and remember certain knowledges and devalue and forget others.' What we cannot tell ourselves we know, what we have to repress of ourselves in the process of becoming educated, become the 'sanctioned ignorances' of our knowledge."[86] It is impossible to read these words without thinking of the vita, of the role it plays in producing "sanctioned ignorances," its disciplining force—but, equally importantly, its role in paving the way to inclusion.

The web offered an escape, though a necessarily incomplete one, from sanctioned ignorances. And here too Behar is exemplary. As early as 1998, she had a professionally designed personal website. It did not include her vita. Rather, she drew selectively from it, weaving a biography in which the personal served the professional and entrepreneurial. Her personal website, as updated in 2000, included a personal photo, the covers and links to each of her books, and a long, linked "Bio." That bio began, "RUTH BEHAR was born in Havana, Cuba and came to live in New York with her family in 1962." "Since her youth, Ruth Behar has had a strong attachment to the Spanish-speaking world. . . . She has written about her experience of crossing cultural borders as a poet, essayist, fiction writer, editor, and ethnographer." And accompanying the bio were photos of Behar that reinforced the narrative of a border-crossing woman and scholar.[87] But interwoven with this personal narrative were her educational credentials and honors and awards, including a "MacArthur Foundation 'genius' award" and a Guggenheim Fellowship. In *Translated Woman*, Esperanza says at one point of Americans' likely response to the stories of her life, "I say that they won't believe it."[88] That feeling was one that many who came to intellectual life as outsiders understood and shared. And so, while they might have sought to escape the constrained identity of the vita, they, as much as others, maybe more, needed the vita and the recognition signaled by credentials and honors and awards listed there.

A. Hunter Dupree had described the "research contract"—a World War II US creation by which the federal government funded academic research—as "revolutionary" because it made research itself the product.[89] What entrepreneurial scholars voluntarily embraced to further their individual recognition and reputations, to connect with new and broader audiences, to break free in some measure from the constraints universities, disciplines, and the vita placed on ways and ends of knowing, was simultaneously grasped by universities as a tool to further their own recognition, reputation, and prestige.[90] As "the road to preferment" in academia shifted to research, *and* the culture of academia favored the entrepreneurial, *and* universities hungry for recognition and external funding competed for academic stars who brought in huge grants and contracts or won major prizes—"newsmakers"—*and* as others strived to themselves join the elect, there was a way in which academics themselves became the product. And so, it is not surprising to discover that universities took it upon themselves to post faculty vitae online. By 2001, for example, elite law schools had a link for every faculty member that included their "Resume/CV."[91]

There came to be, as well, an expectation that one's vita, or at the very least some form of current individual research bio, would be available online. Critiques of the "surveillance state" and of social media seem apposite here. As John Gilliom and Torin Monahan write, "To what extent are we truly willing participants when a nearly universal architecture of communication . . . dominates our social world and becomes necessary for keeping a job, attending a school, or having a life? Can you really opt out? Can you really even *imagine* opting out?" Or, as Julia Angwin writes, "In a culture where people judge each other as much by their digital footprints as by their real-life personalities, it's an act of faith to opt out of sharing your data."[92] In a world where recognition was "the coin of the realm," as Robert Merton dubbed it, a failure or decision not to have an online professional self was effectively a choice not to trade in the coin of the academic realm.

Recognition "the coin of the realm." The history I was coming to understand pushed up uncomfortably on my own professional life. I began my academic career in 1995, just as the World Wide Web was beginning. I had two small children, a commuting professional spouse, and was focused on just keeping my chin above water. But I also was not attuned to the web, and I shy away from self-promotion. As I worked on this book, I knew my faculty bio was long out of date. Reluctantly, I searched the Internet Archive for myself and discovered that in 2006, the College of Liberal Arts at the University of Minnesota posted on the university's website a vita I had submitted in a required faculty annual review.[93] It feels strange to look for oneself this way and find the record one has and has not left, the record one has created and that others have created of you.

What happens when you unexpectedly find yourself in the story? You have been there all along, you say to me. And, of course, you are right. Having made others the subject of history, histories that they had lived but did not know—both in the history of the vita and the cowboy suit tragedy—I too discover myself a subject of this history, a subject in time. In sharing excerpts of my letters to Frances, in the structure of this book, and in its claim to personal knowledge, I have been here all along. But tracing the history of the curriculum vitae as an academic form and bringing that history to the present, I discover the course of my life in it. It is uncomfortable.

When I first turned to my letters to Frances in a lecture a year after her death, it was because I could not speak about losing her, about how hard I was finding it to live, so I let excerpts from my letters voice what I could not speak to directly. I was not thinking of how sharing parts of my letters fit into a culture in which people share deeply personal things about themselves on social media or about the mushrooming of memoir as a genre. Having never had a social-media profile, did I think I was living somehow outside the broader culture? So too, the history of the proliferation of prizes and recognition and their role in the transformation of the vita and individual identity cast in a new light prizes, awards, and other recognitions on my vita. "My vita," we say, obscuring the institutional, professional, and disciplinary forces, the history that has in a sense produced it. But in the vita's ordered form there is not only a broader set of forces at work, not only an expression and pursuit of institutional and individual power, privilege, and belonging, but also a particular expression of a deeply human struggle for meaning and control—a struggle to define the course of a life in the face of events and forces beyond our control.

· PART VI ·

Precarity

time

Dear Frances,

The sun seems to be shining. I haven't gotten out of bed yet. Don't really want to, but I have to do better with today than I did with yesterday. Last night after I stopped writing, I found myself thinking that I know the future and that is what makes living so hard. That's one of the things that marks death—we know in death what the future holds in a way that we do not in life. Next week you will have been gone for a year and the week after that you will still be gone. It's that knowing the future that makes it hard to get out of bed.

...

I have been beginning to understand that Dad and I have to start to chart a future, to plan for the future, not just make it from one day to the next, to model for Wilder that planning for a future, that living, not just existing is what we all—him included—have to do. . . . I never thought though that I would have to model this: how to live when one of my children could not, did not get that chance. I feel like I'm being pulled toward a cliff in a river that is engorged with water. And I know already that I am going to be washed over the cliff, because I already have been.

...

Last year you spent this day sleeping late and then doing nothing at all, just relaxing all day, looking forward to your last [high school] choir concert. I wish I'd taken time to look nicer that night so that in the last picture we have of you and me together I looked nicer. You looked beautiful, radiant. So now I'm going to get out of bed, get my slippers and robe on, brush my teeth, and try to remember that on this day you were full of life.

...

Yesterday, I finally took your corsage from the choir concert out of the frig. It's been there since the night of your concert last year. For a long time it was very important to me to keep it. It was a link to you. I panicked one day in early winter when I didn't see it and thought someone must have thrown it out. I felt such relief when I discovered it still there. Sometime, a bit ago, I realized that it now felt different to have it there. It was dry and the rose shriveled. It was dead and felt like something lost and gone. But I wasn't sure what to do with it. Yesterday I had an idea for it and it feels good: I took all the petals from the yellow rose and put them in one of the small pots you made in pottery in middle school and set it on the table next to the couch in the family room right next to your glasses. The dried yellow petals look beautiful in the glossy brown pot and they fill it perfectly. Now, rather than a dead rose, it's like having beautiful dried petals and it feels very good to have this reminder of you and your final concert in the family room.

. . .

What is time like where you are Frances? As we retrace the hours and days of this week in April from last year, do you too retrace them? In 'Requiem for a Friend' the poet Rainer Maria Rilke describes death as "wrench the till-then from the ever-since — / this concerns us: setting it all in order/ is the task we have continually before us." His phrase "wrenching the til-then from the ever-since" speaks so powerfully to me. Is there, for you, Frances, an "ever-since"?

. . .

Why must I relive this week? There is a sense that this is the last week we get to live together, because this time last year you were alive and though we knew you had had a massive stroke neither we nor the doctors knew yet why or just how bad it was. And so today holds the memory of great fear, but also love and hope. And it's because of this, I think, that I am swept into the current of that week, of this day. This time last year I believed without being fully aware of thinking about the future that we would be returned to our lives and the belief that you could have been returned to your life as it was—even though things did not turn out that way—means that I must be in this day fully again.

. . .

What a hard scrabble day this has been. I got the letter done that I told you I had to get done, but then I was at a loss; I could not work, but I also could not write you. I felt emotionless, like I was waiting, but also knowing that there is no waiting—I can wait, but you cannot come back. I find myself waiting or alternately feeling moments of peace only to have them slip away with the realization that this cannot be overcome or waited out.

...

I'm not looking forward to the Walk for Animals. The idea that I have to spend the first anniversary of the final morning of your life surrounded by hundreds of people at a festive fund-raiser is enough to make me want to scream. But then we will take Wilder back to school and it will be the same deafening quiet that we faced last year when suddenly we were home and everyone had left and a hush descended over the house: no doctors, no hallways, no other patients, no beeping, no drips, no flashing lights, no you.

...

Because it is April 28th it is Wednesday in my mind. This was the day that [one of the doctors] put the pressure monitor in your brain. . . . There's a hypnotic quality to machines in a hospital room. You find yourself staring, straining, studying, looking to them for signs that you cannot read in the still body of your child.

...

Dad and I saw our first barge on the river this morning as we walked Sam. I've always liked seeing our first barge—it marks the change in seasons here along the Mississippi River in the Upper Midwest. I might have texted you with the news. Not sure how you would've replied, but somehow I expect sweetly.

...

Went to buy flowers to do for the planters. It is another activity I associate with you. For as long as I can remember, you were the one who always went with me. Thinking about that today, I remembered the wonderful times of you and me shopping for plants in the spring together. And though you weren't much on being involved in the planting itself, you often kept me company as I planted or spread out wood chips—another purchasing activity we generally did together. Reminds me of the time a few years back when we were at Home Depot together and you were just standing behind our cart as I heaved bags of soil and wood chips onto the cart and some woman walked by full of disgust at how lazy today's teens were and made some snarky comment about maybe "the princess" doing nothing should be doing the lifting.

I was just delighted to have you along and very happy to do the lifting myself which I viewed as exercise. I remember you and I laughed a bit about it.

. . .

It was about this time on the 29th last year when the Dr. on duty for the night in Intensive Care told us the results of the CT scan they'd done that evening: the scan showed that you'd had another stroke, this one on the other side of your brain and that the swelling from the first stroke was worse. We sat there next to him at a computer screen as he showed us the images and told us the news. I remember sitting there tears streaming down my face and Dad asking if you would make it through the night. . . . I want to have this one last night with you, a night in which though you were slipping away, your skin was still warm, your heart still beating, the respirator keeping you going. Oh, Frances—I can see you there and I feel so desperate to be with you again. Good night, sweetheart.

. . .

Today is April 30th. I don't remember what the weather was like last year on this day. It has been so important to me all year to tell you about the weather "here." I've wanted you to know the days, the seasons. Today has dawned dark gray, cold, with a steady rain falling. Today last year was your last day Frances. I "gave" you a poem for Christmas and one for your birthday and plan to continue that for the rest of my life. The third event I plan to recognize each year with a poem to you is April 30th. This year I wanted to give you the poem that Frau Crowder first gave you last May. It's by the German poet Goethe. I'm going to write it first in German and then in English:

> *"Es rauschen die Wasser, die Wolken vergehen,*
> *doch bleiben die Sterne, sie wandeln und stehen.*
> *So auch mit der Liebe der Treuen geschiecht:*
> *Sie wegt sich, sie regt sich und äudert sich nicht."*
>
> *"The waters are rushing away, clouds go by,*
> *but the stars remain, they wander and they stand*
> *That is also what happens with loyal love:*
> *It moves, it stirs and it does not change."*

. . .

It has now been one year, Frances. It does not seem possible: either the fact of your being gone or the time passed. I suppose this is how one year becomes two and two years become three, and so on. There is both the absoluteness of the thing and the incomprehensibility of it. I think the death of a child is like this and so we can know it is so, but the searing physical pain gives way to flashes of heartbreaking knowing, but in between there's a gauzy unreality that I suppose allows one to carry on in a fashion. . . . Writing to you this year has gotten me through this year. Has it done the same for you, Frances? This day last year, Frances, we thought we were saying our final goodbyes to you. But you were already gone then. Without knowing it we were beginning the transition to a new relationship that each of us individually would continue to have with you. I didn't understand that then and only gradually and still incompletely understand that now. I know now that you'll never be gone to me. . . . I love you, sweetheart.

chapter twenty · "for the rest of his natural life"

"I sort of remember coming home," Gaither Bates Jr. said to me. "It was, you know, it seemed like a joyous occasion."[1] And it was, for the parents and families of children who survived. But the joy was mixed with other emotions. Households had changed. Some dramatically. Casimir Krzeczkowski's brother, Stanley, had died from his burns. Casimir was now an only child. His parents had divorced. Other couples would also. The Viands household had shattered. Home for Robert Viands and his oldest brother became a shifting series of foster "homes" and then an orphanage for all four boys. Far less dramatic changes nonetheless left a powerful imprint. In the three years that Tommy Habina was in the hospital, his family moved, his mother had another child, and whether because she thought he would have outgrown them or that he was not going to survive, she threw his clothes and toys away. Then there was the disruption that an injured—what could seem to siblings and spouses, now a favored—child brought to a household. "I kind of disrupted the whole family," Jack Lockhart said. "Everything was geared around me, you know."[2] And looming over the present was a future rendered uncertain in new and profound ways.

This certain uncertainty was captured in the phrase that appeared in some way in the legal claims of every family whose child had survived: *for the rest of his natural life*. The phrase was common to civil claims for damages for physical injury. It posited a future rendered uncertain by the defendants' wrongful actions. It contained its own analogue—a certain future, a natural life. These children's and their families' future unfolded in the same broad historical context as the "road to preferment." The realm of life accounted for by law was as incomplete as life reflected in the vita, even as each, law and the vitae, shaped the course of lives.

By Easter 1948, when Jackie Izzo's mother brought her home—"she just checked me out and never took me back," in Jackie's words—skin had yet to grow over the stumps where Jackie's legs had been amputated at the hip. Even had it already done so, there was so little left to her legs that she had no support to balance and sit upright. Her mother was terrified that she would do something that would cause Jackie to die. But soon enough her parents must have looked ahead trying to imagine what sort of life she could have. Who would care for her when they were gone? Would there be money for her support? Could she be self-supporting? They had only learned that January about the *McCormack* verdict. About the same time that Jackie's mother brought her home from the hospital, they filed suit. But whether they would get anything from the lawsuit, whether there would be money for Jackie's support when she was no longer a child, was unclear. Remember that long before the first settlements or even cases were filed, families of children burned in the early years had been living with the uncertainty of what their child's injuries would mean for their and their child's future.

For Scott Timberlake's parents, was there even joy in the homecoming? The high fever that the burns produced had left him unable to speak, unable seemingly to comprehend even basic things, his right arm drawn up against his body, his hand loosely clenched. Only a few months earlier he had proudly dressed himself and ridden his tricycle. Now, without words or comprehension, he screamed, pinched, bit, and scratched. He ripped the wallpaper next to his bed off the wall; anything that could be knocked over and broken in their home—tables, lamps—was, in his many falls and when he lashed out in frustration. Whether he might with intensive, expensive therapies regain even part of what had been lost was unclear.[3] Things they had taken for granted—dressing and feeding oneself, toileting, following rules, speaking—all things their five-year-old son had done before he was injured—were now uncertain. And their dreams for his future? That there were things they had taken for granted, dreams they had had, was exposed to all these parents in the same moment in which those assumptions and dreams were cast into shadow and doubt.

The headline in the *Tampa Bay Times* above the photo of a boy sitting on a tricycle, his feet on the pedals, his smiling face looking into the camera, read "Pat Peterson Rides Again."[4] The article proclaimed he was home and "well," "*able to run and play like any other seven-year-old*." The truth was more complicated. He was out of the "crippled" children's hospital that he had hated.[5] And he was home. That a child burned so grievously lived was itself something to celebrate. He could walk again, though with difficulty.

A recent operation had revealed permanent damage to the tendons of his left ankle, meaning that he would never be able to touch that heel to the floor and would always walk on the toes of that foot.[6]

But there were other injuries that were not visible. The terrors came unbidden in the night. At the children's hospital in Umatilla there had been a boy—Pat?—who needed whirlpool treatments. Other boys would float lit matches on wax toward him in the whirlpool as he screamed, unable to escape, desperately trying to keep the matches from reaching him. In Pat's nightmares, the matches were coming toward him, floating, lit.[7] "I was having all kinds of um, issues, mentally when I first came home," Jack Lockhart Jr. said to me. He and his brother had shared a room before he was injured, but when he was brought home from the hospital, unable to walk, he was placed in a hospital bed in the living room. "I tore the wallpaper just about off that wall," he said. There were also the day terrors. "Any kind of fire would throw me into a panic," he recalled. Even a controlled burn of tall grasses along the railroad tracks that abutted their home was a source of terror for him, trapped in his wheelchair, unable to move himself.[8]

For two and a half years after he got out of the hospital, Jack Lockhart could not walk, his legs fixed in a bent position. "I used to scoot," he explained. "That's how I'd get around the neighborhood."[9] "Do you remember friendships from that time?" I asked. "Uh, not really. I uh, I didn't have any friends."[10] But he explained that as a child he thought, "'It's a temporary hiccup. I'll be up and running, you know, again.' Because that's what a kid thinks. He's looking forward. 'I'm invincible. I'm a kid. I will get better.'"[11]

Burned when she was six and a half, Jackie Izzo was ten when her mother "checked her out and didn't take her back." Other children her age were in school, and so her playmates became preschool-age children. She remembered the little kids taking her everywhere: "They had my mother put me in their little red wagon." Laid on her back on a bed of pillows. But, as she explained, "we didn't like that. I was too low. So, they took the baby bassinet and put me in that." She chuckled. "We went to Albosta's Hardware and those poor little kids'd lift that up the curb into the store, it was like a step. Guess where Jackie was? On the cement!" I gasped. "They dumped you out? Not on purpose—" "No!," she exclaimed, laughter in her voice. "They're scared to death! But they were smart enough, those little kids: 'Mrs. Izzo!' They're yellin', cause our house was like kitty-corner . . . [S]he come running, pick everything up, put me back in, and help 'em to get in." When the older kids were out of school for the day, there were adventures by bicycle, the kids collectively lifting Jackie and putting her in the basket on the handlebars, strongest kid pedaling the bike, others alongside on their

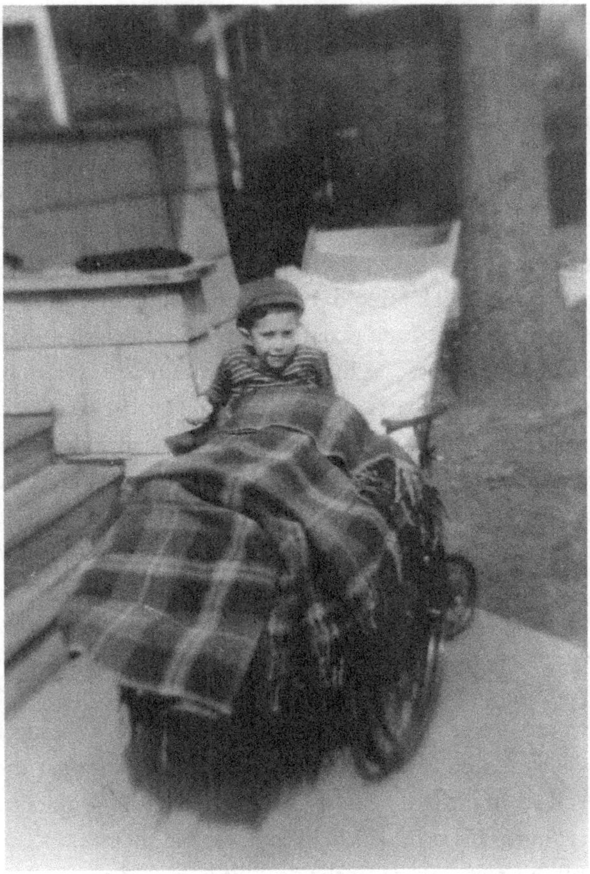

own. "Kids were awfully wonderful to me," she remembered.[12] *Happy in her predicament.* Those were the lawyers' words as they sought a judge's approval of the terms of the settlement. *She was a child*, is my retort. One can be thankful for, recognize the power in a child's acceptance and joy without, as they did, using it against her interests.

Their parents' reactions undoubtedly played a role in how they felt about their circumstances, shaped in some measure the rest of their lives. There were children whose fathers made them feel responsible for what happened to them. "Shouldn't have been playing with fire," Gaither Bates Jr. said to me; "I mean my father said that to me many times."[13] It was hard to hear, hard to know that he and others had grown up with this unjust burden.[14] But others found acceptance. "I wanted a pair of saddle shoes when I finally got out of the hospital," Jackie told me, "with the red soles, black and white." "Wait a minute, even though you didn't have feet?" I asked. The question came unbidden, unthinking, inexcusable. "Right!" Jackie agreed. Her mother hadn't questioned her desire. She wanted them and that was enough. "So, my mother went to Granville's and bought me a pair. Brought them home in a box, says, 'Is this what you want?'" And Jackie remembers saying, "'Thank you! Thank you!' I took them out and set them in my closet, on the floor, and just looked at them. . . . My mother was one hell of a lady," she remembered. "The first reason none of this stuff bothered me, it didn't stop her."[15]

But accepting their children did not mean that parents thought the ordeal was over. It was not. Their parents knew this in ways the children could not. When Jack Lockhart was first released from the hospital, his parents knew that any hope of his walking depended on another surgery; they knew that whether that surgery would succeed was uncertain. Two and a half years later—years that Jack Jr. remained out of school—there was another surgery and in turn another year in the hospital, this time in traction. On his return home, his father—a sheet-metal man at Ford—built a traction device with a weighted pulley connected to hooks in the bottom of a pair of Jack's shoes. Each night at bedtime the shoes went on, the attached weights hung down over the end of the bed, pulling. When he could no longer endure the pain, Jack would untie the shoes, and the weights with the shoes attached would drop to the floor with a thunk. They—who? his father?—began to tie the shoes in such a way that Jack could not get them off by himself. And so, in the bed he now again shared with his older brother, he would bargain for his brother's help to undo the shoes, on the condition that Jack rub his feet. "That was the deal," Jack Jr. said to me.[16]

The article with the headline "Pat Peterson Rides Again" had described him as "well." But through age sixteen, Pat had more surgeries, stretching over ten years of his life starting at age six.[17] For many of these children, additional skin grafts and surgeries extended not only through their childhoods but through their teenage years and long after. Tom Habina, burned at age five, was eight before he was home. For the next eight years, until he was sixteen, his summers were spent having and recovering from skin grafts.[18]

The risk of a breakdown in the skin was always there. What would be a minor injury for someone who had not suffered second- and third-degree burns represented a serious threat to those who were burned, a threat they carried through their lives. Seven years after being burned, Casimir Krzeczkowski Jr. was still regularly undergoing treatments.[19] And in the years after, ulcerations on the sites of earlier grafts necessitated more surgeries. As had been the case for all these children from the start, some grafts took; many did not.[20] *Periodically. From time to time. Difficult to heal. For the rest of their natural lives.*

Skin is an organ of the human body. Many of the things that skin does, the areas where they had been burned no longer did: cooling the body through sweat and blood rising to the surface (gone); skin cells replenishing (gone); nerve endings for feeling pain (gone for at least many). This loss of function meant that day in and day out, year after year, their legs required special care. But beyond this concern, there were abrasions or small cuts that would not heal; ulcerations; infections that required hospitalization and surgeries; new grafts from donor sites from their bodies; the slow, uncertain process of healing; and—looming in their futures—the threat of cancer.

"I got to tell you this story right now, so I don't forget it." Jackie Izzo and I had been talking for hours. "They come"—governmental social-service sorts—"wanna know how the Izzo girl's doing now that she's finally home and out of the hospital, is she able to go to school? My mother's standing on the front porch talking to 'em. And she's 'well, Jackie didn't feel so good today, she's sleeping.'" But as Jackie explained, "I was setting in a rubber tire, swinging from a tree trunk," put there to swing by either her mother or the little kids in the neighborhood. Referring to her mother, Jackie noted, "She thought for sure they would come and get me then. . . . Oh my God! The biggest worry my mom had was the Social Services coming to take me way from her."[21]

There were children who missed only a few months of school and returned in the same grade as their peers, others who repeated a grade, but for many, as was true for Jackie, it was years before they returned to or started school, and for others even once they returned to school their condition meant more interruptions, more time lost. What the delays in returning to or starting school and their injuries meant for how they felt about school, friendships, activities; how far they got in school; how well they did, varied as much as the time away from school did. James Baer—injured in April 1946, near the end of first grade, when he was six—was in the hospital from April through mid-August, but he started back to school with his peers that fall. Though John Sansbury had to repeat first grade, his classmates did not know it because his family had moved to a new state. Roy Cizek was three when he was burned in 1946 and left not only with all the complications and compromises of third-degree burns over 40 percent of his body but also blind in both eyes and deaf in one ear. Had he not been injured, he likely would have started first grade in 1949. He started school only a year late in 1950: The School for the Blind connected with the Riley Hospital, a division of the University of Indiana.[22]

But for others, when or whether they might return to school was uncertain. In 1950, four years after David Gagnon was burned in Westport, Maine, at age seven from his ankles to his waist, he was still bedridden, unable to walk, and able to stand only with the aid of a four-legged walker.[23] Jackie Izzo did not return to school until she was fifteen years old. It was her younger sister who insisted that Jackie had to return to school. As Jackie remembered her saying, "'She can't just set home and play games with all the neighborhood kids. We gotta find out if she can walk or we gotta get her back in school and get her educated. She gotta work.'"[24] By the time she was brought home from the hospital, Jackie's classmates from first grade were in fifth grade. By the time she returned to school, they were in ninth grade. She returned to school not with them but in a school for children with physical disabilities and hearing impairments. Jackie graduated from high school at age twenty only with the pressure of her mother on teachers and the principal to pass her.

Being significantly older than one's classmates made one out of place, and that experience impacted one's education and life in more profound ways. "It was just, like I say, a lot of rehab—and it was a long time 'til I got back to school," Gaither Bates Jr. explained. "How old were you when you graduated?" I asked. "I didn't," he said. "I didn't get out of grammar school. See, I lost so much time in school." It wasn't only the injuries, hospitalizations, and rehab, but also the hardships of a working-class family of nine in the postwar years. "My family moved a lot. I mean we went from East Paterson to Florida, and then back again . . . And when I turned sixteen, I applied for my working papers. I was sixteen in the eighth grade."[25] The school that Robert Viands attended in Union Mills, North Carolina, was part of the orphanage to which he and his brothers were sent after the collapse of their family. The orphanage allowed him to stay when he turned eighteen, but only to graduate. He then was not only out of school but no longer had a home.[26]

Scott Timberlake, in kindergarten when he was burned, never returned to school. His parents had tried placing him in a school for "crippled children" but were told at the end of one term that unless he made dramatic improvements over the summer he could not return. Two and a half years after he was burned, Scott's parents placed him full-time in institutionalized care. Family life took on new patterns. Every Sunday after church they went to visit Scott or, on occasion, brought him home for a few hours. When his sister, Kay, was eleven, her parents had another child. Kay's father threw himself into his job as vice president of a large midwestern paint company; he began volunteer work with the Cerebral Palsy Foundation. Her mother, who had first returned to teaching in 1950 in part because of the expense of private institutional care for Scott, continued teaching. Years passed this way. Scott's sister Kay found she could not remember her and her brother's lives before he was burned.[27]

And Scott? What were these years to him? In the same deposition in which the doctor said that it was impossible to determine whether Scott was comfortable, he was asked whether there was a possibility of improvement, whether it was worth continuing the intensive therapy routines. He replied that in his experience, there was some possibility of improvement to age fifteen. And if there was no appreciable improvement, then less-intensive therapy might still be worthwhile to age twenty. Lacking significant improvement, at that point, appropriate care would mean "adequate custodial care of some type, commensurate with what his family would like to provide for him." A family could expect "deterioration . . . in that the individual takes less and less care of himself as he loses the motivation to do anything for himself." The Timberlakes did not ultimately face these later decisions. On January 26, 1956, Scott died of pneumonia. It had been seven years since he was burned. He was thirteen years old.

The legal cases focused on the individual burned, but injury did not happen only to the individuals; it radiated out to every member of a family and beyond, like the ripples in a pond from a stone thrown in the water. "Did your family change with Scott's death?" I asked Kay Timberlake. There was a pause before she spoke. She had told me she was lonely after her brother was injured. She no longer had her brother as a playmate, and thinking back on it, she also noted being alone because her parents were occupied by her brother's injuries. By the time her brother died, Kay was fourteen. "Was there this different kind of hole in your life after he died?" I asked. "I don't know," she said. "For me, he died a long time ago." Her brother's death held its own meaning for her parents. "My father," she explained, "became a spokesperson for cerebral palsy, and I think it was cathartic for him. I think it was part of how he healed, was doing whatever he could to help other people go through what he had, he, not necessarily my mother, but what he had gone through." Her mother never found such consolation. "My mother, I don't know," Kay said. "She never, ever, 'til the day she died, could talk about Scott without crying or the lip quivering." And so Kay never raised the subject of her brother. Throughout her own life she felt, "I just cannot, I cannot fail."[28]

All the lawsuits referred in one way or another to the burden of being "disfigured for life." That burden was real even as children. "As a boy did you wear shorts?" I asked Jack Lockhart. "No, never," he replied. And though he insisted that it was not a big deal because everybody wore jeans, his wife, Angela, reminded him about swimming. "But, when you did go to the gravel pit and all the kids were swimming," she said, "you wouldn't go swimming." "No, nay, I would never go," he admitted.[29] When I asked that same question—"Did you ever wear shorts?"—to Gaither Bates Jr., he replied, "No. Never. . . . I wouldn't go swimming, you know, things like that. Just uh, to hide the fact." Because of his family's many moves, other kids did not know that he had been burned. When I started to ask if he ever told them, he jumped in. "Oh no! That's the last thing I'd ever bring up. In fact, I took steps to hide it. . . . Yeah. Because they would feel less of me if they knew. I, I always, that's what I always thought, you know."[30] Like so many others, Michael Felton, as he grew up, avoided activities that would allow others to see his legs. "Why?" I asked him. "Because I thought that it would revolt them. It's ugly, it's not normal. And uh, I thought, you know, it's like you go to the circus to see, uh, abnormal things like that."[31]

Looking through high school yearbooks and news clippings, none of this burden is apparent. There is Michael Felton as a high school senior in a football uniform, class president, dedicating a new scoreboard, during halftime of a game. In high school yearbooks, pictures of others who were burned as children in Gene Autry cowboy suits. Team pictures—baseball, basketball, football, tennis, and wrestling teams; Future Farmers of America; a high school rifle club. Individual portrait-style photos by high school class. How is one to read these photographs? There is relief in finding a number of the children, now teens. Alive. In school. Active in school groups. Clearly some as teens played sports, even contact sports.[32] There is relief in a *Tampa Morning Tribune* article from 1955 with a photo of Pat Peterson in his scout uniform with the headline, "Once Near Death by Burns, Boy Wins Eagle Scout Rank."[33] But even as I read these stories and look at these photos, I know better than to assume they represent the experience of all those burned who survived. I think of Tom Habina telling me he had wanted to do gymnastics but the school not letting him because of his legs, of Casimir Krzeczkowski's mother petitioning the court for permission to buy her son a television because his injuries meant he could not play outdoors like others his age.[34] I know too that they do not reveal an inner life.

Most of the yearbooks are from the 1950s. A photo of Gerald Palmateer, fourth row, eighth from the left, in a group picture of the rifle club in a 1957 high school yearbook in Washington, DC. Burned when he was four

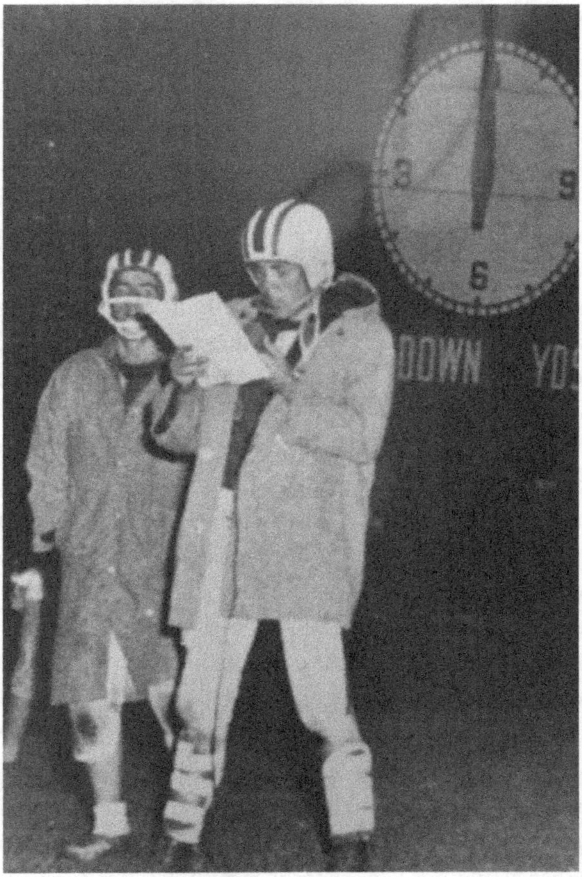

years old in 1946, now fifteen. Nice-looking kid.[35] The photo dates from three years after the US Supreme Court's decision in *Brown v. Board of Education* holding that racial segregation in education is unconstitutional. And here are white and Black teenagers together in a high school rifle club. Dramatic contestations and transformations in American life in the 1950s and 1960s swirled in and about these children, now teens, as they grew up. These transformations too must be considered in attempting to trace the course of their lives.

One year later, in 1958, Gerald Palmateer drowned in Tampa Bay, Florida. He was sixteen years old.[36] I turn back to his photo in his high school yearbook from the year before and understand that nothing about *the rest of their natural lives* can be assumed from those photos.

The legal settlements that, however inadequately, were intended as compensation for injuries understood to impact their future employability, marriageability, health, and happiness themselves reshaped the course of these children's and their families' lives. The children's portions of the legal settlements was intended for after they reached age twenty-one. But the realities of working-class families' lives, deepened by the burden that these injuries placed on family finances, meant that many families could not wait. Hardly more than a year passed after the settlement in Casimir Krzeczkowski's case before his mother was petitioning the court for money from the settlement for her son.[37] She earned less than a $1.00 an hour at her factory job, and the boy's stepfather had been out of work.[38] Casimir Jr., now fifteen, signed an affidavit, as he would with each of his mother's requests to the court, saying the petition was brought at his request. And the court granted his mother's petition. Other petitions followed, the court granting each one.[39] Like Casimir's mother, with courts' permission, families drew on the settlements for their children for a broad range of expenses, some immediately for the child—such as medical expenses for additional skin-grafting operations, or things like a heating lamp for a child's legs, a wheelchair, a typewriter and desk, or private school tuition—but also for things that benefited the family as a whole, like a rental for a family summer trip to the seashore, a rental of a lakeside cabin, or the purchase of a house.[40]

The extent of court oversight of the settlement funds varied dramatically.[41] "I never got a strict cash settlement out of it," William McMaster Jr. told me. He was eight years old when the case settled in 1948, $13,000 of the settlement set aside for him.[42] It would be thirteen years before he turned twenty-one. He never saw that money. But, as he said to me, he was sure his father would not have spent it foolishly.[43] Not everyone had that same confidence. $19,700 of the $41,000 settlement for Pat Peterson's injuries had been set aside for him. "He never got it," his widow, Ellen Peterson, flatly told me. When I asked if she thought he knew about the settlement, she said, "If he did, he would say 'It's water under the bridge.'"[44] There were other cases still in which parents treated the money as belonging to the family. Charles Baragona Jr. described his mother telling him that while it was his money, since they were a family, it was the whole family's money. Without ever telling him how much the settlement had been, she said they used it to buy the mill house they lived in. So, in a way, she explained, it was "his house," but even as she said this, she repeated that because they were a family, it was the family's house.[45]

Money could be corrosive and simultaneously a salvation. In Jackie Izzo's case, it was both. Only a matter of months after the settlement, Jackie's father asked the lawyers to "fix things up" so that he could invest $25,000 of the settlement in a local saloon. The lawyers told him that the Probate

Court would never allow it. They claimed it was only then that Jackie's parents began to express dissatisfaction with their lawyers, including with the lawyers' fees.[46] The Izzos hired new lawyers to challenge the amount of the fees. And when the judge denied their motion for rehearing, they appealed.[47] A wound began to grow in the Izzo household. Jackie was told that her case had been worth a million dollars. She and her parents came to believe the settlement and the attorneys' fees were a gross injustice. Jackie's father blamed her mother as much as the lawyers. He drank more. He became violent, and they were afraid of him.[48] Jackie was seventeen years old before the Circuit Court took up the case in 1954.[49] It was 1959, one week after Jackie's twenty-third birthday, before the Michigan Supreme Court issued its opinion effectively upholding the original fee agreement.[50] The decision closed the case, but it did not, maybe could not close the wound that had festered now for so many years.

Maybe that wound in part explains Jackie's memories about the house. "The worst house in the whole world!" she called it.[51] A few months after her parents had hired new lawyers to challenge the attorneys' fees, they had petitioned the Probate Court to spend $15,000 of Jackie's money to buy a house in Saginaw. When Jackie was injured, like so many Americans in the 1940s, they were renters, living in an upstairs flat in a Polish neighborhood. Maybe, like Charles Baragona Jr.'s mother, Jackie's parents felt the money was the family's. They might have been even more inclined to feel that way because their own claim for damages had been barred by the statute of limitations. The house they proposed to buy was a ranch located, the petition said, in a good neighborhood, with a school and church nearby. The Probate Court authorized the purchase, on condition that title to the house be in Jackie's name and that her parents pay the costs of taxes and ordinary repairs.[52]

The house did not prove to be the "desirable" house they had described. The steam boiler and plumbing were old and in poor condition. The school it was near had no wheelchair accessibility, so when Jackie returned to school, she had to take a taxi, miles each way every day, another expense on the funds set aside for her in adulthood.[53] We might ascribe Jackie's feelings about the house to its having been a bad investment bought with her money. But that is not my sense. The house became the site of years of simmering tensions—the festering anger over the attorneys' fees; her father's "chasing and drinking"; the violence that the anger and drinking brought into their home—that traced their roots in some measure to the cowboy suit that left Jackie severely disabled.

Ultimately, that money also, though, enabled their escape from Jackie's father's violence. As she said, we were "afraid that he'd kill us, all of us . . . and take the money and go to Mexico." "Was your getting the settlement money, this $33,000, important to your ability for you and your mom and all to leave your dad?" I asked. "Yes," Jackie said. "That money was a big change over. It made us very brave." First, they bought a car, a station wagon that they could get Jackie's wheelchair into that gave them a way to escape the house when he would come home drunk. And one weekend, when he was away on a fishing trip, they left altogether.[54]

Many of those burned knew of the money as they grew up and anticipated collecting it when they turned twenty-one. Whether it was what they expected and what it meant in and for their lives is a different question. "That money?" Michael Felton said when I asked him about what had happened to the settlement money for him. His father, a lawyer, had been in charge of investing it and when Michael turned twenty-one, he explained, "we kept it invested." "How did you feel about that money?" I asked. "I was proud of it."[55] And because he did not need it, did not touch it, it continued to grow. But most were not in a position like Michael Felton. Casimir Krzeczkowski Jr. petitioned for the release of the funds the day after turning twenty-one. Tom Habina was told not once, "but all the time," through all the hardships his injuries brought, "You've got $100,000 when you become twenty-one years old."[56] And so that was what he came to expect. It would have taken a fantastical sixfold increase over twelve years, after taxes on the gain, for the $15,000 set aside for him to have grown to $100,000 by the time he turned twenty-one.[57] But there had been the summer trips to the seashore and bad investments by the trust, and what he got when he turned twenty-one in 1960 was not $100,000 but $19,000. For a young working-class man, engaged to be married, it was a lot of money. But it was a far cry from what he had grown up believing would be his for the injury he suffered and would live with for life.

Gaither Bates's father had twice been granted permission to withdraw money for medical expenses for his son, but when Gaither Jr. turned twenty-one, the original $22,000 had nonetheless grown to $26,929.56.[58] Gaither Jr., who had been supporting himself since age sixteen and was engaged to be married by the time he was twenty-one, described going with his fiancé to each of the savings banks where the money for him had been deposited. "Had you ever seen that kind of money in your life?" I asked. "No," he quickly replied. He spent $19,000 to buy and furnish a house. "What did that mean to you?" I asked. "It meant a lot. It meant, uh, people of my ilk would have to save and strive for years to get the down payment of a house. And here I just stepped right in and bought one free and clear. And it meant a lot."[59]

"All six of us kids graduated college."[60] Charles Baragona Jr. made this announcement within five minutes of our beginning to talk. While their injuries contributed to some who survived not completing high school, for others those injuries were equally bound up in lives of educational achievement, including college and advanced degrees in a range of fields.[61] Again, there were broader forces in play—the economic prosperity of the postwar era, the Cold War, the dramatic expansion of higher education.[62] Like Charles Baragona, neither of Roy Cizek's parents had gone to college.[63] But at age eighteen, Roy graduated from the Indiana School for the Blind; went to Indiana University, where he majored in music and music theory, minoring in physics; and from there went on to MIT, where he earned a degree in engineering.[64] Richard Szumita's expression is serious, looking out from the University of Rhode Island yearbook in 1969. He was twenty-seven years old by the time he graduated with a degree in business management. The headline in a news clipping read: "Big Day for Richard Szumita: Man Battles Handicaps to Earn URI Degree."[65] One can recognize in his college yearbook photo the face of the boy of six from photographs taken almost a year after he was burned, when his life still hung in the balance.[66] The child of textile mill workers, he was the first member of his family to go to or graduate from college; the only one of his four siblings who did.[67] Others, whose parents' background included some college or advanced degrees, also went to college. Michael Felton followed his father into law. Herbert Ulick, the boy whose mother had described changing over a dozen pus-filled sheets a day, graduated from UCLA in 1958 and from medical school at the University of California, Irvine, in 1965. John Devens, the boy whose grandmother seeing him in flames in the distance had screamed at him to roll, graduated from Belmont College and earned a PhD in audiology at Wichita State University.

Others died as young adults. And their deaths too reflected broader transformations, here the dramatic rise in automobile fatalities, and the limits of knowing, of saying that this or that aspect of their lives was linked to, caused by their burns. James Ikner, burned at age eight in 1945 in Saginaw, Michigan, had graduated from high school and served in the US marines. He was killed in a car accident in Sacramento, California, in 1964. He was twenty-six years old.[68] Two years later, in 1966, James Baer was killed in a car accident in Akron, Ohio. He too had graduated from high school—a private boy's school. He had started college at the University of Michigan;

it is not clear whether he graduated. The story in the *Akron Beacon Journal* of Baer's death was shaped by his father having been a leading banker and Akron citizen. It was also shaped by the circumstances of the accident: The car Baer was driving had slammed into a tree at high speed, tearing it in half and throwing him nearly eighty feet.[69] Like Ikner, he was alone at the time. He too was twenty-six years old. Both men were single. The same year that Baer was killed, Congress passed the Highway Safety Act and the National Traffic and Motor Vehicle Safety Act.[70]

Looking at a photo of one of the burned boys in spring 1948, Judge Knox had said, "A kid that is scarred up something like that, he is going to get married some day and the effect of those scars on his wife is something to take into account, and his own humiliation from it." As a boy of nine, Michael Felton remembered his dawning interest in sex and with it the thought, "I don't see how I could ever be accepted by a female to have sex. Because of the way I look."[71] As Jack Lockhart Jr. explained to me, "Every woman I ever went out with, that'd be the first subject. You know, because I was embarrassed to take off my pants. Still am."[72] Their fears were shared by others. Andrew Szumita told me that his father's greatest fear had been that he would never find a woman willing to marry him because of the scars on his legs and torso. "I worried about her too," Tom Habina said, referring to his wife Dorothy. They had met at a dance. He was twenty-two; she was twenty-one. At some point in their dating, he pulled up his pants and showed her his legs. As he remembered it, he told her, "'I probably will never be in a way to do things with you. I don't know what I'm going to be like in life.' And she says, 'Do you love me?' I says, 'Yeah.' So she decided to take me on."[73]

"I still wonder how she handles it," John Sansbury said of his wife about the scars on his legs and chest from the burns and grafts. "That, that thought comes in now and again." His wife Kristen, laughing, said, "I never saw him without his clothes"—that is, before they were married. She had known him since childhood; knew that he had been burned. They grew up together, went to the same church, fell in love. As we talked, she jokingly said, "I was glad it didn't harm anything important." And we all began laughing. John saying, "Me too!" And Kristen, added, "That would've been a deal-breaker!" And the three of us laughed.[74] There was warmth, love, a playful intimacy expressed in that moment. And though we laughed together, it was not funny, really. Judge Knox had assumed those who were burned would marry. But not all did. And given the fears expressed by those who did marry, it seems possible, likely even, that for those who did not, their burns played a role.

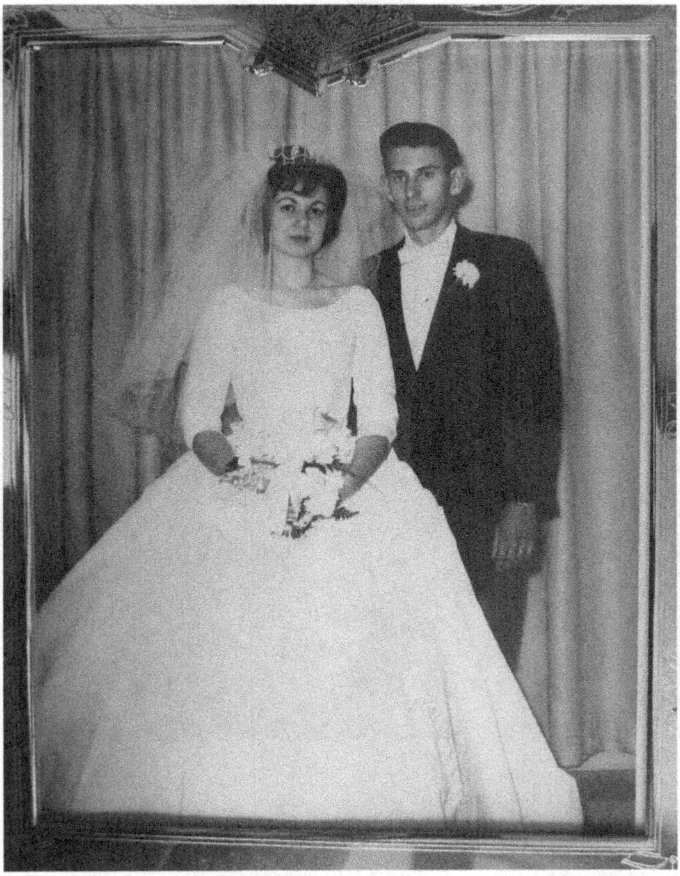

The fears carried over to having children. "I always used to think all of the time when I talked to the doctors, I said 'If I have children by my wife, are [their] legs going to be deformed?'" And the doctors assured Tom Habina that they would not be. But when he and Dottie had their first child, a boy, he went to the nursery and said, "'I'm Tom Habina, and I'd like to see my son.' She says, 'There he is right there.' I says, 'would you mind pulling off the cover off of him?' And she pulled it off and held it up. And I looked at him and says, 'Thanks God.'" However unreasoning, he could not shake the fear that his children would be born with legs like his. "Deformed." Looking back on this, he said, "I don't know what the hell was wrong with me." But he was not alone in his thinking. "One thing I wanted to tell you," Judy Felton began, "is when our son was born, our first child, um, it was Mike's senior year in law school, and the first thing he said was, 'He doesn't have any scar tissue.' . . . That was one of those aha moments," she explained,

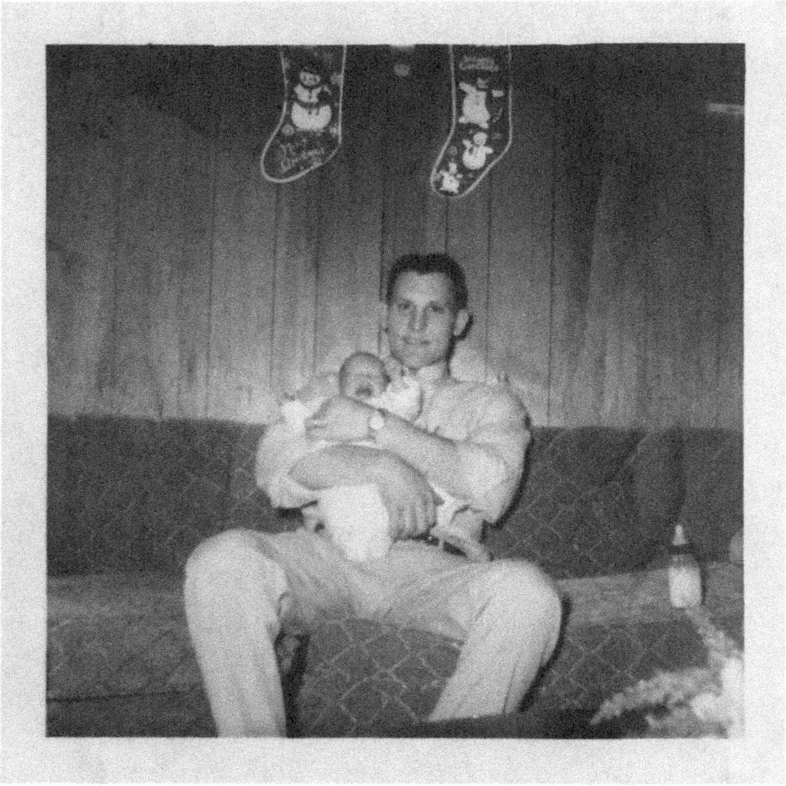

"when it brought to me—" And Mike interrupted, to finish her thought, "How deep-seated the concern."[75]

For some, having and raising children was important to achieving a greater acceptance of themselves. "It was when we had our children," Cathy Viands said. They lived in Florida and their daughters, as she explained, wanted to be in the swimming pool all the time. "You know, they didn't, they never saw the scars because their little eyes were used it, you know? . . . They just thought that was the way he was made, you know . . . and they really were the ones that helped him overcome his scars and his life."[76]

I cannot help but wonder whether their earlier losses shaped that change as well. Cathy Viands had had a series of miscarriages, and they had had a stillborn child. "When I had my first full-term live birth," she said, "you know, we were just rejoicing."[77]

But the intimacies of marriage and children did not change how many men felt. I expect this may have been truer for men for whom the burns and grafts left their legs, as Tom Habina described them, "deformed." As he explained, "I was even ashamed with my own kids. I would never go in the water with them either. . . . Dottie would take them and then I would stay up there and have my long pants on." Avoiding sunburn was important because of the earlier burns, the fragility of the skin on his legs, and the risk of cancer. But shame was a powerful force. There was a cream he had to put on his legs every day. One of his daughters, as a child, would say, "'I'll do that for you, Pop-Pop.'"[78] Hearing that story from this man who had carried so much, I loved that little girl.

Some of those who married young remained married to the same person for a lifetime. Richard Szumita—who had feared that because of his legs he would never find someone who would marry him—had to ask four times, but it was not his legs that held Sally up; it was the question first of whether he had been baptized Catholic (a necessary condition for her) and, secondly and somewhat contradictorily, of her not wanting to live the hard life her mother had had with five children. She finally said yes when Richard promised her, "It will just be the two of us." Five children later, a handwritten note taped to the refrigerator that read "just the two of us," they were still married.[79] Sarah Catherine Viands, who had married Robert when she was sixteen years old—"a marriage of convenience," she called it, enabling her to escape the orphanage in which she too had grown up—introduced herself to me saying, "I married Robert Viands on March the sixteenth, 1961 . . . and we've been happily married, for the most part, for fifty-six years." And then she and Robert both laughed.[80] *For the most part.* Their marriage, as I learned, survived great hardships. Many of these marriages did. And some of those hardships related back to the trauma these individuals had faced as children and carried with them.[81]

But many first marriages of those who had been burned did not survive.[82] Roy Cizek's first marriage survived less than two years.[83] He would ultimately marry three times, his first two marriages ending in divorce.[84] Their childhood traumas and the complex legacies they left on and in their lives shaped their intimate relationships. But the end of these marriages also fit within the postwar rise in divorce that began in the early 1960s.[85]

Whatever the cause for the end of a marriage, it meant facing again the gauntlet of potential rejection. Ron King's first marriage had ended with the death of his wife to Lou Gehrig's disease. He was forty when he met Rosanne Solimine; she was seven years younger and had never been married. After they had been going out for several months, she remembered he said to her, "'I want to show you something.'" "Did you know it was going to relate to his body?" I asked. "No," she replied. "And uh, he sat me down, and he pulled up his pants and he said, 'What do you think?' And I said,

'Well, what do you mean, what do I think?' 'You know.' He says, 'Would you still marry me if my legs look like this?' I says, 'I'm not marrying your legs. I'm marrying you, not your legs.' But he was hesitant, you know, in showing me and telling me. . . . He wanted to make sure that I didn't, you know, that you know, you're disfigured or something, but I didn't see it that way."[86] "The only one that sees them," Jack Lockhart Jr. said to me, referring to his legs and nodding toward his second wife, Angela, "are her. . . . And my doctors," he added. "That's it."[87] That many could hide the scars and misshapen legs did not lessen the ways in which the injury shaped their sense of self, the not completely dismissible questioning of even the acceptance of intimates, the fear that exposure would, might, bring rejection.

Those burned in Gene Autry cowboy suits were not among Erving Goffman's research subjects for his 1963 book *Stigma: Notes on the Management of Spoiled Identity*.[88] What was for Goffman a research topic, a signature publication on a curriculum vitae that marked his road to preferment, was for those who survived being burned in Gene Autry cowboy suits central to the course of their lives. The management of stigma had broad implications for adulthood. As children, their parents or others had been responsible for them. As adults, they were responsible for their own support and—for many—the support of a family. That injury interrupted and for some ended their education short of even a high school degree. It contributed to others not going on to college in a context in which access to and the benefits of higher education dramatically compounded the burden of these injuries in their lives. Gaither Bates, who had dropped out of school in eighth grade, began work in 1957 as a "floor boy," at $1.00 an hour, barely over $2,000 a year. "What did a floor boy do?" I asked. "Anything he was told," was his reply. He ultimately landed in plastics and packaging, working his way up at a series of firms to foreman, then plant manager, vice president of operations, president, and CEO. He and his wife had three children. They raised them in the house he had bought with the legal settlement. But Bates was among the lucky ones.

Those burned in Gene Autry cowboy suits came of age well before there were meaningful employment protections for those with disabilities and a social movement demanding their enforcement. Workmen's compensation laws, a response to the crisis of industrial injuries in the early twentieth century, paradoxically increased discrimination against workers who had prior injuries, health conditions, or disabilities that would make a subsequent injury more expensive for an employer under the law. The first disability civil rights law would not come until the 1970s, mid-life for those burned in Gene Autry cowboy suits, and the Americans with Disabilities Act (ADA) would not be passed until most of those burned had reached retirement.[89] Tom Habina had been in his job in the shipping department at a printing company for only a few months when he got hurt.[90] He had been told to get into a huge dumpster and pack the paper down by jumping on it. Someone had thrown some banding wire in the dumpster, and it stabbed into his ankle. When he mentioned it a day or two later, they sent him to a doctor, who immediately sent him to the hospital where he had to have surgery. He was out for three or four months. The day after he returned, they fired him. The doctor had told them he "had problems," that he could "get bumped at any time" and would then need skin grafts "so they said that's why they were letting me go. . . . I was a hinder to their company." Like any number of others among those burned, he went into business for himself.[91] Doing so meant not being denied a job or fired because he was a risk, "a hinder" to a company. But it also meant that when he was laid up by further surgeries—and he would be—there was no pay coming in.

For those lucky enough to get a union job, there were protections against dismissal. Jack Lockhart Jr. was twenty years old, married, and expecting a first child when his brother-in-law got him on at GM. He had taken the civil service exam for the post office and might have gone there—the pay was higher—but he worried about what would happen if he got laid up and could not carry mail. He was lucky to get the GM job; had they known of his injuries he likely would not have. But with the protection of the union, when the skin on his legs broke down and he needed other surgeries—and there were many—he did not lose his job.

Those whose disability was apparent faced even greater difficulties. Jackie Izzo had dreamed of being a teacher, but the inaccessibility of schools meant it was years before she even returned to school. And once she was out of high school, as she explained, "See, nobody would [hire me]. Bell Telephone wouldn't. Consumers' Power wouldn't. Shop wouldn't." Shop? General Motors.[92] She got her first job only because a classmate, a kind girl whose father was the manager of the Sears store in Saginaw, pressured her father to hire Jackie. They put her out of sight in the catalog department. But this did not matter to her; she was thrilled to have a job.[93] The work was important to her sense of self-worth. She might well have continued at Sears, but for the violence in her household that had to be escaped. Later, she worked in a dress shop her mother established, a job that meant she was not subject to the barriers to hiring and the risk of firing she would otherwise have faced throughout her working life. She worked for thirty-three years, an accomplishment in which she took pride.

The economic and social advantages of having a college or more advanced degree in the post–World War II era were manifest. But for those burned in the Gene Autry cowboy suits, like others with disabilities, the importance of education was like compound interest. It meant far less likelihood of not being hired or fired, because their prior injuries made them a "hinder" to a company. It meant far less risk of the kinds of injuries that were so debilitating because of their prior injuries. And it meant pay and benefits that made covering the costs of necessary surgeries less of a burden.

As a child, Jack Lockhart Jr. had thought of his injuries as "a temporary hiccup." But for many it never ended. Fifteen years after he had been burned, the skin on Michael Felton's legs was still tissue-paper thin. There were scabs and spots that bled and oozed. As his wife, Judy, explained, his legs were "raw-looking." Almost every morning she had to change their bedding because his legs bled and oozed in the night.[94] Thirty-six years after he had been burned, fighting ulcers on his legs was still an unremitting battle in Ron King's life. He and Rosanne had married in 1980. "From the time you knew him," I asked her, was "medical care for his legs an issue?" Her response was immediate. "Yes. All the time."[95] Roy Cizek was left deaf in one ear and blind, but he considered his legs, which never fully healed and had to be soaked every day throughout his life, his worst affliction.[96]

And then there were the continuing surgeries. A tube graft surgery when he was twenty-eight kept Jack Lockhart Jr. out of work for a year and a half.[97] Even though he was protected from being fired by the union, time off from work meant less pay, years of service and benefits reduced, and facing the suspicion of co-workers. "I don't believe they thought I was on sick leave for a year and a half," Jack Lockhart told me of the tube graft surgery. A home visit from his supervisor, ostensibly in support, was really a way of checking the truth of his claims. "He comes over, stands right there, you know, looks down and sees it." After that there were never questions asked in the years and surgeries to come. But he never shook the humiliation of having his supervisor see him this way.[98] Others faced unsuccessful experiments, skin grafts with cow or pig tissue.[99] The appeal was that the skin did not have to come from their own bodies. But every surgery meant time lost and the problem of healing. They lived with the fear of having any injury to the areas that had been burned, not only because of what a surgery would mean but also because doctors were reluctant to treat them at all, given the risks their skin posed.[100]

As the years went on, there was a growing sense of resignation. "Well, gotta go get another one done," Jack Lockhart remembered. "And go get it done. I'd have to drop everything. . . . everything." Without really recognizing it at the time, he explained, "I'd have to go into, because I went into a world of my own when that happens. . . . I didn't realize I was doing it, but I do it. And I know why. It protects me. It gives protection emotionally and mentally. I have to go into a state that—accepts that I've got to go through this period of time. I've got to take that out of my life, and deal with this problem."[101] And as they did so, there were family events missed; plans cancelled. As Jack said, "it affects everybody. It affects everybody in the whole family. I know it does."[102]

Take that out of my life. The time preparing for, undergoing, recovering from surgeries as *time lost from a life* had greater consequence still because many of those burned died in middle age.[103] Edward Bradley died at age thirty-seven. Casimir Krzeczkowski was forty-five. Herbert Ulick and Richard Szumita, forty-nine. Joseph Powell, Roy Cizek, and William Pritchard, all fifty. There were undoubtedly others. Whether their early deaths were directly or indirectly linked to their childhood trauma and its enduring legacies or not, they were connected in this way for their families and the communities in which they had built lives, if only in the fact of this person having borne what seemed yet another unjust burden with strength and dignity. Richard Szumita's family established a scholarship in his name. The idea began with Richard's brother Bob, who had been with him as a boy when Richard was burned. The scholarship for a student at the high school, as one of Richard's sons explained to me, was not for "the kid with the highest grade-point average. It was the kid who worked hard. Had a sense of community, he'd had a struggle of some kind."[104] William Pritchard Jr. had been one of the "late" cases the defendants quietly and quickly settled, the burns so deep they exposed one of his hip bones. He never married. Following his death in 1992, the high school in Pasadena, Maryland, where he had been a longtime art teacher and football and baseball coach renamed its gym the William E. Pritchard Gymnasium. The dedication recognized his "courage to face life challenges with personal strength, dignity and leadership."[105]

All these individuals were shaped by these injuries in ways that burdened their lives physically, mentally, emotionally, and economically, burdens shared in some respects at least by parents, siblings, spouses, children, and others. Their injuries were isolating. But they also led them to forge connections with others. After college and a master's degree, Pat Peterson enlisted in the second cohort of the Peace Corps and after he returned completed a PhD at the University of Wisconsin in agricultural economics, providing the foundation for a career with USAID and service in Jamaica, Bangladesh, Pakistan, and Yemen.[106] Ellen Peterson said of her husband, "Bottom line, he wanted to help people."[107] Roy Cizek solved problems in the production of sound that had mystified others, building systems that made it possible to hear through a speaker as though one were seated in the concert hall listening to a live performance.[108] John Devens went on to use his training in audiology to provide speech and hearing services to families in remote Northern villages in Alaska, and as mayor of Valdez, Alaska, when a giant Exxon oil tanker spilled hundreds of thousands of gallons of crude oil in the waters of Prince William Sound in 1989, fought for environmental justice.[109] Family members too of those injured or who died found connection with others life-affirming. In a quiet moment in my conversation with Scott Timberlake's sister, Kay Bryant, she said to me, "I feel most alive when I make people laugh."

mornings and ends

Dear Frances,

The first day of the second year. Last May I could not have fathomed that we would face a second year.

. . .

I found myself thinking this morning about how fundamentally morning & ends (of the semester, year, project) have been transformed. It used to be that almost no matter how down or defeated I felt by the end of a day or in the wakeful hours of the night, I woke feeling again that all things were possible. Now I wake each morning to the reality that you are gone and my limbs and heart feel heavy, my mind slows, the joy and possibility drain from the day. So too with endings. I used to feel a new energy at the end of a term, especially in May with summer beyond. I don't feel that now. Try as I might, the world is less bright without you in it.

. . .

I wake every morning to the fact that you are gone. It is an impossible way to begin.

. . .

It seems like such a very long time since last summer. At this point last summer, we weren't even two weeks into living without you. . . . I was talking to [a friend] today about you, telling her about those moments your senior year where you'd agreeably say sure to going to dinner or something else at a place other than the one you initially suggested, and then say, with a touch of marvel in your voice, "See, I'm being flexible" and we'd all laugh.

. . .

I try to focus on the time we had with you, not the time we aren't having, the time you aren't having as a living being to chart your own course. But months ago I thought about the fact that come May your classmates would be coming home, excited to be back home for the summer, grown up in a new way through their year away, newly confident in their success at independence. I had thought about this moment months ago, but now it is here and I can't help but cry for what is not. In every milestone for others we will face knowing that these are milestones we'll never celebrate with you. Our future with you is different. . . . We thought we knew at least the beginning of the path to your future. It's funny how we do this: imagine/plan for/speak about a future that sometimes we find ourselves in or are not even conscious of how the script changed until we're in a different future than we once imagined. But here the loss of the future was so abrupt. And yet, even as I say that, I realize it's a particular future that is lost. Last year, at this point, I could not imagine, there was no such thing as time, I was out of time. But I see now you still have a future. I also think I can begin to see that your future is no more or less certain now than it was last April. We just need to stay open to new futures for you. I am working to find a way to do this thing with you, even if it's not the thing either of us, any of us, imagined we'd be doing with you.

. . .

I finally went for a physical this morning. I have, apparently, gone through the menopause. . . . Maybe it seems strange to wish I could share this with you, but . . . I can imagine saying to you, "Frances, it seems that I've gone through the menopause and didn't even know it." And we might joke about how old I am. Or, you might say how nice you thought it would be not to have to have a period each month or cramps. And I would say I kind of miss having periods—they were part of the rhythm of life for my whole remembered life. And you'd tell me that was really weird, that you wouldn't miss not having periods. And so the conversation would go. And how good that sharing would have felt. So, I tell you here because it's the only place I have to tell you.

. . .

As I started to write you this morning, I realized that all the things that have structured time in my life—not really all, but two of the really important ones—have gone and now I am left to find structure in some other way. Since I was 13—so for close to 40 years—having a period provided a biological, monthly rhythm to my life. And then there is no longer a need to get up to get you and Wilder to school. For the last 21 years, every morning I had to be up because I had children. Your body clocks as babies and toddlers was my clock—24 hours a day. And then your school clock became my clock. So that even once you were old enough to be up on your own, on school days, I was always up with you. And so here I now find myself without the two most fundamental structures that have established structure in my life. It is a sort of female/motherhood retirement. So, realizing this I see I need to begin to find/establish new structures. I have found myself not wanting to get started with my day because I'd rather be with you. But I also see that my life has been structured for so many years around/according to other clocks that I have no idea how to get started because I am, in a sense, waiting for the starting point that has disappeared. You know, even if you weren't gone, I'd be having this clock problem because you'd be away at school. And I would have told you about it, and you might have laughed and said, "well then stay in bed if you want" perhaps not fully grasping the darker side of staying in bed.

. . .

It upsets me that last summer I didn't want to live and couldn't imagine that I could; I wanted to be with you and felt also that if you couldn't live, as your mother I couldn't. And yet here I am now just over a year later working at living. I have pushed myself to take steps: getting up every day, teaching, finishing the play, and then more personal things related to living in my body—yoga, going to the doctor, the dentist, and now a trip, a long weekend away with Dad. And I have managed all these things. I feel hollow, I don't laugh much, joy and happiness and being carefree still escape me, but I am alive and it upsets me to be so. How is it, Frances, that the very thing that I've worked so hard to do, that I felt like I owed to you since you did not get to live, now feels so bad? I am left feeling, questioning how could my love for you have been my whole being and yet I am alive and you are not.

. . .

This past year I spent the year, or much of it, at least, looking backward. But now, even though I still cannot fully grasp that you are gone, forever, I feel like I can no longer simply look past—"this time last year," the thought process I spent so much of the last year in no longer brings the reward of your laugh, your joy, your loving encouragement, your achievements—but I don't know how, feel so little, no interest in looking forward knowing that you too are not able to look forward. I don't know how to proceed.

chapter twenty-one · the vita of precarity

We need to go back. One last look at the academic world beginning from the late 1960s and 1970s. As was true in the American economy more generally in the 1970s, in academia a precarity that to that point had been limited became more widely shared.[1] Precarity ran alongside preferment. In many respects, it made the world of preferment possible. But what was not initially understood was that the crisis that began in the late 1960s and early 1970s was not just a temporary employment crisis. It was, in fact, the beginning of a new era in which precarity in academia and more generally would become more and more the norm, preferment the exception. Precarity generated its own history of the vita. But the *vita* of precarity—that is, the life of precarity—was so much more than this.

The "seller's market" of the mid-1960s had become by 1969 "a 'time of troubles.'" John J. Rumbarger, assistant executive secretary of the American Historical Association, began his annual report, "The year 1969 was a 'time of troubles' for the fledging historian: jobs were in short supply."[2] In 1965, the AHA Professional Register had had 1,200 registrants; a year later it had 1,600.[3] The number of registrants continued to climb. Jobs did not keep pace. At the AHA annual meeting in January 1971, well over two thousand people struggled to connect with "somewhat over 100 active recruiters, in less than seventy-two hours."[4]

A University of Michigan history PhD candidate named Henry Bryant Avery, writing to AHA President David Potter a month later, introduced himself as "one of the thousands of persons around the country with Phds. in history (or close to it) who are searching for positions for next year."[5] He acknowledged his good fortune in a range of respects: His field (Chinese history) had fewer individuals competing for positions; he had an "exceptionally diligent adviser"; and he was at an institution with a strong placement service. He wrote, as he explained, not because he had yet to secure a position, although that was true, but rather to register his embitterment at the indignity, uncertainty, and unforgivably chaotic process for securing a position. "Can't the AHA do something about this mess? . . . [W]e are all alike in feeling unnecessarily traumatized by the way these matters are settled now."[6]

The field of history reflected a broader reckoning. The flush academic hiring market of the mid-1960s had evaporated almost as quickly as it had materialized.[7] In 1955, the Committee of Fifteen wrote in panicked tones of a projected shortfall in PhDs. In fact, in that time, American universities had awarded almost one hundred thousand more doctorates than the Committee of Fifteen had projected.[8] Between 1960 and 1970 alone, American universities awarded 191,697 doctorates.[9] The "production" of PhDs outstripped available positions. And it was not as though the spigot—the pipeline of graduate students in the system—could just be turned off.[10]

Henry Bryant Avery's plea to the AHA was echoed in other disciplines. But the truth was that professional societies could do little about "this mess" because they had no control over the number of positions—or, for that matter, the number of PhDs produced by graduate programs. The response of some professional associations to scenes like that at the 1971 AHA convention was to terminate their role as intermediaries in facilitating interviews arranged at their conventions. In April 1972, the AHA council announced the end of the convention's Professional Register. The AHA would continue to advertise vacancies in a newly named *Employment Information Bulletin* and provide space for interviewing at the annual meeting, but it would no longer act as the intermediary between hiring institutions and candidates.[11]

In stepping away from the role of intermediary, the AHA followed the lead of the Modern Language Association. "Do not . . . come to Chicago expecting to arrange interviews when you get there," the October 1971 MLA *Job Information List* announced. "MLA no longer operates the frustrating and generally unsuccessful faculty exchange or matching service."[12] The MLA's assessment was shared more generally. Professional societies' job exchanges had never met the hopes of their creators, much less those of the candidates who had used them. Their end alleviated the public indignity and chaos that had characterized professional registers as at the 1971 AHA annual meeting.[13] But the end of the scramble for interviews at conventions did not solve the problem of the mismatch between the number of candidates and positions. It simply made that pain and the search for employment more private. "The time for hysteria and action is upon me," wrote a

Columbia PhD student in sociology in October 1973. "I am in the process of sending out those desperate and humiliating pleas for employment to every place that resembles an institution of higher learning in the San Francisco area, and it is a painful and lonely procedure."[14]

What is today known by terms like "flexible," "contingent," or "gig" labor had always been part of the economy of higher education. Where smaller or less elite institutions hired other institutions' PhD candidates in temporary positions, large public and private institutions hired their own graduate students as they worked toward degrees. The dramatic expansion in the number and size of PhD programs in the postwar era facilitated the reduction of tenured and tenure-track faculties' teaching load, freeing them to spend more time on the research that brought recognition to them and their institutions. Nor was teaching the only field of contingent labor in academia. In the post–World War II era, the flood of federal dollars funding research in the sciences and social sciences fed the need for full- and part-time researchers and technical staff with advanced training—graduate students, postdocs, researchers—employed under federal contracts and private foundation grants.

Precarity had long included those who had completed their advanced training. Women with PhDs, largely closed out of tenure-track appointments by sex discrimination before the 1970s, had long provided a flexible, cheap, immobile labor pool on which universities and colleges relied.[15] They were, as sociologist Jessie Bernard termed it, "fringe benefits." They were "on the fringe of the profession" and simultaneously "of great benefit to the institutions where the work is done."[16] What happened in academia in the 1970s was that a precarity that had been limited became more widely shared.[17]

The advertising of academic positions that had created an academic job market now meant that the market collapse was public. The visibly palpable shortfall of positions fueled candidates' frustration and anger. The MLA had begun publishing its *Job Information List* in 1965. Its organization of job listings and those of other professional societies by zip code, or alphabetically by state—or, worse still institution name—rather than field, meant that candidates had to scour entire issues to discover whether there might be positions in their field; it laid bare the grim prospects.[18] The October 1971 MLA English Edition *Job Information List*, the first in which it hinted at the shortfall in positions, for example, was eighty-five pages long and listed 1,562 departments.[19] But close to half the listings read: "No Information Received by Press Deadline / See December List." And in the first thirty-three pages alone, there were another 130 departments that said in one way or another that they would not be hiring for the next year. The most common verbiage was: "No vacancies anticipated for 1972. Please do not write."[20] Some announcements said that cuts were in store.[21] Departments that held out some possibility of a hire hedged their language: "we hope," "at most we might," "if circumstances allow," "possibility of," "may eventually have openings for." As the English Department chairman at Notre Dame put it, "Situation normal: uncertain."[22] Until budgets were clear, which would only happen later in the academic year, few departments firmly stated they were hiring.[23] And as the number of full-time tenure-track positions shrank, the "just in time" employment that colleges and universities had long practiced expanded: temporary replacement hiring, part-time, and non-tenure-track year-by-year appointments teaching entry-level courses.[24]

The same patterns applied equally in other disciplines. So, for example, the AHA's *Employment Information Bulletin* had the same hundreds of listings that read only, "No Information Received by Press Deadline. See [next] List." There were hundreds more that said, in one way or another, "No expectation of adding to staff for 1972–73 year"—or, more plainly, "I can't hire; don't write." And departments that noted some possibility or hope of hiring voiced the same budgetary uncertainty.[25] Issue after issue of the AHA's *Bulletin* voiced the grim prospects for employment. "Of the 207, or minimum number of jobs to be filled this year"—that is, for 1973–1974—"nearly 50% are either temporary or part-time." As the AHA noted, "the figures bode ill for the profession. Neither does the economic situation outside academia offer much promise of relief."[26] Facing its own budgetary crisis, the AHA stopped listing institutions from which it received no reply as to whether they were hiring and grouped "no vacancy" listings together at the end of the *Bulletin*, and then it dropped that list as well. The *Bulletin* visibly shrank. Early issues had run to sixty-five pages. The October 1974 issue of the *Bulletin* was only seven.[27] Much of the reduction came through eliminating listings for institutions that had sent no information or had no vacancy. Still, there was a larger symbolism.

The collapse of the job market was not limited to the humanities and social sciences. In the sciences, too, there was a new precarity; in fact, it began there.[28] Long gone were the flush years, for example, in which physicists were in short supply.[29] Correspondence to the AIP placement service in 1971 ran well over a thousand pages, the stack of letters over a foot high, most from those searching for positions. Many voiced anguish, desperation, and frustration. "Another soon to be unemployed physicist writes for help!" began a representative letter. For the past two years, the writer had been an assistant professor at the Firelands campus of Bowling Green State University. But economic circumstances meant his position was being eliminated. "I knew I'd never get rich in Physics," he closed, "but this is ridiculous!" Others shared his plight. "I am an assistant professor of applied mathematics," wrote a man who had been teaching at Centre College in Danville, Kentucky, since completing his PhD in Physics at Vanderbilt in June 1970. "This position is being taken over by the Dean of the College." And yet another, "This market is more brutal than last year. Peter Gibbs of Utah had a thousand applicants. Most seem to have several hundred." The letter closed, "The federal government deliberately tried to produce more physicists than would have been freely produced. Now those of us on the market face a very real possibility of no employment at all in physics. This is irresponsibility." And enclosed with their letters were vitae, resumes, or both.[30]

Three years later, prospects had not improved. The AIP's revised "Classification and Search Form" was dense with categories and boxes to check, casting in sharp relief the specialization that characterized physics by the last quarter of the twentieth century. The form enabled registrants to identify every subspecialty in which they were trained or had experience, to express preferences in their work interests, and to self-identify their skills. But as registrants understood, each box they checked, or did not, contributed to a composite identity that would determine whether they were even considered for a position and from which who they were in any individual sense had been extracted as irrelevant.

Finding a position with the promise of economic security in a locale rich with research collaborators was no guarantee for the future. "Single, Age 34, Excellent Health," began the two-page resume of a woman who had completed her PhD in physics four years earlier at Harvard. She had gone to college on a New York State Regents Scholarship and began her PhD at Harvard in 1961 with a three-year NSF Graduate Fellowship. Her PhD took ten years, during the final two years of which she taught physics as an assistant professor at Framingham State College in Massachusetts. From 1971–1974, she was an assistant professor of Physics at Wellesley College, spending the summers of those years as a research associate at Harvard in her former PhD advisor's experimental high-energy physics research group. That work led to minor publications, each with many authors, among whom she was listed last. What was implicit on her resume was explicit on the registration form she completed with the American Institute for Physics in 1974. Under "Present Employment" she checked the final box: "unemployed."[31] More than many others in the huge pile of registration forms, resumes, and vitae filed with the AIP in 1974, she had seemed to have found a position that offered a path to the road to preferment. But she, like so many others, found herself among the many PhDs and near-PhDs caught in the economic downturn, desperately seeking a secure foothold in a world that suddenly offered far fewer of them, part of a larger phenomenon of women and racialized minorities gaining inclusion just as the prize's value—here, a secure tenure-track position—is diluted.

As the academic job market collapsed, professional societies worked to protect department chairs from a flood of desperate applications. That had been one of the goals, in fact, of the AIP's revised registration form.[32] Other societies were more direct. The MLA directed candidates to assess their chances in "light of the total 'market,'" write only to institutions that invited letters for which they were "qualified," and enclose "a carefully prepared one-page vita sheet. . . . Do not write letters to chairmen who have stated in this issue that they have no openings, or whose openings or interests would not apply to you. . . . chairmen understandably do not want to receive applications from candidates who could not possibly fit their hiring plans, and especially so if there are no hiring plans."[33] The sentence at the top of the AHA's May 1974 *Employment Information Bulletin* "No Vacancy" list read simply: "Please do not write to them."[34]

Professional societies' admonitions to those in search of positions reflected in part an effort to save job candidates from wasting their time, energy, and money on fruitless applications.[35] Equally important though, they reflected the fear that a flood of "unwanted" letters and vitae would lead departments to retreat from their tentative and still-incomplete embrace of an open job market.[36] But since hundreds of departments did not respond to professional-society inquiries into whether they were hiring, and other disciplines had no organized job listings at all, candidates were left with little choice than to send out those "desperate and humiliating pleas for employment" at large.

Life choices made in one set of circumstances had unanticipated consequences as straitened budgets in the early 1970s led to restructurings and reductions in staff. "Our plans for the fall are very much up in the air," wrote a Columbia sociology PhD candidate seeking a letter from Robert Merton in August 1973: "The department Bob was teaching in here has just been completely changed in purpose and reduced in size from 11 to four men. He will no longer be teaching here. We are, therefore, considering relocating where one or both of us can obtain jobs." Her vita listed her field as "the sociology of occupations and professions, or more generally, sociology of work." Her own work history, which resembled that of so many others in this era, would have been a worthy subject of study. Like graduate students more generally, her graduate work had been funded through a mix of teaching, research assistantships, and "fellowships" on sponsored research in which faculty were the PIs. At some point, she married a fellow PhD student and moved with him to North Carolina, where he had found a teaching appointment. Like so many women in similar positions, more than a decade passed in which she did not finish her dissertation. And now it was too late.[37]

The work of supporting oneself in part-time and year-to-year positions as one worked toward a degree, the dismal prospect for tenure-track positions, was compounded by the broader cultural and political context. And this too contributed to many never finishing their degrees. Henry Bryant Avery, the University of Michigan PhD candidate in Chinese history who had written AHA President David Potter in February 1971, found a teaching appointment later that year at Lafayette College in Eastern Pennsylvania. It was one of those insecure, year-to-year appointments that had long provided the cheap, flexible labor pool on which institutions of "higher education" depended and through which many graduate students supported themselves.[38] But finding the time, energy, and discipline to finish a dissertation was harder in the 1970s in part because the chance of finding a secure position on completion was so uncertain.[39]

For many, as well, the Cold War that in part had provided the funding for their professional training laid the seeds of their disillusionment. Avery noted the "deep irony": "There I was, a 1960s version of a green, aspiring professional scholar, going to Asia to learn the language of my government's enemy, courtesy of National Defense Foreign Languages (NDFL) grants and a Fulbright scholarship. And what I learned, besides a bit of Chinese, was the meaning of imperialism, the face of rich versus poor peoples and class politics, and the filter down effects of the Vietnam War with its 'R&R' prostitutes in the best sections of Taipei." For Avery and many others like him, the Vietnam War changed the course of his life. As he wrote, "By 1976 I, like others on the amorphous left of U. S. academic life, was also permanently scarred by the Vietnam War. I had lost no limbs to the war, nor even a close relative or friend. But the guilt and embarrassment—the fury that grew—as millions of us watched the nightly slaughter of Asians and Americans had pierced like nothing else in my life." Avery taught at Lafayette College for five years. But not having finished his dissertation by 1976, he was done. As he later wrote, "Without the doctoral parchment, and because there were dozens of eager junior candidates to fill my teaching slot. . . . I was not going to be rehired, there or anywhere. Not in academe."[40]

The postwar years are known, as Richard Freeland dubbed the era, for "the triumph of the professoriate." That triumph included higher salaries, lower teaching loads, retirement benefits, and—most important of all in academia—the expansion and consolidation of tenure.[41] Tenure, with its guarantee of employment, economic security, and academic freedom, was the academic parallel of the postwar American Fordist economy. But what David Harvey, Margot Canaday, and others have noted of the broader economy was just as true in academia. In fact, Canaday might have been describing academia when she wrote, "When heightened competition and labor surpluses made it possible to do so in the 1970s, employers began to look for an escape from these expensive, lifelong commitments to primary workers and their families. In the ensuing years, the 'core' who could still rely on such permanent full-time employment continued to shrink, and part-time, temporary, and subcontracted work became far more prevalent."[42] This was the vita of precarity.

In academia, limitations on the number of tenured appointments and an increasing reliance on various forms of part-time and full-time non-tenure-track appointments emerged early in the 1970s. The AAUP took its first formal stand on the crisis in 1973 in a statement assailing the imposition of tenure quotas. A 1978 report documented and condemned the dramatic increase in the number of full-time, non-tenure-track appointments.[43] There were what the report dubbed "folding chair" appointments of two to three years, the holders of which taught introductory-level classes; annual appointments renewable for up to two, three, or four additional years; and annual appointments with unlimited renewals. And there were many institutions with no policy at all but in which full-time, non-tenure-track appointments were widespread.

Institutions offered similar explanations for their practices. As the report noted, "the same words and phrases appeared again and again. . . . The institution (it was said) needed the flexibility with which to face shifts in student interests and shrinking enrollments; the institution needed a 'buffer of term faculty'; the institution would otherwise soon be 'tenured in.' . . . One senior administrator wrote to his faculty that an increase in 'temporary faculty' would serve as a protection for tenure." Nor were nontenured faculty appointments limited to teaching; many of those responding to the inquiry noted themselves as "research faculty," supported in whole or part by external funding, on indefinitely renewable contracts. The practices and policies represented an end run around and an erosion of the institution of tenure, a threat to academic freedom, and the creation of a second class. They in no way fit the exception of temporary appointments. These were appointments often in subjects that were a regular, ongoing part of the curriculum. "The teachers who must go, hat in hand, every year (or every two years, or every three years), indefinitely into the future, to ask if they may stay, are not teachers who feel free to speak and write the truth as they see it." And those holding "folding chairs" and limited renewable appointments were even more vulnerable because in their case "such systems impose no requirement to give reasons for nonreappointment." Near the close of its report, the subcommittee raised a grim, but prescient, question: "If having some non-tenure-track positions gives an institution some flexibility, will not having more such positions provide more flexibility?"

Two years later, in 1980, an AAUP subcommittee took up the question of the status of part-time faculty.[44] The report began with the dramatic growth in reliance on part-time faculty in both relative and absolute terms. Figures from the National Center for Education Statistics indicated that "between the years 1972 and 1977, the rate of faculty growth was 50 percent for part-time staff and 9 percent for full-time staff." At some community colleges, "almost the entire faculty serves on a part-time basis." But part-time faculty were not limited to community colleges. As the report noted, approximately 24 percent of faculty at four-year liberal arts colleges and 20 percent of faculty at research universities were part-time. And this tally was independent of graduate students teaching at the institutions where they were students or those who held "part-time" positions but whose appointments at a single institution were equivalent to a full load.[45]

That reliance marked the beginning of a new era. Noting that "the primary motivation for many of these appointments has been to reduce the cost of instruction," the MLA was one of the first discipline-specific professional societies to issue a statement on the use of part-time faculty. Decrying the "dramatic increase" in the use of part-time faculty in many departments of English and foreign languages, the statement noted, "The very conditions under which most temporary and permanent part-time teachers are employed define them as non-professionals. Often they are hired quickly, as last minute replacements, with only hasty review of their credentials. They receive little recognition or respect for their contributions to their departments; in many instances they are paid inequitably."[46] That statement and guidelines for departments, adopted by the MLA Executive Council in 1982, came a decade into the academic employment crisis. In 1994, the MLA adopted a new statement on the use of part-time and full-time adjunct faculty that began, "The expansion of the adjunct ranks in language and literature departments over the past two decades threatens the integrity of the profession and instructional programs."[47] English and foreign languages represented one point in a larger shift, the equivalent in STEM fields being ever-lengthening postdoctoral and research appointments.

The economic crisis in academia and the American economy more broadly that began in the 1970s frustrated other kinds of change. Departments and universities used the constriction in budgets as an excuse for their failure to make progress on hiring and promoting women and racialized minorities—academia's parallel to last-hired, first-fired policies in employment generally.[48] Recall Hofstra's denial of tenure to Natalie Allon in 1977—a decision framed in terms of declining enrollments, a highly tenured faculty, and the administration's responsibility for the fiscal integrity of the university.[49] Precarity similarly slowed the elimination of personal data from vitae. The law prohibited discrimination; it did not prohibit individuals from electing to include their age, sex, and marital and parental status on their vitae.[50] As the MLA's 1985 *Career Guide for PhDs and PhD Candidates in English and Foreign Languages* noted, it was "inappropriate and indeed in most instances illegal, for potential employers to ask candidates" about their age, marital status, number of children, health, ethnicity, national origin, religious affiliation. But the guide acknowledged that it was not illegal for a candidate to include them. "Obviously, however, if most candidates provide such information as a matter of course, the purpose of the policies and laws—to prevent unfair discrimination—will be frustrated."[51]

Precarity is a powerful disciplining force. In that same 1985 MLA *Career Guide*, the first sentence of "General Advice for Job Seekers" read "You have already begun." It continued: "As soon as you begin specializing in a course of study with the intention of making a career in that field, you also begin establishing a record of your abilities and accomplishments." Reading this statement in 2023, I understood its truth—I had watched, listened for two decades as PhD students worked to "fill out" their vitae—but I also found it chilling. What of free exploration, reflection, the pursuit of knowledge for its own sake, following interests and ideas where they led, serendipity? In its place: a disciplined construction of a professional identity and its paper-double: the vita. Every course, paper, conference interaction an opportunity—nigh a command—"for generating content to put into a vita or resume." As the MLA guide directed, "Your vita is an ideal use for word processing. Not only can you produce letter-perfect copy, but also you can update it constantly."[52] *Content. Update it constantly*. In 1996, an expanded and updated MLA *Career Guide* noted, "Remember, your reader will be looking at hundreds of vitae; be sure that your reader can take in your qualifications at a single glance. If your vita requires a second look or demands extra effort, you will in all likelihood stand at a severe disadvantage."[53] This too was the vita of precarity. The vita became the focus for constructing one's identity. What it should include shaped and drove intellectual inquiry from the moment a prospective student entered a graduate program. When did it end? Noting that finding an initial position might take years, the MLA guide noted, "None of this time need be considered wasted or lost; use it to gain experience and to build up your vita."[54] The hard truth, as the MLA and other professional societies knew, was that many who remained in academia would do so as adjuncts in one form or another, never hired into tenure-track positions at all.[55]

Precarity came to shape intellectual life generally. It began with the start of graduate training, fundamentally shaping the character, content, and quality of intellectual inquiry through tenure if one got there and so became bound up with the intellectual DNA of one generation after another. As a 1977 University of Chicago history PhD—part of the so-called "lost generation" of those who completed PhDs in the late 1970s and early 1980s—put it in 1990 in a letter to *The Chronicle of Higher Education*, "The tight job market militated against intellectual risk taking. Anything too outlandish might threaten tenure or promotion. Safe topics and established methods filled the journals. Such conservatism was natural and sensible in any field where the means of livelihood were threatened, but it has not necessarily made for better-quality research."[56] The writer referred to tenure and promotion, but the point began much earlier with college and graduate training. The vita of precarity in this sense referred not simply to a document, nor only to lives and livelihoods, but to intellects and ideas shaped in precarity's shadow.

With the birth of the World Wide Web in the 1990s, the search for security increasingly played out online. New disciplines like computer science that were integral to the revolution in computing not surprisingly embraced what was for them a native habitat. In 1997, the Department of Computer Science at Columbia University listed seventy-one PhD students; all had home pages.[57] So too PhD students in the Department of Computer Science at Michigan, but here there were two hundred students.[58] Other disciplines were explicit in their embrace of the web as a tool for job placement. Economics departments had long placed students in industry and government as well as academic positions. The web offered a sort of made-to-order medium for reaching all three simultaneously. The home page of the Department of Economics at Columbia, for example, created on December 5, 1995, and updated a year later, announced, "We have a table of graduate students on the job market which lists their fields of specialization. We also have their CV's available on-line as well." Nor was Columbia alone in this respect. The home page of the Department of Economics at the University of Chicago prominently included a link to "Job Market Candidates," which in turn led to a list of "Students on the Job Market" with their names, emails, primary and secondary fields, links to their faculty references, and—for the students who had created them—individual home pages. Moreover, as the site directed, employers could contact students directly or get a "packet of CV's" from the Student Affairs administrator.[59]

In the 1930s, some departments at elite institutions, desperate to place their PhD students in the midst of the Depression, had mailed circulars to other universities with brief student bios.[60] Was there any real difference here other than the mode of communication and its public character? Faculty receiving the 1930s-era lists dismissed them, literally threw them out. In the era of personal placement, any candidate on a list was treated as not first-class. What is unsettling in the lists of job market candidates with linked CVs on the web at century's end is the sense that the job candidates were viewed by their departments—and had been trained to view themselves—as being just like any other commodity. Moreover, whereas the state of affairs in the 1930s had been seen as a temporary crisis, the norms of this new era were accepted as the way things worked. The shift reflected just how dramatically the academic economy had changed by century's end.

Departments were anxious to place their students. Students were anxious to secure jobs. Advice on vitae now extended to whether one needed and what made for an effective home page. As the authors of a 1998 article in *The Chronicle of Higher Education* noted, "Since more and more candidates and employers are using the Internet for everything. Yes, it's a good idea." They closed with a piece of advice: "A good way to test the effectiveness of a C.V. is to show it to someone for 30 seconds and ask them what they saw. If your strongest qualifications stood out, you did a good job. Have several people take a quick look at your home page. Then ask what impression it made. If they say what you hope to hear, you've got a good home page which will work for you 24 hours a day."[61] Time had a new meter.

But the early web was not only a tool for job placement or a mode of professional communication and connection between those sharing a field. *Curriculum vitae*, in its classical Latin meaning, had referred to the lived course of life, not to an academic form or a life reduced to a form. Early on in the life of the web, the actual course of lives broke through the disciplined form. In a world where jobs and security were scarce, self-defense alone suggested that one avoid defining oneself solely through them. The University of Michigan Economics Department, like other prominent economics departments, was early in embracing the web. But where universities like Chicago and Columbia were explicit in marketing their job candidates, the Michigan Economics Department offered simply to include home pages of students who elected to create them.[62] Many did. And though some were entirely professionalized, many were not. "Welcome to my homepage!" announced Carolyn Fischer, on a page she had created in May 1996 and updated in August 1997.[63] "Get to know me and some of my interests—if you want useful information, you might want to go elsewhere." Two lines near the top of the page were announced as "NEW" (bold, all caps, bright red edged with yellow—a sort of textual neon sign without the blinking lights): "I'm employed!" began one of the new announcements, and the second, "I'm buying a house [link]!" And in the upper right-hand corner, a small photo of a joyful-looking woman.

Fischer included her vita in the section under the heading "Professional Information": "I do work in environmental and natural resource economics, as well as public finance, particularly taxation. You can look at my CV [link] if you're interested."[64] She included links to papers she had written, with a brief, breezy explanation of their focus, and noted her current funding and past experience. But everything on the page was conversational. Here was a new way of connecting. "If you are also an economist with a web page, my friend John S. Irons [link] is compiling a list [of] us ecgeeks." And under "Personal Background": "When I'm not working on my dissertation, I'm usually playing guitar. I play a Takamine G Series EG-10C [link]. . . . I'm in a duo called Strange Affliction [link] with a guy named Dave." And on it went.

Carolyn Fischer was not alone. Another Michigan economics graduate student described his current research and recent publications but also offered a link to a page titled "Fun Stuff": "In my spare time, I love to play ultimate frisbee, a fast paced and exciting team sport that's rapidly growing in popularity. . . . Here's a neat on-line version of The Tortoise and the Hare [link] adapted by my fiancée Rebeccah Kamp for the Internet Public Library's children story page."[65] On these websites, conventionally framed vitae were background, literally, on a foreground that was personal even when it was professional.

But this moment of unabashed freedom and uncalculated openness passed quickly. The personal siphoned off, perhaps, by social-media start-ups like Facebook. Or reined in by the growing professionalization of the academic web. As Mary Morris Heiberger and Julie Miller Vick from the Career Service Office at Penn had directed job market candidates considering creating home pages in their 1998 *Chronicle* article, "Don't include personal material unless you're truly willing to be rejected on account of it."[66] One could appreciate the dark humor of a PhD candidate at the University of Chicago's Graduate School of Business, whose link to his curriculum vitae read, "My life compacted into a two page document."[67] As he wrote on his personal home page "So what about my life?? . . . I'm trying to find a position as a professor. Don't worry, I'm taking a correspondence course in refrigerator repair in case things don't work out."[68]

The Chronicle of Higher Education marked the new century with an "Advice" column featuring a series of life stories from the job market. Some writers used their actual names, others used pseudonyms. They came from a variety of disciplines, including biology, history, and sociology. Some were just finishing their degrees, others had already spent several postdoc years in someone else's lab; some were single, others were navigating what they called the "two-" or "three-" body problem, dual academic couples, some with a child. Their stories had titles like "My First Invitation to the Dance," "The End of an Academic Affair," and "On the Market: To Rule in Hell or Serve in Heaven."[69] Their posts fit the larger confessional culture, but their willingness to share their job search trials openly also reflected a sort of rebellion against the private desperation that had prevailed for so long.

Daniel Kowalsky, a PhD candidate in history at the University of Wisconsin, was one of those who chronicled his life in a series of posts from October 2000 to July 2002. The narrative arc of the course of his life in this moment is hinted at in the titles to his posts: "On the Market: Diary of a Would-be Historian," "What I Saw at the Job Conference," "My Narrow Escape From a Life Without Letterhead," and "Next Stop: Cairo."[70] In a post from February 16, 2001, he wrote, "I'm spending a lot of time these days listening to the soundtrack from A Chorus Line." As he described it, the 1975 Broadway musical "is about a group of aspiring dancers," but "it's really about a job search" and the "anxieties and self-doubt that one experiences in trying to land a job in a tight market." One could see why the soundtrack was running through his head. His thirty-fifth birthday and dissertation defense were imminent, and he had just spent four days interviewing at the AHA's annual conference. His favorite song from the musical was "the opening number," which he recalled as "'I Hope I Get It.'" He focused on the lines, "I really need this job. Please, God, I need this job. I've got to get this job!"[71]

It was not until summer, as Kowalsky described in a post with the title

"My Narrow Escape from a Life Without Letterhead," that he secured a tenuous hold on academic employment: a one-year appointment at Washington University in St. Louis to begin that fall. But even as he began that appointment, he wrote, "a dark cloud hung over me; to wit, the fleeting status of my position. Almost as soon as I settled into a routine of lecturing and getting to know my students, I was already scrambling to line something up for the following year." He had finished his degree, but he also shared that the stresses of the job market and the prospect of living for many years or permanently in a different city than his spouse (who had secured a tenure-track appointment) had led him and his wife to formally separate and divorce. The upside? He was no longer limited geographically in his job search.

With degree in hand and learning just before the 2002 AHA conference that his dissertation had been awarded a prestigious prize that included a publication contract with Columbia University Press, he thought his prospects now for a tenure-track position at a research university would be good. But whether because the prize came too late or otherwise, he found himself facing, as he described it, "the cruelest irony of them all": The book contract that might have earned him a shot at a research university position effectively disqualified him in the eyes of the teaching-intensive institutions that had offered him interviews. The reward? Another temporary appointment. "Next Stop: Cairo" was how he titled his post. Here's how he spun the result for himself and readers: "I'll be living in the middle of a bustling, exotic city, where I will be teaching European history to an entirely different pool of students. I'll get to study a new language and experience what day-to-day life in the Arab world is like. Yes, it is true: I had no choices this year; Cairo was the only option. It also happens, however, to be my dream job."

And maybe it was. That year, like the preceding year at Washington University in St. Louis and the year after at the University of Bristol, a succession of one-year appointments, became lines on Daniel Kowalsky's vita. In 2004, Columbia University Press published his interactive e-book, titled *Stalin and the Spanish Civil War*, the product of the E-Gutenberg Dissertation Prize he had been awarded in 2001. And in 2005, he landed a more permanent position as lecturer in the School of History, Anthropology, Philosophy and Politics at Queen's University Belfast (where, as of 2025, he remained).[72]

But many, increasingly most in fact, never found that security in the United States or elsewhere. Marginality on various axes of difference had long defined American academic life. Even as social movements mobilized law in the 1960s and 1970s to open academia to those who by virtue of sex, race, and other elements of identity had been excluded or marginalized, the new defining axis of marginality became contingency. By 2008, 68.8 percent of faculty in American universities and colleges were "contingent" faculty.[73] No discipline escaped it, no institution—public or private, large or small—had clean hands. Universities and colleges facing tight budgets meant that even many who taught for years on annual appointments suddenly faced nonrenewal. Even tenure did not guarantee security.[74]

There was stigma in contingency. And because the vita was by the early 1970s the gateway form of American academic life, that stigma was visible, which made escape from it more difficult.[75] And so, perhaps it is not surprising that just as those who had seen their entitlement in the era of bald-faced exclusion and discrimination as the product of merit finding its own place, in this new era, the age of the vita, in which the specter of contingency grew, those with vitae that documented their security held fast to the belief, the hope, that it reflected their merit. And here too the vita served universities' ends by individualizing preferment and precarity.

Near the end of the opening song from *A Chorus Line*, one of the auditioning dancers plaintively sings, "Who am I anyway? Am I my resume? That is a picture of a person I do not know."[76] Those whose lives we have glimpsed here were no more their vitae than the dancers in *A Chorus Line* were their resumes. Or the children burned in Gene Autry cowboy suits only that. Or my daughter Frances only a girl who died at age eighteen.

on being

Dear Frances,

The backyard is littered with apples from the tree that you and I planted when you were still in lower school. Last year was the first year it had apples. Does an apple tree only bear fruit once it has matured? It was strange last summer—the first summer you were gone—to have it suddenly have fruit when it never had before.

. . .

I started an article in The New Yorker *today by a philosopher named Derek Parfit. I need to finish the article, but I found it very hopeful. His first book was titled* Reasons and Persons *and in it he argues for a more impersonal (in the sense of personhood being embodied in a single body), non-physical, self-less view of human life. It gives me a way to understand my sense that you continue to be, to understand my writing to you, and even to understand the sense that when you died I died too. So that you continue to live unembodied and I continue to live embodied, though also gone. As he wrote, "My death will break the more direct relations between my present experiences and future experiences, but it will not break various other relations." As the author of the article explains, "Some people will remember him. Others may be influenced by his writing, or act upon his advice. Memories that connect with his memories, thoughts that connect with his thoughts, actions taken that connect with his intentions, will persist after he is gone, just inside different bodies." It is a wonderfully hopeful view. It doesn't make me think about myself, but rather of you and of the many bodies in which you continue to live.*

. . .

When I first began writing you my focus was on trying to understand what had happened, trying to find a way to go back, to change the course of events, to tell you how much we loved you and needed you. And I told you about the weather. I didn't talk about news because I was unaware of anything that was happening in the world, unable to listen to the radio or look at a newspaper. And so I didn't find myself wondering if I had already told you something or whether I was repeating myself. But now that there is more of the everyday in my notes to you, I do find myself hesitating—"Did I already tell Frances . . ." I could, I suppose look back at what I've written, but although they are right there, they are, in my mind, sent off to you. There's something unnerving about looking back, a recognition that they haven't been sent (and hence not received), unsendable/unreceivable, at all. And so I don't look. So, if I repeat myself, forgive me.

. . .

Tonight when Dad and I were getting dinner together, he had an itch on his back and went over to the door frame to use as a scratching post. It was something you did on occasion. I had forgotten until he reminded me. But once he did, I could see you in that long blue, oversize t-shirt with the otter on the front, and a pair of long, dark blue gym shorts standing there in the kitchen, a big smile on your face and explaining as you used the corner of the door-jam to scratch your back that you had an itch. It's a sweet, endearing memory.

. . .

Dad told me tonight as we walked that the world's population is expected to reach 7 billion people on October 31st, that population is once again a major issue among people who worry about the future. I found myself thinking about how devastating it is to be without you—just one person—and then I tried to think about what it meant that the earth had 7 billion people. Somehow the two didn't fit together.

. . .

[I am at a conference.] Yesterday at the panel I was on one of the other presenters—a scholar whose work I had read and admired—focused her talk on "children's archiving." The panel was about sources and methods in the History of Children. What she meant by "children's archiving" was looking at the things that children put on the walls and doors of their room. The rooms she has access to are those of the wealthy or significant in some historical way. They share one other feature: the children died as children. Their parents preserved their child's room just as it was when the child died. And it has remained and become accessible to historians because of the family's sta-

tus. I sat there looking at the images, listening to her analysis, thinking about you and your room. I imagine that I was the only person in the room who understood what those rooms meant to those families, the only one who had lost a child, the only one who had a room in my house that preserved a child's room just as it was. Should these families' heartache be part of how she approaches these "sources"? Should she find in these children's early, premature deaths an opportunity that as a historian she is delighted by without some sort of acknowledgment, registering of the loss that in a sense produced this archive? Do we only, as historians, register "biases" in "the archive"? Can she write this history without registering, without considering the love, the hopes and dreams, the loss that is there in the words, pictures, things on those walls?

chapter twenty-two · growing old

"I just want to be shod of this whole thing. . . . But I can't outlive it. . . . You know. It's just too many memories, you know. From time to time, I revert back to these feelings, and I just can't, uh, shake 'em. I'm just going to have to live with it, that's all."[1] Gaither Bates Jr. was seventy-six years old and had lived with it for seventy years.

Before I spoke with those who had been burned as children in Gene Autry cowboy suits, I had not understood this. My worry had been dredging up a long-past trauma. Now that I better understood the experience and meaning of this injury in their lives, I found myself thinking of Robert Smithson's giant earthwork sculpture *Spiral Jetty*. A great counterclockwise spiral, 1,500 feet of mud, salt crystals, and basalt rocks, extending far out into the Great Salt Lake in Utah. Like the Spiral Jetty, there had been times in these lives when the injury was fully present—there in daylight and in darkness—above the surface of the water, and times when it was wholly or partially submerged.[2] Like the Spiral Jetty, time and its elements changed the injury, changed its meaning in their lives. But even as it did, the injury would always be there.

The experience of these injuries that had been so much a part of the course of their lives changed again as they aged. Part of this change was a function of their aging bodies. Severe burns are perilous because skin is part of the organ system of the human body. And like other organs, skin loses capacity with age. Our skin gets thinner, drier; healing slows. For those who were burned, their healed and grafted skin was already compromised, their risks of cancer greater, and so aging brought new meaning to the injury in their lives.

Like many of those burned, Ron King had fought ulcers on his legs through much of his life. When he was in his late sixties, the ulcers on his right leg developed into cancer. For eight years he fought it, until finally, in 2014, his right leg was amputated. Because of the burns and skin grafts, his legs were misshapen—which meant that he could not use a prosthesis that would have enabled him to walk. And so, the burns that cost him his leg in turn transformed what would have been a partial disability into full disability. His wife Rosanne remembers saying to him, "It's not the end of the world, you know. So, I wheel you in a wheelchair, you know, it's not like, you know— " But, she admitted, "he felt self-conscious." The impact of having his leg amputated was compounded by his diagnosis two years earlier with Parkinson's disease. He had had to quit his job at a company where he had worked throughout his adult life and that he had played an important role in building. His doctors had suggested that the Parkinson's may have been linked to his earlier burns, but whether it was or not, the combination of the two meant that the orbit of his life was dramatically circumscribed. Wheelchair-bound, his speech too became increasingly impaired. He "suffered his later years." Rosanne King loved her husband deeply, would have done anything for him and did. But "it was hard," she explained. The day before we were scheduled to meet, Ron King was admitted to the hospital. He died three weeks later, on December 24, 2016. He was seventy-six years old.[3]

For those who lived into their sixties and seventies, the meaning of their injuries changed also because as they grew older their sense that time was limited sharpened. Jack Lockhart Jr. was seventy-six years old when we met in 2015. He was the youngest child in his family and had only one sibling still alive. He and his wife, Angela, were both retired and had moved from Michigan to Florida. The day we met, he sat in a recliner, his legs stretched out in front of him, the summer having been lost to another surgery and recovery. They had had two trips planned for the summer. But then one trip had to be cancelled because he needed another grafting surgery and the second cancelled because the recovery had been slow. In the thirty-six years they had been married, his wife, Angela, said that he had had surgery "at least, probably on the average, once a year. . . . There were a couple years that we made it two years, but then it seemed like the next year was twice in a year. . . . I've accepted it," she said. "It's part of my life." But she admitted that it was different for him. As he got older, the recoveries were longer and less certain. There seemed no end to it. He got angrier, his fuse shorter, the time lost from life with each surgery seeming more precious. "Will it never end?" he asked. And then he answered his own question: "And it won't. So. And I'm getting less patient with it, let's say, the older I get."

As they grew older, there were other losses in their lives, and the meaning of their injury changed in the face of those losses. Despite having had her legs amputated as a child and being in a wheelchair, Jackie Izzo had lived independently throughout her adult life. She had worked for thirty-three years. Driven her own car. Done her own grocery shopping, cooking, and housekeeping. When Jackie was forty-eight years old, her mother died of lung cancer. Her mother, who Jackie described, as "one hell of a lady," about whom Jackie had said, "The first reason none of this stuff bothered me, it didn't stop her." After her mother's death, Jackie still had her brother, John, and sister, Jeannie. It had been her sister who demanded that Jackie be in school, had searched for jobs for Jackie, had tried to get her outfitted with prosthetics, had made it possible for her to drive. "She was always there!" Jackie said. When Jackie developed lung cancer and had to have a lung removed, Jeannie was there. Though she too was suffering from lung cancer, she put Jackie's needs before her own. When Jackie needed another surgery, this one for an open sore that would not heal on one of her stumps, Jeannie told her, "Go have your surgery," assuring Jackie that she was fine. But while Jackie was in the hospital, her sister died, two days before Jackie's seventy-fifth birthday. "She lied to me," Jackie said.

Over the course of these individuals' lives, I expect there were many such lies in many families.[4] The negligence of those who made the Gene Autry cowboy suit did not cause Jackie's sister's death. But that Jeannie did not tell her to postpone the surgery, that she was deprived of Jackie's presence at the end of her life, and Jackie deprived of the opportunity to say final farewells, was inextricably bound up with that negligence. The loss of her sister, in turn, compounded Jackie's loss of her right lung, which itself was disabling in a way that it would not have been but for the injuries she suffered as a child. Now independent living for Jackie required caretakers; it meant no longer being able to drive, not being able to do all the things she had done for herself. She continued to live alone and yet was dependent in new and hard ways that limited her world.

What was true for Jackie Izzo was true for others: Illnesses and deaths of family members mingled with this injury from their childhood and changed its meaning in their lives. For so many of those burned, there had been earlier losses, and these too had shaped the meaning of their own injury in their lives. But earlier losses had mingled with joys, had come in the midst of the striving of mid-life. Losses in old age bore more heavily. Gaither Bates was sixty-seven when his youngest daughter died of cancer. Her husband had died of a heart attack six months earlier. "Hell of a year," was how he put it.[5] Art Cumberledge lost his sister; he and his wife Jenny lost a grandson to cancer who lived with them the final year of his life and died in their home; his wife Jenny had macular degeneration and was losing her sight. A few months after Jack Lockhart retired, his only son died unexpectedly. "I was a very protective parent," he said. "And then to lose my son, the one I was most protective of, that uh, that made it even worse."[6] When his only brother—whom he had negotiated in the dark with to help him get the weighted shoes off his feet—died, Jack missed the funeral because of another surgery. He learned afterward that his brother had donated his skin to a burn center. "I didn't know he was gonna do—" and he stopped mid-sentence, unable to continue.[7] For some, my sense is that the significance of their own injury, loss, and suffering receded in the face of losses that felt greater to them. For some, my sense is that their suffering left them with less resilience in facing other losses and increased their anger at not being able to be fully present for others.

But other hardships, other losses in their lives also became part of their understanding of what had happened to them: It was just part of life. "In the wrong place at the wrong time, that's all," Jack Lockhart said of being burned.[8] "It's, it's life? You know?" his wife, Angela, said. Many—most, I now expect—of those burned in Gene Autry cowboy suits, including those in families that pursued lawsuits, had gone through life not knowing the true cause of what had happened to them and—beyond that—not knowing that many other children had similarly been injured, suffered, died. One has to pause to absorb this fact. It seems improbable. I had assumed that even though the history of this tragedy was not known today, those to whom it had happened had known it for what it was. But they did not. Any number of those I talked with—Charles Baragona, Mike Felton, Jackie Izzo, William McMaster—had not known that other children had been burned. I now believe that what was true for them was true for most others.

There were some who, by the circumstances of the event, knew that they were not the only child to have been burned while wearing a Gene Autry cowboy suit. Brothers or friends playing together in their Gene Autry cowboy suits—Casimir Krzeczkowski Jr. and his little brother Stanley; Joey Intelisano and his friend Gerald Sukinik; Joseph, Donald, and James Powell—all of them burned. But even they did not know the role of their clothing in what had happened. And since in each instance only one of the children survived, they were left in the event more alone. Some children burned in Gene Autry cowboy suits had met other children similarly burned in the hospital or through the lawsuits their parents brought. Tom Habina had been in Temple University Hospital in Philadelphia at the same time as two other boys burned in Gene Autry cowboy suits. They had had wheelchair races down the hospital corridors. "Well, we always believed that, uh, the three of us were burnt, that was it. We never knew about nobody else," Tom Habina explained to me.[9]

For most of those I met, their first awareness that others had been burned as they had was a letter through their mail slot decades later that began, "My name is Barbara Welke and I am a historian at the University of Minnesota. I am working on a book focused on a set of incidents from the early 1940s through the 1950s in which children across the United States were severely burned, a number of whom died, when the Gene Autry cowboy suits they were wearing caught fire." I had not anticipated, but perhaps should have as a historian, how little they would know of the history of this event, a history it had taken me years, after all, to piece together. Their not knowing was part of this history. But their not knowing also brought for me the agonizing realization, in one conversation after another, of being the agent, a participant in a conversation that disturbed long-unquestioned events, settled understandings, and hard-fought acceptances, conversations that had the potential to rewrite, in some measure, the course of a life.

What was shared, that is, common to the experience of individuals impacted in this tragedy, was divided along many axes of difference: age, sex, class, race, status, personality, region, and time. The experience of mothers was different from that of fathers; both were different from the experience of their children who were burned. Part of the difference was that at least those parents who brought suit learned that what had happened was not just an accident. Why did they not tell their children what they knew? There are so many possible explanations for their silence. They were themselves caught up in the trauma of the event, their knowledge incomplete and, for many, delayed by years. But the reasons for parents not telling their children go beyond the fog of traumatic injury. Most of the incidents had happened during a war that had brought suffering, disability, and loss of unfathomable proportion, others in its immediate wake. And then there was the boundary adults drew—far sharper in the 1940s and 1950s than it would be in later decades—between matters for adults and matters for children. Perhaps some did not tell their children out of a desire to protect them, others because they believed their child was at fault. The warning that children should not play with fire carried greater, not less, weight for parents in the face of what had happened. After all, had there been no fire, there would have been no harm. And, finally, what had happened had happened. What would be gained by dwelling on what could not be undone?

The burned children who survived and the siblings of those who did not filled the space left by their parents' silence. Jackie Izzo explained to me that she had never questioned what happened. She wondered about that now. But, as she explained, she had been too busy. "Fighting for an education. Fighting to keep my younger brother and sister from getting killed [by their father]. . . . That's what worried us. See, stuff like that was on my mind."[10] Though the circumstances of every household were different, I expect Jackie was not alone in not having questioned what happened. Age most certainly played a role. Some of those burned or who lost siblings lived their lives believing that what had happened was an accident, just part of life.

Others, including those who were told it was their fault, men like Gaither Bates, carried the burden of personal responsibility for their suffering through their lives. That burden extended to those who had bought the cowboy suit for the child and to siblings and playmates who were with a child when burned. An unexplored legacy of settlements in personal-injury actions involving hazardous products is the cover they give to the narrative of personal responsibility. Settlements mean that the burden of responsibility is never laid in the hands, hearts, and minds of those who are the agents of the harm.

Others still came to accept the trials of their injuries as an all-powerful God's test of their faith. Through his years of acute suffering, Ron King had steeled himself to accept that suffering without complaint, saying to his wife, "God never gives you more than you can handle."[11]

Trauma, pain, injury, and loss are isolating. What did it mean for survivors to now discover that others had been burned in Gene Autry cowboy suits, some far worse than they, some of whom had died? Robert Viands's response was to be newly appreciative that he was alive. For this man who had had so much hardship in his life beyond the trauma of being burned, here, he learned, was an instance of his having won what seemed life's lottery.[12] He had lived where others had died; he had had no ongoing medical issues where others had had a life of surgeries. "I feel great," he exclaimed. "What happened to me versus what happened to some of these kids . . . I, you know, I feel great, I'm lucky, I am lucky, lucky, lucky." Jackie Izzo voiced a different set of emotions in learning that there were others. We had laughed together as she told stories about her childhood, but now, hearing that she had not been the only one, that other children had suffered, she said, "Oh my God, I wasn't the only one that had nightmares nights and days and not wanting to go to the next skin graft and go under."[13]

Would it have mattered, had these children known as they grew up that they were not alone? Would that knowledge have changed the experience and meaning of this injury in their lives? Recognizing polio's important differences from injury and death caused by another's negligent or intentional actions, the experience of polio victims suggests it could have mattered to the course of their lives. William "Skip" McMaster Jr., one of those burned in a Gene Autry cowboy suit who had also had polio, had, as a young adult, been part of athletic teams that traveled across the United States, precursors to the Paralympics. He had met on one of those trips the woman—a physical therapist along to assist the team—who became his second wife, and to whom, when we met, he had been married for forty-five years. Those teams were normalizing; they created community. As an adult, he was active in post-polio groups that again created community.[14]

Those burned in Gene Autry cowboy suits never had this kind of community in their lives, a community of others who shared their experience, from whom they might learn important medical information, with whom they might develop deep bonds grounded in a shared experience, and to whom they could talk openly about their feelings about what had happened, what it meant to live with this injury, with whom they could share feelings of anger, frustration, being fed up without their listener feeling guilty or taking them to mean that they wished they had a different life.[15] That they did not have this community was another kind of loss, another facet of this tragedy.

Such a community likely also would have meant learning much earlier in their lives that their injury had not been an accident. That knowledge would have changed the meaning of this injury in their lives, relieved them from the unjust burden of feeling they were responsible. It might have allowed them to see what had happened as an injustice, to have a focus for their anger, to channel that anger collectively to seek change. Women's challenge to sex discrimination in academia, as traced in this book, grew out of such a collective recognition that their exclusion from and subordination within higher education was a product not of personal failings but of injustice based on their sex. As this history suggests, another unexplored consequence of legal settlements, and not just those in product liability actions, is their impact in undermining collective action by not only keeping wrongs from coming to light but also dividing those who might otherwise have come together.

There is a difference between sharing with someone what you know of a history from your own research and asking them to reflect on their own life. "Do you think it makes a difference that it didn't have to happen?" I asked Jack and Angela Lockhart. It was a hard question. Why did I ask it? What did I expect by way of answer? How are such questions important to history, important to a life? My question came in part from my surprise in learning that Jack Lockhart, the first individual I spoke with, someone who had reached out to me through the internet, had not known of the defendants' responsibility for what had happened, an unknowing replicated in my conversations with others. The cause of trauma and injury matters to its lived meaning in a life. They had lived their lives not knowing that cause. But there were also so many other hardships and losses in these individuals' and families' lives, many for which no one was to blame, others that were bound up with larger structural forces of inequality. I was not asking whether Jack Lockhart or any of these individuals wished they had had a different life; I was trying to comprehend the significance of causation not in law, but for a life. It was a question that I understood individuals would answer differently, if they could consider the question at all.

Jack Lockhart's reply to my question was immediate. "That's wasted, that's wasted energy. It happened. That's it. You live with it, and you learn to live with it. That's it."[16] Maybe the immediate circumstances—in which he was still recovering from surgeries that once again meant time lost from life, as he saw it—shaped his response. There were conversations as with Jack and Angela Lockhart where I asked the question directly; in others, the question arose unasked from my description of what the defendants had known. Jackie Izzo expressed a raw anger when I explained what the defendants had known. "All from the legs from these damn chaps. Ooch! Why don't you get a gun with me, we'll go find these people and shoot their grave." We both laughed. We weren't laughing because it was funny, but out of a sense of a raging helplessness. *Get a gun and shoot their graves.* "You know what I mean? God!" she said.[17] As we continued to talk, she turned to the solace that had long provided comfort in her hard life. "Oh, it just really gets me now." She laughed sadly, "I'll have to see the Lord for a couple days to get over this. I just can't, I just can't believe it."[18]

Their answers not only reflected their present circumstances but were filtered as well through class position, professional training, and political and religious perspectives. Their answers might well have been different at other life stages. But more than stage of life shaped their answers. I completed the bulk of my interviews in the months following the 2016 presidential election, in which Donald Trump was elected president. The political climate was one suffused with outrage and the rhetoric of personal responsibility. Mike Felton, an Idaho lawyer, expressed the view that the defendants should have been punished "much more severely than they were." But he insisted, "I still think that, um, that I have to bear the lion's share of the responsibility for putting myself in a position where their negligence could harm me." It wasn't, he explained, like he had just been "walking down the street and a spark on the breeze ignited my stuff." He had, he said, willfully chosen to do something he had been told not to, that is, to "play with fire."[19]

But many children burned in Gene Autry cowboy suits had been doing the equivalent of just walking down the street. Moreover, Mike Felton's statement suggested that he held himself—and effectively others—to a standard to which no court, then or today, held a child of six. Perhaps, as he grew up, he had been held to that standard for what had happened to him; there were children who had been so held. None of these children was responsible for what happened to them. None of them should have been burned because their clothing, a child's playsuit, should never have been made from this fabric. Had Milton Henry not sold the remaining cowboy suits he had on hand after he learned that children had been burned and died, Mike Felton and many others, children like Charles Baragona Jr. and John Sansbury, would never have been burned even though they had played with matches, and other children who had not been playing with matches—children like James Hummel, who died at age seven an hour after being burned; Scott Timberlake, who died at age thirteen having been rendered mentally incompetent and institutionalized for the remainder of his life; Gerald Palmateer, who died at age sixteen; James Ikner who died at age twenty-six; and Pat Peterson—would never have been burned.

"Well, the way that would affect me," John Sansbury, a retired engineer said, as though we were discussing a hypothetical situation, "was it would make me mad. Because something, something could have been done. . . . If not for me, for certainly, 'til 1954, when you said that . . . [it] pissed me off, it sort of did. I thought, how can anybody do that when they know . . . they know, and still didn't stop it?"[20] John Sansbury was burned in April 1947, four and a half years after the first deaths of children and two full years after the defendants knew that children had been injured and died. But even if he had been one of the first children burned, his question—"how can anybody do that when they know?"—applied. The defendants had known. But there were also other possibilities in seeing the broader history of this event, even if only late in life. "It might bring closure to it," Gaither Bates said of this thing he had lived with for seventy years; this thing he could not shake. "That's what I'm hoping."[21]

Learning there were others, even and perhaps especially late in life, held out as well the possibility of alleviating some of the aloneness. Jack Lockhart had known from his boyhood that there were at least a couple of other boys in Michigan who had been burned like he was. In the two years before we met, he and his wife, Angela, had begun to search the internet for oth-

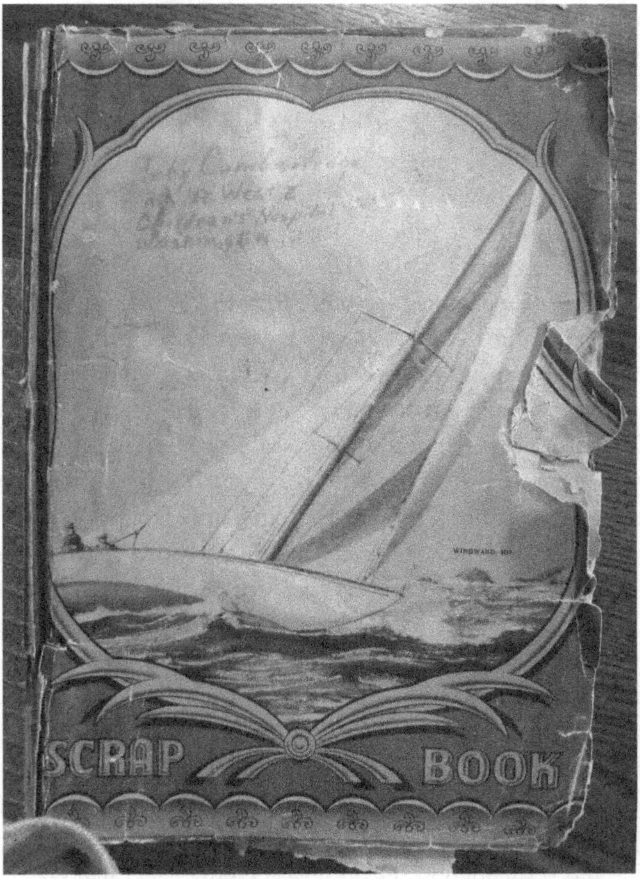

ers burned in Gene Autry cowboy suits. He wondered if their doctors had found a way to bring an end to the cycle of surgeries that would work for him. But whether they had done so or not, he hoped to find others, to talk with them so that, as he explained to me, they would know that they were not alone.[22] And though he did not say it directly, perhaps also so that he would feel less alone.

A flimsy paper scrapbook with tattered edges. A drawing of a sailboat on a sunny windswept sea. The promise of adventure and happy memories. In a neat hand on the blue sky, the words "Toby Cumberledge Rm. A West II Children's Hospital Washington, D.C."[23] Opening the cover, page after page of homemade and store-bought cards from children and adults. One can trace time through the cards. Easter. A birthday. And after the cards, page upon page of news clippings from Washington, DC, papers—the *Times-Herald* and *Evening Star*—the newsprint brittle with age, the edges tattered, the lines of words at the bottom of many articles long since broken off. The news clippings: extended, urgent news stories with photos of children, some in hospital beds, others who had died from their burns, smiling in family snapshots. Art Cumberledge Jr., "Toby," is one of the boys shown in a hospital bed. He is mentioned in the text of some of the stories along with others. Most of the clippings are from early April 1945, when the news first broke. Then a leap in time to 1954. A clipping from the *Nippon Times*. A paragraph underlined in red pencil. And at the top, in the same neat hand as the writing on the scrapbook cover, "Toby will be interested." "Who put this together?" I asked. "I don't know," Art Cumberledge Jr. replied. "Probably my mother, I imagine; it's the kind of thing she would do."[24]

Other parents too, mothers mostly I imagine, had clipped news articles, saved letters and family photographs, and passed them on to their children, who also saved them. Charles Baragona Jr.'s mother had saved every letter—from the nuns, from the hospital, from Charles—from the period that her son was in the Shriners' Hospital in Shreveport, Louisiana.[25] Tom Habina's mother had carefully saved the article written by one of the doctors at Temple University Hospital about their course of treatment of Tommy and two other boys burned in Gene Autry cowboy suits. Pat Peterson's mother had clipped dozens of stories from the newspaper about Pat being burned, his injuries, the skin grafts, the Elks fundraising campaign, his going from the hospital to the Elks home in Umatilla, Florida, and finally his homecoming. Joseph Intelisano's mother had saved the photograph of "Joey" from the Passaic *Herald-News* in a hospital bed, his legs wrapped in bandages and suspended in the air. Every family I met had saved things; some had been lost over time or were in a box that could not now be found, but someone had saved things marking this moment.

But there was no more a single meaning to be drawn from these items being saved than there was a single meaning in the lived experience to which they related. History, the mysteries of an all-powerful God, the miracle of modern medicine, life, love—in every case, love. The news broke of the hazard the Gene Autry cowboy suit posed two weeks after Toby Cumberledge was burned in Washington, DC. His mother, Mary Louise Cumberledge, had clipped articles from the *Times-Herald* and *Washington Evening Star* the first three days of the coverage. The coverage had continued after April 11, 1945, including articles with Toby's name in them, but her clippings had stopped.[26] The reason is not hard to imagine: Four days into the breaking story about the hazard, President Roosevelt had unexpectedly died, leaving the nation stunned and military families like the Cumberledges especially so.[27] Mary Louise Cumberledge may well have begun clipping the articles from the papers because her child was one of those burned, because they documented the hazard that caused his injuries, because he was alive where others had died.

But was there also, perhaps, the sense that in this too their lives were bound up in a larger history? Nine years later, the Cumberledges were stationed in Japan. The final article in the scrapbook, from the Tokyo *Nippon Times* on March 3, 1954, was titled "U. S. Legislation Prevents Use of Inflammable Cloth." Its focus was on the passage of the Flammable Fabrics Act, which was set to go into effect that year. The underlined paragraph read: "Officials said the legislation came into being because certain American manufacturers were making so-called 'torch sweaters' and cowboy chaps of children's playsuits from dangerously flammable materials. They recalled several cases in which such clothing was set on fire, seriously injuring the wearers." The historical arc of the scrapbook changes with this as the final article: Toby was horribly burned in a hazardous cowboy suit; friends and neighbors gathered to support him; the hazard was now guarded against.[28] The personal arc of the scrapbook changes as well—"Toby will be interested"—her child had survived and was by that point almost seventeen years old.[29] Within a year he would have dropped out of high school to marry the girl he was dating when she got pregnant, "do the right thing" as he put it.

But there were other meanings in families' saving things related to this trauma in their lives. Tommy Habina had languished on the verge of death at the first hospital he had been in. The doctors at Temple University Hospital had saved his life; they also had told the Habinas that the cowboy suit was responsible for their son's injuries and had recommended that the family bring a lawsuit. For the many deeply religious families, saved news clippings, letters, and religious symbols were testaments to God's grace. These families had faced a trial and their child had lived. The news clipping Joey Intelisano's mother saved of him in the hospital with the caption "He is in Pain" was the third image in a photo montage his stepchildren created for his funeral. Saving letters, news clippings, and artifacts of this trial served as a reminder of that place, as a reminder to them to place their trust in God.

Parents saved things because this was their trial too. "I tell you something," Jack Lockhart said. "My mother's friends told her, all of her lady friends, because she belonged to a lodge"—Daughters of Scotia Lodge—"they all said that [she] was blessed that this happened to [her] son." And then he stopped to gather his composure so that he could keep talking without breaking down. "Because of me getting hurt, she was blessed from that. Now [she had] a place in heaven."[30] Newspaper accounts of these children's injury, suffering, and battle for survival held warning for other parents and adults and—as often as not—sought their support in blood drives and monetary donations. But for the children's parents these battles had been their lives. They were the kinds of people who, for the most part, would never be the subjects of "news"—but here was their child, his or her story, their story, written in the paper.

A historian clipping these stories would have noted the date, page, and newspaper on each, perhaps noting the surrounding coverage. Mothers were caught up in the moment. And so Pat Peterson's mother, like so many others, noted none of these things. Her son had been horribly burned. It was unclear if he would live, and once it seemed he would survive, it was unclear what lasting injuries he would have. She had clipped the stories from the paper each day not knowing what the future held. He had miraculously survived. They had lived this event from the day of his accident to his joyful homecoming and long after. Years passed. Pat grew to adulthood, married, and had children of his own. "Dad and I wanted to fix this for you before he got so sick," Pat's mother wrote in the Christmas greeting card she included with the album. "I know he would be pleased to know you have it now." Pat Peterson's mother was sixty-nine when she made the album, his father already gone; Pat was forty-three and married with two children. Glued into a family photo album, the news clippings securely situated this brush with death in the course of a life—not just an individual's but a family's life. "Hope you enjoy this Family Photo tree as much as I enjoyed fixing it for you," she wrote. "There is 4 Generations in here and Room for you to add pictures of you and Ellen and Megan & Shannon which will make 5 Generations."[31] For all these families, saving physical documents was part of making sense, giving meaning to this event in their lives, marking it as part of the course of their lives.

Pat Peterson's mother closed her note, "May God bless and keep all of you in his tender love & care always. Love—Mother."[32] In all these families, love was part of the saving. And it was love that was at the heart of the children, now themselves growing old, keeping and treasuring these things that their mothers had saved. Whether a scrapbook, a single news clipping, a photograph, or a set of letters, these items held a love strengthened in the face of trauma. Parents whose child died might also have saved cards, letters, and news clippings from before their child had died, holding time suspended, preserving that moment when a different outcome was still possible, and, from after death, the news clipping of an obituary or death notice or funeral, or notes of condolence, that could be read and reread, part of making real the fact of the death of one's child.

In 1998, Art Cumberledge's sister, Jayne, wrote a letter to Gene Autry asking if he would send an autographed picture for her brother's sixty-first birthday. She explained that Art was one of those who had been seriously burned in Washington, DC, in spring 1945, that Autry had visited them at home when Art was recovering, "which meant a lot to us." A photograph had been taken at the time. Their brother had torn up that photograph many years before in a moment of spite. She said it had been "lost." She said that though the doctors had said "he would never walk again," Art "walks, dances and is a wonderful human being."[33] Her letter hangs framed in Art and Jenny Cumberledge's den on a wall crowded with family photos. Next to it is a framed photograph of Autry dressed in his signature cowboy hat, shirt, pants, and boots, alongside two horses, the one saddled up to ride—the photo that Jackie and Gene Autry's executive assistant had sent in reply to Jayne's letter.[34]

Looking at the framed letter and photo together with Art Cumberledge, in spring 2017, he said "Jayne was always protective of me." "Is that memory from before the accident or after, do you think?" I asked. And, his voice quiet, he replied, "From after." They had been children playing on a spring Sunday afternoon in the nation's capital in the midst of the war when the small paper bag a neighbor boy had lit on fire as part of a science experiment began to flare and Jayne had told Toby to stomp on it and then he was on fire. "I think it had a big effect on her," Art said. There was a long pause. His voice quiet, he continued: "She always—I didn't find out 'til later, she thought she was responsible."[35] It was only a year or two before she died that she told him. He was visiting her in Virginia. They had gone to lunch together "and she was talking about how bad she felt about it." "And do you feel like that was something she had carried with her through her life?" I asked. And he said, "Yes. I think so." And he held his lips together tight, the edges of his mouth quivering. I started to ask him whether he remembered what he had said in response, but before I could finish, he said, "I told her that it, you know, it wasn't her fault."[36]

The conversations I had with individuals and families were long and intimate. They were also hard and draining. "I didn't realize this would be so hard to talk about," Jack Lockhart said early in our conversation. "We've never really talked about it," his wife, Angela, added. At many points as we talked, he paused to gather himself. There were moments when tears ran down his face, others when he held the corners of his mouth with his hand so as not to break down. At one point, he got up and left the room and did not come back for some time. Near the end of our conversation, he said again, that he had not realized how hard talking about this would be on him. "I'm sorry," I said. And he replied, "It's not your fault, it's not your fault at all. It's something maybe I've never addressed. . . . I've probably talked more than I ever have," he said. "I think it's done me some good."[37]

Every one of these conversations had such moments. They brought long-buried, never-fully-acknowledged events and emotions to the surface. They involved not just sharing factual details and memories but also thinking together about memory, trauma, injury, loss, and love. In telling stories about their lives to which they had never given voice, in seeing themselves as a part of history, those I spoke with knew themselves and their lives differently. Others who were part of the conversations—a man's wife, his son, brothers and their wives, a man's daughter—too knew their loved one differently through these conversations. I could see in the intensity of their faces that they were hearing stories they had never heard. The conversations rewrote a life they had in part shared. They changed me and the history I was writing.

I had long referred to this history as the "cowboy suit tragedy."[38] And it was a tragedy—in the carelessness of life in pursuit of profit, bringing terror, pain and suffering to so many children and taking the lives of some. There is tragedy in the injustice of the burdens it imposed on the lives of all the children and their families. And there is tragedy in the refusal of those responsible for the harm to own their responsibility that in turn brought more suffering and death. But there is not only tragedy. My daughter Frances's death had led me to seek out individuals and family members of those burned to give them the opportunity to speak to this event in their lives. In so doing, I have come to understand that we can never fully know a life. But it has also reaffirmed for me the importance of the attempt. *Curriculum vitae*, the course of life. Here, both in the moment—the life-affirming actions of so many, strangers and kin, and of the children themselves—and in the lives they made in the years after, there is something greater than tragedy. This is a history not only of wrongs done that brought trauma, anguish, suffering, and loss, but also of striving, hope, love, and acceptance. Reaching this conclusion does not lessen the wrong done or absolve those responsible for the harm; if anything, it sharpens it.

Many of the children burned in Gene Autry cowboy suits died within hours, days, or months of being burned. It was left to their parents, siblings, extended family, and childhood friends to remember that they had lives, to carry them forward in their lives. Others who survived died premature deaths but had built lives despite and with their injuries. And others still lived to grow old. Jackie Izzo was one of these. She was eighty years old when we met in December 2016. As she said of her life, "I adjusted. . . . I've had a good life. . . . You see, too many normal things in life I've had."[39] Were I writing a poem, her words would form a verse.[40]

a gentle rain

Dear Frances,

It has been raining all day. A steady, gentle rain . . . I took Sam for a walk in the rain. We had the paths to ourselves. Last week I found your bright green umbrella in your suitcase. And so today I walked in the rain shielded by your bright umbrella.

afterword, 2025

Curriculum vitae. The course of life.

I long resisted colleagues, friends, and finally my editor's suggestion that this book could not have been written by anyone but me. My resistance reflected in part the disciplining power of our training and of structures like the vita which reinforce it. It reflected, as well, my commitment that the stories of others be the center of this book. But they were right. It was my daughter Frances's death that tangled these two histories in my life. And it was through Frances that I returned to the work of thinking. This book has been part of the course of my life.

At the end of the preface, I described this book as a journey. It has been that for me. My hope is that it is that for readers as well. Journeys are personal. And so, readers will take from this book their own meaning. It is part of what makes this an unconventional history or something both more and less than history. With that understanding in mind, I had planned to end the book with the final chapters and letter to Frances. But a dear friend said to me, "Readers will want to know something of what you saw in this journey." I am grateful for that push because it led me to see things that otherwise would not have come fully into focus.

Time. Work. Knowing. Each multiplies in meanings in this book. Those meanings are bound up with the course of our lives and bound anew in what we call the course of a life.

time

The cowboy suit tragedy and the history of the vita unfolded together over the course of the twentieth and now twenty-first centuries. But even as they share a time, they are profoundly separated in time. In braiding these histories together with my letters to Frances, I found that I was disrupting how I and we commonly think about and account for time, how easily we assume the linearity and singularity of time.

Many years ago, I wrote about the national and global standardization of time, beginning in the 1880s, made possible and driven by technologies like the railroad and the international telegraph. Public time was standardized. But as this book highlights, time remains, in a deeper sense, fundamentally fragmented, a cacophony of times. Many registers of time run through this book. Hard times. War time. Work time. Tenure clocks. God's time. Over the course of an individual life, too, there are many metrics of time. Time differs at distinct life stages: childhood, adolescence, young adulthood, middle age, old age. The meter of time too shaped distinctly by sex, gender, class, education, marriage, religion. Trauma, injury, and loss change time. Not only in the moment but in lasting ways. Falling out of time. Lost time. Memory and reflection.

Is it any wonder, in this cacophony of times, that intellectual disciplines, professions, and state apparatuses define their own times? Academic history has its own distinct meter of time: moments, eras, ages, periodization. So does law: statutes of limitation, strategies of delay, trial calendars, trial dates. So does news: the news cycle. So does medicine. Think back to Scott Timberlake's doctor describing the long-term prognosis for a child with his condition. So do universities. So does the vita. Consider here the reverse chronology of the curriculum vitae; the fragmentation of time in divisions by category; the registering of completion/publication and not the time that goes into the work itself; annual reviews; the different times by which elements of the vita operate; all the things that are part of a life, even a thinking life, that drop out; all the things that are excluded by convention or academic norms or in defense of being known as an individual, or in defense of retaining some realm of life that is private.

My letters, written in the year and a half after Frances's death, are simultaneously in and outside time. They are "in time" in the sense of the very fact of my writing. The families to whose loss my letters are a bridge lived in a time in which no one encouraged them, as my son Wilder encouraged me, to write to their dead child or grieve through writing. And yet my letters also reflect what David Grossman so powerfully described as "falling out of time."

When I began writing to Frances, the fact of her death was set against a future that we had thought we knew, a future both imagined and planned. The future is a composite of time and knowing. I do not think I had reflected before on how fundamentally bound up the future is with the present. It was only after Frances died that I saw that I had assumed many things about her future. Most fundamentally, that she would have a future. Life in the present is as bound up with imagining, planning for, and producing the future as it is with grappling with the past. Strangely, what seemed concrete elements of the future—things that were dates on the calendar, like Frances going to college—offered a sort of lifeline for me in the face of her death. They were, it seemed, a way of knowing what she would have been doing, the future beyond that a terrible lacuna. Only gradually did I recognize that we did not, could not, know even that immediate future. What is interesting to me now is that even as I recognized my inability to know the future of what Frances's life would have been, I was sure I knew what the future of her death meant. And then I quickly replaced that—a void—with another future: knowing she would never be gone to me. A sense of a future as necessary as a past to life in the present.

It was in part my imagining the future—of what would and would not now appear on my curriculum vitae and what those who read it would think they knew about me—that led me to question the vita. But the future is everywhere in the history of the vita. How could it not be? Its origins as a form were bound up in producing a new future: the modern research university, staffed by PhD-trained scholars who would produce the future of knowledge. Throughout this history, the future was a looming presence. It is there in the Depression and the flight of European scholars and the response to them, in the war emergency, in postwar planning, in the feared shortfall of PhDs, in social movements, in the dramatic expansion of higher education and its equally spectacular contraction. The vita is a form for projecting and predicting the future and in so doing sometimes makes it.

The families of the children in the cowboy suit tragedy had imagined futures for their children that this event cut short or changed in ways both small and profound. Thinking of the children themselves in the midst of what Arthur Cumberledge Sr. described as his son's "siege," I am drawn back to Emily Dickinson's words: "Pain has an element of blank . . . It has no future but itself." When they were through the worst of it, did the past become the time before they were burned, the future an imagined time when they would be better? Some of the children's dreams for the future, like Jackie Izzo's dream of becoming a teacher, were ended by their injuries because those injuries happened in a time in which, to adapt Alice Kessler-Harris's term, an ableist imaginary assumed they were incapable, or a risk, and law, social assumptions, and the construction of physical space reinforced that assumption.

Their injuries also troubled the future in the most intimate aspects of life, shaping their lives in the present. Remember the anxiety that so many men expressed that they would never find a woman who would accept them, have sex with them, love them, marry them. And when they did marry, for some the fear that their children's bodies would be scarred like theirs.

The future too ran through the legal cases. The phrase in virtually every legal proceeding about the impact of these injuries: "for the rest of his natural life." It is there in Perry Caparco's lawyer Edmond Butler accusing the defendants of stalling in hopes that the boy would die. It is there in Judge Knox looking at a photo of a boy's injuries, noting, "Someday this boy will marry and the humiliation of these injuries, must be taken account." It is there in the settlements imagining of the future that in its terms shaped these children's future. Consider too, the change over time in how those who were burned imagined the future of these injuries for their lives. As a child Jack Lockhart imagined that he would be up and running again in no time; in old age, the future he imagined was one in which the cycles of surgery and the ever-lengthening recoveries would never end.

work

Work has so many distinct yet overlapping registers, meanings, and spaces: livelihood, identity, a unit of time, a physical place, productivity, striving, emotion, failure, adjustment. This book speaks to the work of living, to the ways in which individuals in the face of events, forces, and structures beyond their control nonetheless worked to define and give meaning to the course of their lives.

Creation, livelihood, identity, family, survival, grief, and loss run through the cowboy suit tragedy. There was the work that went into creating and manufacturing the fiber, the fabric, the Autry "brand," the chaps of the cowboy suit bearing his name. The work of selling and buying. The work of bystanders, neighbors, parents, doctors, nurses, others to save, or attempt to save, children's lives. The livelihoods of the families that made them part of Autry's market audience—and that meant, in the face of this tragedy, that they had fewer resources to meet a demand they should never have faced. The work of the defendants in trying to avoid liability, to pay less, to not have families find out. The pride of Judge Knox and of the lawyers for Autry, Du Pont, Henry, Timme, and Woonsocket in the work they had done settling or avoiding altogether families' legal claims. And all the while, the work of parents, siblings, and others living loss and trauma. All the while, the work of the children themselves—child labor—of dying, of steeling themselves for another skin graft, of relearning how to walk, of concealing one's shame in being years older than one's classmates. Throughout their lives, the stigma and the work of covering. The kinds of work as adults from which they were excluded by virtue of this childhood injury, and the work they turned to and its consequences for their livelihoods. The work of steeling themselves for rejection in the search for intimacy. The work of marriage, of raising children of their own, all with this injury shaping their daily lives, identity, and fears. The work embedded in Jackie Izzo's simple phrase, "I adjusted." This was not a history that I had thought of as about work when I began. But that I had not, that perhaps you had not, highlights the limited registers in which we too often think when we credit what counts as work, when we write the history of work.

You likely understood from the start that the curriculum vitae would necessarily be a history of work. I did not. It shows how fundamentally the origin point of a project can shape our initial sense of it. It was the juxtaposition of Frances's death and my own professional milestones that made me question the curriculum vitae. Those professional milestones were the result of years of work, work that was bound up with my identity. But in the face of Frances's death, that work was rendered suddenly meaningless. And so, as I began my search for how the curriculum vitae had come to be, I was thinking about love and loss, about what is not on our vitae and how a form that bore the heading *curriculum vitae* excluded most of what really matters in a life. It was only once I was immersed in the research—the work and the lives of others—that I began to see the obvious: This was a history of work, and academia was a workplace. The individual and collective human stakes of that workplace pressed in on me as I traced the desperate flight of German and other European scholars in the 1930s and 1940s for whom the curriculum vitae became a sort of lifeline in securing academic positions in the US qualifying them for non-quota visas: escape, livelihood, and life bound up together. The individual and collective stakes pressed in on me as I traced the demands of women, racialized minorities, and others to be judged on their own capabilities. Thinking deeply about the meaning, the work, in a name at the top of a vita, or the phrase "married, two children" immediately beneath a man's or woman's name, I understood how the personal came to be a part of this history of work and its gendered readings. It was only as I realized how the academic workplace mirrored the precarity of the broader work world by twentieth century's end that I recognized how well this individuating form that presents our work—"my vita," we say—serves universities.

Work, too, runs through my letters to Frances. There is work in the sense of employment, both livelihood and sense of identity. I write letters of recommendation, attend workshops, host scholarly events, teach. I refer to Bill having been a good provider. The work of parenthood, intimately intertwined with livelihood for Bill, for me a separate sphere. In the wake of Frances's death, I seek solace in the domestic labor that was long mine: cleaning closets, attempting to create household order, cleaning Frances's room. And then there is grief, the hardest work of all. *This is work I never dreamed I would have to do*, I wrote Frances. Working to understand, working to survive, working to live. And, finally, I write to Frances about the work of producing knowledge. It was through Frances that I returned to the work of thinking. The seeds of this book germinated in a keynote lecture, "Telling Stories: Love, Loss, History and Who We Are," that I gave the year after her death braiding together the cowboy suit tragedy, the curriculum vitae, and my experience of our loss.

knowing

Knowing too is vital to living. It runs through this book. How we know, the consequences of knowing or not knowing, the elusiveness of knowing, knowing a thing, knowing oneself, being known by others, the known world, the pursuit of and efforts to forestall knowing, personal knowledge, producing knowledge.

Though I never would have made the connection had I not been writing these two histories together, the cowboy suit tragedy was linked from its start to the knowledge world of higher education. The properties of the fiber and fabric that underlay this tragedy were produced in labs led by highly trained PhD chemists, part of the twentieth-century synthetic revolution in fibers, furnishings, and clothing. From the start of my research, part of my search for understanding was seeking to discover why it had taken so long for this hazard to be known for what it was and the consequences of not knowing. My anger was in part driven by learning what the defendants had known about the hazard, how hard they had worked to keep families and courts from knowing both what and when they knew, their efforts aided by the known world, reinforced by news coverage: what happens when children play with fire. In depositions, children like Cecil

D'Wayne Warnick were asked if they knew the difference between right and wrong, between telling the truth and telling a lie, what happens to people who do not speak the truth. Law played a crucial role in the construction and bounding of knowing: legal doctrine, statutes of limitations, rules of evidence, the structure of legal proceedings, settlements, court filing rules. And, finally, the unknowing that survivors carried through their lives and the guilt, isolation, and misplaced sense of personal responsibility this unknowing left them with.

The curriculum vitae, from its birth as a form, shared an origin story with the modern research university and the worlds of knowing that that institution has fostered, for better and worse. The curriculum vitae as narrative attestation to the foundations of one's knowledge, attached to and a requirement for the PhD, was part of the creation of the Doctor of Philosophy as "authorial persona." Seen in this light, it would seem almost a given that scholars would have become known through their curricula vitae. But in fact, in the US it was only when other ways of knowing failed, when the system of personal placement broke down, that the curriculum vitae became a job placement form and the form through which we know others and ourselves. A world that celebrated itself as based on the life of the mind, had rested, in fact, on knowing the man. For women and others long excluded from or subordinated within academia, the vita held out the promise that one might be known and judged on one's merit rather than on one's sex, race, disability, or any other category of unjust discrimination. But the revolution for which they fought was slow and incomplete. Universities used this new tool to their own ends, knowing and judging their faculty in new ways. Incomplete as well because even as the vita became the foundation of academic life, a vital tool in the creation of a new individualizing identity—"research scholar"—the shadow of precarity extended over academic lives and livelihoods. Here, as in the cowboy suit tragedy, law played a vital role in producing and simultaneously limiting knowledge of and recourse for wrongs done. How ironic that in a world that for so long rested on personal knowledge of a man, personal knowledge would be seen as an oxymoron, antithetical to "objective" knowledge production.

Knowledge is not always sought. Sometimes it is forced upon us. Again and again in my letters to Frances, I write to her of the crushing weight of the knowledge that she is gone. And again and again I write to her of how that surety of knowing in one moment slips away from me in the next, only to again crash over me. My letters speak of being haunted by the weight of failing to know that her life was at risk, by the weight of whether she would be angry at us for not knowing and somehow saving her. I describe my deepest desire that if we cannot have her back, I hope at least that she did not know the end was coming. The incomprehensible desire on my part that through my letters she will know the days, the seasons, our love for her. Being in what we know are our last days with her alive last year. Coming to know for the living what is on the other side of final goodbyes. Coming to know my daughter in new ways.

From my first reading of the trial record in which Tommy McCormack's parents retraced the final months of their youngest child's life, I was shaken by every injury, every death in this tragedy. Many of those burned died within hours, days, or—like Tommy McCormack—months of their injuries. Others who survived died in their teens, or as young adults, or in midlife. When I found and talked with some of them about their lives, they were in their seventies, or, like Jackie Izzo, eighty. I knew that it was possible, likely even, that some would die before I completed this work. Ron King was hospitalized the day before we were scheduled to meet and died several weeks later. I talked with his widow, Rosanne King, about her husband's life just months after his death. As she said, it would be important to him. Jackie Izzo died on February 21, 2017, two months after we finally met in person. Others, too, have died in the years since they opened their lives to me. Robert Viands, who had told me, on learning that others had been burned, many far more severely than he, that he felt "lucky, lucky, lucky," died on August 5, 2022, at the age of seventy-six. Gaither Bates who had said, "I just want to be shod of this whole thing. . . . But I can't outlive it," died on October 1, 2022, at the age of eighty-one.

The death of my daughter, Frances, had led me to seek them out, to see the importance of their having the opportunity to speak for themselves about the meaning of this event in and for their lives. But even then, it was only through the conversations—conversations that I undertook thinking they were about the past, history—that I realized they were something more. One such moment came after a draining conversation with the sister of a boy who was burned at age six and died in a car accident, alone and at high speed, at age twenty-six. In this moment and many others, I realized that my taking these journeys with these individuals and families was itself part of this project.

Some of those I spoke with knew before we met that I had lost a child. They had done their research too. With others it came up in our conversation. But even for those who did not know, it was a silent presence in every conversation because it is part of who I am. It enabled me to be with them in their loss. But what I have also realized is that taking this journey with them became part of my grief journey. Those who were burned as children in Gene Autry cowboy suits, their siblings, and spouses are older than me, mostly born in the late 1930s and early 1940s. I was born in the late 1950s. But in my first encounter with them through legal records and newspaper stories, our age positions were reversed: They were children burned in a terrible tragedy, their parents mostly younger than me. It was in one of those awakenings to the obvious in the midst of my oral histories that I realized their parents and they had long since traveled the ground that I was only beginning to travel of learning to live in the face of profound loss and grief. I had undertaken these conversations as a historian, but they brought me strength and healing as a person. And this too speaks to the work of history in our lives.

The course of life. *Curriculum vitae.*

acknowledgments

Acknowledgments used to come at the beginning of books, a recognition of the fundamentally collaborative character of creative and intellectual work, the sustaining, fruitful interplay of the personal, professional, and intellectual. The relegation of acknowledgments to the end of books in recent years is in keeping with much that you have read here of the vita. And yet in this case—a book that has been over two decades in the making, the time extended, the project itself recast by personal loss—it seems appropriate that thanks and gratitude be the final word. As these acknowledgments attest, though this book will appear on my vita, it is in fact a tribute to a rich, wonderful, and sustaining intellectual collectivity.

Historians depend for their work on the experience of those who lived the events we hope to write into history and on the documentary and material traces of the past preserved in archives, libraries, courts, businesses, and more private collections. I could not have written this work without the generosity of those who opened their lives to me and the rich documentary collections in a broad range of archival, court, university, and other records. I first read the long record on appeal in the case of *McCormack v. M. A. Henry Co., et al.* in 2003, with thanks to the archival staff at the New York State Library in Albany, New York. Access to the case files for cases filed in Federal District Court in New York was facilitated by Gregory J. Plunges and others at the National Archives and Records Administration (NARA)–Northeast Region in NYC. For cases filed in New York state court, NY County, I am indebted to Erlon Hodges, Joe Antonelli, Mickie Ruiz, and others staffing this busy court who combed their indices for cases on my list. The incomplete data I had in terms of family names and when cases were filed meant there were many records they could not find, but that they found as many as they did was crucial to this work. I am indebted also to conversations with Eric Janus, Carolyn Chalmers, and fellows at the American Bar Foundation (ABF) about sealed court files; and for the assistance of the late Norman Goodman, county clerk and clerk of the Supreme Court; Steven J. Kubinec, court clerk specialist and deputy chief clerk, Supreme Court NY County; and the Hon. Jacqueline W. Silbermann in securing a court order to unseal sealed state court Gene Autry cowboy suit case files. My thanks also to the archival staff at the National Archives–Pacific Alaska Region (Seattle, WA), the National Archives–Kansas City, and the University of Michigan Law Library.

Legal records are generally public. Not so with corporate, business, and individual collections. I am grateful to have had access to two business collections critical to this project. At the Hagley Library, Margorie G. McNinch, research archivist, Lynn Catanese, and Carol Ressler Lockman helped me find my way to relevant records in the vast collections of Du Pont. The recommendation of Susan Rugh, historian and dear friend of many years, led me to the papers and business records of Gene Autry at the Autry National Center. I am deeply appreciative to Marva Felchlin, director, Autry Library; Michael Duchemin; and Karla Buhlman for access to Autry's papers and business records, which remain the property of Gene Autry Enterprises, Inc.

Tracing the history of the curriculum vitae required work in other kinds of collections, including university archives, the papers of individual scholars and professional societies, and collections holding the papers of Jewish émigré scholars and professionals. I am glad to be able to thank by name some of those who worked to give me access to these collections. At Princeton University, Daniel J. Linke, university archivist and curator of public policy papers; at Columbia University, Jocelyn K. Wilk, university archivist, and Joanna Rios, records manager; at the University of Minnesota, Rebecca Toov, collections archivist, Erin George, assistant archivist, and Daniel Necas, IHRCA archivist; at the AHA Washington, DC, Executive Director James Grossman; and at the Leo Baeck Institute, Michael Simonson. My appreciation also for the remarkable collections, archivists, and staff at Harvard University, the University of Chicago, the University of Kansas, the University of Pennsylvania, the Library of Congress, the American Center for Physics, and the Schlesinger Library. And finally, my thanks to librarians and staff at the University of Minnesota Law Library and in Interlibrary Loan at the University of Minnesota Libraries.

But for the COVID-19 pandemic, I might still be digging in the immense collections of university archives. The pandemic forced me to find new avenues to sources. It made me especially grateful for digitized collections that proved enormously important to this project, including the digitized collections of the Leo Baeck Institute and Archives, the Hathi-Digital Trust, and the Internet Archive. For permission to quote from the papers of Sigmund A. Cohn, given to the LBI by his daughter Marianne Freeman, my thanks to Cohn's grandchildren Anita Hopkins, Stan Freeman, and Roger Freeman.

I spent years in legal, newspaper, and archival research to recover the cowboy suit history, but as I noted in the preface, it was only the silencing of Frances's voice that led me to see the importance of at least trying to find survivors and other family members. Finding survivors of an event from almost three-quarters of a century before is not an easy task. I am indebted to the meticulous research of Laura Luepke, who was at that point working on her own dissertation in history at the University of Minnesota, for what became not just addresses and phone numbers for survivors and other family members in which I could have confidence, but an expansive genealogical database on over one hundred families.

My first interview with a survivor was with Jack Lockhart and his wife, Angela, in August 2015. Between August 2015 and August 2017, I had extended in-person conversations with sixteen survivors and other family members. I am deeply indebted to Charles J. Baragona Jr. and his daughter Rebecca Griffiths; Gaither R. Bates Jr.; Arthur Cumberledge Jr. and his wife, Jenny; Michael Felton Jr. and his wife, Judy (including their hospitality in hosting me overnight at their home); Thomas F. Habina and his wife, Dorothy; Joseph Intelisano's sisters Camille Intelisano and Patricia Cerrigone; Jacqueline Izzo; Ron King's widow, Rosanne King; William K. McMaster; John R. ("Jack") Lockhart Jr. and his wife, Angela; Pat Peterson's widow, Ellen Peterson; John R. Sansbury and his wife, Kristin; Richard Szumita's brothers Ken and Bruce Szumita, Ken's wife Denise, and Richard Szumita's son, Andrew, and his wife, Lisa; Scott Timberlake's sister Kay Bryant; Robert F. Viands and his wife, Cathy; and one person who wished to remain anonymous. These conversations changed this book. They led me to see the impact of this event not simply on their childhoods but on the course of their lives and to see meaning beyond tragedy.

The transformative impact of those conversations led me to also undertake oral histories for the CV strand of the book. I would have loved to do more of these. My thanks to Laura J. Cooper, Suzanne Gossett, Stanley N. Katz, Linda K. Kerber, and William J. Tuttle Jr. for thinking deeply and openly with me about their intellectual, professional, and personal lives.

This project took me into new and foreign research terrain. I could not have done my work without the assistance of multiple generous interlocutors. Kevin Murphy, Dominique Tobbell, and Margot Canaday shared their expertise in the field of oral history. Over a very early morning coffee in Princeton, Anthony Grafton thought out loud with me about the curricula vitae I had found appended to early German written dissertations. Ben Hansen was my expert guide to Latin usage from and scholarship on the ancient world through the sixteenth century. Sheer Ganor introduced me to the rich collections at the Leo Baeck Institute. Kirsten Fischer provided crucial translations of handwritten German correspondence from those collections. Steve Ruggles introduced me to the rich depositories of the Internet Archive. Lucy Salyer shared her expertise in writing narrative history.

Over the many years this project took, many University of Minnesota graduate students assisted me with a broad range of tasks. In addition to Laura Luepke and Ben Hansen, my thanks to Eliana Chavkin, Robert Gilmer, Melissa Hampton, Heather Hawkins, Nate Holdren, Scott McDowell, James McElroy, Chantel Rodriguez, and Allison Schwartz.

Many aspects of academic life have come in for strong criticism in this book, but intellectual life and community were crucial to my carrying on living after Frances died and to the book I have written. I have been fortunate to spend my professional academic life at two large public research universities, beginning with the University of Oregon and, for the last twenty-seven years, the University of Minnesota. In the wake of Frances's death, I was surrounded by students close to her age, immersed in their hopes, dreams, crises, joys, and intellectual and personal becoming. That may sound excruciating, and you can hear in my letters to Frances that I was often overwhelmed and exhausted. But students, both undergraduate and graduate, were a life-affirming gift. So too, my colleagues. The many departmental events we had hosted at our home meant that my colleagues knew Frances, Wilder, and Bill. Loss is isolating. These elements made it less so.

I am grateful for the generous and supportive department culture created and nurtured by colleagues over decades, all of whom have supported this project in countless ways, including Sarah Chambers, Sara Evans, Elaine Tyler May, MJ Maynes, and Ann Waltner. The deep commitment to interdisciplinarity, the openness to new fields and methods of historical and legal inquiry, the strong supportive workshop culture for sharing work in progress, and smart, intellectually open, creative, and generous colleagues and former and current graduate students provided fertile ground for this project. That I had tenure, moreover, gave me the time and security to grieve and intellectual freedom to write a book that challenged disciplinary, institutional, and structural norms.

Equally important have been relationships from the field of legal history.

The American Society for Legal History (ASLH) has provided a sustaining disciplinary home for me for over thirty years. Friendships grounded there provided a critical mooring in the wake of Frances's death. But long before that, at the beginnings of my work on the cowboy suit tragedy and as the project evolved, they were the source of invitations to share work in progress at legal-history and other workshops, join conference panels as at the ASLH, and (on multiple occasions) share pieces of the project at the Hurst Summer Institute. I benefited immensely from the conversations and colleagueship at the ASLH; the University of California–Berkeley; Brandeis University; the Cleveland-Marshall College of Law; the University of Chicago; Columbia University; Duke University and its Triangle Legal History Seminar; Hebrew University; the Hurst Summer Institute (2007, 2011, 2017); the University of Michigan; the Midwest Law and Society Retreat; the University of Minnesota; Northwestern University and the ABF; the Ohio State University; the University of Oregon; the University of Pennsylvania; the American Studies Workshop, the Davis Seminar, and the Program in Law and Public Affairs at Princeton; the University of Virginia; the University of California–Irvine; the University of Tel Aviv; Vanderbilt University; the University of Vermont; and Williams College. I am indebted to those who extended these invitations, including Ed Balleisen, Binyamin Blum, Ari Bryen, Martha Chamallas, Anne Cheng, Kathy Conzen, Ariela Dubler, Laura Edwards, Howie Erlanger, Peter Garlock, Risa Goluboff, Sally Gordon, Tom Green, Michael Grossberg, Dirk Hartog, Jacquelyn Jones, Roy Kreitner, Sophia Lee, Michelle McKinley, Rebecca McLennan, Serena Mayeri, Ajay Mehrotra, Cynthia Nicoletti, Bill Novak, Nicole Phelps, Mitra Sharafi, David Stebben, Yael Sternhell, Karen Tani, Chris Tomlins, Kim Welch, Michael Willrich, and Scott Wong. My notes remind me of the depth of commitment they and other participants in these workshops brought to their reading. I am deeply appreciative to all those who participated, some of whom appear by name in the notes I took at the time, others only by the thoughts they shared. One example speaks for many. A comment by Jane Kamensky at Brandeis—that the cowboy suit history was its own book—began the first evolution of this project.

At each stage of this project, the affirmation, financial support, and time away from teaching provided by academic fellowships, research grants, and awards were critical. That I had these opportunities began with generous colleagues who nominated me, read drafts of proposals, and wrote in my support. My thanks to Margot Canaday, Nancy Cott, Laura Edwards, Mike Grossberg, Dirk Hartog, Linda Kerber, Danny LaChance, Sophia Lee, Elaine Tyler May, and Chris Tomlins. My work on the cowboy suit history began as part of a socio-legal history of product liability supported by a McKnight Land-Grant Professorship awarded by the University of Minnesota and in turn by two fellowships from the William Nelson Cromwell Foundation. Later, recognitions with funding from the University of Minnesota—a CLA Scholar of the College Award and Distinguished McKnight University Professorship—held special importance because of their timing. The first of these came less than a year after Frances died. It was unexpected. It reminded me of this other element of who I was. It was a nudge (carrot, not stick) to re-engage. Two research grants—one from the Friends of the Princeton University Library and the other, the Joan Challinor Research Grant from the Schlesinger Library—seeded my CV research.

I have seen, time and again in this project, how an invitation and event can be both emotionally sustaining and intellectually generative. Less than three months after Frances's death, Carole Srole invited me to give the 2011 keynote lecture at the Western Association of Women Historians (WAWH) annual meeting. That invitation was a gift. I had not imagined that I would ever think again. And yet, not long after accepting the invitation I had an idea for the lecture. It was like taking a giant gulp of air after not breathing. That invitation and the lecture I wrote became the seed for this book. Neither could have been written without the extraordinary support, intellectual honesty, and critical engagement of many people. When I settled down to write the WAWH lecture, I reached out to a small circle of scholar friends—Margot Canaday, Linda Kerber, Elaine Tyler May, Jennifer Pierce, and Chris Tomlins—to ask if they could be honest interlocutors. It was a huge ask. They were true to their word. They, together with professional invitations, the pressure to say yes, and the support I found there meant I could not simply retreat into myself.

Each of the audiences for "Telling Stories: Love, Loss, History and Who We Are" paved a path for me. I delivered a practice of the lecture at the longstanding Workshop of the Comparative History of Women, Gender, and Sexuality (WCHGWS) in the Department of History at the University of Minnesota. I remember the room as being crowded. I am sorry that I cannot remember all who were there. But I do have my notes from those who offered comments: Kirsten Fischer, Tracey Deutsch, Riv-Ellen Prell, MJ Maynes, Helena Pohlandt-McCormick, Susanna Blumenthal, Nate Holdren, Anna Clark, Ruth Karras, Alex Wisnoski, and Libby Sharrow. Linda Kerber and Elaine Tyler May came to the WAWH at the Huntington Library for my keynote. Their presence helped me steel myself to publicly share this loss. I am deeply appreciative to the audience for the keynote lecture at the WAWH and equally so to the audience at the Committee on Women Historians (CWH) Breakfast at the AHA in January 2012. For the CWH event, my special thanks to Leora Auslander, Kathy Conzen, and Alice Kessler-Harris. I did not know the history of either of these groups when I gave those lectures. It was only as I dug into the history of women's challenge to sex discrimination in academia in writing the history of the CV that I learned that these two groups grew out of women's experience of and challenge to sex discrimination in academia.

Audiences at both events encouraged me to publish the lecture, something that at that stage I could not imagine. An invitation to present at the American Studies Workshop at Tel Aviv University, in May 2012, became the first time I shared the paper itself for an audience to read—and there, again, a remarkable conversation and encouragement to publish the paper for a larger audience. I submitted "Telling Stories: Love, Loss, History and Who We Are," to the *American Historical Review* (*AHR*) in fall 2012 and learned that even rejection can open doors. Replying to my submission, editor Robert Schneider began by speaking personally as a parent, embracing me and our family's loss. Only then did he speak as an editor, saying that the piece was not right for the *AHR*. His letter thoughtfully engaged the questions my essay raised, noting the need and the importance of addressing them and suggesting a book-length essay. The book I have written is different from what I think he imagined. It is certainly longer. But just as the encouragement of those who heard or read the lecture led me to imagine it as a published essay, Robert Schneider's supportive, embracing rejection gave me the first push to think of this project as a book.

There are so many stages in this project where a different response might have brought it to a halt. But in each such moment, I was greeted instead by interest, probing questions, and encouragement. Two residential writing fellowships gave me critical time away from teaching. A semester-long fellowship at the University of Minnesota Institute for Advanced Study (IAS) in fall 2016 was the first fellowship I received for this project, then conceived as a braided narrative titled "The Course of a Life." The affirmation of the fellowship itself mattered. It was also in that semester that I wrote and presented the first sketch of the book and undertook the first oral histories with survivors. As I explained to the other IAS fellows that term, my goal for the semester was to learn how to talk about this project in a way that opened up rather than shut down conversation. My thanks to Jennifer Gunn, director of the IAS; the IAS staff; and my IAS cohort. Later, a yearlong residential fellowship from the Shelby Cullom Davis Center for Historical Studies, Princeton University, offered not only the riches of Princeton's library and archival collections but my first experience of what Virginia Woolf called a room of one's own, the freedom to work for hours on end uninterrupted, without family obligations, the solitude complemented by a wonderful cohort of Davis fellows and postdocs and many Princeton faculty and past and current graduate students.

The sustained support and critical engagement over many years of other scholars who were willing to be honest, critical readers who took time, many repeatedly, from their own work was crucial at each stage of the evolution of this project. As first imagined, this book had twenty-six substantive chapters. The book you have read has twenty-two, but I wrote all twenty-six. And generous readers read and gave me written comments on all those chapters. Some read as I finished each draft. Their encouragement and questions kept me going. Kirsten Fischer read and commented on all twenty-six chapters. Her confidence in this book, long before I could articulate how the strands fit together, sustained me. The list of those who read and gave me comments on chapters is long. Many read and gave me feedback on multiple chapters. They include Susanna Blumenthal, Dan Bouk, Jon Connolly, Angela Creager, Michael Grossberg, Jennifer Gunn, Aaron Hall, Dirk Hartog, Nate Holdren, Linda Kerber, Regina Kunzel, Serena Mayeri, Erika Milam, Riv-Ellen Prell, Dan Rodgers, Karen Tani, and my husband, Bill Welke. Others gave me feedback on particular chapters, including Carol Chomsky, Brooke Depenbusch, Tracey Deutsch, Kellen Funk, Sheer Ganor, Ben Hansen, Jill Hasday, Will Jones, Danny LaChance, Laura Luepke, Elaine Tyler May, Lary May, Kay Reyerson, Evan Taparata, and Keith Wailoo. I am deeply indebted to all these readers.

I owe a special debt to readers of full drafts of the manuscript. I wrote my way through the chapters of each historical strand before putting them together with the Dear Frances segments to attempt to make a book. 260 pages into that attempt, I questioned whether to continue. Serena Mayeri read and urged me to keep writing. Nate Holdren and Aaron Hall read what was the second full draft. When my editor, Tim Mennel, said I needed to cut the manuscript by another 30 percent, their belief that the three strands had become truly a book made it possible for me to do so. Dan Bouk and Serena Mayeri read the next full draft. They told me I was done, but they also gave me targeted, written comments relating to both style and substance. All of these readers have continued to be extraordinary intellectual partners and supporters. Chris Tomlins and Martha Hodes read the manuscript for the press. And here too, I am grateful for both their critical comments and their enthusiasm. All these readers helped me complete this book; their comments made it a better book.

I have concentrated here on formal sites of input into this project. But for every one of these there were other informal exchanges in hallways or office doorways, at conferences, over coffee, a drink, or dinner, some with those I have already named, but also many others. For a very long time, my sense that the three strands belonged together was more felt than understood. Informal conversations were as essential as written comments in helping me find my way.

We are lucky to still have physical books in our lives. By the time I had a first sprawling draft, I thought of this as a University of Chicago Press book. That is not the same as saying that the press would think so. My colleague Elaine Tyler May introduced me to Executive Editor Tim Mennel, who enthusiastically responded to my initial brief email with the words "weird and wonderful." He asked to see the sketch and then fearlessly tackled the unwieldy first draft of the manuscript. He has been exactly the editor I had hoped for. I am grateful to him. I am also grateful to many others at the University of Chicago Press for their commitment and craft in producing beautiful books and helping them find their way to readers. My thanks to Andrea Blatz, Annie Leue, Lindsy Rice, Anne Strother, and Jess Wilson. And on the index, special thanks to Enid Zafran.

You have been waiting to hear of my family. They have been here all along. Frances, Wilder, and Bill, individually and collectively, have been critical to this book coming into being. It was through Frances that I returned to thinking. But I could do so because Wilder, Bill, and I had each other, supported by our extended families and many dear friends. Our families do not expect to appear in our books beyond acknowledgments. Wilder had first encouraged me to write to Frances after her death. Wilder and Bill trusted me in drawing on my letters to Frances in which they both appear. This book has long sustained me; it has also been a heavy weight. Bill has carried that weight with me.

The thinking life I treasure would not be whole without the supporting circle of love and respite my family provides. I wish I could remember exactly when it was that Frances announced that when she got married, she wanted to find someone like Dad. I thought then that she was wise beyond her years. I still do. Bill and I met in law school and married the summer we graduated. This summer we will have been married for forty-three years. I am thankful for his steadiness, sense of humor, and intellectual curiosity, and for his bottomless well of love, support, and respect. He makes all things possible.

We had our children, Wilder and Frances, when I was in graduate school, working on my dissertation. In the years I have worked most intensively on this book, Wilder has grown to adulthood. We often joked that he should be credited with hauling research boxes up and down the stairs for me (something Bill deserves credit for also). But more seriously, Wilder has always been remarkable. I admire his deep empathy and emotional intelligence and his values for what matters in a life. I hope these qualities, about which I have learned so much from him, are in evidence in this book.

When my second book, *Law and the Borders of Belonging*, was published in March 2010, Frances said she wanted the first copy. She took the book, flipped to the acknowledgments, and hungrily searched for her name. She did not like what she saw. "Why do I have to share sentences with Wilder?" she asked. "Dad gets his own sentences. I want my own sentences." It was such a sweet moment. I laughed warmly and assured her that in my next book she would have her own sentences. A month later, she was gone. Dear Frances, I hope you hear your sentences in this book.

This April it will be sixteen years since Frances died. The sharp edges of that loss have smoothed. Part of that is the passage of time. But it is also because we carry Frances with us; she continues to shape our lives, thoughts, and way of being in the world. Bill, who has retired from practicing law and now creates breathtaking wildlife and landscape photographs, has Frances, who loved to travel and loved his photographs, with him on every journey. Wilder has now been a hospice social worker for a decade. Frances is with him in the support and comfort he gives to families. He married a wonderful woman named Jamie who has come to know Frances well through us and whom Frances would have loved as much as we do. Frances loved that I was a teacher and took pride in my books. Her support and belief in me continue to sustain me. I still teach at the University of Minnesota, where I daily see in my students things that remind me of Frances—the intensity of emotions of young adulthood, the excitement (and anxieties) of charting life and career paths—and with whom I share the joy of discovery, thinking, and learning.

St. Paul, Minnesota
December 2025

note on methods and sources

Writing with Fire is written in a personal voice and includes a personal, epistolary strand, but it otherwise rests on traditional research methods and sources. This note describes my methodology and key sources in each strand.

1. cowboy suit strand

Five basic types of primary sources ground this strand: legal case files and court opinions, newspapers, business records, genealogical sources, and oral histories.

COWBOY SUIT LEGAL CASE FILES. This history relies heavily on the case files from lawsuits involving the Gene Autry cowboy suit. As I explain in the book, we will never know just how many children were burned in Gene Autry cowboy suits, but over one hundred families took some kind of legal action against either the retailer from whom the suit was purchased or, more commonly, against those involved in making or marketing the fiber, fabric, or cowboy suit. Except for lawsuits against local retailers, the lawsuits were overwhelmingly filed in New York City, in either state or federal court, for the simple reason that this was the one place where a court had jurisdiction over the principal defendants. The most important exception was Gene Autry, whose residence and place of business was California. But he could be served in a lawsuit when he made appearances in New York—as, for example, at the rodeo. This was what made New York appearances so dangerous to him during the years of litigation.

I was able to locate case files in seventy-five cases. Of these, forty-nine were brought in federal district court in New York and twenty-five in New York state court.[1] It is important to note that in New York, the "supreme court" is the trial court, and the New York Court of Appeals is the highest state court. Filing suit required local counsel and individual lawyers, many of whom represented multiple families. Edmond Borgio Butler, of O'Connell & Butler, and Elliot Paley, of Nemeroff, Jelline, Danzig & Paley, represented more families than any others and were both involved in the litigation from the start. Paley's firm represented the McCormack family. Butler's firm represented most of the first families from the Washington, DC, metropolitan area to bring suit. Butler almost uniformly filed in federal court, whereas Paley uniformly filed cases in state court.

The difference in the number of cases I was able to find in federal versus state court may have as much to do with filing systems as anything else. The records in cases filed in the Southern District of New York (SDNY) are held by the Northeast Region–New York branch of the National Archives in New York City. Their index for case records is by defendant last name and is open to researchers. In litigation of this character involving the same defendants, I was able to have some confidence of finding all the cases filed in the SDNY that named any of the principal defendants. The New York Supreme Court for New York County, by contrast, indexed cases by year and within a year by plaintiff's last name only. The case files remain part of the court's records, and the index is not public. In other words, I needed to know a potential plaintiff's name and the year suit was filed and was dependent as well on the good offices of clerks to search their index in a very busy court system. All these elements contributed to my finding fewer state court cases. Without the Autry records that included lists of pending legal claims identified by the family's last name, I would have found even fewer.

The fact that there is much of a legal record at all was shaped by at least two factors. First, the defendants' resistance meant that, with very few exceptions, families had to file suit to secure a settlement. Second, because the cases involved children (minors), legally enforceable final settlements required court approval.

But access to records was shaped by another characteristic of this litigation: sealed files. As I explain in the book, the defendants were anxious to prevent publicity about cases that might lead more families to bring suit or otherwise adversely impact their reputations. The defendants were most anxious to have files sealed in cases involving late sales, late injuries, especially severe injuries that did not lead to death, and large settlements. Both judges in federal and state court readily approved defendants' requests to seal records. But what portion of a case record they sealed and what happened to those records differed dramatically between federal and state court. In the SDNY cases, Judge Knox, who oversaw settlement of the vast majority of cowboy suit cases brought there, only allowed for the Order of Compromise, which set out the financial terms of the settlement, to be sealed; other material in these files remained open. The one exception was *Izzo*, which importantly was before a different judge. The parties asked to have the file as a whole sealed and told the judge that Judge Knox had agreed to this in other cowboy suit cases; Judge Leibell sealed the entire file. I could find no record of the Izzo case in the federal archives, but I was able to recover some material in the case through proceedings before the probate court in the state of Michigan, including the transcript of the settlement hearing before Judge Leibell and the records in the litigation the Izzos later brought in Michigan challenging the attorneys' fees. In the SDNY cases where the Order of Compromise was sealed, the docket sheet notes that the final order was "impounded" and notes "in vault." As I learned, whatever once may have been in a vault is now gone.

In contrast, in cases filed in the New York Supreme Court New York County, in which defendants requested to have a file sealed, the court sealed the entire file. Those files remained sealed when I received them over fifty years later—literally bound with a pink ribbon, a stamp, and a note that the file was sealed to all but the parties involved. With the assistance of Norman Goodman, county clerk and clerk of the Supreme Court, County of New York, and a court order signed by Judge Jacqueline W. Silbermann (June 28, 2006), the sealed files were officially unsealed. But it is also important to note that when I later sought to see some of those records again, the clerk's office was unable to locate them. As they explained it, this was probably because of a reorganization of the filing system of old records that had taken place since I first saw files. It is easy to be suspicious. I will note only that professional colleagues at Columbia Law School were amazed in the first instance that the clerk's office in this busy court had been willing to search its indexes for a historian and even more surprised that the office found as many of the case files as they did.

Only two cases against the principal defendants were fully tried. The McCormack case was the only case brought by a family against the Henry Company, E. F. Timme & Son, and Woonsocket Falls Mill that went to trial (Autry and Du Pont were not named in this suit). The only other case against the principal defendants, here including Du Pont, that was tried was brought by a retailer, Louis and Ida Lutz, doing business as Lou's Auto Stores. Lutz had been sued by and paid judgments to three families (Detrick, Flesher, and Warnick) who brought suit in state court in Maryland. Both the *McCormack* and *Lutz* records are voluminous, including trial transcripts, extensive exhibits, and lawyers' briefs. The Lutz case was tried before a jury over two weeks in March 1949, Hon. J. Waties Waring presiding. The transcript is 1,660 pages. The Henry Company had brought Du Pont into Lutz as a third-party defendant, and there is extensive testimony documenting Du Pont's actions and long relationship with Timme. In addition to the transcript and related materials, the record in Lutz includes depositions, taken in December 1948, in Cumberland, Maryland, of James Edmond Detrick and both his parents, Cecil D'Wayne Warnick and both his parents, and Robert Flesher's parents (Robert died from his injuries).

But the case files in other suits, though not uniform in their contents, are also rich depositories. All the case files from the SDNY include docket sheets that record every filing and order in the case; there were no docket sheets in the state court files. A second major difference relates to basic pleadings (complaints, amended complaints, answers, and similar documents). This kind of material is uniform in the SDNY cases and largely absent from the state court records. As I discovered, the reason for the difference rests in the New York practice rules. As George Carpinello notes, "because there is no general filing requirement in New York, all pleadings can be served and discovery proceed to completion without the filing of any papers with the court. In contrast, most other states and the federal system require the filing of all papers before service is made." Carpinello also notes that "the lack of such a filing requirement results not only from administrative necessity, due to the huge volume of cases, but also from the underlying assumption in New York that the pretrial process, absent court intervention, is the litigants' business rather than the public's."[2] With the sole exception of the SDNY cases in which the order of compromise was sealed, all the case files include the Order of Compromise, laying out the financial terms of the settlement and often including supporting affidavits from lawyers, parents, and doctors. Other materials found in the files include: petitions and orders for appointment of guardian ad litem; interrogatories and answers to interrogatories; depositions of the children burned, their parents, neighbors and others who witnessed the incident, doctors and other hospital personnel, and major actors among the defendants, including William E. Roschen, Arthur Robertshaw Jr., and Milton Henry; bills of particulars; affidavits from lawyers, children's parents (mostly fathers), and doctors; hospital records; photographs of the children's injuries for the lawsuits; motions for preference and supporting affidavits; plaintiffs' lawyers' brief summaries of case details and "asking" prices; stenographer's minutes of hearings before the judge for approval of settlement; and following settlements, petitions, and affidavits to withdraw settlement funds set aside for the child, as well as petitions from the children when they reached the age of majority for the settlement funds set aside for them.

A few files include materials that extend beyond that case. The transcript of the proceedings before Judge Knox in the consolidated "trial" [settlement] in May 1948 are in *Richard Johnson v. M. A. Henry Co., Inc., Civ. 35-454*. The consolidated proceedings included the following cases: *Adams*; *Baer*; *Bates*; *Berry*; *Bradley*; *Burke*; *Cumberledge*; *Detrick*; *DiTrapani*; *State of Maryland (Flesher)*; *Gates*; *Jones*; *King*; *Klinck*; *Lockhart*; *McMaster*; *Stultz*; *Tetla*; *Warnick*; and *Wilks*. The case file in *Richard Johnson* also includes pre-trial depositions of William E. Roschen (September 26, 1946) (general partner, E. F. Timme & Son and treasurer, Woonsocket Falls Mill) and Arthur Robertshaw (September 27, 1946) (manager, vice president, and secretary, Woonsocket Falls Mill). Portions from these depositions were later read into the record in the *McCormack* trial in January 1948 and the *Lutz* case in March 1949. The case file in *Klinck* includes answers to interrogatories by Milton Henry that include an exhibit with a list of pending actions against the M. A. Henry Co., and an exhibit of the number of cowboy suits sold to Philadelphia Wholesale Distributors during or before December 1944. The case file in *Habina* includes a list of sales made in 1942 and 1943 to one major retail chain that sold the cowboy suit (McCrory). The *McCarthy* case file includes an affidavit from William W. Heiberger, the lawyer representing the McCarthys, with an itemized, dated listing of all his activities on the case, one of the few instances of a full itemized accounting of a plaintiffs' lawyer's time. Only two depositions were taken of Autry in these proceedings. The first deposition was taken on October 29, 1947 (signed by Autry on February 14, 1948) in the *Weatherell* case. But that deposition is not in the *Weatherell* case file. It is in the *Peterson* case file, the case in which a second deposition of Autry was taken in fall 1949. The second Autry deposition was not filed with the court in *Peterson* but is in the Autry Collection. *Timberlake* is a voluminous file, including several hundred pages of depositions, and was an especially important late case involving sales by the Henry Company of the cowboy suit after it knew as fact that children had been burned and after it said it had destroyed the remaining suits on hand.

In addition to the cases in which I found legal case files, my accounting of instances of children being burned in Gene Autry cowboy suits and of families who pursued legal action against a retailer, property owner, or the principal defendants includes cases identified through three sources:

Milton Henry's November 1947 response to interrogatories in the Habina case listing actions pending against him (see Habina case file); correspondence between Autry, his lawyer William Martin, and his agent Mitch Hamiburg (see Autry Collection); and newspapers. Whereas the Henry interrogatory included plaintiff full name, court and docket number, and date of accident, with the result that I was able to find all but one of these cases (Harry W. Griffin (child John), Supreme Court NY County, #9706, burned January 12, 1946), many of the references from the Autry correspondence list the child's last name without other identifying details, with the result that I was not able to find these cases (Appleby, Frevelle, Hutchinson, Irarius, Roland, Slater, Travis, and Trimabli). The Autry Collection also includes correspondence relating to three cases that the defendants settled without suit being filed (Bobby Grosch, Philip Hooper, and Verbonitz [no first name given]) and correspondence in 1951 and 1952 with a mother (Lenore Bair) relating to her son Ronald, who was burned in Pennsylvania and whose action was barred by the statute of limitations. Finally, newspaper coverage reported legal actions by the parents of Philip Contino (burned in Passaic, NJ, on March 15, 1943), Joseph Porreca (burned on March 30, 1945, in Providence, RI), Richard Kropp (burned in 1945 in Chicago, IL), Robert Smith Jr. (burned in June 1945 in Dubuque, IA), Elizabeth Jane Hooper (burned on March 11, 1946, in East Liverpool, OH), Michael Tender (burned on November 21, 1946, in Paterson, NJ), and James Mistretta (burned on October 29, 1948, in Hackensack, NJ).

COWBOY SUIT PUBLISHED OPINIONS. The cowboy suit litigation produced at least fourteen published legal decisions. The decisions relate to published trial court opinions on particular contested legal issues in a case (e.g., *Blessington*), appeals of cases dismissed as barred by statutes of limitations (e.g., *Duffy*, *Moore*), interlocutory appeals in pending cases of orders relating to dismissal of a party or claim (e.g., *Blessington*, *Devens*, *Donahue*) or denial of a motion to add a party (e.g., *Timberlake*), and, finally, the appellate decision in *McCormack*.

COWBOY SUIT ORAL HISTORIES. Determining clear contact information was my first priority and required extensive genealogical and address research. Based on these findings, I mailed an initial letter to nineteen individuals (or family members), followed up with a phone call, and then traveled to talk with individuals in person, conducting sixteen (taped) extended oral histories between August 2015 and May 2017. Ten of the interviews were with individuals burned as children (five of these interviews also included a spouse; one included a daughter), four of the interviews were with siblings (and one that included as well children), and two of the interviews were with spouses of men who had died. The interview subjects included individuals burned from 1944 to 1948. All but one of the families pursued a lawsuit that resulted in a settlement. The one family that did not had filed a suit against the retailer, but then withdrew, their suit. Many of those I interviewed shared material records from their lives, including news clippings relating to their injuries, treatment, and fundraising efforts; scrapbooks and photo albums; letters; family photographs from across their lives; and memorials. Only one of those I interviewed asked that their name not appear in the book.

BUSINESS RECORDS. Unlike court records, which—apart from sealed records—are public, corporate and other business records are private. Even where a business, corporation, or—here—public personality establishes an archive, what they deposit in that archive and the terms of use remain under the control of the creator. Two collections were especially important in my research of the cowboy suit tragedy: the collections of Du Pont, held at the Hagley Library (Wilmington, DE) and the Gene Autry Collection, on temporary loan to the Autry National Center (Los Angeles, CA). Quoting from the Autry Collection requires written permission from Gene Autry Entertainment (Studio City, CA).

NEWSPAPER RESEARCH. A foundational source for my newspaper research was *N. W. Ayer & Son's Directory of Newspapers and Periodicals*, published annually beginning in 1880. A comprehensive directory for advertisers, organized alphabetically by state and city, it includes newspaper names, circulation numbers, and publishing information, as well as basic data relating to the cities themselves. For every incident that I knew of, I searched local newspapers around the date of the incident, when a child was released from the hospital, when suit was filed, and when a settlement was reached, as well as other dates identified through case files. To look for coverage of the hazard more generally and to find incidents I did not otherwise know about, I searched indexed newspapers, including the *New York Times* and *Washington Post*; used the commercial digitized database Newspapers.com; and searched other indexed periodicals.

GENEALOGICAL RESEARCH. I began genealogical research for the purpose of locating individuals for oral histories, but the research became a rich source of data for over one hundred families. My genealogical database includes US manuscript census, marriage, divorce, birth, military, immigration, and death records; city directories; and high school and college yearbooks, as well as address and other records. Ancestry.com and FamilySearch.com were especially important tools. I am indebted to the meticulous work of Laura Luepke for much of this research.

VARIANT SPELLINGS.

Krzeczkowski: As with many immigrant names, the spelling of "Krzeczkowski" ranged widely in different sources, including in this instance in the cases filed for Casimir's injuries and Stanley's death. When quoting or citing case file names, I use the spelling from the source. Otherwise, I use "Krzeczkowski," the spelling that appeared on Stanley's death certificate.

DiTrapani: As with many immigrant names, the spelling of "DiTrapani" ranged widely in different sources. When quoting or citing newspaper articles, I use the spelling from the source. Otherwise, I use "DiTrapani," the spelling that appeared in the family's court filing.

Intelisano: As with many immigrant names, the spelling of "Intelisano" varied in different sources. When quoting or citing the court filing, I use "Intelisana." Otherwise, I use "Intelisano," the spelling that the family currently uses.

Du Pont: The authors of a major work on Du Pont (David A. Hounshell and John Kenly Smith Jr., *Science and Corporate Strategy: Du Pont R&D, 1902–1980* [Cambridge University Press, 1988]), use "Du Pont" throughout. However, case filings referred frequently to "DuPont." I use "Du Pont" unless quoting directly from the filings.

Toby Cumberledge: In the deposition, Arthur Cumberledge Jr.'s nickname was spelled "Tobey." But the spelling his family used was "Toby." Except where quoting from a source that spells the name otherwise, I use the spelling his family used.

II. dear Frances strand

This strand of the book is composed of excerpts from letters I wrote to my daughter Frances after her death.

On the night of Sunday, April 25, 2010, Frances went to bed a happy, apparently healthy girl. Sometime before morning, she suffered a massive stroke. Over the course of the week that followed, she had two more strokes, all caused—we later learned—by a rare abnormality in the structure of her brain that she had likely lived with for years or possibly been born with. She died at the end of that week, on Friday, April 30, 2010. Frances was eighteen years old. She died on what would have been her last day of classes in her senior year of high school. She would have been a freshman at Carleton College that fall. Frances was our only daughter, our youngest of two children.

I began writing to Frances on May 30, 2010, one month after her death. I dated and noted the time of each entry and began each entry "Dear Frances." I wrote my letters in lined journals. On many days I wrote to her more than once. I first decided to use excerpts from my letters for a keynote lecture to the Western Association of Women Historians in April 2011. For the lecture, I had decided to write a braided narrative, incorporating my research on the cowboy suit tragedy, preliminary research on the CV, and my experience of traumatic loss of a child. But I was still deep in grief; I did not have the distance or composure to speak directly to my experience. In deciding to draw from letters I had written to Frances, it was important to me not to change my relationship with her or the character of my ongoing letters to her. My writing was to her only; it was imperative to me that it remain so. With that in mind, for the lecture I did not use any entries from after the date I had the idea to draw on my letters. I continued to write to Frances, but I did not again read any of my letters to her until February 2020, close to ten years later for purposes of this book. This book incorporates excerpts from letters I wrote to Frances from June 3, 2010, to December 14, 2011. Any stopping point has an arbitrariness to it. But I thought it important to go beyond February of that first year and also felt that ending with the one-year anniversary of her death imposed a neatness on grief that did not reflect my experience. In some respects that second year was harder than the first in part because there was no "this time last year" to look back to in which Frances was alive.

In selecting excerpts from letters, I have attempted to capture the range of my experience. Several aspects of my letters are important to understand in that regard. My letters were not a personal journal; they were letters to my daughter. This shaped their tone, voice, and substance. Had I been keeping a personal journal of my experience, it undoubtedly would have been different. But these were letters to Frances written from within the experience of unexpected, traumatic loss of a teenage daughter. This also means that the character and extent of references to even other family members are different than they would have been had I been writing to and for myself. Finally, because the decision to use excerpts from my letters in this public way was mine, I have limited excerpts referring to my husband Bill and son Wilder.

I have retained here the order and exact text and punctuation. The only changes I have made are to replace personal names of non–family members with general descriptive references (e.g., "the minister"). Each entry in the book includes excerpts from letters from multiple days. I signal a new entry by a new paragraph. My letters include references to Frances's father/ my husband ("Dad"); our son Wilder, who was in college at the time; and our dog, Sam. The letters include references to our home in St. Paul, Minnesota, as well as to a cabin that we had bought in Northern Minnesota on Burntside Lake in fall 2009. The letters also include references to my work. I was (and remain) an academic, a professor of history and law at the University of Minnesota.

Apart from the excerpts used in this book, my letters remain private.

III. curriculum vitae strand

Researching the history of the vita required a different research methodology than for the cowboy suit history. The cowboy suit history involved a specific event unfolding over less than two decades. Though children were burned across the United States, law effectively corralled the bulk of the legal sources into two courts. The number of principal actors was also finite, even as I carried the story forward through genealogical research and oral histories. In contrast, the history of the curriculum vitae traced here stretches from the classical Latin meaning of *curriculum vitae*, to the birth of the modern research university in Germany in the early nineteenth century, and from the late nineteenth century through the early twenty-first century in the United States. It would have been easy to enter the essentially inexhaustible domain of university archives and individual scholars' papers and never emerge, to have become tangled up in distinctions between disciplines, to have gotten caught up by a particular moment. Whereas the cowboy suit tragedy required recovering an event in time and tracing across time its lived meaning in the lives of individuals impacted by it, the vita required looking across time and considering the meaning in the lives of distinct individuals in the many moments I mark as turning points.

With these differences in mind, seven basic types of primary sources ground this history of the curriculum vitae: American university archives (including presidential papers and other administrative records, university placement office records, departmental records, individual scholars' papers, committees/commissions on the status of women, and university records relating to legal challenges to instances of discrimination), papers and journals of professional associations, dissertations (for the earliest curricula vitae) and curricula vitae, émigré scholars' papers and records of organizations relating to émigré scholars, oral histories, and the Internet Archive (the Wayback Machine).

I learned early that collecting vitae without knowing when and why they were created offered little to my understanding of the evolution of the vita. It was essential to see vitae in context.

My university archival research centered on six research universities: Chicago, Columbia, Harvard, Minnesota, Penn, and Princeton, plus extensive research in the collections of the Schlesinger Library. I worked in departmental collections in disciplines in the humanities, social sciences, and sciences, including especially chemistry, English, history, physics, politics, and sociology. Intra- and inter-collegiate/university correspondence gave me a good sense of the broader landscape not only at research universities but far down the ladder. Four chapters that I ultimately cut from the manuscript—on the personal placement system that largely prevailed through mid-century and well after; university placement offices; tenure; and early professional-society placement efforts—of which only slivers remain, were important nonetheless for my ability to speak with confidence about the evolution of the vita in purpose and form.

Discipline-specific professional associations were important actors throughout this narrative. From their formation in the late nineteenth and early twentieth century, they were concerned about placement of scholars trained in their field and also the standing of their field. I relied on the publications of professional societies including the American Association of University Professors (AAUP) and American Council on Education (ACOE), and discipline-specific professional societies in the fields of anthropology, chemistry, economics, English, history, mathematics, philosophy, physics, political science, sociology, and others. I worked in the papers of the American Historical Association, the American Institute of Physics, the American Political Science Association, and two women's professional organizations, Sociologists for Women in Society (SWS) and the Coordinating Committee for Women in the Historical Profession (CCWHP), as well as committees at Chicago and Harvard.

If the scale of available sources was in one sense inexhaustible, in another laws limiting access to student records posed a real roadblock. Legal restrictions on access to student records as incorporated into archival policy by various universities range from fifty to one hundred years. The restrictions made especially important here open collections of more recent individual scholars' papers. Although I conducted only a few oral histories for this strand, they too proved an important resource in accessing the history from the 1960s forward. Equally important were collections related to the women's rights movement, committees and women's professional organizations, legal records in cases of denial of tenure, and papers of professional associations. Of special importance are the papers of the Women's Equity Action League (WEAL) and Bernice Sandler, held at the Schlesinger Library. A final resource, one I had not even known existed, proved especially important for seeing into the most recent evolution of the vita: the Internet Archive, also known as the Wayback Machine. Its collections are massive, comprising hundreds of millions of captures from 1996 to the present.

A final set of archival collections was vital to the vita strand of the book. Anyone doing research in university archives in the 1930s, 1940s, and 1950s will find correspondence from and about and vitae of émigré scholars. But in addition to university administrative, departmental, and individual scholars' papers, two other archival collections were especially important: the Leo Baeck Institute, Center for Jewish History (digital collections), and the American Council for Emigres in the Professions IHRCA Records, at the University of Minnesota.

notes

abbreviations

For cowboy suit source abbreviations, see cowboy suit case files, published legal opinions, and oral histories.

ACEPR, IHCRA, UMN. American Council for Emigres in the Professions Records, Immigration History Research Center Archives, University of Minnesota, Minneapolis, MN.

AIP Papers. American Institute of Physics Papers, Neils Bohr Library and Archives, American Center for Physics, College Park, MD.

AHA Papers (LoC). American Historical Association Papers, Library of Congress, Washington, DC.

AHA Papers (headquarters). American Historical Association Papers, held by organization, Washington, DC.

CUA. Columbia University Archives, Columbia University, New York, NY.

HUA. Collections of the Harvard University Archives, Harvard University, Cambridge, MA.

LBI. DigiBaeck Digital Collections at the Leo Baeck Institute—New York/Berlin for the Study of German-Jewish History and Culture. https://www.lbi.org/collections/digibaeck/.

PUA. Princeton University Archives, Department of Rare Books and Special Collections, Princeton University Library, Princeton University, Princeton, NJ.

Schlesinger. Schlesinger Library, Radcliffe Institute, Harvard University, Cambridge, MA.

UA, UMN. University of Minnesota Archives, Elmer L. Andersen Library, University of Minnesota, Minneapolis, MN.

UChicago. Hanna Holborn Gray Special Collections Research Center (SCRC), University of Chicago Library, University of Chicago, Chicago, IL.

UKansas. Kenneth Spencer Research Library, University of Kansas, Lawrence, KS.

UPenn. University Archives and Records Center, University of Pennsylvania, Philadelphia, PA.

preface

1. Ruth Behar, *The Vulnerable Observer: Anthropology That Breaks Your Heart* (Beacon Press, 1996), 18.

chapter one: child's play

1. Habina Interview.
2. Deposition of Cecil D'Wayne Warnick, Cumberland, MD, December 30, 1948, Record in Lutz.
3. The Warnicks lived in Potomac Park, MD, five miles south of the city of Cumberland. In 1944, when Cecil was burned, there were no named streets or house numbers in Potomac Park. For population data in 1940, see US Census Bureau, *Sixteenth Census of the United States: 1940* (Government Printing Office, 1942), https://www.census.gov/library/publications/1942/dec/population-vol-1.html.
4. For children in this era, see William M. Tuttle Jr., *Daddy's Gone to War: The Second World War in the Lives of America's Children* (Oxford University Press, 1993), 236–53.
5. Tuttle, *Daddy's Gone to War*, 148; Studs Terkel, *"The Good War": An Oral History of World War Two* (Pantheon Books, 1984), 136.
6. See Howard Chudacoff, *Children at Play: An American History* (NYU Press, 2007), 99–100; James D. Schmidt, *Industrial Violence and the Legal Origins of Child Labor* (Cambridge University Press, 2010); Michael Grossberg, "A Protected Childhood: The Emergence of Child Protection in America," in *American Public Life and the Historical Imagination*, eds. Wendy Gamber, Michael Grossberg, and Hendrik Hartog (University of Notre Dame Press, 2003), 213–39; Kriste Lindenmeyer, *"A Right to Childhood": The U. S. Children's Bureau and Child Welfare, 1912–1946* (University of Illinois Press, 1997); Viviana A. Zelizer, *Pricing the Priceless Child: The Changing Social Value of Children* (Basic Books, 1985), esp. 77, 79.
7. See Kriste Lindenmeyer, *The Greatest Generation Grows Up: American Childhood in the 1930s* (University of Chicago Press, 2005), 156–205; Lisa Jacobson, *Raising Consumers: Children and the American Mass Market in the Early Twentieth Century* (Columbia University Press, 2004); Tuttle, *Daddy's Gone to War*. On radio, see Susan J. Douglas, *Listening In: Radio and the American Imagination, from Amos 'n' Andy and Edward R. Murrow to Wolfman Jack and Howard Stern* (Times Books, 1999); Michele Hilmes, *Radio Voices: American Broadcasting, 1922–1952* (University of Minnesota Press, 1997); J. Fred MacDonald, *Don't Touch That Dial! Radio Programming in American Life from 1920 to 1960* (Nelson-Hall, 1979). On movies, see Robert Sklar, *Movie-Made America: A Cultural History of American Movies* (Random House, 1975, 1994); Gregory A. Waller, *Moviegoing in America: A Sourcebook in the History of Film Exhibition* (Blackwell Publishers, 2002). On department stores, see Vicki Howard, *From Main Street to Mall: The Rise and Fall of the American Department Store* (University of Pennsylvania Press, 2015);

William Leach, *Land of Desire: Merchants, Power, and the Rise of a New American Culture* (Pantheon Books, 1993). On Gene Autry, see Holly George-Warren, *Public Cowboy No. 1: The Life and Times of Gene Autry* (Oxford University Press, 2007).

8. See, e.g., Deposition of Mary Louise Cumberledge, San Diego, CA, April 12, 1948, 63–64, Cumberledge Case File; Deposition of Cecil D'Wayne Warnick, Record in Lutz.
9. Zelizer, *Pricing the Priceless Child*, 3; Habina Interview.
10. Chudacoff, *Children at Play*, 98.
11. Deposition of Mrs. Gertrude Cunningham, Washington, DC, December 30, 1945, 42, Bradley Case File.
12. Baragona Interview. As Charles Baragona remembered, "If you fell and scratched yourself any one of the neighbors would take you in and give you a Band-Aid, and if you were over there they'd set you at the table and you'd have a sandwich with them or whatever."
13. Deposition of Mary Louise Cumberledge, 100, Cumberledge Case File.
14. Deposition of Evelyn Fox, Terre Haute, IN, September 12, 1949, 86; Deposition of Kenneth Fox (eight), Terre Haute, IN, September 12, 1949, 102, both in Cizek Case File.
15. Deposition of Kathryn Timberlake, Kansas City, MO, September 15, 1950, 270, Timberlake Case File.
16. Izzo Interview. See also Deposition of Kathryn Timberlake, 271–74, Timberlake Case File.
17. Izzo Interview.
18. Izzo Interview.
19. Deposition of Helen C. DiTrapani, Washington, DC, July 11, 1946, 9, DiTrapani Case File; Deposition of Evelyn Fox, 79, Cizek Case File; Interrogatories William A. King, Fort Lauderdale, FL, November 17, 1947, 6, King Case File; Deposition of Mary Louise Cumberledge, 83, Cumberledge Case File; "Playing With Fire Costs Boy His Life," *Herald-News* (Passaic, NJ), November 2, 1943, 1. See Ruth Schwartz Cowan, *More Work for Mother: The Ironies of Household Technology from the Open Hearth to the Microwave* (Basic Books, 1983); Susan Strasser, *Never Done: A History of American Housework* (Pantheon Books, 1982).
20. Tuttle, *Daddy's Gone to War*, 70–71, 78, 89.
21. Testimony of James McCormack, 81, McCormack Record on Appeal.
22. Tuttle, *Daddy's Gone to War*, 31.
23. Stenographer's Minutes, Consolidated Trial, Hon. John C. Knox, DJ, May 17, 1948, 72, Richard Johnson Case File.
24. See also Deposition of Cecil D'Wayne Warnick, Cumberland, MD, December 12, 1947, Warnick Case File.
25. David Nasaw, *Children of the City, at Work and at Play* (Anchor Press/Doubleday, 1985), 19; Mergen, *Play and Playthings*, ch. 5.
26. McMaster Interview.
27. Bates Interview. See also Baragona Interview. "And were there lots of kids?" I asked Charles Baragona. The answer was, yes:

> This lady had six, sev—eight kids. . . . And one kid was one year older and one kid one year younger, my best friend here was born four days after me and he had a brother the same age as my sister Theresa Mary, and this guy over here moved in a little bit later, but he was the same age, had a brother two years younger, and over here was a Catholic family of five kids, and so right there, was a number of kids. We could always get a crowd just within our neighborhood because there was two, four, six, eight, and then a couple of girls there were ten of us plus my family.

See, as well, Habina Interview. "Were there lots of kids in your neighborhood?" I asked. "Yes. There was lots of children."

28. "Boy, 5, Burned to Death Roasting Marshmallows," *Herald-News* (Passaic, NJ), June 13, 1946, 1 (Gerald Sukinik (five) died; Joseph Intelisano (four) was seriously injured); Petition, William McMaster Jr., June 11, 1948, 4–5, McMaster Case File.
29. I have not found a general history of fire in everyday American life. But for parts of this history, see Priscilla J. Brewer, *From Fireplace to Cookstove: Technology and the Domestic Ideal in America* (Syracuse University Press, 2000); David E. Nye, *Electrifying America: Social Meanings of a New Technology, 1880–1940* (MIT Press, 1990).
30. Affidavit of Edward McFadden Jr. (counsel to Andrew Javinsky and his father Paul Javinsky), 2–3, Javinsky Case File; Deposition of Evelyn Fox, 77–78, Cizek Case File; Deposition of William A. King, Fort Lauderdale, FL, November 17, 1947, 7, King Case File.
31. Bates Interview.
32. Petition of John A. Touhill, 1, Touhill Case File; "Girl, 4, Burned Badly by Yule Tree Bonfire," *Herald Statesman* (Yonkers, NY), January 10, 1949, 3.
33. "Another Passaic Boy Burned When Cowboy Suit Ignites," *Herald-News* (Passaic, NJ), October 10, 1946, 1.
34. Habina Interview.
35. Deposition of Ben Rittmaster, Kansas City, MO, September 15, 1950, 308, Timberlake Case File.
36. Deposition of Kenneth Fox, 102–3, Cizek Case File.
37. Affidavit of Edward McFadden Jr., 2–3, Javinsky Case File.
38. Deposition of Evelyn Fox, 77–78, Cizek Case File.
39. Deposition of Mary Louise Cumberledge, 86–88, Cumberledge Case File.
40. Deposition of Kathryn Timberlake, 283–84, Timberlake Case File.
41. "Son of Meyers Coach Is Seriously Burned at Play," *Wilkes-Barre Record*, March 31, 1945, 1.
42. Lockhart Interview; "Boy, 5, Burned; Playsuit on Fire," *Daily Tribune* (Royal Oak, MI), January 14, 1944, 1.
43. Baragona Interview.
44. See Mergen, *Play and Playthings*, 103–23; Chudacoff, *Children at Play*, 116–22.
45. Deposition of Edward Alexander, Cumberland, MD, December 30, 1948, n.p., Record in Lutz.
46. Deposition of Edward Alexander, Record in Lutz.
47. Deposition of Evelyn Fox, 91–92, Cizek Case File.

48. Deposition of Evelyn Fox, 94, Cizek Case File; Deposition of Edward Alexander, Record in Lutz.
49. Deposition of Arthur A. Cumberledge Jr., San Diego, CA, April 12, 1948, 11–12, Cumberledge Case File.
50. Deposition of Mary Louise Cumberledge, 84–85, Cumberledge Case File.
51. Deposition of Arthur A. ("Toby") Cumberledge Jr., 11, Cumberledge Case File.
52. Deposition of Arthur A. Cumberledge Jr., 3, 12–18, 32, Cumberledge Case File; and Deposition of Jane Cumberledge, San Diego, CA, April 12, 1948, 37, 44–45, 46, 53, Cumberledge Case File.
53. John Elwyn Jones, Answers to Interrogatories, 4a, October 14, 1947, Jones Case File.
54. Felton Interview.
55. See, e.g., Testimony of James McCormack, 121, McCormack Record on Appeal; Deposition of Calvin Lee Sibley, Washington, DC, September 19, 1949, 96–97, Sibley Case File (U. S. Dist. Ct. SDNY).
56. Allan M. Brandt, *Cigarette Century: The Rise, Fall, and Deadly Persistence of the Product that Defined America* (Basic Books, 2007), 30. See also Robert Sobel, "The Match," in *They Satisfy: The Cigarette in American Life* (Anchor Books, 1978), 64–71.
57. National Board of Fire Underwriters with the assistance of the United States Bureau of Education, *Safeguarding the Home Against Fire: A Fire Prevention Manual for the School Children of America*, 7th ed. (National Board of Fire Underwriters, 1939), 11–18.
58. Sansbury Interview.
59. Izzo Interview.
60. See Tuttle, *Daddy's Gone to War*, ch. 9. On newsreels, see Maggie Valentine, *The Show Starts on the Sidewalk: An Architectural History of the Movie Theatre, Starring S. Charles Lee* (Yale University Press, 1994), 128–36. On movie theaters in small towns, see John Margolies and Emily Gwathmey, *Ticket to Paradise: American Movie Theaters and How We Had Fun* (Little, Brown and Company, 1991), 78.
61. Baragona Interview.
62. Tuttle, *Daddy's Gone to War*, 154.
63. Richard White, "Frederick Jackson Turner and Buffalo Bill," in *The Frontier in American Culture: An Exhibition at the Newberry Library*, ed. James Grossman (Newberry Library, 1994), 7–66; Ray White, "The Good Guys Wore White Hats: The B Western in American Culture," in *Wanted Dead or Alive: The American West in Popular Culture*, ed. Richard Aquila (University of Illinois Press, 1996), 135.
64. Theaters were not always safe, see Magda Fahrni, "Glimpsing Working-Class Childhood Through the Laurier Palace Fire of 1927: The Ordinary, The Tragic, and the Historian's Gaze," *Journal of the History of Childhood and Youth* 8 (2015): 426–50.
65. White, "Good Guys Wore White Hats," 135, 146–47.
66. Izzo Interview.
67. Deposition of Helen C. DiTrapani, Washington, DC, July 11, 1946, 9, DiTrapani Case File.

68. "Charge Inflammability of Garment Resulted in Boy Suffering Serious Burns," *Times Leader* (Wilkes-Barre, PA), April 17, 1948, 3.
69. Bates Interview.
70. Testimony of James McCormack, 81–86, McCormack Record on Appeal.

chapter two: curriculum vitae

1. Charlton T. Lewis and Charles Short, *A Latin Dictionary* (Clarendon Press, 1979), under "curriculum." Lewis and Short's is one of two principal dictionaries for Latin translation. Founded on Andrews's edition of Freund's Latin dictionary, it was revised, enlarged, and in great part rewritten by Charlton T. Lewis, PhD, and Charles Short, LLD. The second is P. G. W. Glare's *Oxford Latin Dictionary*, 2nd ed. (Oxford University Press, 2012). Both rely heavily on Cicero's speeches and texts. Throughout the book, *vita*, *curriculum vitae*, etc., are only italicized when referring to the classical Latin meaning of the terms; they are not italicized (except in direct quotations) when referring to the academic form.
2. Glare, *Oxford Latin Dictionary*, 2nd ed. under "vita." See also Lewis and Short, *Latin Dictionary*, under "vita."
3. For two examples from Cicero, consider first his adaptation of Plato's *Timaeus*, circa 45 BCE, in which he writes, "And he who justly and honorably completes the course of his life [*curriculum vivendi*] which was given to him by nature, to that astral realm, which fits his nature, he shall return." (See Cicero, *Timaeus/De Universitate* ["On the Universe"], trans. Benjamin Hansen, referenced in abbreviated form in Lewis and Short, *Latin Dictionary*, under "curriculum.") In his philosophical magnum opus *De Natura Deorum* ("On the Nature of the Gods"), written circa 45 BCE, Cicero, in discussing the opinions of the radical skeptics of Greek philosophy, wrote: "They held that human faculties were limited, minds were faulty, the span/course of life [*curricula vitae*] was brief . . ." (See Cicero, Acad. 1.44, trans. Benjamin Hansen, referenced in Lewis and Short, *Latin Dictionary*, under "curriculum.") Cicero and others also often used *cursus* rather than *curriculum*, as in *cursus vitae* or *vitae cursus*; the two Latin words are often treated as synonyms. In surviving classical texts, *cursus* appears more frequently than *curriculum*. See Lewis and Short, *Latin Dictionary*, under "cursus"; the entry includes seven examples from Cicero of vitae cursus. *Cursus honorum*, translated in the *Oxford Classical Dictionary* as "career path," had a particular meaning: a system of advancement in public office, developed in the early Roman republic, most important in the second and first centuries BCE. The concept continued into the Roman Empire, with diminished significance. See Simon Hornblower, Antony Spawforth, and Esther Eidinow, eds., *Oxford Classical Dictionary*, 4th ed. (Oxford University Press, 2012), under "careers."
4. In the 1559 edition of the *Institutes*, Calvin used the phrase *vitae curriculo* five times. He also used *vitae cursu* and *vitae cursum*; see Joannis Calvini, *Institutio Christianae Religionis* (Apud Guilelmum Thome, 1846), https://catalog.hathitrust.org/Record/008567922. See also David Hamilton, *Towards a Theory of Schooling* (Falmer Press, 1989), 8. The first usage of *curriculum* to mean a course of study listed in

the *Oxford English Dictionary* dates from 1633. See *Oxford English Dictionary*, under "curriculum," accessed December 8, 2025, https://www.oed.com/dictionary/curriculum_n?tab=meaning_and_use#7556257.

5. William Clark, *Academic Charisma and the Origins of the Research University* (University of Chicago Press, 2006), 36.
6. Walter Rüegg, "Themes," *A History of the University in Europe*, vol. 3: *Universities in the Nineteenth and Early Twentieth Centuries (1800–1945)*, ed. Walter Rüegg (Cambridge University Press, 2004), 3. Of the 143 European universities in existence in 1789, only eighty-three remained in 1815.
7. Clark, *Academic Charisma*, 197. In the wealth of scholarship on the history of universities in Europe and the United States, William Clark's work is the only book in which I have found a reference to the curriculum vitae. Clark's attention to the vita is limited to two mentions. But the chapter on the doctor of philosophy in which they appear and the narrative arc and argument of the book are critical for contextualizing the emergence of this first formulaic vita. Through chapters on key forms and practices in university life—the lecture, the exam, the granting of doctoral and masters' degrees, the library catalog—Clark traces the bureaucratization and commodification of academic practices from which the research university emerged. The character of the Prussian state and the fact that universities were state institutions is critical in the history he traces. As he notes in the opening chapter, "a German Protestant academic had to pass muster with bureaucratic or rationalized criteria for appointment, which included productivity in publication, diligence in teaching, and acceptable political views and lifestyle. But to achieve success, one also had to acquire fame, be in fashion, and display 'originality,' a spark of genius, in writings. This became a new sort of academic charisma tied to writing for 'applause' and 'recognition.'" (3–4). For additional evidence of the curriculum vitae as a requirement for obtaining a *DPhil* (PhD) at many German universities in the nineteenth century, see Clark, *Academic Charisma*, 500–508 (appendix 5). Clark used the vita for purposes of documenting the number of known "classics" majors who transferred from other universities. In other words, they were, in this respect, a source of information not a subject of interest in and of themselves. Clark's data relates to the years 1815–1837 and refers to students' vitae at the University of Berlin, University of Bonn, University of Breslau, and University of Halle-Wittenberg. For later in the nineteenth century, see the Harvard University Library Accession Records, which include complete bibliographic detail for each item, including vitae. Between January 1890 and January 1894, Harvard's library documented accessions of 287 dissertations, the vast majority of which were from German universities. Although variously titled, over two-thirds (198 of the 287) included a vita. See *Harvard University Bulletin* 6, nos. 1–8 (1892) and *Harvard University Bulletin* 7, no. 105 (1894), https://catalog.hathitrust.org/Record/008373186.
8. George Bancroft, quoted in Paul G. Buchloch and Walter T. Rix, eds., *American Colony of Göttingen* (Vandenhoeck and Ruprecht, 1976), 122–25 (the book includes both the handwritten Latin document and its translation). Bancroft's vita was exceptional in one respect: He did not include his parents' names. Most nineteenth-century German curricula vitae, continuing into the twentieth century, did. See, e.g., Francis John Curtis, "An Investigation of the Rimes and Phonol-

ogy of the Middle-Scotch Romance Clariodus" (PhD diss., University of Heidelberg, 1894), *Curriculum Vitae*: "I, Francis John Curtis, was born on January 2nd, 1861, at Blandford, in the County of Dorset, England, as the 3rd son of Charles Thomas and Marianne Bennett Curtis," https://books.google.com/books/about/An_Investigation_of_the_Rimes_and_Phonol.html?id=Ty0lIyCUa6kC. For examples from the early twentieth century, see ch. 4, "letters from strangers."

9. Jurgen Herbst, *The German Historical School in American Scholarship: A Study in the Transfer of Culture* (Cornell University Press, 1965), 16.
10. Frederick A. P. Barnard, quoted in William F. Russell, ed., *Rise of a University* (Columbia University Press, 1937), 376.
11. Some stayed for only a term, others for a year or two, many studied at multiple universities—part of the challenge of tracking exact numbers; not everyone sought or completed a PhD. See Anja Werner, *The Transatlantic World of Higher Education: Americans at German Universities, 1776–1914* (Berghahn Books, 2013); Daniel T. Rodgers, *Atlantic Crossings: Social Politics in a Progressive Age* (Belknap Press of Harvard University Press, 1998), 76; Konrad Jarausch, "American Students in Germany, 1815–1914: The Structure of German and U. S. Matriculants at Göttingen University," in *German Influences on Education in the United States to 1917*, eds. Henry Geitz, Jürgen Heideking, and Jurgen Herbst (German Historical Institute, 1995), 195–211; Buchloch and Rix, eds., *American Colony of Göttingen*; Jurgen Herbst, *The German Historical School in American Scholarship: A Study in the Transfer of Culture* (Cornell University Press, 1965), 1–22; Laurence R. Veysey, *The Emergence of the American University* (University of Chicago Press, 1965), 125–33; Daniel Bussey Shumway, "The American Students of the University of Göttingen," *Americana Germanica* 8, nos. 5–6 (1910): 171–246.
12. George Ticknor, Edward Everett, and Joseph Cogswell, all of whom went on to become distinguished scholars in their fields, preceded Bancroft in studying at Göttingen. See Buchloch and Rix, *American Colony of Göttingen*, 133–36, 158–59; Shumway, "American Students of the University of Göttingen," 171–73.
13. The establishment of graduate education in the United States is well-traveled ground. See especially Veysey, *Emergence of the American University*; Richard J. Storr, *The Beginnings of Graduate Study in America* (University of Chicago Press, 1953), which focuses on the pre–Civil War history that laid the foundations for an experiment like Hopkins to happen; as well as more general accounts, including John R. Thelin, *A History of American Higher Education*, 3rd ed. (Johns Hopkins University Press, 2019); Roger L. Geiger, *To Advance Knowledge: The Growth of American Research Universities, 1900–1940* (Oxford University Press, 1986). There are also numerous helpful works on individual institutions; see, e.g., John W. Boyer, *The University of Chicago: A History* (University of Chicago Press, 2015); James Axtell, *The Making of Princeton University* (Princeton University Press, 2006); Morton and Phyllis Keller, *Making Harvard Modern: The Rise of America's University* (Oxford University Press, 2001); Richard Norton Smith, *The Harvard Century* (Simon and Schuster, 1986); John C. French, *A History of the University Founded by John Hopkins* (Johns Hopkins University Press, 1946). See also autobiographies and memoirs of American university presidents in the era in which graduate education first flourished in the United States, including Daniel Coit Gilman, *The*

Launching of a University (Dodd, Mead and Company, 1906); Nicholas Murray Butler, *Across the Busy Years*, 2 vols. (Charles Scribner's Sons, 1939).

14. Francesco Cordasco, *The Shaping of American Graduate Education: Daniel Coit Gilman and the Protean Ph.D.* (Rowman and Littlefield, 1973), 28–29.
15. Cordasco, *Shaping of American Graduate Education*, appendix 2, 147–49. Columbia, by contrast, awarded twenty-two PhDs in its first decade of granting doctoral degrees and by the end of the 1880s had still only granted sixty-five PhDs. See *Theses, Doctor of Philosophy, 1872–1910* (Columbia University, 1910), CUA.
16. Gilman, *Launching of a University*, 49. It would be an exaggeration to say that "to a man" the founding figures of graduate education in the United States were influenced by the German model, but only a slight exaggeration. See Veysey, *Emergence of the American University*; and Cordasco, *Shaping of American Graduate Education.*
17. Working from *Theses, Doctor of Philosophy, 1872–1910*, CUA. I used the HathiTrust Digital Library to determine whether, before 1893 (the year Columbia published its first catalog to include degree requirements), dissertations had included vitae (they had not) and when, after 1893, the (new) policy began to be followed (1896).
18. As Francesco Cordasco notes, prior to 1887, "theses were returned to the candidate." See Cordasco, *Shaping of American Graduate Education*, 87–88, 90, 147–49 (appendix 2).
19. *Twelfth Annual Report of the President of the Johns Hopkins University, 1887* (Johns Hopkins University, 1888), 46, https://babel.hathitrust.org/cgi/pt?id=hvd.hnawks&seq=105&q1=1887.
20. In 1913, American universities awarded 465 PhD degrees in the arts and sciences. Three institutions accounted for close to one-third of that number (Columbia [63], Harvard [52], Chicago [46]), and eight institutions accounted for 68 percent of PhDs awarded (in addition to Columbia, Harvard, and Chicago were Yale [39], Cornell [35], Johns Hopkins University [32], the University of Pennsylvania [31], and the University of Illinois [20]). See Clarence J. Wes and Callie Hull, comp., *Doctorates Conferred in the Arts and the Sciences by American Universities, 1921–1922*, Reprint and Circular Series of the National Research Council (National Research Council, 1923), 4–5. *Catalogue, 1893–94, Columbia College in the City of New York* (Columbia College, 1893), 110, CUA; *The Regulations of the University of Chicago* (University of Chicago Press, 1903), 44, https://babel.hathitrust.org/cgi/pt?id=uiuo.ark:/13960/t1vd8m197&seq=5; *Annual Register, July 1910–July 1911* (University of Chicago Press, 1911), 126–27, https://catalog.hathitrust.org/Record/010308519; *General Announcements of the Catholic University of America, 1909–1910* (Catholic University of America, 1909), 25–26, https://babel.hathitrust.org/cgi/pt?id=uiuo.ark:/13960/t0tq75697&seq=3; Johns Hopkins University Department of Philosophy, Psychology, and Education, *Announcement of Graduate Courses and General Information for 1911–1912* (Johns Hopkins University, 1911), 10, https://ia800608.us.archive.org/19/items/announcementofgr00john/announcementofgr00john.pdf.
21. Microfilming of dissertations began in 1938.
22. My evidence for this point has two sources: a conversation with Jocelyn Wilk, Columbia University archivist, February 2020; and a reference in Arnold H. Trotier

and Marian Harman, eds., *Doctoral Dissertations Accepted by American Universities, 1949–1950*, vol. 17, comp. Association of Research Libraries (H. W. Wilson Company, 1950), iii (noting that it had come to their attention that Columbia only reported dissertations for a given year that had met the publication requirement of Columbia and have been deposited in final form in the Columbia University Libraries).

23. Proquest Dissertations and Theses and the HathiTrust Digital Library were key to checking the breadth of practice regarding vitae appended to dissertations. The principal disadvantage of Proquest is that dissertations from the most prominent research universities are not available through it for the early years. But it did give me a sense of the pervasiveness of the practice of dissertation vitae before 1950. In order to access dissertations that did not include vitae as well as those that did, I searched not for *vita* (or similar terms) but for the language that the title page was required to include (e.g., "Submitted in Partial Fulfillment of the Requirements for the Doctor of Philosophy, in the Faculty of [Pure Sciences/Philosophy/Political Science], Columbia University"). These searches produced hundreds of results. For example, my search for dissertations prior to 1950 in the "faculty of Philosophy" yielded 1,594 hits of which 802 were fully viewable. I did not look through all of these. My goal was to get a sense of patterns and the range of expression, not complete a quantitative review. That vitae were attached to dissertations coming out of universities ranging from the University of Chicago to the University of Illinois, University of Nebraska, and Northwestern University, from the first decade of the twentieth century, suggests the range of the practice.
24. Of sixteen JHU dissertations added to the Harvard University Library collections between January 1890 and January 1894, five included a biographical statement titled variously "life" (2), "autobiography" (2), and "biography" (1). See *Harvard University Bulletin* 6 (1892) and *Harvard University Bulletin* 7 (1894). PhD requirements at Johns Hopkins were first comprehensively set in 1878.
25. *Catalogue, 1893–94, Columbia College in the City of New York*, 108–9.
26. John Angus MacVannel, "Hegel's Doctrine of the Will" (PhD diss., Columbia University, 1896), https://archive.org/details/hegelsdoctrineof00macvuoft/page/n5/mode/2up, 103.
27. For other examples, see, e.g., Arthur Beatty, "Browning's Verse-Form: Its Organic Character" (PhD diss., Columbia University, 1897), n.p.; Ludwig Bernstein, "The Order of Words in Old Norse Prose" (PhD diss., Columbia University, 1897), 62, https://archive.org/details/orderofwordsinol00bernrich; Ernst Freund, "The Legal Nature of Corporations" (PhD diss., Columbia University, 1897), n.p. https://archive.org/details/legalnaturecorp00freugoog; Francis R. Stark, "The Abolition of Privateering and the Declaration of Paris" (PhD diss. Columbia University, 1897), 165, https://archive.org/details/abolitionofpriva00staruoft/page/n5/mode/2up.
28. *Catalogue and General Announcements, 1910–1911, Columbia University in the City of New York* (Columbia University, 1910), 188, CUA.
29. The heading "Vita" reflected German trends. In Germany, by the 1890s, *Vita* or *Lebenslauf* had largely supplanted the longer title *Curriculum Vitae* for the doc-

ument appended at the end of German dissertations. See, e.g., the list of dissertations, most from German universities, purchased by Harvard between 1890 and 1894. *Harvard University Bulletin* 6, nos. 1–8 (1892) and *Harvard University Bulletin* 7, no. 105 (1894).

30. Palmer Cobb, *The Influence of E.T.A. Hoffman on the Tales of Edgar Allan Poe* (University of North Carolina Press, 1906), vita, https://archive.org/details/jstor-4171648/mode/2up. Perhaps at the Catholic University of America, which specifically required that the "biographical sketch" appended to the dissertation show the candidate's "whole academic record and stating under which professors of this University he pursued his studies," the older form carried forward, but if so, it was an outlier. See *General Announcements of the Catholic University of America, 1909–1910* (Catholic University of America, 1909), 25, https://babel.hathitrust.org/cgi/pt?id=uiuo.ark:/13960/t0tq75697&seq=3.

31. They did not though completely disappear. See, e.g., Louis Weisner, "Groups Whose Maximal Cyclic Subgroups Are Independent" (PhD diss., Columbia University, 1923), https://catalog.hathitrust.org/Record/000464365: "The writer welcomes this opportunity of expressing his appreciation of the valuable counsel and encouragement received from Professor Cole and of the inspiration afforded by his lectures on the Theory of Groups."

32. See, e.g., Freund, "Legal Nature of Corporations." In some respects, the departure in Freund's dissertation was all the more striking because he was German-born and educated. But other Columbia PhD candidates under the faculties of political science beginning in 1897 also eschewed narrative for the list. See, e.g., Milo Roy Maltbie, "English Local Government of To-Day: A Study of the Relations of Central and Local Government" (PhD diss., Columbia University, 1897); F. H. Noble, "Taxation in Iowa: Historical Sketch, Present Status and Suggested Reforms" (PhD diss., Columbia University, 1897), https://catalog.hathitrust.org/Record/100515770; Charles Franklin Emerick, "An Analysis of Agricultural Discontent in the United States" (PhD diss., Columbia University, 1897). The first vita appended to a dissertation in the pure sciences at Columbia, Gary N. Calkins's 1898 dissertation, too was formatted as a list and included another innovation: the author's name, centered in all caps and a larger font at the top. See Gary N. Calkins, "Mitosis in Noctiluca Miliaris and Its Bearing on the Nuclear Relations of the Protozoa and Metazoa" (PhD diss., Columbia University, 1898), https://onlinelibrary.wiley.com/doi/10.1002/jmor.1050150306.

33. This too was a likely element in the shift of vitae from the first to the third person and in the disappearance of details of coursework and expressions of gratitude.

34. See the Harvard University Library Accession Records published in the *Harvard University Bulletin*. The listings include complete bibliographic detail for each item, including vitae, variously labeled "vita," "lebenslauf," "curriculum vitae," "life," "autobiography," and "biography." Between January 1890 and January 1894, Harvard's library documented accessions of 287 dissertations, the vast majority of which were from German universities. Over two-thirds (198 of the 287) included a vita. See *Harvard University Bulletin* 6, nos. 1–8 (1892) and *Harvard University Bulletin* 7, no. 105 (1894).

35. The burden of the printing requirement meant that many PhD candidates published their dissertations before their PhD was formally conferred. For example, Francis Bertody Sumner's dissertation included a vita; the original publication did not. Compare Francis Bertody Sumner, "Kupffer's Vesicle and Its Relation to Gastrulation and Concrescence" (PhD diss., Columbia University, 1900), https://catalog.hathitrust.org/Record/100781047, with *New York Academy of Sciences Memoirs* 2, part 2 (October 15, 1900): 47–83. (Note that the *Memoirs* were made digitally available to researchers during the COVID-19 pandemic but are now only available by request: https://www.nyas.org/ideas-insights/publications/new-york-academies-digital-archive/.) For other examples where a dissertation included a vita but the published version did not, see, e.g., A. L. Kroeber, "Decorative Symbolism of the Arapaho" (PhD diss., Columbia University, 1901), https://archive.org/details/DecorativeSymbolismOfTheArapaho; A. L. Kroeber, "Decorative Symbolism of the Arapaho," *American Anthropologist* 3 (April–June 1901), https://archive.org/details/sim_american-anthropologist_april-june-1901_3_2; Leon Elmer Woodman, "A Study of the Multiple Reflections of Short Electric Waves Between Two or More Reflecting Surfaces" (PhD diss., Columbia University, 1910), https://babel.hathitrust.org/cgi/pt?id=njp.32101054768773&seq=1; L. E. Woodman and H. W. Webb, "A Study of the Multiple Reflections of Short Electric Waves Between Two or More Reflecting Surfaces," *Physical Review* 30, no. 5 (May 1901): 561–93, https://archive.org/download/crossref-pre-1923-scholarly-works/10.1103%252Fphysrev.7.442.zip/10.1103%252Fphysrevseriesi.30.561.pdf; Arthur Waldorf Thomas, "The Influence of Certain Acids and Salts upon the Activity of Malt Amylase" (PhD diss., Columbia University, 1915), https://catalog.hathitrust.org/Record/008430601; H. C. Sherman and A. W. Thomas, "Studies on Amylases. VIII. The Influence of Certain Acids and Salts upon the Activity of Malt Amylase," *Journal of the American Chemical Society* 37 (1915): 623–43, https://pubs.acs.org/doi/10.1021/ja02168a024; and Marjorie O'Connell, "The Habitat of the Eurypterida" (PhD diss., Columbia University, 1916), https://babel.hathitrust.org/cgi/pt?id=nnc1.cu56095287&seq=5; Marjorie O'Connell, "The Habitat of the Eurypterida," *Bulletin of the Buffalo Society of Natural Sciences* 11, no. 3 (1916): 1–278, https://en.wikisource.org/wiki/The_Habitat_of_the_Eurypterida.
36. Elsie Oschrin Bregman, "Studies in Industrial Psychology" (PhD diss., Columbia University, 1922), reprinted from *Archives of Psychology* 59 (1922): 1–65, https://catalog.hathitrust.org/Record/001633271. Curiously, though a vita is listed in the table of contents in the journal, it is missing from the scan on which it appears in the dissertation. But the point is that it did appear originally in both the journal publication and the dissertation.
37. Clark, *Academic Charisma*, 202, 211.
38. The term *authorial persona* is William Clark's (see *Academic Charisma*, 197–202, 203, 207–11). His term derives from the fact that in the Middle Ages, the award of degrees both presumed a certain moral subject and literally created a new juridical person ("juridical persona"). I see the vita as a critical element in creating the public authorial academic persona.

chapter three: "a circle of flame"

1. Testimony of James McCormack, 86–89, McCormack Record on Appeal.
2. Testimony of James McCormack, 90, McCormack Record on Appeal.
3. Testimony of James McCormack and John ("Jackie") McCormack, 86, 122, McCormack Record on Appeal.
4. The McCormacks lived at 126 E. 98th Street, NY, NY.
5. James McCormack was a doorman at 15 W. 81st Street, NY, NY.
6. Testimony of James McCormack, 74–75, 81–82, 85–86, McCormack Record on Appeal.
7. Testimony of James McCormack, 102, McCormack Record on Appeal.
8. Testimony of Catherine McCormack, 247–50; Testimony of Dr. Ernest E. Arnheim, 201, McComack Record on Appeal.
9. Joan Didion, *The Year of Magical Thinking* (Vintage International, 2005), 3.
10. Lockhart Interview.
11. Bates Interview.
12. Edward Alexander, Answers to Interrogatories, December 30, 1948, Record in Lutz.
13. Deposition of Jane Cumberledge, San Diego, CA, April 12, 1948, 38, Cumberledge Case File; "Saved Lad, 8, from Burning in Play Suit," *Times-Herald* (Washington, DC), April 22, 1945, 1.
14. "'Cowboy,' 6, Badly Burned," *Wilkes-Barre Record*, April 30, 1946, 1.
15. Felton Interview.
16. Lockhart Interview.
17. Sansbury Interview.
18. Habina Interview.
19. Lockhart Interview.
20. "Boy Burns to Death," *Indiana (PA) Evening Gazette*, September 17, 1946, 9.
21. "Playing with Fire Costs Boy His Life: Eastside Brothers Set Grass Ablaze—Both Become Human Torches," *Herald-News* (Passaic, NJ), November 2, 1943, 1.
22. Habina Interview.
23. Bates Interview.
24. Felton Interview.
25. Christina Crosby, *A Body, Undone: Living On After Great Pain* (New York University Press, 2016), 13.
26. Deposition of Israel Edmond Detrick Jr., Keyser, WV, October 15, 1947, 6, Detrick Case File.
27. Deposition of Helen C. DiTrapani, Washington, DC, July 11, 1946, 9, DiTrapani Case File.
28. Elwyn Jones, Answers to Interrogatories, October 14, 1947, 3a, Jones Case File.
29. Lockhart Interview.
30. Baragona Interview.
31. "Clothing Ablaze, Boy Badly Hurt," *Philadelphia Inquirer*, August 27, 1944, 3B.
32. Deposition of Edward Gaines, Washington, DC, December 30, 1948, 20–22, Greatorex Case File.

33. "Playing with Fire Costs Boy His Life"; "Eastside Brothers Set Grass Ablaze," 1.
34. "Playing with Fire Costs Boy His Life"; "Eastside Brothers Set Grass Ablaze," 1.
35. Frances Flesher, Answers to Interrogatories, December 30, 1948, Record in Lutz.
36. "William Augustus Strong III," *Winston County Journal* (Louisville, MS), November 9, 1945.
37. Deposition of Laura C. Bradley, Washington, DC, December 4, 1947, 7–10, Bradley Case File.
38. Deposition of Mrs. Winifred Cunningham, Washington, DC, December 30, 1947, 41, Bradley Case File.
39. The timing of these incidents fit into an emerging awareness among doctors and professionals in the National Safety Council that the home posed serious hazards to children. By the end of World War II, accidents in the home had dramatically surpassed childhood diseases as the leading cause of death among children. On mothers'/wives' responsibility for home safety, see Joel A. Tarr and Mark Tebeau, "Housewives as Home Safety Managers: The Changing Perception of the Home as a Place of Hazard and Risk, 1870–1940," in Roger Cooter and Bill Luckin, eds., *Accidents in History: Injuries, Fatalities and Social Relations* (Rodopi, 1997), 196–233; Joel A. Tarr and Mark Tebeau, "Managing Danger in the Home Environment, 1900–1940," *Journal of Social History* 29 (Summer 1996): 797–816; and John C. Burnham, "Why Did the Infants and Toddlers Die? Shifts in Americans' Ideas of Responsibility for Accidents—from Blaming Mom to Engineering," *Journal of Social History* 29 (Summer 1996): 817–37.
40. Testimony of Catherine McCormack, 247–50, McCormack Record on Appeal.
41. Testimony of Catherine McCormack, 247–50, McCormack Record on Appeal.
42. Oliver Wendell Holmes, *The Common Law*, ed. Mark DeWolfe Howe (Little, Brown, 1881, 1963), 23. See also Elaine Scarry, *The Body in Pain: The Making and Unmaking of the World* (Oxford University Press, 1985), 294–96.
43. Testimony of Catherine McCormack and James McCormack, 247–48, 86–89, McCormack Record on Appeal.

chapter four: letters from strangers

1. "Methods of Appointment and Promotion in American Colleges and Universities: Report of Committee B," *Bulletin of the AAUP* 15, no. 3 (March 1939): 179.
2. In the 1920s, especially the latter half of the decade, the size of universities and colleges—and, with them, faculties—grew dramatically. So did the size of graduate programs and the number of PhDs awarded. In the 1921–1922 academic year, forty-one institutions conferred a total of 739 doctorates, the vast majority of which were conferred by just ten universities. Just over a decade later, the number of dissertations accepted had grown more than threefold to 2,630, and the number of PhD-awarding institutions almost doubled at eighty-one. The expansion of university and college faculties in the latter half of the 1920s absorbed the growing number of PhD-trained scholars, concentrated at the lower ranks. But as the emergence of the practice of men seeking appointments on their own suggested, even before the depression, the dramatic expansion in the number of PhDs was outstripping avail-

able positions. See Clarence J. West and Callie Hull, eds., *Doctorates Conferred in the Arts and the Sciences by American Universities, 1921–1922* (National Research Council, March 1923), 1–5; Donald B. Gilchrist, ed., *Doctoral Dissertations Accepted by American Universities 1933–1934* (H. W. Wilson Company, 1934), table 3.

3. The rules the AAUP advocated for tenure in 1915—a shared understanding between faculty member and university administration of the terms (in writing) of every appointment; permanent tenure independent of rank after a probationary period of not more than ten years; procedural protections in cases of dismissal—were followed nowhere in the United States. As Laurence Veysey notes, of the late nineteenth/early twentieth century, "throughout this period the concept of permanent faculty tenure, though not entirely unknown, was forthrightly accepted by very few university presidents even of leading institutions, and professors were at the mercy of their superiors to a far greater degree than would be true at the better universities a half-century later." Noting that "demand for professorial tenure was in large measure a quest for security," Veysey quotes from Henry Seidel Canby's memoir, *Alma Mater*: "Our strongest desire was to be made safe, to stay where we were on a living wage, to be secure while we worked. . . . No scrimping, no outside earning, could safeguard us. We were dependent upon the college, which itself was always pressed for money, and could not be counted upon to be either judicious or just." See Veysey, *The Emergence of the American University* (University of Chicago Press, 1965), 305, 387; Henry Seidel Canby, *Alma Mater: The Gothic Age of the American College* (Farrar and Rinehart, 1936), 153. On Harvard, see Richard Teichgraeber III, "The Arrival of 'Up-or-Out' Tenure: James B. Conant and the 'Tempest at Harvard,' 1936–1939," in *Shaping the American Faculty*, ed. Roger L. Geiger (Transaction Publishers, 2015), 79–112; Roger L. Geiger, *To Advance Knowledge: The Growth of American Research Universities, 1900–1940* (Oxford University Press, 1986), 225–28.
4. See, e.g., Enclosure, T. S. Taylor to E. D. Duffield, box 13, folder 1, Physics (ACC 133), PUA; Wilmond W. Parker to head of History Department, December 1, 1930, letter and enclosure, box 7, folder 1, University of Chicago Department of History Records, UChicago; Robert L. Baker Jr. to Prof. Schmitt, "Enclosure," September 21, 1939, box 7, folder 1, University of Chicago Department of History Records, UChicago; J. Thomas Field to Owen L. Shinn, "Information Sheet," April 4, 1930, letter and enclosure, box 4, folder Applications for Assistantships and Instructorships, 1930–1931, Department of Chemistry, UPenn.
5. Alice D. Duschak to S. C. Lind, March 11, 1934, box 6, folder Personnel DO-FOR, School of Chemistry Records (UAR 915), UMN.
6. Lloyd B. Ham to George W. Pierce, January 23, 1932, box 8, folder I, Physics (UAV 691), HUA. The desperation to place their PhDs led elite departments to circulate lists of bios of available candidates, as in Yale's "Who's Who of Candidates Available in 1932." See E. S. Furniss to William E. Dodds, December 9, 1931, box 8, folder 1, University of Chicago Department of History Records, UChicago. For the broader context of showing during the years of the Depression that job losses or straitened economic circumstances were through no fault of one's own, see Michele Landis Dauber, *The Sympathetic State: Disaster Relief and the Origins of the American Welfare State* (University of Chicago Press, 2013).

7. T. S. Taylor to E. D. Duffield, February 26, 1933, box 13, folder 1, Princeton University Physics Department Records (AC 133), PUA; Leland G. Boardman to Harvard University, May 30, 1932, box 7, Students and Jobs B (1930–1932), Harvard University Physics (UAV 691), HUA.
8. M. Blumer to Dr. A. L. Shinn, May 26, 1930, box 4, folder Applications for Assistantships and Instructorships, 1930–1931, Department of Chemistry, UPenn. Blumer's letter was one of many sent to the Department of Chemistry at the University of Pennsylvania by men completing their PhDs in chemistry in 1930.
9. D. R. Blumer, Pittsfield, to S. C. Lind, September 7, 1931, and Lind to Blumer, September 9, 1931, folder Personnel Bed-Bl, School of Chemistry Records (UAR915), UMN. Letters from strangers offer the barest glimpse into the desperate search for academic employment in the years of the Depression. Correspondence between department heads and advisors and their former students flesh out that picture. The correspondence between Blumer and Lind, stretching over four and a half years, is one such example.
10. Norris W. Goldsmith to Prof. E. P. Adams, February 25, 1933, box 13, folder 1, Princeton University Department of Physics Records (ACC 133), PUA.
11. "Academic Unemployment," *Bulletin of the AAUP* 19, no. 6 (October 1933): 354.
12. See, e.g., Frederick A. Saunders to F. T. Holmes, February 8, 1932; to Lloyd B. Ham, February 15, 1932; and to Maurice L. Huggins, February 15, 1932, box 8, folder I, Harvard University Physics (UAV 691), HUA; Frederick A. Saunders to Dr. Charles M. Gewertz, June 24, 1932, box 8, folder G, Harvard University Physics (UAV 691), HUA.
13. The replies of Assistant Chairman E. P. Adams, Department of Physics, Princeton, are representative in this regard. See box 13, folder 1, Princeton University Department of Physics Records (ACC 133), PUA.
14. As the first generation of American men with PhDs secured positions in elite institutions, Thomas Haskell notes, they established a pipeline for others who also held PhDs. He notes that Herbert Baxter Adams, who would go on to establish the American Historical Association, and who was one of John Coit Gilman's early hires at Johns Hopkins, "kept a map on which the location of each Hopkins graduate was marked with a pin like a display of colonial outposts." See Thomas L. Haskell, *The Emergence of Professional Social Science: The American Social Science Association and the Nineteenth-Century Crisis of Authority* (University of Illinois Press, 1977), 179, 236–37.
15. See, e.g., *Columbia University Bulletin* (June 1898): 247–48, box 269, folder 5, Appointments Office—Clippings, 1910s–1930s, Historical Subject Files, CUA; Board of Vocational Guidance and Placement, annual survey 1927–1928, box 1, folder 1, Board of Vocational Guidance and Placement minutes, 1927–1938, UChicago.
16. Penn and Colorado, for example, both established placement offices in the 1930s. See *Bulletin B: Rules Which Govern Registration and Negotiations*, University of Pennsylvania Placement Service, effective July 1, 1931, box 57, Corres. with other Colleges/Univ. re Placement—Rules of Placement Offices, Harvard University Office of Career Services (UAV 262), HUA; Colorado to Walker W. Daly, Jan-

uary 24, 1936, letter, box 57, Corres. with other Colleges/Univ. re Placement—Role of Placement Officers, Harvard University Office of Career Services (UAV 262), HUA.

17. As Thomas Haskell notes, the late nineteenth and early twentieth centuries' founding of professional societies like the American Historical Association (AHA), American Economic Association (AEA), American Political Science Association (APSA), and American Sociological Society (renamed the American Sociological Association [ASA] in 1959) was inextricably bound up with the pursuit of academic employment. See Haskell, *Emergence of Professional Social Science*, 236–37. The AAUP's prioritization of employment was marked by its committee structure: Committee A, Academic Freedom and Tenure; Committee B, Methods of Appointment and Promotion; Committee C, Methods of Recruiting the Profession. See "Committees of the Association," *Bulletin of the AAUP* 2, no. 2 (April 1916): 20–21.

18. The AAUP *Bulletin* published the first "Appointment Service Announcements"—divided between "Vacancies Reported" and "Teachers Available"—in March 1929. See "Appointment Service Announcements," *Bulletin of the AAUP* 15, no. 3 (March 1929): 260–62. On preparation for the new service, see "Notes and Announcements" and "Committee on Placement Service," *Bulletin of the AAUP* 14, no. 7 (November 1928): 494; "Notes and Announcements" and "Appointment Service," *Bulletin of the AAUP* 14, no. 8 (December 1928): 568. On the services established by the American Sociological Society (ASS) and AEA, see "Personnel Exchange" and "News and Notes," *American Journal of Sociology* 37, no. 5 (March 1932): 781; "Academic Vacancies and Applications for Teaching Positions," *American Economic Review* 29, no. 3 (September 1939): 663. The American Political Science Association took a different tack. Beginning experimentally in 1928–1929 and then continuing through the Depression, it created a list of bios of those completing their degrees and circulated the list to departments. See APSA Personnel Service, *Report on Nine Years of the Personnel Service*, 7–8, box 6, folder APSA, William Anderson Papers (UAR 0360), 1928–1937, UMN.

19. Appointments offices at both private and public research universities commented on faculty resistance. See Paul Brissenden, "The Scope and Functions of the Columbia University Placement Office," in *Annual Reports, 1923* (Columbia University, 1924), appendix 3, 277, box 60, folder 5, Historical Subject Files, CUA; R. A. Walker, director of placement, University of Wisconsin, "A Program for Placing College Teachers," in *Current Practices in Institutional Teacher Placement* (National Institutional Teacher Placement Association, 1941), 91–93.

20. The services explicitly deferred from making recommendations. The American Economics Association was typical. See "Academic Vacancies and Applications for Teaching Positions," *American Economics Review* 29, no. 3 (September 1939): 663. But what hiring officials wanted in making appointments was a trusted, personal, recommendation.

21. See, e.g., Registration Blank, Harvard University Appointment Office, Student Records: Samuel Flagg Bemis, 1914, HUA; Registration Blank, Princeton University, Bureau of Personnel and Appointments, Department of Teaching Appoint-

ments, Graduate School Alumni Records, box 29, Ben Edwin Perry, ca. 1926, PUA; Registration Blank, Appointments Office, Columbia University, box 269, folder 4, Appointments Offices, 1920s–1930s, Historical Subject Files, CUA.

22. See, e.g., examples from the Department of History Records at the University of Chicago (1930): John G. Hazam to Bernadotte E. Schmitt, May 26, 1930; G. Adolf Koch to Dr. Frederick Woodward, March 4, 1929; Frances E. Baldwin to W. E. Dodd, February 17, 1930, box 7, folder 1, University of Chicago Department of History Records, UChicago.
23. Enclosure in L. Wilmond W. Parker to Head of History Department, University of Chicago, December 1, 1930, box 7, folder 1, University of Chicago Department of History Records, UChicago.
24. See, e.g., Robert L. Baker Jr., to Prof. Schmitt, "Enclosure," September 21, 1939; J. Thomas Field, "Information Sheet," enclosure in J. Thomas Field to Owen L. Shinn, April 4, 1930, box 4, folder Applications for Assistantships and Instructorships, 1930–1931, Department of Chemistry, UPenn.
25. See, e.g., Ben Edwin Perry, registration blank completed July 19, 1926, Department of Teaching Appointments, Bureau of Personnel and Appointments, Princeton University, box 29, folder Perry, Ben Edwin (AC105), Grad School Alumni Records, PUA.
26. W. B. Ross to W. E. Dodd, November 9, 1932, box 7, folder 1, University of Chicago Department of History Records, UChicago.
27. See, e.g., C. F. Huth to John Rothenstein, June 14, 1926 ("Your letter of June 1 with the interesting inclosures [*sic*] about your preparation and capacity has been received by this Department."), box 7, folder 1, University of Chicago Department of History Records, UChicago.
28. There is an immense scholarly literature on the refugee scholars of the 1930s. It has, in the main, focused on the most prominent and successful refugees, their intellectual contributions, and the organizations and foundations that aided them. More recent scholarship offers a critical counterpoint to the earlier celebratory literature. See notes that follow for specific references.
29. Laurel Leff, *Well Worth Saving: American Universities' Life-and-Death Decisions on Refugees from Nazi Europe* (Yale University Press, 2019), 26–28. As an example of the news of dismissals circulating quickly and broadly, consider an article in the *Manchester Guardian*, "Nazi 'Purge' of the Universities, a Long List of Dismissals," dated May 19, 1933, and—drawing from the German press—listing professors dismissed between April 13 and May 4, 1933, by date of dismissal, name of institution, and name and field of scholar. It notes: "Most of the professors have been dismissed because of their Jewish origin, a few because of their liberal sentiments." Reprinted in Gabrielle Simon Edgcomb, *From Swastika to Jim Crow: Refugee Scholars at Black Colleges* (Krieger Publishing Company, 1993), 6–16.
30. The law applied even to those who had converted to another religion and was later extended to those whose spouse was Jewish or of Jewish descent.
31. See Maurice R. Davie, *Refugees in America: Report of the Committee for the Study of Recent Immigration from Europe* (Harper and Brothers Publishers, 1947), 5–8; Laura Fermi, *Illustrious Immigrants: The Intellectual Migration from Europe*, 2nd ed. (University of Chicago Press, 1968, 1971), 42, 51.

32. On compiling lists and opportunity, see Fermi, *Illustrious Immigrants*, 71–76; Judith Friedlander, *A Light in Dark Times: The New School for Social Research and Its University in Exile* (Columbia University Press, 2016), ch. 7; and Tibor Frank, "Organized Rescue Operations in Europe and the United States, 1933–1945," in *In Defence of Learning: The Plight, Persecution, and Placement of Academic Refugees, 1933–1980s*, eds. Shula Marks, Paul Weindling, and Laura Wintour (Oxford University Press, 2011), 143–60. See also the brief bios of "300 Notable Emigres" included in Donald Fleming and Bernard Bailyn, eds., *The Intellectual Migration: Europe and America, 1930–1960* (Belknap Press of Harvard University Press, 1969), 675–718. On the persistent concern that appointments for émigré scholars not deprive Americans of positions in the Depression, see Leff, *Well Worth Saving*, 87–90; Stephen Duggan and Betty Drury, *The Rescue of Science and Learning: The Story of the Emergency Committee in Aid of Displaced Foreign Scholars* (MacMillan Company, 1948), 173–76, 186; Davie, *Refugees in America*, 302. See also "Proposed Program for Joint Action by the American Universities to Provide Asylum for Those Refugees from European Countries Who Are Distinguished Members of the International Community of Scholars," box 142, folder 9: Refugee Problem, 1938–39, Office of the President Records (ACC 117), PUA. On antisemitism, see Daniel Kevles, *The Physicists: The History of a Scientific Community in Modern America* (Harvard University Press, 1995), 211–12. And for an all-too-representative example, consider an exchange relating to a potential appointment in history at the University of Chicago in 1936 between the chair of the department, Bernadotte Schmitt, and Sidney Fay at Harvard. Fay noted that he had learned something "I had never suspected": One of the men he had recommended was "a Jew." He added, "He doesn't look it and doesn't have any of the undesirable characteristics of one, so that it had never occurred to me; but I mention it in case it would make any difference with you." Schmitt replied that he was sorry to learn this fact since the candidate otherwise better filled their requirements. But "inasmuch as we already have two Jews in the Department it seemed to us inadvisable to add a third even though he may not look like a Jew or have the undesirable characteristics of one. Our two members who are Jewish happen also to lack those characteristics and we get along with them admirably but for various reasons it seems wiser not to appoint another." Schmitt and Fay wrote each other as peers with a long relationship. And it was these relationships and the world these men shared that allowed discrimination full expression and full play. See Bernadotte M. Schmitt to Sidney B. Fay, July 13, 1936, and reply July 14, 1936, box 6, folder 2, University of Chicago Department of History Records, UChicago.
33. The first organizations established specifically for aid of displaced scholars were the Emergency Committee for the Aid of Displaced German Scholars (US); the Academic Assistance Council (AAC), renamed the Society for the Protection of Science and Learning (SPSL; Great Britain); and the *Notgemeinschaft der Deutschen Wissenschaft* (Zurich, relocated to London in 1936). See Gerald Kreft, "'Dedicated to Represent the True Spirit of the German Nation in the World': Philipp Schwartz (1894–1977), Founder of the Notgemeinschaft," in *In Defence of Learning*, eds. Marks et al., 127, 129, 137. On the Emergency Committee and the AAC/SPSL, see Duggan and Drury, *Rescue of Science and Learning*; David Zimmerman,

"'Protests Butter No Parsnips': Lord Beveridge and the Rescue of Refugee Academics from Europe, 1933–1938," and Georgina Ferry, "Max Perutz and the SPSL," both in *In Defence of Learning*, eds. Marks et al., 29–44, 87–100.

34. Fermi, *Illustrious Immigrants*, 17.
35. Immigration to the United States from China had been restricted beginning in 1882, and from Asia more generally, it had been completely barred under the Immigration Act of 1917—a restriction again incorporated into the 1924 Act. But it was only with the 1924 Act that a system of quotas was adopted limiting migration from Europe. See Erika Lee, *At America's Gates: Chinese Immigration During the Exclusion Era, 1882–1943* (University of North Carolina Press, 2004); Mai Ngai, *Impossible Subjects: Illegal Aliens and the Making of Modern America* (Princeton University Press, 2004).
36. From almost the first national law restricting immigration to the United States, the Chinese Exclusion Act of 1882, an exception was carved out for, among others, students and teachers.
37. Section 4(d) provided a non-quota visa to "an immigrant who continuously for at least two years immediately preceding the application for admission to the United States has been, and who seeks to enter the United States solely for the purpose of, carrying on the vocation of minister of any religious denomination, or professor of a college, academy, seminar, or university; and his wife, and his unmarried children under 18 years of age; if accompanying or following to join him."
38. On Alvin Johnson and the New School for Social Research, see Friedlander, *Light in Dark Times*; on the Institute for Advanced Study, see Abraham Flexner, *I Remember: The Autobiography of Abraham Flexner* (Simon and Schuster, 1940). See also Fleming and Bailyn, *Intellectual Migration*.
39. On not extending offers to men over fifty-five, see Leff, *Well Worth Saving*, 84–90; Frank, "Organized Rescue Operations," 145, 151.
40. The Leo Baeck Institute Digital Archives provide a rich source of collections of émigré Jewish scholars. For examples of German curricula vitae in the 1920s, see, e.g., Arthur Prinz Lebenslauf (ca. 1923), Arthur Prinz Collection, AR5103, LBI; Walter Benjamin (1925 habilitation application); Josef Soudek Lebenslauf (ca. 1928), dissertation CV and "Career of Life" (ca. 1935), Josef Soudek Collection, AR 6285 LBI (hereafter Soudek Papers, LBI). Lists of publications were separate from vitae. See, e.g., "Prof. Dr. Theodor Plaut Publications" (ca. 1930, 1932), Theodor Plaut Collection, AR 5019, LBI (hereafter Plaut Papers, LBI). It was routine as well for men to gather "testimonials" at each juncture of their professional life. See, e.g., "Testimonials I" (February 25, 1914; July 29, 1920) and "Testimonials II" (May 29, 1933), Prof. Dr. Theodor Plaut, Plaut Papers, LBI.
41. See, e.g., Fermi, *Illustrious Immigrants*, 72 (re: letters in files of Robert M. Hutchins, chancellor, University of Chicago).
42. Friedlander, *Light in Dark Times*, 91.
43. See, e.g., Lucie Adelsberger to Prof. A. Carrel, August 26, 1938, box 1, folder 15, ACEPR, IHRCA, UMN; Dr. Werner Worms to Dr. Farmer, May 25, 1938, and to the Emergency Committee in Aid of Displaced German Physicians, NYC, May 25, 1938, and Curriculum Vitae, box 26, folder W.W., ACEPR, IHRCA, UMN; Sigmund Cohn to the president of the New School for Social Research, October 3,

1938, Sigmund A. Cohn/Suzanne Lewy Cohn Collection, AR 11084, LBI (hereafter Cohn Papers, LBI); Theodor Plaut to the Emergency Committee in Aid of Displaced Germany Scholars, January 12, 1934, Plaut Papers, LBI.

44. R. S. Hearns to Sigmund Cohn, August 25, 1938, Cohn Papers, LBI.
45. Alan W. Stayne to Mr. Jacob Billikopf, April 16, 1934, Richard G. Salomon Collection, AR 3862, LBI (hereafter Salomon Papers, LBI).
46. Reprinted in Edgcomb, *From Swastika to Jim Crow*, 23–24.
47. Duggan and Drury, *Rescue of Science and Learning*, 186–87. Initially a temporary commitment was enough, but as the true stakes emerged and with them the need for longer-term appointments, aid societies required firmer commitments from universities and colleges.
48. Josef Soudek, "Career of Life" (ca. 1935), Soudek Papers, LBI.
49. I found especially helpful, for seeing the points noted here, the following collections in the LBI: Ernst Kantorowicz Collection, AR 7216 (hereafter Kantorowicz Papers, LBI); David Baumgardt Collection, AR 797 (hereafter Baumgardt Papers, LBI); Cohn Papers, LBI; Hermann Gundersheimer Collection, AR 25546 (hereafter Gundersheimer Papers, LBI); Plaut Papers, LBI; Salomon Papers, LBI; Eduard Strauss, AR 7192 (hereafter Strauss Papers, LBI). All these collections include vitae; many include extensive correspondence and other documentation. Also important for my work were the ACEPR, IHRCA, UMN, which include many doctors who were research scientists.
50. See, e.g., Lebenslauf (ca. 1935), Eduard Strauss: "In that year [1922] he followed a call . . . to the Georg Speyer Haus research institute, of which he remained a member until 1935. At the end of this year he was given leave of absence, on 1.1 1936 his retirement." In folder I.A. Curriculum Vitae, Strauss Papers, LBI; Werner Worms to Dr. Farmer, May 25, 1938, and to the Emergency Committee in Aid of Displaced German Physicians, NYC, May 25, 1938, and Curriculum Vitae. Written as a narrative, Worms's vita—like many of those written by scholars while still in Germany—was not explicit about his termination; only the dates and the context make it clear: "From January 1925 to March 1933 . . ."
51. Aid organizations like the Emergency Committee and AAC, foundations like the Rockefeller Foundation, and individual universities like the New School limited offers to those who had lost their appointments under Germany's racial laws or similar laws adopted in other countries over the decade. See Friedlander, *Light in Dark Times*, 91; Frank, "Organized Rescue Operations in Europe and the United States, 1933–1945," 143–60; Duggan and Drury, *Rescue of Science and Learning*, 186. Compare Eduard Strauss's *Lebenslauf* (ca. 1935, in German, while still in Germany), with his curriculum vitae (ca. late 1939–1940, in English, re: his parents ["both of German-Jewish extraction"] and his research position ["I lost my membership in the institute in 1936 as a result of the racial legislation"]), Strauss Papers, LBI. For other examples, see the vita that David Baumgardt wrote in England in English (ca. 1937, referring to his loss of his professorship at the University of Berlin "which I lost January 1st 1936, according to the Nurnberg Laws"), Baumgardt Papers, LBI (the collection also includes an earlier vita (ca. 1932) before he lost his appointment that is in German); and Dr. Hermann Gundersheimer's curriculum vitae (ca. 1939, in German: "This intention [re: getting his habilitation] has become

impossible because of my dismissal as a Jew in March 1933"), Gundersheimer Papers, LBI.

52. "Of course, the first thing that your friend must do, is perfect himself in English, with which he is apparently familiar, but does not speak fluently. For us to help him before he is perfect in English, will be very difficult." Leo M. Frenkel to Kurt E. Lande, October 4, 1938, "Re: Sigmund Cohn—Genoa", Cohn Papers, LBI. In a second copy of the letter sent the same day, Demuth typed in a new sentence: "A thorough knowledge of English is necessary." See F. [Fritz] Demuth to Ernst Kantorowicz, July 27, 1938, Kantorowicz Papers, LBI.

53. See Kantorowicz Papers, LBI, and Robert E. Lerner, *Ernst Kantorowicz: A Life* (Princeton University Press, 2017). Kantorowicz is a complex figure to use in illustration here. His biographer challenges the charge that Kantorowicz "would have been a Nazi had he not been Jewish" (Lerner, 159), but he also acknowledges that Kantorowicz began as a right-wing nationalist and was a fervent disciple of Stefan George. His reluctance to leave Germany so long as he was able to travel and do research look different in light of these facts. He lived lavishly and was deeply misogynist and elitist. However erudite and significant as a scholar, he does not emerge as an appealing human being. But Nazism cost him, as it did so many others, his academic position and had he not escaped in late 1938 he would undoubtedly have been arrested, sent to a concentration camp, and very possibly killed. His mother, Clara, died in Theresienstadt on February 10, 1943 (Lerner, 260). Throughout his life, he staunchly defended academic freedom, a commitment which cost him his position at Berkeley. Part of what makes him fascinating is his intellectual and political shift to the left after he left Germany. But for all his particularity, Kantorowicz's redrafting of his vita and pursuit of "friends" to support his case for an academic position in the United States mirrored the pattern of others. The completeness of the documentary record in this respect provides a rich illustration of broader patterns.

54. His appointment in history was full of anomalies: he had not studied history; he had never completed a habilitation, a fundamental requirement for an appointment as a professor in Germany; his religious background made his appointment to teach history, a "national" subject, surprising; his unfootnoted biography of Frederick the Second, though popular, was considered unscholarly. As Lerner notes of his original appointment as an honorary professor in 1930, "it is unlikely that the philosophical faculty of any other contemporary university [in Germany] would have granted the controversial outsider Ernst Kantorowicz a professorial position, even an honorary one." See Lerner, *Kantorowicz: A Life*, 145–46, 151–52. None of this context is evident in the vita he wrote between July 1938 and July 1939, as he desperately sought a teaching appointment in the United States. See Kantorowicz Papers, LBI.

55. See Ernst Kantorowicz, "Curriculum Vitae," July 29, 1938, Kantorowicz Papers, LBI, for Kantorowicz's description. See also Lerner, *Kantorowicz: A Life*, 158–68, 171. An exception in the Civil Service Restoration Act for those who had fought for Germany in the First World War initially protected Kantorowicz's teaching position. But the Nazification of the University of Frankfurt, effectively barring

him from the classroom, led to his forced retirement in November 1934, though he retained his pension until he left Germany in 1939.

56. "When you write me that you don't easily want to leave as long as you still have possibilities for living and work in Europe, of course, I naturally understand that," Mommsen wrote in a letter to Kantorowicz in May 1938, adding: "About the longevity of these conditions I of course can make no judgment from here." As to Kantorowicz's claim to have "a certain line of retreat in Oxford," Mommsen replied, "That too is very difficult to judge from here since always people are coming here who have been there a short while but are not taken up there on duration, but instead with very sound letters of recommendation get sent on to the U. S. A." See Theodor Mommsen to Ernst Kantorowicz, June 13, 1938 (in German), Kantorowicz Papers, LBI. By 1938, most scholars were only admitted to Great Britain with assurance that they had a commitment from an American university, so that their stay in Britain would not be more than a few months, a stopgap in their wait for an American visa.
57. Dr. F. [Fritz] Demuth to Ernst Kantorowicz, July 27, 1938.
58. Kantorowicz, "Curriculum Vitae," July 29, 1938, attached to Ernst Kantorowicz to Fritz Demuth, box 5, folder 3, Kantorowicz Papers, LBI (Kantorowicz's letter was written in German, but the attached vita was written in English).
59. Kantorowicz, "Curriculum Vitae," July 29, 1938. Other vitae too spoke to this closing off. See, e.g., Josef Soudek, "Career of Life" (ca. 1935), and Soudek, "Career of Life" (ca. 1935, in English shortly before his emigration in 1936), Soudek Papers, LBI.
60. Ernst Kantorowicz, "Curriculum Vitae," ca. March 1939, box 5, folder 3, Kantorowicz Papers, LBI.
61. Ernst Kantorowicz to [Austin L.] Poole, August 8, 1938, and Ernst Kantorowicz to Dr. [William E.] Dodd, n.d., box 5, folder 3, Kantorowicz Papers, LBI. It is clear from the file that others had/were writing in support as well: Bowra, George Haskins, H. A. L. Fisher—all in August 1938.
62. Fritz Demuth to Ernst Kantorowicz, August 6, 1938; Fritz Demuth to C. M. Bowrs, August. 11, 1938, both in box 5, folder 3, Kantorowicz Papers, LBI.
63. Theodor (Ernst) Mommsen to Eka [Ernst Kantorowicz], May 8, 1938; Theodor (Ernst) Mommsen, to Eka [Ernst Kantorowicz], June. 13, 1937 (handwritten in German, noting "You should do a lecture trip here"), both in box 5, folder 3, Kantorowicz Papers, LBI.
64. Ernst Hartwig Kantorowicz, "Document 1," curriculum vitae attached to visa application, July 20, 1939, Kantorowicz Papers, LBI.
65. Lutz Hamburger to Sigmund and Suse Cohn, September 2, 1938, Cohn Papers, LBI.
66. See Sigmund Cohn to Dr. Jacobson, August 15, 1938 (Jacobson had been a lawyer in Germany and had immigrated to the US ca. 1933), and Sigmund Cohn to the American Jewish Joint District Committee Inc., August 19, 1938, Cohn Papers, LBI.
67. Hamburger to Cohn and Cohn, September 2, 1938; Sigmund Cohn to Lutz Hamburger, September 11, 1938 ("Now to your no-quota idea. It is undoubtedly very

good and very respectable. For three years I have been assistant to Professor Attilio Cabiati for national economics as the national economy [although not with the official title. . . .]" [in German]), Cohn Papers, LBI.

68. Sigmund Cohn to Prof. M. Ch. F. Remer, October 1, 1938, Cohn Papers, LBI. Cohn wrote numerous letters of application, and each included some version of this statement and his curriculum vitae. See, e.g., S. Cohn to "the President of the 'New School for Social Research, NY,'" October 3, 1938; S. Cohn to Dr. Demuth, October 7, 1938; Sigmund Cohn to the Carnegie Foundation, October 11, 1938; S. Cohn to the Rockefeller Foundation, NY, October 11, 1938; S. Cohn to the National Coordinating Committee for Aid to Refugees and Emigrants coming from Germany, NYC, October 11, 1938; and S. Cohn to Nathan Isaacs, Harvard University, October 15, 1938, all in the Cohn Papers, LBI. The only copy of Cohn's curriculum vitae in his papers is incomplete (first page only) and not dated. See Sigmund Cohn, curriculum vitae, Cohn Papers, LBI.

69. Sigmund Cohn to Rudolph Hearns, December 18, 1938; Cecilia Rasovsky to Sigmund Cohn, December 9, 1938, both in the Cohn Papers, LBI.

70. "Harold Hirsch's Funeral Here Being Planned," *Atlanta Journal*, September 24, 1939, 1, 4.

71. The first aid organizations had recognized from the start that the ability of universities and colleges to make temporary appointments for displaced scholars would require external financial assistance, assistance that came from foundations, aid organizations, Jewish groups, and individual benefactors. This was true across the ranks of universities and colleges. For a list of the institutions that received Emergency Committee grants, see Duggan and Drury, *Rescue of Science and Learning*, 197–204 (appendix 6, "Institutions Which Received Grants from The Emergency Committee," and appendix 7, "Geographical Distribution of Emergency Committee Scholars, Rosenwald Fellows, and National Research Associates"). The Emergency Committee's funding came almost exclusively from prominent Jewish foundations. See Duggan and Drury, *Rescue of Science and Learning*, 188. On Hirsch's connections to the University of Georgia and, a few months after Cohn's arrival in the US, his sudden death, see "Harold Hirsch's Funeral Here Being Planned," 1, 4. When Harold Hirsch had first suggested Cohn to the president of the University of Georgia, the president had explained that state law prohibited the payment of state funds to non–US citizens. Harold Hirsch assumed responsibility for paying Cohn's salary. Following Hirsch's unexpected death, his widow and son committed to continuing the monthly payments, but their final payment was in July 1941. Only when Cohn became a US citizen in spring 1944 could the University of Georgia pay his salary. See Cohn Papers, LBI.

72. Female scholars' best opportunity of legal exit was as domestic servants in Great Britain. Female academics who reached the US on non-quota family visas also found themselves with few alternatives other than domestic service. See Leff, *Well Worth Saving*, 92–98; Susan Cohen, "In Defence of Academic Women Refugees: The British Federation of University Women," in *In Defence of Learning*, eds. Marks et al., 161–76.

73. Adelsberger's vita was three pages, written in English as a chronology beginning

with her birth on April 12, 1895, at Nuremberg, Germany. Her list of publications was an additional three pages and included twenty-seven entries dating from 1921 to 1937. Her initial letter, dated August 28, 1938, to Prof. A. Carrel, Esq. at the Rockefeller Institute and her enclosed curriculum vitae were both written in English. All her other correspondence was written in German. See Adelsberger, Lucie, box 1, folder 15, ACEPR, IHRCA, UMN.

74. For the reference to the importance of being personally known, see Robert A. Lambert to Laurence Farmer, December 5, 1938; for the Harvard appointment, case notes (LF:CS), December 23, 1938, box 1, folder 15, ACEPR, IHRCA, UMN. For a fuller biography of Adelsberger including her international reputation, her pioneering contributions as an allergist, her unsuccessful attempts to escape Germany to the US (1938) and Great Britain (1939), and her life and medical work in Auschwitz, see Lucie Adelsberger, *Auschwitz: A Doctor's Story* (Northeastern University Press, 1995), introduction by Deborah E. Lipstadt, xv; and Benjamin Kuntz, *Lucie Adelsberger, Doctor—Scientist—Chronicler of Auschwitz* (Hentrich and Hentrich, 2021).

75. The atomizing character of the non-quota visa exception for academics and their spouses and children under age eighteen forced individuals to make an impossible choice: Accept an appointment in hopes of then finding another route to safety for parents and other family members, or remain together and search for a shared route to security. There was no sure or right decision. Adelsberger spoke to this impossibility and the guilt it produced in her memoir, published first in German and only much later in English. See Adelsberger, *Auschwitz*, xx–xxii, 3–5, 10–12. See also Kuntz, *Lucie Adelsberger*, 34–39.

76. Lucie Adelsberger to Mr. Dr. E. Libman, January 5, 1941, box 1, folder 15, ACEPR, IHRCA, UMN. On discrimination against women in medicine in Germany, see Adelsberger, *Auschwitz*, xiv–xvi.

77. Theodor Adorno to Walter Benjamin, July 16, 1940; Walter Benjamin to Theodor W. Adorno, August 2, 1940, reprinted in *Theodor W. Adorno and Walter Benjamin: The Complete Correspondence, 1928–1940*, ed. Henri Lonitz, trans. Nicholas Walker (Harvard University Press, 1999), 337–41.

78. For examples of letters in which Benjamin discussed US immigration law and its implications for his case, see, e.g., Walter Benjamin to Gerhard Scholem, April 8, 1939; Walter Benjamin to Gretel Adorno, January 17, 1940; and Walter Benjamin to Max Horkheimer, June 16, 1940, all reprinted in *The Correspondence of Walter Benjamin, 1910–1940*, eds. Gershom Scholem and Theodor W. Adorno, trans. Manfred R. Jacobson and Evelyn M. Jacobson (University of Chicago Press, 1994), 600–601, 626–27, 635–36.

79. Benjamin to Henny Gurland [and Adorno?], September 25, 1940, reprinted in *Theodor W. Adorno and Walter Benjamin: The Complete Correspondence 1928–1940*, ed. Henri Lonitz, trans. Nicholas Walker (Harvard University Press, 1999), 342. See also Howard Eiland and Michael W. Jennings, *Walter Benjamin: A Critical Life* (Belknap Press, 2014), 669–76.

80. Three of Benjamin's vitae are included in translation in the four-volume *Walter Benjamin: Selected Writings*, published by the Belknap Press (1996–2003). For

all six vitae in the original, including the purpose for or context in which they were written, see *Walter Benjamin Gesammelte Schriften*, vol. 6 (Suhrkamp Verlage, 1981), 215–28, 771–77.

81. Lebenslauf, in *Walter Benjamin Gesammelte Schriften*, vol 6, 215–16, 771. For an English translation, see *Walter Benjamin: Selected Writings, Vol. 1: 1913–1926*, eds. Marcus Bullock and Michael W. Jennings (Belknap Press of Harvard University Press, 1996), 422–23. For the full list of the elements of the application, see *Walter Benjamin Gesammelte Schriften*, vol. 1, part 3, 898.
82. Walter Benjamin, "Curriculum Vitae Dr. Walter Benjamin" (no. 6), 6 in *Walter Benjamin, Selected Writings Vol. 4: 1938–1940*, eds. Howard Eiland and Michael W. Jennings, trans. Edmund Jephcott et al. (Belknap Press of Harvard University Press, 2003), 382.
83. Lucie Adelsberger to Mr. Dr. E. Libman, January 5, 1941, box 1, folder 15, ACEPR, IHRCA, UMN. For a brief discussion of the "emergency visitor visas" and the work of Varian Fry in assisting about two thousand refugees to escape before the State Department pulled Fry's visa, see Leff, *Well Worth Saving*, 200–201.
84. Harry D. Biele, Physicians' Committee, to Miss Mayerson, Migration Department, interoffice memorandum re: Luci Adelsberger, July 21, 1941; Dr. Emmanuel Libman, chairman of the Emergency Committee in Aid of Displaced Foreign Medical Scientists, to Dr. Adelsberger, unsent draft letter [n.d.]; Augusta Mayerson, Migration Department, to Carolina Sundheimer, Physicians' Committee, interoffice memorandum "Re: Dossier Enclosed of Dr. Lucie Adelsberger, Berlin Germany," August 14, 1941, box 1, folder 15, ACEPR, IHRCA, UMN.
85. "Case Notes for Lucie Adelsberger," November 14, 1946, Lucie Adelsberger, box 1, folder 15, ACEPR, IHRCA, UMN. Her file was closed in 1947. On hostility to competition from émigré physicians and state medical licensing barriers, see Davie, *Refugees in America*, 257–86. The digitization of medical and scientific journals makes it possible to trace in rough outline the course of Adelsberger's life as a medical research scholar, beginning from articles in German journals in the 1920s, identifying her affiliation with the Robert Koch Institute, coming to an abrupt halt in the mid-1930s, and resuming in 1951, now written in English and published in American journals, identifying her institutional affiliation as the Laboratory Division of the Montefiore Hospital, NY, NY. The last article I have found is from 1965. A March 1946 article in *The Lancet*, identifying her as an MD in Amsterdam, begins to fill in the gap for the war years. Her 1959 memoir would do so more fully. Adelsberger died in New York City, in November 1971, well before that memoir was translated into English and published in the United States.

chapter five: "made to man's order"

1. "Police Probe Cowboy-Suit Tragedies," *Times-Herald* (Washington, DC), April 9, 1945, 17; Interrogatory of Elwyn Jones, October 14, 1947, 1a, Jones Case File.
2. The phrase "land of desire" was first used by John Wanamaker, the founder of the department store bearing his last name. See William Leach, *Land of Desire: Mer-*

chants, Power, and the Rise of a New American Culture (Vintage Books, 1994), xiii–xv.

3. On the American toy industry, the commercialization of childhood, and the commodification of play, see Leach, *Land of Desire*, 85–90; William Leach, "Child-World in the Promised Land," in *The Mythmaking Frame of Mind: Social Imagination and American Culture*, ed. James Gilbert, Amy Gilman, Donald M. Scott, and Joan W. Scott (Wadsworth Publishing Co., 2003), 209–38; Howard P. Chudacoff, *Children at Play: An American History* (NYU Press, 2007), 116–22; Lisa Jacobson, *Raising Consumers: Children and the American Mass Market in the Early Twentieth Century* (Columbia University Press, 2004); Gary Cross, *Kids' Stuff: Toys and the Changing World of American Childhood* (Harvard University Press, 1997); Bernard Mergen, "Made, Bought, and Stolen: Toys and the Culture of Childhood," in *Small Worlds: Children and Adolescents in America, 1850–1950*, eds. Elliott West and Paula Petrick (University of Kansas Press, 1992), 86–106; Stephen Kline, "Toys, Socialization and the Commodification of Play," in *Getting and Spending: European and American Consumer Societies in the Twentieth Century*, eds. Susan Strasser, Charles McGovern, and Matthias Jundt (Cambridge University Press, 1998), 339–58; Bernard Mergen, *Play and Playthings: A Reference Guide* (Greenwood Press, 1982).
4. *The Playthings Directory of the Toy Industry, 1925–1926* (McCready Publishing Co., 1925), 8–9; Leach, *Land of Desire*, 85, 328.
5. On the point that the advent of radio advertising in the 1930s extended the commercial reach of the new child world to rural and working-class children, see Jacobson, *Raising Consumers*, 2, 7.
6. In summer 1935, *Playthings* published an article titled "A Well Balanced Toy Department," a guide to buying based on sales figures for a toy department with total annual sales of $50,000. It was the sort of accounting that claims to represent but that in its very publication produces. Dolls (and related accessories) garnered over one-quarter of the sales at 26.3 percent ($13,150), mechanical toys 16.2 percent ($8,100), "wheel goods" and games 15 percent ($7,500) each, and sporting goods 4.4 percent ($2,200). Play suits made the list. Barely. Of the $50,000 in sales, play suits accounted for 3.6 percent ($1,800). Republished in *The Playthings Directory of the Toy Industry, 1936* (McCready Publishing Co., 1936), 30–32.
7. In 1933, the company was named the Feinberg-Henry Co. The name was changed in 1943 to the M. A. Henry Co. See *The Playthings Directory of the Toy Industry, 1934–1935* (McCready Publishing Co., 1934–1935), 60, 213; *Playthings Directory of the Toy Industry, 1936*, 63, 171, 232.
8. *Playthings Directory of the Toy Industry, 1938*, 228.
9. The date of the contract between Autry and Feinberg-Henry Mfg. Co. was December 22, 1940, with a starting date of April 21, 1941. See Interrogatories of Gene Autry, 1949, Peterson Case File; *The Playthings Directory, 1939* (McCready Publishing Co., 1939), 228.
10. The Melody Ranch radio program began broadcasting in 1939. See Holly George-Warren, *Public Cowboy No. 1: The Life and Times of Gene Autry* (Oxford University Press, 2007), 188–89.

11. Testimony of Milton A. Henry, 265, McCormack Record on Appeal.
12. "New Firms," *Textile America* 1–2 (November 6, 1897): 9.
13. Testimony of William E. Roschen, 702, McCormack Record on Appeal.
14. "Otto Timme" (obituary), *Women's Wear Daily*, August 11, 1937, 29.
15. When Otto's father, Edward, had died at the age of seventy in 1919, the firm was well enough known in the fabric business that an obituary appeared in the trade journal the *Upholsterer and Interior Decorator*. See "Edward F. Timme," *Upholsterer and Interior Decorator* 61 (May 1919): 79.
16. William E. was the son of William Roschen and Emilie Timme—one of Edward Timme's daughters.
17. Testimony of William E. Roschen, 704–5, McCormack Record on Appeal.
18. Testimony of William E. Roschen, 140, 702–6, 726, and Testimony of Arthur Robertshaw Jr., 851–52, McCormack Record on Appeal; Memorandum of Agreement, January 1, 1942, between the Estate of Otto Timme, doing business as E. F. Timme & Son, and Woonsocket Falls Mill (Plaintiff's Exhibit 17), 1154–58, McCormack Record on Appeal. Prior to the war there had apparently been some variation in the contract rate Woonsocket paid to Timme, but with the war, Timme and Woonsocket signed a contract for a flat 7 percent rate on net sales.
19. Testimony of William E. Roschen (examination before trial), 174–76, Testimony of Arthur Robertshaw Jr. (examination before trial), 193–97, 512–17, Plaintiff's Exhibit 17 (Memorandum of Agreement between E. F. Timme & Son and Woonsocket Falls Mill), 1154–59, McCormack Record on Appeal.
20. In contrast to the textile industry in the United States more generally, rayon production was highly concentrated in a few firms. See David A. Hounshell and John Kenly Smith Jr., *Science and Corporate Strategy: Du Pont R&D, 1902–1980* (Cambridge University Press, 1988), 162; Grace Hutchins, *Labor and Silk* (International Publishers, 1929), 63–65; Paul David Blanc, *Fake Silk: The Lethal History of Viscose Rayon* (Yale University Press, 2016), 58–59.
21. The major producers in the US were Viscose, Glanzstoff, and Bemberg. See Hutchins, *Labor and Silk*, 65.
22. On Du Pont's transformation from a firm focused solely on the manufacture of explosives to a highly diversified chemical company, see Hounshell and Smith, *Science and Corporate Strategy*; and Alfred D. Chandler Jr., *Strategy and Structure: Chapters in the History of the Industrial Enterprise* (MIT Press, 1962), 52–113.
23. Hounshell and Smith, *Science and Corporate Strategy*, 163–67.
24. Testimony of Arthur Robertshaw, 205, Testimony of William E. Roschen, 240–41, Testimony of P. F. Brown (Director of Sales, Rayon Division, Du Pont), 161–64, Record in Lutz; "Du Pont Rayon" trademark 207, 203, registered December 22, 1925, acc. no. 500, series 2, part 2, v. 611, 11, E. I. Du Pont de Nemours and Company Archives, Hagley Museum and Library Archives, Wilmington, DE. Hereafter Du Pont Collection.
25. E. F. Timme & Son Invoice to Feinberg and Henry Mfg Company, March 18, 1942, Plaintiff's Exhibit 16; Testimony of William E. Roschen, 710, 736, Testimony of Arthur B. Robertshaw Jr., 853, 911, McCormack Record on Appeal.
26. Testimony of Arthur B. Robertshaw Jr., 853, McCormack Record on Appeal.
27. Exhibit 49, compilation of Du Pont sales of viscose rayon yarn to Woonsocket Falls

Mill, 1940–1945, 159–60, Stenographer's Minutes, Record in Lutz (before Hon. J. Waties Waring).

28. "This Magic Called Rayon," *Harper's Bazaar* (October 1939): 92–93, 110.
29. "This Magic Called Rayon." For more technical descriptions of the "viscose process," see Hounshell and Smith, *Science and Corporate Strategy*, 163; Rutledge Scrapbooks, acc. no. 500, series 2, part 2, v. 611, 5, Du Pont Collection; and Robert B. Evans, "Survey of Development and Use of Rayon and Other Synthetic Fibers," October 1944, United States Department of Agriculture, Agricultural Research Administration, Bureau of Agricultural and Industrial Chemistry, Southern Regional Research Laboratory, New Orleans, LA, 5–6. Hounshell and Smith do not address the toxicity of carbon bisulfide, the chemical key to producing the yellow viscous liquid in the first stage of the process; Paul David Blanc does. In *Fake Silk*, Blanc shows that manufacturers knowingly exposed workers to the hazards of carbon bisulfide.
30. Hounshell and Smith, *Science and Corporate Strategy*, 164–65.
31. Hounshell and Smith, *Science and Corporate Strategy*, 162.
32. For Charch's biography, see Herbert T. Pratt, "William Hale Charch," in *American Chemists and Chemical Engineers*, ed. Wyndham D. Miles (American Chemical Society, 1976), 76–77; Robert E. Ellsworth, "Personality. They Do Something About Ideas! It's W. Hale Charch and His Investigators Who Dream Up Promising New Textile Fibers," *Modern Textiles Magazine* 34, no. 7 (July 1953): 36, 45, 78–79; Hounshell and Smith, *Science and Corporate Structure*, 175–76, 180–82. The only lab that included some women as researchers was Hale Charch's Pioneering Research lab. See Hounshell and Smith, *Science and Corporate Strategy*, 287–97.
33. Hounshell and Smith, *Science and Corporate Strategy*, 309.
34. See Hounshell and Smith on the "innovation strategy" adopted by the management of Du Pont in the 1920s (*Science and Corporate Strategy*, 119–20).
35. For an example of an exchange that captures both the internal corporate conversations in the development of new fibers and the interactions with the "trade" (manufacturers who wove Du Pont fibers into fabrics)—in this case, E. F. Timme & Son—see the following series of letters, each titled "Fibers for the Plush Industry": B. H. Bossidy to Dr. W. H. Charch, May 9, 1939, box 14, folder PV-4B Viscose: Fiber D Field & Fabric Tests, January–June 1939, series 1: Pioneering Research Division, sub-series A: Chronological Files, acc. no. 1771, Du Pont Fibers, Du Pont Collection; Manfred Keller to Charch, May 9, 1939, also in box 14; Charch to Keller, May 11, 1939, box 14; and Waldemar Kuenzel to Charch, September 18, 1940, box 16, folder PV-8 Viscose: Fiber E, 1940, series 1: Pioneering Research Division, sub-series A: Chronological Files, acc. no. 1771, Du Pont Fibers, Du Pont Collection.
36. Du Pont men in the development and research divisions knew what fabric manufacturers were making from their fibers. The collaborative character of R&D assured that. But even apart from the visits, the phone conversations, the written correspondence, and buyers' uses were meticulously recorded on corporate "Trade Reports" forms. See, e.g., "Trade Report, 3/20/41, Buyer E.F. Timme & Son, Person Interviewed Mr. William Roschen," box 14, folder PV-4 Viscose: Fiber D, 1941, series 1: Pioneering Research Division, sub-series A: Chronological Files, acc. no.

1771: Du Pont Fibers, Du Pont Collection. Corporate letters nominally from one man in the Development Section to one man in Pioneering Research included not only a long list of "ccs" but also a stamped list of other individuals to whom the letter had been circulated. Scribbled initials and checkmarks signified that a letter had been received and read. "Progress and Status Reports" provided regular updates on the range of fabrics for which a fiber was being considered and used for and by which buyers. See, e.g., "Progress & Status Report Fiber D Carpet Development, PN-124," February 10, 1940, box 16, folder PV-VB Viscose Fiber D, Field & Fabric Tests, 1940, series 1: Pioneering Research Division, sub-series A: Chronological Files, acc. no. 1771, Du Pont Fibers, Du Pont Collection.

37. In the late 1930s, Timme was on the verge of breaking into the lucrative automobile upholstery market. Correspondence between Manfred Keller of the Development Section; Dr. W. H. Charch, director of Pioneering Research, and Roschen illustrates the collaborative character of product development. See Manfred Keller to Dr. W. H. Charch, July 18, 1939, box 14, folder PV-VB Viscose: Fiber D Field & Fabric Tests, July–December 1939, series 1: Pioneering Research Division, sub-series A: Chronological Files, acc. no. 1771, Du Pont Fibers, Du Pont Collection. For other correspondence with Timme re: automobile upholstery, see Manfred Keller to Dr. W. F. Underwood, January 5, 1939; W. F. Underwood to Manfred Keller, January 5, 1939, both also in box 14.
38. Woonsocket made its first high-pile fabrics with rayon in 1938. The fabric that Henry settled on was one that Woonsocket first began making in 1940. See Testimony of Arthur B. Robertshaw Jr., 865–66, McCormack Record on Appeal; W. H. Charch to Manfred Keller, "Subject: Fibers for the Plush Industry," May 11, 1939 (referring back to Woonsocket's first test in 1938 and noting the excitement at Du Pont of producing a fiber that Timme could use in "certain types of plushes, particularly the long pile plush where we obtain a very woolly effect," which would be a "unique fiber without competition."), box 14, folder PV-4B Viscose, Fiber D Field & Fabric Tests, January–June, 1939, series 1: Pioneering Research Division, sub-series A: Chronological Files, acc. no. 1771, Du Pont Fibers, Du Pont Collection.
39. Testimony of Dr. Lester S. Sinness, director, Viscose Rayon Research Section, Du Pont, 176, 182–83, Record in Lutz.
40. William J. Novak, *The People's Welfare: Law and Regulation in Nineteenth-Century America* (University of North Carolina Press, 1996), 51–82.
41. On the Triangle Shirtwaist Fire, see Leon Stein, *The Triangle Fire* (Lippincott, 1962).
42. See ch. 7, "Playing with Fire."
43. On the increase in product liability claims, see "Product Liability Becoming Big Program for Retailer," *National Underwriter*, June 25, 1936, 30.
44. "Flameproofing of Textiles," May 1936, letter circular LC 467, Department of Commerce, National Bureau of Standards, Washington, DC.
45. The bibliography was compiled by Emily Williams Akin as part of her MA thesis in home economics and was published over two issues of the journal. See Emily Williams Akin, Prof. Lilly H. Spencer, and Dr. A. R. Macormac, "Bibliography on Flameproofing of Textiles," *American Dyestuff Reporter*, August 19, 1940, 418–20;

September 2, 1940, 445–51. Reflecting the gendered division of academic departments in this era, her home economics professor (Spencer) was female; her chemistry professor (Macormac) was male.

46. Testimony of Arthur B. Robertshaw Jr., 214–29, McCormack Record on Appeal.
47. Testimony of Philip P. Brown, director of sales, Rayon Division, Du Pont, 174, Record in Lutz.
48. On the pattern of businesses shifting the costs of injury and death, see, for example, Allan M. Brandt, *The Cigarette Century: The Rise, Fall, and Deadly Persistence of the Product That Defined America* (Basic Books, 2007); Sarah S. Lochlann Jain, *Injury: The Politics of Product Design and Safety Law in the U.S.* (Princeton University Press, 2006); Sally H. Clarke, *Trust and Power: Consumers, the Modern Corporation, and the Making of the United States Automobile Market* (Cambridge University Press, 2007); Gerald Markowitz and David Rosner, *Deceit and Denial: The Deadly Politics of Industrial Pollution* (University of California Press, 2002); Laura Nader, *The Life of the Law: Anthropological Projects* (University of California Press, 2002), esp. 158–211; Ralph Nader, *Unsafe at Any Speed: The Designed-In Dangers of the American Automobile* (Grossman, 1965).
49. Manfred Keller to Dr. W. H. Church, April 28, 1939, box 14, folder PV-4B Viscose: Fiber D Field & Fabric Tests, January–June, 1939, series 1: Pioneering Research Division, sub-series A: Chronological Files, acc. no. 1771, Du Pont Fibers, Du Pont Collection.
50. W. H. Charch to Manfred Keller, May 2, 1939, box 14, folder PV-4B Viscose: Fiber D Field & Fabric Tests, January–June, 1939, series 1: Pioneering Research Division, sub-series A: Chronological Files, acc. no. 1771, Du Pont Fibers, Du Pont Collection.
51. E. W. Spangel to G. P. Hoff, March 20, 1945, box 74, Du Pont Fibers, folder Technical Information Files—Flammability, 1941–1945, 1949, 1983, series 3: Technical Service Section, acc. no. 1771, Du Pont Fibers, Du Pont Collection.
52. For a description of the process by which the Woonsocket Falls Mill produced the high-pile fabrics from Du Pont rayon, see Testimony of Arthur B. Robertshaw Jr., 855–62, McCormack Record on Appeal.
53. Testimony of William E. Roschen, 800–817, McCormack Record on Appeal.
54. Testimony of Milton A. Henry, 355; M. A. Henry to E. F. Timme & Son, February 19, 1942, Defendants Timme and Woonsocket's Exhibit TW4; and Henry Bullwinkel to M. A. Henry, February 20, 1942, Defendants Timme and Woonsocket's Exhibit TW5, 344–45, 1190–92; all in McCormack Record on Appeal.
55. It is not entirely clear whether Henry was seeing which fabric customers liked best or ordering what he could get most quickly from Timme at the moment, but in the first six months (March–September 1942) Henry worked with Timme, he used several different fabrics, two that were high-pile but of slightly different color and two that were of a lower pile, all of which were rayon with cotton backing. From October 1942 to March 1945, all Henry's orders were for Peachfox Fluffy. Defendants Timme and Woonsocket's Exhibit TW3, 1188–89, McCormack Record on Appeal.
56. Deposition of Gene Autry (in Weatherell), October 29, 1947, 8, Peterson Case File; Deposition of Gene Autry (in Peterson), October 1949, 5, box 1, Agents & Licensees, T94-45-30, folder M. A. Henry Legal 1948–1949, Autry Collection.

57. George-Warren, *Public Cowboy No. 1*, 204.
58. Testimony of Milton A. Henry, 278, McCormack Record on Appeal.
59. This number is from Louis Lutz who sold the suits in his Lou's Auto Stores in 1944 and 1945. It also fits evidence from other cases. See Testimony of Louis P. Lutz, 106–7, Record in Lutz.
60. Ralph Merle Hower, *History of Macy's of New York, 1858–1919: Chapters in the Evolution of the Department Store* (Harvard University Press, 1943), 237–44, 403. The author's preface details Hower's access to Macy's records. For a brief, broad gloss on department stores' response to the war and its impact on their inventories, practices, and profits, see Vicki Howard, *From Main Street to Mall: The Rise and Fall of the American Department Store* (University of Pennsylvania Press, 2015), 114–31.
61. Hower, *History of Macy's of New York*, 403. The year cited here is 1939. Hower was an assistant professor of business history and administration at the Harvard Graduate School of Business when he began work in 1938 on his study of Macy's. As was true for so many, the war changed his direction in life. As part of the staff of the chief quartermaster for the European theater of operations, he worked on final plans for the Normandy invasion, received multiple commendations, and by the time he was discharged held the rank of colonel. In the years after the war, his work turned to developing schools of business administration abroad and consulting for large companies, including Esso, Shell, Eli Lilly, and Du Pont. His consulting took his scholarly work in a new direction. He never returned to his second planned volume on Macy's. "Ralph Hower, 69, of Harvard, Dies," (obituary), *New York Times*, August 4, 1973, 26.
62. I have wondered whether Macy's didn't sell the suit because it did not fit its clientele or possibly because it did not pass muster with the Macy's Bureau of Standards. Macy's established a Bureau of Standards in 1927. Hower suggests it was "probably the first one to appear in a retail store" in the US. And explains that by the early 1940s, the bureau was testing goods at the rate of over two thousand analyses per month. See Hower, *History of Macy's*, 403.
63. Testimony of Milton A. Henry, 409, McCormack Record on Appeal.
64. Godfrey M. Lebhar, *Chain Stores in America, 1859–1962*, 3rd ed. (Chain Store Publishing Corporation, 1963), has data for major individual chain stores by years, including the years of the war (see appendix, "Growth of Leading Chains in Selected Categories," 391–415) and also a table ("Retail Census, 1929, 1939, 1948, 1954 and 1958," table 15, 74–77) that provides collective numbers for retail sales and also by category (e.g., "Variety Stores," "Dry Goods and General Merchandise Stores," "Department Stores," etc.) so that one can see the change between 1939 and 1948. Across the board, total sales between 1939 and 1948 rose dramatically.
65. Lebhar, *Chain Stores in America*, 3rd ed., 401 (appendix, "Growth of Leading Chains: McCrory Stores Corporation"). See also Interrogatories of Milton A. Henry, November 4, 1947, Habina Case File (list of Henry Co. Gene Autry Official Ranch Outfit sales to McCrory Stores Corporation for 1942 and 1943).
66. See Interrogatories of Milton A. Henry, November 4, 1947, Habina Case File. For a "comprehensive" history of McCrory's, see *Chain Store Age, Variety Store Edition* (June 1962). McCrory's is also one of the chain stores included in Lebhar, *Chain Stores in America*, 3rd ed.

67. *The Playthings Directory of the Toy Industry, 1925–1926* (McCready Publishing Co., 1925), 5. See also Leach, *Land of Desire*, 329.
68. Testimony of Louis P. Lutz, 70–71, Record in Lutz.
69. Testimony of Louis P. Lutz, 94, Record in Lutz.
70. Testimony of Louis P. Lutz, 29, 83–85, Record in Lutz.
71. Deposition of Ben C. Hamilton, Terre Haute, IN, September 12, 1949, Cizek Case File.
72. Consider also City Hall Hardware Co. in Pawtucket, Rhode Island, which was selling the suit in 1944 and still selling it in 1947. See Affidavit of Edmond B. Butler, February 2, 1951, Caparco Case File; Affidavit of Edmond B. Butler, June 19, 1951, Szumita Case File.
73. Deposition of Kathryn Timberlake, Kansas City, MO, September 15, 1950, 275, Timberlake Case File.
74. See ch. 18, "public cowboy no. 1."

chapter six: global war

1. For examples of émigré scholars appearing in placement files, see box 7, folder 4, University of Chicago Department of History Records, UChicago; box 9, folder 81, University of Minnesota Department of Political Science, and box 11, folder Faculty Candidates with PhD, 1943–1946, School of Chemistry Records, UA, UMN; box 12, folder 12 (vitae in this file date from 1938 to 1947), Princeton University Department of Politics, PUA. The field of physics represented a distinct case. But this was because by 1941, as Daniel Kevles notes, "more than one hundred foreign physicists, including eight past and future Nobel Prize winners, had found academic posts in the United States." See Daniel Kevles, *The Physicists: The History of a Scientific Community in Modern America* (Harvard University Press, 1995), 281.
2. Eric Fischer, "Memoir" (unpublished, ca. 1984), part II, "Years of Wandering," 1, 3, Eric Fischer, AR 5534, LBI (hereafter Fischer Papers, LBI).
3. Fischer, "Memoir," part II, 34 ("Job Applications"). For other examples of vitae in files in the war years, with or without a cover letter, with no evidence of a reply, see, e.g., John Hornbostel to H. D. Smyth, April 11, 1940, box 2, folder 2, Princeton University Department of Physics Records, PUA; Kurt Wohl, "Curriculum Vitae of Kurt Wohl," ca. 1943, box 11, folder Faculty Candidates with PhD, 1943–1946, UMN School of Chemistry Records, UA, UMN; Rudolf Ernst Freund, vita, ca. 1946, box 7, folder 4, University of Chicago Department of History Records, UChicago; Richard Sallet, "Qualifications Dr. Richard Sallet," ca. 1938, and Walter Schiffer, "Personal History and Qualifications," ca. 1945, box 12, folder 12, Princeton University Department of Politics Records (AC 166), PUA.
4. Eric Fischer, "Autobiographical Statement" and "List of Publications," with cover letter to Bernadotte E. Schmitt, February 29, 1944, and to William T. Hutchinson, March 10, 1944, box 7, folder 4, University of Chicago Department of History Records, UChicago.
5. See, e.g., Franz Landsberger, PhD. vita, ca. 1939, Franz Landsberger Collection, AR

2318, LBI; David Baumgardt, vita, ca. 1939, David Baumgardt Collection, MF 553, LBI; Ernst Hamburger, "Curriculum," ca. 1940, Ernst Hamburger Collection, AR 7034, LBI.

6. Eric Fischer, *Memoir*, part II, 47 ("jobs in wartime Washington"), Fischer Papers, LBI.
7. See Cornelia Visman, *Files: Law and Media Technology* (Stanford University Press, 2008), 168–70; Nicholas Blomley, "Making Private Property: Enclosure, Common Right and the Work of Hedges," *Rural History* 18, no. 1 (2007): 1–21. I see the curriculum vitae as doing something akin to the hedge for the self.
8. Fischer, "Autobiographical Statement" and "List of Publications."
9. The mobilization of higher education for war began in advance of the US declaration of war. See American Council on Education Studies, *Organizing Higher Education for National Defense: The Report of a Conference Called by the National Committee on Education and Defense, Held in Washington, D.C., February 6, 1941*, series 1, vol. 5, no. 13 (American Council on Education Studies, March 1941). On the mobilization of science for war, see A. Hunter Dupree, "The *Great Instauration* of 1940: The Organization of Scientific Research for War," in *The Twentieth-Century Sciences: Studies in the Biography of Ideas*, ed. Gerald Holton (W. W. Norton and Company, Inc., 1972), 443–67.
10. "Memo to Graduate Students re Teaching/War Research for Academic Year 1941–42," n.d. (ca. early March 1941), box 2, folder 1, Princeton University Department of Physics (AC 133), PUA.
11. On the history of resistance to government funding and applied research, see Roger L. Geiger, *The History of American Higher Education: Learning and Culture from the Founding to World War II* (Princeton University Press, 2015); and Geiger, *To Advance Knowledge: The Growth of American Research Universities, 1900–1940* (Routledge, 2004).
12. Wayne W. Johnson to head, Department of Chemistry, December 21, 1943, box 12, folder Placement File-Academic 1944, University of Pennsylvania Department of Chemistry Records, UPenn.
13. See, e.g., Celanese Corporation of America, "Staff Employment Application," and Monsanto Chemical Company, "Application for Employment," box 12, folder Placement File-Industrial 1943, University of Pennsylvania Department of Chemistry Records, UPenn; Eastman Kodak Company, "Personal Qualification Record," box 11, folder 6, Princeton University Department of Physics Records (AC 133), PUA; Du Pont, "Qualification Record," and Naugatuck Chemical, "Technical Employment Application," box 12, folder Placement File-Industrial 1944, University of Pennsylvania Department of Chemistry, UPenn.
14. See, e.g., Earl C. Spaeth, "Personal Data Sheet of Earl C. Spaeth," January 13, 1946, and Gilbert H. Ayres, "Education and Experience Record of Gilbert H. Ayres," ca. November 1945, both in box 11, folder Faculty Candidates with PhDs, 1943–1946, University of Minnesota, School of Chemistry Records, UA, UMN.
15. For an example of the "Outline of Curriculum Vitae" form from 1940 (before it became part of the registration form), see E. B., box 3, folder 62, ACEPR, IHRCA, UMN. For an example of the four-page registration form, including the "Outline of Curriculum Vitae" blank, as used from 1941 to 1944, see, e.g., A. S. (registered

1941), box 21, folder A. S.; D. A. (registered 1942), box 1, folder 9; J. A. (registered 1943), box 1, folder 12, ACEPR, IHRCA, UMN. For an example of the two-page registration form that the ACEP began using in 1945, see H. M. (registered 1945), box 15, folder H. M., ACEPR, IHRCA, UMN. For examples of curricula vitae in the files more generally, see, e.g., Lucie Adelsberger, "Curriculum Vitae," Berlin, August 26, 1938 (chronological narrative organized by dates on left-hand margin), box 1, folder 15; E. K. (registered 1940), "Curriculum Vitae," March 29, 1940 (one page in English narrative), box 12, folder E. K.; A. S. (registered 1941), "Curriculum Vitae," ca. August 1941 (one page in English, narrative), box 21, folder A. S., ACEPR, IHRCA, UMN.

16. See, e.g., J. A., "Curriculum Vitae," ca. 1939, and "Curriculum Vitae," ca. 1940, box 1, folder 17, ACEPR, IHRCA, UMN. For an example of a narrative "Career of Life" in English by a German medical doctor hoping to emigrate but written while he was still in Germany in 1937 and sent to the ACEP, see A. F., "Career of Life," Hamburg, April 16, 1937, box 6, folder 15, ACEPR, IHRCA, UMN.
17. S. C. Lind to H. S. Brown, October 21, 1945, letter and reply with completed blank enclosed from Harrison S. Brown to S. C. Lind, November 20, 1945, box 11, folder Faculty Candidates with PhDs, 1945, University of Minnesota School of Chemistry Records, UA, UMN. For other examples, see, e.g., Robert B. Duffield to S. C. Lind, November 16, 1945, with completed Request for Information enclosed, and S. C. English to S. C. Lind, April 9, 1945, with completed Request for Information blank enclosed, both also in box 11, folder Faculty Candidates with PhDs, 1945, University of Minnesota School of Chemistry Records, UA, UMN.
18. See box 11, folder Faculty Candidates with PhDs, 1945, and folder Faculty Candidates with PhDs, 1943–1946, University of Minnesota School of Chemistry Records, UA, UMN.
19. I refer to the queries directed to department chairs and other leading men seeking recommendations of candidates for positions, by the shorthand "'we want a man' letters" because this phrase uniformly appeared—indeed, often repeatedly in a single letter. For examples, see the correspondence of the following men: A. C. McLaughlin, chair, History Department, University of Chicago; Ernest Burgess, Sociology Department, University of Chicago; and H. D. Smyth, chair, Physics Department Princeton University—in, respectively, box 15, folder 1, University of Chicago Department of History Records, UChicago; Ernest Watson Burgess Papers, box 17, folder 11, Department of Sociology, University of Chicago, UChicago; and box 11, folder 6 Recommendations, 1935–1936, Princeton University Department of Physics Records (AC 133), PUA.
20. Consider, for example, the Manhattan Project (tasked with building an atomic bomb), located at Los Alamos in New Mexico, and the Research Branch of the Special Services Division of the War Department, based in Washington, DC (tasked with carrying out research on the attitudes of enlisted men in the army), and the OSS. See Kay Bird and Martin J. Sherwin, *American Prometheus: The Triumph and Tragedy of J. Robert Oppenheimer* (Alfred A. Knopf, 2005); Kevles, *Physicists*; Samuel A. Stouffer, Edward A Suchman, Leland C. DeVinney, Shirley A. Star, and Robin M. Williams Jr., *The American Soldier: Adjustment During Army Life*, vol. 1 (Princeton University Press, 1949), xi–xii (list of the professional and

administrative personnel), ch. 1; John A. Clausen, "*The American Soldier* and Social Psychology: Introduction," *Social Psychology Quarterly* 47, no. 2 (1984): 184–85; Joseph W. Ryan, *Samuel Stouffer and the GI Survey: Sociologists and Soldiers During the Second World War* (University of Tennessee Press, 2013); and Ellen Herman, *The Romance of American Psychology: Political Culture in the Age of Experts* (University of California Press, 1995).

21. Historian of education scholar V. R. Cardozier refers to a series of studies of various institutions and within them of various disciplines relating to faculty drawn into war service in one way or another. Resignations and leaves of absence were not evenly distributed among institutions or across disciplines, but many institutions lost 20 to 25 percent of their faculty to military service, the government, war industries, and other positions. See V. R. Cardozier, *Colleges and Universities in World War II* (Praeger, 1993), 183–210.
22. L. H. Farinholt to Dean S. C. Lind, April 30, 1943, University of Minnesota School of Chemistry Records, box 9, folder Requests for Recommendations for Positions Available in Other Institutions or Industry, UA, UMN.
23. Fischer's appointment at Bard offers another example of the importance of émigré networks in learning of and securing academic appointments.
24. For a description of the Army, Navy, and Air Force programs, see Cardozier, *Colleges and Universities in World War II*, ch. 2, 3, 4, and 6. Military services college training programs cushioned the loss in nonmilitary enrollments, but their distribution was uneven: Large institutions nationally and northeastern colleges benefited far more than others. See Henry G. Badger and Benjamin W. Frazier (US Office of Education), "Effects of the War upon Colleges and Universities, 1943–44," *Bulletin AAUP* 30, no. 2 (Summer 1944): 265–83; Walter Crosby Eells, "The Plight of the Colleges," *Bulletin AAUP* 29, no. 4 (October 1943): 508–17.
25. For a cursory sketch of the broad range of academic fields from which faculty were drawn into the OSS, see Cardozier, *Colleges and Universities in World War II*, 20–4 (anthropology, geography, language experts, geology, political science, history, music (for cryptology work), chemistry, engineering, and physics). As historian Ellen Herman notes, far more is known about the Research and Analysis Branch of the OSS headed by historian William A. Langer from 1942 to 1946, than is known about the Psychological Division directed by University of California psychologist Robert C. Tryon, the names of those employed by the latter after 1942 remaining confidential. Langer's operation gives one a sense of the scale. It employed "around a thousand researchers in Washington and another five hundred around the world by the end of the war: mainly historians with a sprinkling of social scientists." See Herman, *Romance of American Psychology*, 43–47, 328–29 (n. 102 and 103).
26. Bernadotte Schmitt, of the University of Chicago's History Department, offers one example of a senior scholar who held a tenured appointment to which he could and did return at the end of the war. But the war also proved an engine of academic mobility more generally. Two senior geographers with whom Eric Fischer worked offer examples. Preston E. James was a full professor at Michigan when he was drawn into war service as a geographer. In 1945, rather than returning to Michigan, he accepted a position at Syracuse University. The position he took had been held by Sidman P. Poole before the war. Poole, trained at Syracuse, had been on the

faculty there since 1921, working his way up from instructor to full professor. From 1940 to 1946, he was in government service: chief of the Topographic Bureau of the War Department. In 1946, he became chair of the Department of Geography at the University of Virginia, a position he held until his death in 1955. See "Biography," Preston E. James Papers, Syracuse University Archives, accessed September 28, 2025, https://library.syracuse.edu/digital/guides_sua/html/sua_james_pe_prt.htm; "Dr. Sidman Poole, Geographer, Dead; Department Chairman at U. of Virginia Was Head of Army Topographic Unit" (obituary), *New York Times*, October 30, 1955, 88.

27. F. W. Loomis, associate director, Radiation Laboratory, MIT, announcement, August. 14, 1945, box 11, folder Recommendations for Positions Outside of I.T., University of Minnesota School of Chemistry Records, UA, UMN.
28. F. W. Loomis to S. C. Lind, September 24, 1945 (with enclosure "Assistant Professorship at the University of Minnesota"), box 11, folder Recommendations for Positions Outside of I.T., University of Minnesota School of Chemistry Records, UA, UMN.
29. G. B. Kistiakowsky to L. H. Reyerson, November 2, 1945 (plus enclosures), box 11, folder Faculty Candidates with PhDs, 1945, University of Minnesota School of Chemistry Records, UA, UMN. Correspondence of this sort did not take the place of more individualized promotion of candidates. John Clausen describes the operation of these networks after the war as a boon to young scholars' careers and quotes one of his former colleagues, Nathan Maccoby: "'The Research Branch not only established one of the best old-boy (or girl) networks ever, but an alumnus of the Branch had an open door to most relevant jobs and career lines. We were a lucky bunch.'" Clausen notes that each of the senior scholars in the branch took with them or later hired colleagues and students from the branch. See John A. Clausen, "Research on the American Soldier as a Career Contingency," *Social Psychology Quarterly* 47, no. 2 (June 1984): 210–12.
30. Paul C. Cross to S. C. Lind, October 29, 1945, box 11, folder Faculty Candidates with PhDs, 1945, University of Minnesota School of Chemistry Records, UA, UMN.
31. Cross to Lind, October 29, 1945.
32. "Information Concerning: Paul M. Fye," n.d., box 11, folder Faculty Candidates with PhDs, 1945, University of Minnesota School of Chemistry Records, UA, UMN.
33. S. C. Lind to Dr. Paul C. Cross, November 9, 1945, box 11, folder Faculty Candidates with PhDs, 1945, University of Minnesota School of Chemistry Records, UA, UMN.
34. War research laboratories on university campuses like the Metallurgical Laboratory at the University of Chicago, the Jet Propulsion Laboratory at Caltech, and the Radiation Laboratory at MIT, along with the Manhattan Project, offer the most obvious examples. But senior scholars recruited into war work that required them to relocate also took with them prized students, as for example, physics students at Princeton joining Princeton physics faculty in work on the Manhattan Project or students joining faculty in the War Research Branch, Special Services Division, US Army.

35. Thomas L. Jacobs to Lee Irvin Smith, January 10, 1946; Earl C. Spaeth to Lee Irvin Smith, n.d. (enclosure "Personal Data Sheet of Earl C. Spaeth"), box 11, folder Faculty Candidates with PhDs, 1943–1946, University of Minnesota School of Chemistry Records, UA, UMN.
36. Harold W. Dodds to George Graham, interoffice correspondence, "Subject: Letter of Dec. 31 from John Stevens in re Position for James M. Burns," January 6, 1947, box 12, folder 12, Princeton University Department of Politics Records (AC 166), PUA.
37. George A. Graham to Harold W. Dodds, interoffice correspondence re: "The Letter of John Stevens Recommending James M. Burns," January 14, 1947; and George A. Graham to James M. Burns, January 14, 1947, both in box 12, folder 12, Princeton University Department of Politics Records (AC 166), PUA.
38. James M. Burns to George A. Graham, January 17, 1947 (with enclosure "Personal History"), box 12, folder 12, Princeton University Department of Politics Records (AC 166), PUA.
39. George A. Graham to James M. Burns, March 13, 1947 (job offer), and Burns's reply to Graham, March 16, 1947, box 12, folder 12, Princeton University Department of Politics Records (AC 166), PUA.
40. Lee N. Newcomer to William T. Hutchinson, April 3, 1946 (with enclosed "Outline of Record"), box 7, folder 4, University of Chicago Department of History Records, UChicago.
41. Martin Lichterman to William T. Hutchinson, July 16, 1946, box 7, folder 4, University of Chicago Department of History Records, UChicago. For other examples from this file, see Capt. Robert P. Fogerty, June 4, 1945; E. Douglas Webster, July 10, 1946; and Maurice S. Paprin, August 16, 1946. Letters from women are rare, but for one example in the same folder, a woman completing her PhD in history at Clark University, whose "husband has been discharged from the Service and will be at your university," see Roberta Schoenland, July 29, 1946 ("qualifications" included in letter in the format of a vita).
42. For other examples of men writing on their own behalf and including vita qualifications, see Gerald W. Sears to L. H. Reyerson, March 15, 1946, box 11, folder Faculty Candidates with PhDs, 1943–1946, University of Minnesota School of Chemistry Records, UA, UMN; Lt. Comdr. Gilbert H. Ayres to chairman, Department of Chemistry, University of Minnesota, November 30, 1945 (with photograph, "Education and Experience Record," list of publications, and LOA letter enclosed); reply from L. H. Reyerson, December 19, 1945; reply from Gilbert H. Ayres, December 23, 1945 (completed Request for Information enclosed); and "Not Interested" note, n.d., box 11, folder Faculty Candidates with PhDs, 1945, University of Minnesota School of Chemistry Records, UA, UMN.
43. Stouffer et al., *American Soldier: Adjustment During Army Life*, 6.
44. Something of Oppenheimer's defense of salary differentials at Los Alamos (pegged to individuals' previous jobs) speaks to this point. Explaining to a young physicist "why a plumber could earn nearly three times the pay of a college graduate, [Oppenheimer] replied that the plumbers had no idea of the laboratory's importance to the war effort, whereas the scientists did . . . The scientists, at least, were not working for the money." See Bird and Sherwin, *American Prometheus*, 216–17.

45. James M. Burns to George A. Graham, January 17, 1947, box 12, folder 12, Princeton University Department of Politics Records (AC 166), PUA.
46. Clausen, "Research on the American Soldier as a Career Contingency," 210.
47. *Studies in Social Psychology in World War II* (4 vols.): Stouffer et al., *American Soldier: Adjustment During Army Life*; Samuel A. Stouffer, Arthur A. Lumsdaine, Marion H. Lumsdaine, Robert M. Williams Jr., M. Brewster Smith, Irving L. Janis, et al., *The American Soldier: Combat and Its Aftermath*, vol. 2 (Princeton University Press, 1949); Carl I. Hovland, Arthur A. Lumsdaine, and Frederick D. Sheffield, *Experiments in Mass Communication* (Princeton University Press, 1949); and Samuel A. Stouffer, Louis Guttman, Edward A. Suchman, Paul F. Lazarsfeld, Shirley A. Star, and John A. Clausen, *Measurement and Prediction* (Princeton University Press, 1950).
48. Clausen, "Research on the American Soldier as a Career Contingency," 213.

chapter seven: "playing with fire"

1. *Cincinnati Enquirer*, November 5, 1942, 18; *N. W. Ayer & Son's Directory of Newspapers and Periodicals, 1942* (N. W. Ayer & Son, Inc., 1942), 741–43.
2. *Dayton Herald*, November 5, 1942, 18; *Mansfield (OH) News Journal*, November 5, 1942, 1; *Chronicle-Telegram* (Elyria, OH), November 5, 1942, 1; *Delphos Daily Herald*, November 5, 1942, 1.
3. *N. W. Ayer & Son's Directory of Newspapers and Periodicals, 1942*, 741–43.
4. Walter Arm, "Police Reporter," in Joseph G. Herzberg (and members of *The New York Herald Tribune* staff), *Late City Edition* (Henry Holt and Company, 1947), 25–35, at 27.
5. Viviana A. Zelizer, *Pricing the Priceless Child: The Changing Social Value of Children* (Basic Books, 1985), 3, 22–55; Susan J. Pearson, *The Birth Certificate: An American History* (UNC Press, 2021); Kriste Lindenmeyer, *"A Right to Childhood": The U. S. Children's Bureau and Child Welfare, 1912–1946* (University of Illinois Press, 1997); Joel A. Tarmand and Mark Tebeau, "Managing Danger in the Home Environment, 1900–1940" and John C. Burnham, "Why Did Infants and Toddlers Die? Shifts in Americans' Ideas of Responsibility for Accidents—From Blaming Mom to Engineering," *Journal of Social History* 29 (Summer 1996): 797–816, 817–37.
6. "Yule Gift Brings Tragedy to Boy, 11," *Democrat and Chronicle* (Rochester, NY), December 28, 1942, 25.
7. "Geneva Boy, 11, Dies of Burns," *Democrat and Chronicle* (Rochester, NY), December 29, 1942, 24.
8. "Boy's Burns Fatal," *Ithaca Journal*, December 28, 1942, 11; "Gift Causes Tragedy," *Ithaca Journal*, December 30, 1942, 7.
9. "Playing with Fire Costs Boy His Life: Eastside Brothers Set Grass Ablaze," *Herald-News* (Passaic, NJ), November 2, 1943, 1, 2.
10. There were at least two other incidents in Passaic in 1943 in which children were burned when their cowboy suits caught fire: Philip Contino (seven) (March 15, 1943) and John Sondej (nine) (September 30, 1943). Neither incident made the

news at the time. Like Stella Krzeczkowski, John Sondej's mother, Frances, was employed by and had purchased the cowboy suit for her son from the M. A. Henry Co. in 1943. See Complaint, January 14, 1949, 2, Sondej Case File.

11. Documenting absences is challenging, but I have checked the *Bergen News Record* individually and other New Jersey papers through digital databases and found no other coverage of the incident.
12. "Playing with Fire Costs Boy His Life."
13. "Grass Fires Circles 2 Passaic Boys, Burning One to Death," *News* (Paterson, NJ), November 2, 1943, 9.
14. "Condition of Burned Boy Called Poor," *Herald-News* (Passaic, NJ), November 3, 1943, 3.
15. See, e.g., "Boy Fatally Burned," *Daily Tribune* (Wisconsin Rapids, WI), July 20, 1942, 7; "Boy, 4, Fatally Burned After Companion Buys Nickle's Worth of Gas," *Morning Call* (Allentown, PA), August 28, 1942, 1; "Harrison Negro Boy Fatally Burned," *Marshall (TX) News Messenger*, September 30, 1942, 2; "Hazelton Boy Fatally Burned," *Scranton Times*, December 26, 1942, 1; "4-Year-Old Albany Boy Fatally Burned," *Star Press* (Muncie, IN), January 14, 1943, 1; "Boy Fatally Burned," *Star-Gazette* (Elmira, NY), February 1, 1943, 11; "Boy Fatally-Burned by Gas Stove Flame," *Morning Post* (Camden, NJ), February 18, 1943, 4; "Boy Fatally Burned," *Harrisburg Telegraph*, September 15, 1943, 2; "Boy Fatally Burned by Matches," *St. Louis Post Dispatch*, December 13, 1943, 3; "Boy Fatally Burned," *Pittsburgh Post-Gazette*, August 5, 1944, 3; "Boy Fatally Burned in Lighter Mishap," *Standard-Examiner* (Ogden, UT), September 4, 1944, 1.
16. Oswald Garrison Villard, *The Disappearing Daily: Chapters in American Newspaper Evolution* (A. A. Knopf, 1944), 3.
17. Two examples of many include Tommy McCormack, whose injury and death only made the news three years after his death when a verdict was reached in the case, and Michael Blessington, whose death and burial announcement appeared in *The New York Times* but without any reference to the circumstances of his death. See "Deaths: Blessington—Michael," *New York Times*, March 29, 1945, 2.
18. See, e.g., "Boy's Burns Fatal," *Ithaca Journal*, December 28, 1942, 11 (Fred Yerkes); "Child Fatally Burned," *Pittsburgh Sun-Telegraph* (Pittsburgh, PA), May 15, 1944, 2 (Howard Diable); "Clothing Ablaze, Boy Badly Hurt," *Philadelphia Inquirer*, August 27, 1944, 3B (Joseph Moore).
19. See, e.g., "Playmates Take Turns Applying the 'Hotfoot': Girl, Six, Badly Burned," *Saginaw News*, July 22, 1944, 1 (Jacqueline Izzo—referring to "fringe" on cowboy pants igniting); "Two Young Boys Suffer Burns as Bonfires Set Clothing Afire," *Herald Statesman* (Yonkers, NY), March 19, 1945, 5 (Guy Tortenson—"trousers"); "Moscow Boy Badly Burned," *Moscow Idahonian*, May 18, 1946, 2 (Mike Felton—leather breeches); "Boy Burns to Death," *Indiana (PA) Evening Gazette*, September 17, 1946, 9 (James Hummel—"Indian suit").
20. National Board of Fire Underwriters, with the assistance of the US Bureau of Education, *Safeguarding the Home Against Fire: A Fire Prevention Manual for the School Children of America*, 7th ed. (National Board of Fire Underwriters, 1939), 11–18 ("Matches").

21. "Boy, 5, Burned; Playsuit on Fire," *Daily Tribune* (Royal Oak, MI), January 14, 1944, 1.
22. "Burned Boy's Condition Reported 'Much Better,'" *Daily Tribune* (Royal Oak, MI), January 16, 1944, 1.
23. "Freehold Child Is Burned When Clothes Catch Fire," *Daily Record* (Longbranch, NJ), May 2, 1944, 1; "Freehold Boy Dies of Burns," *Asbury Park (NJ) Press*, May 3, 1944, 1.
24. "Lad, 4 1/2, Fatally Burned Playing in His Kitchen," *Freehold (NJ) Transcript*, May 5, 1944, 13.
25. "Playmates Take Turns Applying the 'Hotfoot,'" 1.
26. "Both Legs Amputated in Fight to Save Girl," *Saginaw News*, August 17, 1944, 17; "'Hot Foot' Costs 2 Legs," *Detroit Times*, August 19, 1944, 3.
27. "Clothing Ablaze, Boy Badly Hurt."
28. Henry S. Cohn and David Bollier, *The Great Hartford Circus Fire: Creative Settlement of Mass Disasters* (Yale University Press, 1991).
29. "Big Top Bursts into Flame," *Cincinnati Enquirer*, July 7, 1944, 1; "5 Accused of Manslaughter as Circus Deaths Reach 139," *Herald-News* (Passaic, NJ), July 7, 1944, 1; "Death Toll Is 145 in Big Circus Fire," *Daily Tribune* (Royal Oak, MI), July 7, 1944, 1.
30. Cohn and Bollier, *Great Harford Circus Fire*, 14.
31. "Ringling Says War Barred Safety Material; Five of Staff Charged with Manslaughter; Circus Fire Toll Is 146 Dead, 225 Injured," *Cincinnati Enquirer*, July 8, 1944, 1; "Receiver Named for Circus Assets as Lawsuits Multiply—Death Toll Rises to 162," *Cincinnati Enquirer*, July 13, 1944, 5; "Ringling Circus in Receiver's Hands," *Herald-News* (Passaic, NJ), July 13, 1944, 1.
32. "Two Young Boys Suffer Burns as Bonfires Set Clothing Afire," 5.
33. "Trash Fire Play Burns Boy Badly," *Alexandria Gazette*, March 14, 1945, 8.
34. "Engleside Child Dies of Burns," *Alexandria Gazette*, October 25, 1944, 1.
35. "Burned Boy's Condition Reported 'Much Better,'" *Daily Tribune* (Royal Oak, MI), January 16, 1944, 1.
36. "American Troops Take Fraiture," "Carrier Planes Make Heavy Raids on Japs," "Frank Johnson, 6 Seriously Burned," "Selective Service Orders Induction Deferred Men," *Florence Morning News*, January 7, 1945, 1.
37. "Seen About Town," *Florence Morning News*, March 24, 1945, 6.
38. "Berlin and Other Cities of Germany Wrecked in Unprecedented Raids," *Florence Morning News*, March 24, 1945, 6.
39. "Child Fatally Burned," *Pittsburgh Sun-Telegraph*, May 15, 1944, 2. See also "Boy, 5, Dies of Burns," *Pittsburgh Press*, May 15, 1944, 7.
40. See, e.g., The *Indiana (PA) Evening Gazette*, *Bradford (PA) Era*, *Titusville (PA) Herald*, *Gettysburg Times*, and *Evening News* (Hanover, PA). The cities ranged in size from just under six thousand to almost eighteen thousand.
41. Herzberg et al., *Late City Edition*, 1–2.
42. "D.C. Parents Warned: Inflammable Cowboy Suits Kill One Child Here, Burn 7" and "Fuzzy 'Chaps' Flare Like Torches; Stores Are Notified, Probe Launched," *Times-Herald* (Washington, DC), April 8, 1945, 1, 3.

43. "D.C. Parents Warned" and "Fuzzy 'Chaps' Flare Like Torches," 1, 3.
44. *The Washington Post* ran stories on April 9 and 11; the *Washington Evening Star* ran stories April 9, 10, 11, and 12. See "Cowboy Suits Catching Fire Take Big Toll," *Washington Post* (Washington, DC), April 9, 1945, 1B; "Cowboy Suits Probed as 'Chaps' Catch Fire and Burn Children," *Washington Evening Star* (Washington, DC), April 9, 1945, B-4; "House Group May Probe Play Suit Sale," *Washington Post*, April 11, 1945, B1; "Inquiry Is Promised into Sale of Children's Dangerous Play Suits," *Washington Evening Star*, April 10, 1945, A3; "Preliminary Inquiry Will Open Today on Play Suit Hazards," *Washington Evening Star*, April 11, 1945, B7; "Cowboy Suit Maker's Reply to Hearing Bid Awaited," *Washington Evening Star*, April 12, 1945, A14.
45. "Cowboy Suit Warnings Go All Over U. S.," *Times-Herald* (Washington, DC), April 11, 1945, 17.
46. Rep. John E. Rankin (D. Miss.), Congressional Record, 79th Cong., 1st Sess., microfilm reel 252, April 9, 1945, 3227–28.
47. Dwight Martin and Spence Drummond, "'Most Horrifying Incident': Probe of Cowboy Suit Deaths Demanded by Rep. Rankin; Asks Legislation to Stop Use of 'Fur'; Autry Plans to Visit Victims' Kin Here," *Times-Herald* (Washington, DC), April 10, 1945, 1.
48. Roland Nicholson, "Fire Marshal in N.Y. to Test Cowboy Suits," *Times-Herald* (Washington, DC), April 10, 1945, 17 (using samples of the fabric supplied by E. F. Timme & Son, the manufacturer of the fabric used on the suits).
49. "LaGuardia Asks Full Report on Cowboy Suits Made in N.Y.," *Times-Herald* (Washington, DC), April 11, 1945, 17.
50. William Manchester, *The Glory and the Dream: A Narrative History of America, 1932–1972* (Little, Brown and Co., 1974), 358.
51. *Times-Herald* (Washington, DC), April 13, 1945, 1.
52. Thomas P. Brophy, chief fire marshal, to Hon. Patrick Walsh, fire commissioner and chief of department, "Subject: Flammable Material in Boys' "Cowboy" Suits," April 12, 1945, Fire Department, City of New York, reel 0024, Office of the Mayor, subject files 1934–1945, NY, NY (hereafter Office of the Mayor Subject Files).
53. The two individuals identified as sources in the report were Miss Gloria Henry, the sister of Milton Henry, and William E. Roschen, a partner in E. F. Timme & Son.
54. Brophy to Walsh, April 12, 1945.
55. *N. W. Ayer & Son's Directory Newspapers and Periodicals 1945* (N. W. Ayer & Son, 1945), 4 (table 1, "Estimated Civilian Population of Continental United States by Regions, Divisions, and States: Nov. 1, 1943"), 610 (New York City).
56. The NYC fire marshal's office made quarterly reports to the mayor. The reports were lists, not narratives: number of alarms received, gallons of water used, uniformed forces, intentional fires (arson, juvenile delinquents) and related legal actions, deaths, and injuries—and, for deaths, separate lists identifying age, sex, and cause, as well as the class of buildings where fires occurred. In the first-quarter report of fiscal year 1943–1944, two of twenty-four deaths were to children (one under five, the other between five and ten), both boys. Causes were not correlated in the reports to sex and age, but the number matched the deaths listed as "children playing with matches or fire." In the third-quarter report for fiscal year 1944–1945,

seven deaths were to children (two under age one; five ages five to ten). Four deaths out of forty-one were caused by "children with matches." See, e.g., *Fire Department Report to Hon. F. H. LaGuardia, Mayor of the City of New York*, October 16, 1943; *Fire Department Report to Hon. F. H. LaGuardia, Mayor of the City of New York*, June 18, 1945, NYC Municipal Archives, NYC Hall Library, NY, NY.

57. "Two Young Boys Suffer Burns as Bonfires Set Clothing Afire," 5.
58. For each of these, I checked the New York dailies: *The New Herald Tribune*, the *New York Post*, the *Daily News*, *The New York Times*, and the *New York World Telegram and Sun*.
59. Fiorello H. LaGuardia to Hon. John Rankin, April 12, 1945, Apr–June 1945 Correspondence with House Members, Office of the Mayor Subject Files.
60. The 1940 US census reported the District of Columbia's population as 663,091. War mobilization had dramatically added to those numbers, but in doing so it had likely only made truer what already defined the population. See *N. W. Ayer & Son's Directory Newspapers and Periodicals 1945*, 141.
61. The *Times-Herald*'s weekday circulation in 1945 was 226,596; its Sunday circulation was 273,289, almost fifty thousand higher. The *Washington Evening Star*'s weekday circulation was 192,045. *The Washington Post*'s circulation was 158,051. See *N. W. Ayer & Son's Directory Newspapers and Periodicals 1945*, 147, 148. But while all three papers covered the story, which paper a resident read and how much of the paper they read would have mattered to the depth of their understanding.
62. See, e.g., "Junior Cowboy Suit Warning Given Parents," *Berkshire Eagle* (Pittsfield, MA), April 12, 1945, 11 (notes that the local Chamber of Commerce issued warning to retailers; "it seems that the imitation wool or fur trimming on the chaps is highly inflammable."); "Public Warned Against Certain Type Clothing as Highly Inflammable," *Daily Times-News* (Burlington, NC), April 12, 1945, 9; "Warn Retailers of Inferior Materials Flooding Market," *Dispatch* (Moline, IL), April 14, 1945, 2.
63. Examples of newspapers carrying the UP story on the Gene Autry cowboy suit hazard: "Probe of Fire Deaths Laid to Cowboy Suits Is Urged in Congress," *St. Louis Star-Times*, April 9, 1945, 3; "Cowboy Suits Make Torches of Kids: Rankin," *Daily News* (New York, NY), April 10, 1945, 5C; "Congress Told Cowboy Suits Caused 3 Deaths," *Morning News* (Wilmington, DE), April 10, 1945, 18; "Children in Cowboy Suits Burn to Death," *San Bernadino Sun*, April 10, 1945, 1; "Congress Asked to Probe Reports of 'Tots' Deaths," *Democrat and Chronicle* (Rochester, NY), April 10, 1945, 1; "Cowboy Playsuits Burn Like Tinder Parents Are Told," *Mail* (Medford, OR), April 10, 1945, 2.
64. Examples of newspapers carrying the AP story regarding the cowboy suit hazard: "Play Suit Inquiry Asked," *New York Herald Tribune*, April 10, 1945, 24; "Scores New York Cowboy Suits," *New York Times*, April 10, 1945, 21; "Cowboy Suits Deadly," *Greenville (SC) News*, April 10, 1945, 2; "Rankin Urges Probe of Suit Manufacturers," *Shreveport Times*, April 10, 1945, 8. There was also some non-AP/UP reports on April 12, 1945. See, e.g., "Inflammable Cowboy Suits Take Heavy Toll," *Des Moines Tribune*, April 12, 1945, 30 (two-frame photograph showing test in NYC of how fast the cowboy suit burned; does not identify the suit by name; notes three deaths and eleven injuries in Washington, DC); "Children Die When Play Suits Burn," *Whitewright (TX) Sun*, April 12, 1945, 1 ("Gene Autry" cowboy

suits caught fire). As the brief stories that appeared in NYC dailies on April 10, 1945, highlight, the differences between the UP and AP coverage meant that even in a given city, the news broke unevenly and incompletely. In NYC, only the *Daily News* took its story from the UP.

65. "Governor Signs Urgency Bills," *Los Angeles Times*, January 31, 1945, 12; "Twelve More Measures Get Warren Signature," *San Francisco Examiner*, January 31, 1945, 24.
66. "Legislation Speeds Study of Textile Fire Hazards," *Textile World* 95 (April 1945): 145.
67. "Legislation Speeds Study of Textile Fire Hazards"; "Test to Determine Flammability of Consumer Textiles," *Rayon Textile Monthly* 26 (May 1945): 68; "Inflammability of Consumer Textiles," *Rayon Textile Monthly* 26 (July 1945): 62–63; "Evaluation of Fabrics as to Their Inflammability," *Rayon Textile Monthly* 27 (February 1946): 73.
68. *Times-Herald* (Washington, DC), April 20, 1945, 6; "Congressmen Convinced: Priest Wants Law to Insure Against Inflammable Textile," *Times-Herald* (Washington, DC), April 21, 1945, 17. See also "Law to Control Inflammable Textiles Urged," *Washington Evening Star*, April 20, 1945, B1.
69. See, e.g., "Fire-Hazard Clothing Faces Inquiry in House," *New York Herald Tribune*, April 21, 1945, 7; "Clothing Field Under Scrutiny," *Baltimore Sun*, April 21, 1945, 7; "Fire Resistant Clothes Presage Drive on Hazard," *Daily Oklahoman*, April 21, 1945, 4; "Inflammable Cowboy Suit Points to Probe," *Morning News* (Wilmington, DE), April 21, 1945, 18; "Congress May Open Drive on Clothing Dangers," *News* (Kingsport, TN), April 21, 1945, 3; "Cowboy Suit Starts Heat: Congress May Order Wide Clothing Industry Sift," *Star* (Minneapolis, MN), April 21, 1945, 6; "Probe Begins on Inflammability of Cowboy Suits," *Shreveport Times*, April 21, 1945, 1; "Clothing Probe," *Des Moines Register*, April 21, 1945, 9. All of these were AP stories; none identified the cowboy suit. And the stories appeared on Saturday, the weakest news day of the week.
70. "Victims of Autry Playsuits Shake Hands with Their Hero," *Times-Herald* (Washington, DC), April 21, 1945, 17.
71. "Victims of Autry Playsuits Shake Hands with Their Hero," 17.
72. *Review* (East Liverpool, OH), April 23, 1945, 1. An AP story reporting on the incident appeared in at least one Ohio paper that followed exactly the lines of AP reports from incidents before the "news broke." See "Boy Fatally Burned When Playing Cowboy," *Chillicothe Gazette*, April 23, 1945, 7.
73. The article was exceptional in also describing what made the fabric on the chaps of the cowboy suit so inflammable. Drawing on the Ohio State Safety Council, the article noted that it was the "extremely fine fibers" that made the fabric "burn with almost explosive violence." As the Safety Council explained, "A peculiarity of this material seems to be the ability to ignite without actual contact with flame." But it was the kind of information that appeared in one newspaper, on one day, in a small city.
74. "'Juvenile Booby Traps': Mothers Warned Cowboy Suits May Cause Death of Children," *Cumberland Evening Times*, April 11, 1945, 5.
75. "Booby Traps: Child Burned When Cowboy Pants Ignite," *Cumberland Evening*

Times, May 15, 1945, 1 (reporting on injuries to Bobby Flesher, eight, of LaVale, and Cecil Warnick, eight, of Potomac Park).

76. "Boy Dies of Burns," *Tampa Bay Times* (St. Petersburg, FL), May 2, 1945, 3.
77. Consider David Berry (Muskegon Hts., MI), burned September 15, 1945, and Dennis McCarthy (Brooklyn, NY), burned November 1, 1946. Neither incident was reported in local newspapers.
78. "Funeral Today Chesley Johnson," *Florence Morning News*, August 22, 1945, 8.
79. "Burns Fatal to Son of Coach," *Wilkes-Barre Record*, August 27, 1945, 9.
80. "William Augustus Strong III" (obituary), *Winston County Journal* (Louisville, MS), November 9, 1945.
81. This news clipping was likely from the *Tampa Times* or the *Tribune* on the day or day after Pat was burned, January 2 or 3, 1946. Peterson Interview.
82. "Cowboy Suit Ignites; Boy Badly Burned," *Washington Post*, February 2, 1946, 1B; "Flammable Suit Dangers May Bring Ban," *Washington Post*, February 3, 1946, 11M.
83. "Boy Dies, Brother Badly Burned in Cowboy Suit Fire," *Washington Post*, February 28, 1946, 3; "'Cowboy' Game Ends in Tragedy for Boys," *Charleston (WV) Daily Mail*, February 27, 1946, n.p.; "'Cowboy-Indian' Game Ends in Death of Youth," *News* (Kingsport, TN), February 27, 1946, 1.
84. "Check Stores For Cowboy Suits After Second Child Dies," *Daily Mail* (Hagerstown, MD), February 28, 1946, 1; "Parents Warned on Cowboy Suits" and "Hundreds of Children Are Endangered; Two More Boys Die of Burns," *Cumberland Evening Times*, March 1, 1946, 1; "Cowboy Suit Sales Probed as Second Victim Succumbs," *Washington Post*, March 1, 1946, 10.
85. "Fire Marshal Warns Against Cowboy Suits," *Washington Post*, March 2, 1946, 4.
86. "Boy, 5, Burned to Death Roasting Marshmallows," *Herald-News* (Passaic, NJ), June 13, 1946, 1.
87. "Death Lurks in Boys' Play Suits," *Herald-News* (Passaic, NJ), June 25, 1946, 1.
88. "Death Lurks in Boys' Play Suits." 12.
89. "Stores Remove Original Autry Cowboy Suits," *Herald-News* (Passaic, NJ), June 26, 1946, 1.
90. Edward J. Reardon, "Death Cloth Legislation Bottled Up," *Herald-News* (Passaic, NJ), June 26, 1946, 1.
91. "Praise from the Chief," *Herald-News* (Passaic, NJ), June 29, 1946, 6; "'Can Congress Spare an Hour?' A Camden Editorial on Play Suit Tragedies," *Herald-News* (Passaic, NJ), July 2, 1946, 10.
92. "Another Passaic Boy Burned When Cowboy Suit Ignites," *Herald-News* (Passaic, NJ), October 10, 1946, 1.
93. "Canfield Asks Congress Ban 'Death Suits,'" *Herald-News* (Passaic, NJ), January 7, 1947, 1.
94. "Father of Play Suit Victim Backs Bill to End Tragedies," *Herald-News* (Passaic, NJ), March 5, 1947, 5.
95. Villard, *Disappearing Daily*, 3.
96. "Father, Son Suffer Burns in Trash Fire," *Tribune* (Terre Haute, IN), April 19, 1946, 17 (Roy Cizek, three); "'Cowboy,' 6, Badly Burned," *Wilkes-Barre Record*, April 30, 1946, 1 (Searle Devens, six); "Moscow Boy Badly Burned," *Moscow Idahonian*, May 13, 1946, 2 (Mike Felton, six); "Cowboy Suit Blaze Burns Child, 6, Rescuing

Mother," *Salt Lake Daily Telegraph*, July 28, 1947, 12 (John C. Russell, six); "Boy Burned in Bonfire," *Kansas City Star*, April 4, 1948, 3A (Scott Timberlake, five); "Girl, 4, Burned Badly by Yule Tree Bonfire," *Herald Statesman* (Yonkers, NY), January 10, 1949, 3 (Marion Ormerod, four); "Cowboy Suit Catches Fire; Boy, 4, Dies," *Times Leader* (Wilkes-Barre, PA), October 11, 1952, 13 (Thomas Purcell, four); "Child Burned as Spark Hits Cowboy Suit," *Wellsboro Gazette*, September 9, 1954, 1 (Paul Jaquay, four); "Blazing Boy, 6, Saved from Possible Death," *Courier-Post* (Camden, NJ), December 27, 1954, 3 (Richard Hull Jr., six).

chapter eight: "falling out of time"

Chapter title from David Grossman, *Falling Out of Time*, trans. Jessica Cohen (Jonathan Cape, 2014).

1. "Boy Fatally Burned While Playing Indian," *Harrisburg Telegraph*, September 17, 1946, 11.
2. On Berwick, PA see *N. W. Ayer & Son's Directory of Newspapers and Periodicals, 1945* (N. W. Ayer & Son, 1945), 784.
3. James La Rue Hummel, Certificate of Death, September 16, 1946, file no. 76591, reg. no. 142, in "Pennsylvania (State) Death Certificates, 1906–1963," series 11.90, Records of the Pennsylvania Department of Health, RG 11, Pennsylvania Historical and Museum Commission, Harrisburg, PA, online at *Pennsylvania, Death Certificates, 1906–1963* (database), *Ancestry.com*.
4. See Dan Bouk, *Democracy's Data: The Hidden Stories in the U. S. Census and How to Read Them* (MCD, 2022); Margo J. Anderson, *The American Census: A Social History* (Yale University Press, 1988, 2015); Susan Pearson, *The Birth Certificate: An American History* (University of North Carolina Press, 2021). See also Ian Hacking, "Biopower and the Avalanche of Printed Numbers," *Humanities in Society* 5 (Summer and Fall, 1982): 279–95.
5. Albert Hummel, 1940 US Manuscript Census, Berwick, Columbia, Pennsylvania, ED 19-14, sheet 12A, in US Census Bureau, *Sixteenth Census of the United States: 1940* (Government Printing Office, 1942), https://catalog.archives.gov/id/16660414.
6. Elizabeth Cady Stanton, "The Solitude of Self," in *Elizabeth Cady Stanton and Susan B. Anthony: Correspondence, Writings, and Speeches*, ed. Ellen Carol DuBois (Schocken Books, 1981), 247–54.
7. Only children included James Hummel and Dennis Duffy Jr. Firstborn sons named after their father included Dennis Duffy Jr., Howard Diable Jr., Elwood Athey Leary Jr., Michael Blessington Jr., Willie Wilks Jr., Robert Swalwell Jr., and William Augustus Strong III. Firstborn children included Marco Antonio DiTrapani; lastborn included Tommy McCormack, youngest of four brothers. Howard Diable Jr., Elwood Athey Leary Jr., and William Augustus Strong III were all the only boys in their families. Families in which multiple children were injured included Stanley (died) and Casimir Jr. (survived) Krzeczkowski; Larry and Wayne Meisner (both died; they were their parents' only children); and Donald Clark (died), James Wesley (died), and Joseph Robert (survived) Powell (the three boys were their parents'

only children). Michael Blessington Jr. had a brother and sister. Robert Flesher had a brother and two sisters.

8. Elaine Scarry, *The Body in Pain: The Making and Unmaking of the World* (Oxford University Press, 1985), 4–5; Christina Colby, *A Body, Undone: Living On After Great Pain* (NYU Press, 2017), 31.
9. Testimony of Dr. Ernest E. Arnheim, 199–213, McCormack Record on Appeal.
10. Testimony of James McCormack and Testimony of Catherine McCormack, 103–6, 250–51, McCormack Record on Appeal.
11. William M. Tuttle Jr., *Daddy's Gone to War: The Second World War in the Lives of America's Children* (Oxford University Press, 1993), 44–45.
12. Studs Terkel, *"The Good War": An Oral History of World War II* (Pantheon Books, 1984), 9–10.
13. "Son of Meyers Coach Is Seriously Burned at Play," *Wilkes-Barre Record*, March 31, 1945, 11; "Burns Fatal to Son of Coach," *Wilkes-Barre Record*, August 27, 1945, 9.
14. "William Augustus Strong III" (obituary), *Winston County Journal* (Louisville, MS), November 9, 1945.
15. "Georgia Boy, 9, Fatally Burned at the Stake During Children's 'Cowboy and Indian' Game," *Telegram* (Salt Lake City, UT), December 4, 1944, 1; Clifford D. Longmire, death certificate, August 17, 1945, Texas Death Certificates, 1903–1982, Texas Department of Health Services, Austin, TX.
16. "Two More Cowboy Suit Deaths Are Revealed; Gene Autry, Movie Star Will Join in Probe," *Times-Herald* (Washington, DC), April 9, 1945, 1 (Arthur Lunsford); "Soldier, Formerly Missing, Revealed Dead," *Washington Post*, January 12, 1945, 5 (Howard Lunsford).
17. Robert Swalwell Jr. was born on January 28, 1942; his father entered the service on November 15, 1944, and was released from service on March 3, 1946. Robert Swalwell Jr. was burned on November 1, 1947, and died the next day. See Robert Swalwell Jr., Certificate of Death. November 2, 1947, in "Pennsylvania (State) Death Certificates, 1906–1963," series 11.90, Records of the Pennsylvania Department of Health, RG 11, Pennsylvania Historical and Museum Commission, Harrisburg, PA, online at *Pennsylvania, Veteran Compensation Application Files, WWII, 1950–1966* (database), *Ancestry.com*; "Halloween Cowboy Suit Causes Death of McKeesport Boy," *Charleroi (PA) Mail*, November 3, 1947, 1. On the hardship and loss for children of fathers in the service, see Tuttle, *Daddy's Gone to War*.
18. Intelisano Interview.
19. Intelisano Interview.
20. "William Augustus Strong III."
21. "2 Boys Burned Fatally While at Grass Fire," *Review* (East Liverpool, OH), April 23, 1945, 1.
22. Sister Celeste, St. Mary's Convent, Shreveport, LA, to Teresa Baragona, n.d. (in author's possession), Baragona Interview.
23. Act of Contrition, available at *Catholic Online*, accessed December 8, 2025, https://www.catholic.org/prayers/prayer.php?p=43.
24. Sister Mary Hyacinth, St. Mary's Convent, Shreveport, LA, to Teresa Baragona, n.d. (in author's possession), Baragona Interview.
25. See Robert A. Orsi, *Between Heaven and Earth: The Religious Worlds People Make*

and the Scholars Who Study Them (Princeton University Press, 2005), ch. 1 and 3; and Robert A. Orsi, *Thank You, St. Jude: Women's Devotion to the Patron Saint of Hopeless Causes* (Yale University Press, 1996), 150–51, 252, n. 19.

26. See, e.g., "Deaths: Blessington—Michael," *New York Times*, Mar 29, 1945, 20; and "Burns Prove Fatal to 'Bobby' Flesher," *Cumberland Evening Times*, January 17, 1947, 1 (second section).
27. "Deaths: Blessington—Michael."
28. "2 Boys Burned Fatally While at Grass Fire."
29. "Burns Fatal to Son of Coach."
30. "Burns Prove Fatal to 'Bobby' Flesher."
31. "Funeral Services for Child," *Scranton Times*, June 28, 1945, 1.
32. "Funeral Today Chesley Johnson," *Florence Morning News*, August 22, 1945, 8.
33. "Leary Rites," *Alexandria Gazette*, October 26, 1944, 2.
34. "Richard Crull Johnson," *Harrisburg Telegraph*, August 27, 1945, 7.
35. In the 1850s, one out of six children died before reaching the age of five. See Karen Sánchez-Eppler, *Dependent States: The Child's Part in Nineteenth-Century American Culture* (University of Chicago Press, 2005), 101–48. See also Harold K. Bush, *Continuing Bonds with the Dead: Parental Grief and Nineteenth-Century American Authors* (University of Alabama Press, 2019); Laurence Lerner, *Angels and Absences: Child Deaths in the Nineteenth Century* (Vanderbilt University Press, 1997). On the work of death in the face of the massive scale of loss in the American Civil War, see Drew Gilpin Faust, *This Republic of Suffering: Death and the Civil War* (Alfred A. Knopf, 2008).
36. Reducing infant mortality and accidental child death in the workplace, streets, and homes was central in Progressive Era reforms. See Pearson, *Birth Certificate*; James D. Schmidt, *Industrial Violence and the Legal Origins of Child Labor* (Cambridge University Press, 2010); Kriste Lindenmeyer, *"A Right to Childhood": The U. S. Children's Bureau and Child Welfare, 1912–1946* (University of Illinois Press, 1997); Joel A. Tarmand and Mark Tebeau, "Managing Danger in the Home Environment, 1900–1940," and John C. Burnham, "Why Did Infants and Toddlers Die? Shifts in Americans' Ideas of Responsibility for Accidents—From Blaming Mom to Engineering," *Journal of Social History* 29 (Summer 1996): 797–816, 817–37; Kathryn Kish Sklar, *Florence Kelley and the Nation's Work: The Rise of Women's Political Culture, 1830–1900* (Yale University Press, 1995); Richard A. Meckel, *"Save the Babies": American Public Health Reform and the Prevention of Infant Mortality, 1850–1929* (Johns Hopkins University Press, 1990); Viviana A. Zelizer, *Pricing the Priceless Child: The Changing Social Value of Children* (Basic Books, 1985).
37. Grossman, *Falling Out of Time*, 3.
38. Grossman, *Falling Out of Time*, 62–63.
39. Ps. 23:6.
40. Sánchez-Eppler, *Dependent States*, 102.
41. "Playing With Fire Costs Boy His Life," *Herald-News* (Passaic, NJ), November 2, 1943, 1, 2; Stenographer's Minutes, Settlement Hearing before Hon. John C. Knox, February 3, 1950, 4, Casimir Kresokowski Case File.
42. Szumita Interview.

43. Deposition of Helen C. DiTrapani, Washington, DC, July 11, 1946, 14–17, DiTrapani Case File.
44. Habina Interview.
45. "New Arrivals," *Herald-News* (Passaic, NJ), June 7, 1947, 3.
46. Grossman, *Falling Out of Time*, 192–93.

chapter nine: lost years

1. Deposition of Dr. Jack Savran, Providence, RI, June 26, 1950, 21–27; and Photograph, Exhibit 2, June 27, 1950, both in the Caparco Case File.
2. Deposition of Dr. Floyd Riggs, Terre Haute, IN, September 12, 1949, 32–33, 40–41, 54–55, Cizek Case File.
3. Emily Dickinson, *The Collected Poems of Emily Dickinson* (Barnes and Noble Classics, 2003), 16.
4. Harold Epstein, Settlement Hearing (Hon. John C. Knox) Stenographer's Minutes, February 3, 1950, 2–3, Casimir Kresokowski Case File; Deposition of Dr. Philip Caulfield, Washington, DC, December 30, 1948, 8–18, Greatorex Case File; Bill of Particulars, July 12, 1949, Gagnon Case File; Photograph, May 31, 1949, in Deposition of Dr. Moor and Deposition of Dr. Gerry Hough Jr., Pawtucket, RI, June 22, 1950, Szumita Case File. On articles of clothing providing some protection, see, e.g., Deposition of Mary Louise Cumberledge, San Diego, CA, April 12, 1948, 73 (longer underdrawers and high socks), Cumberledge Case File; Interrogatories of John Elwyn Jones, October 14, 1947, 3a (heavy leather jacket tight at the waist), Jones Case File.
5. Deposition of Dr. Robert E. Moran, Washington, DC, December 30, 1947, 23–28, Bradley Case File.
6. Deposition of Dr. Robert E. Moran, 23–28, Bradley Case File; Cumberledge Interview.
7. See, e.g., Deposition of Dr. Philip Caulfield, 10–12, Greatorex Case File; W. Emory Burnett and H. Taylor Caswell, "Severe Burns from Inflammable Cowboy Pants," *Journal of the American Medical Association* (April 1946): 935–36.
8. Deposition of Dr. Floyd Riggs, 32–35, Cizek Case File.
9. Deposition Dr. Philip Caulfield, 11, Greatorex Case File.
10. See, e.g., Affidavit of H. Taylor Caswell, MD, April 5, 1948, 1–2, Habina Case File; Deposition of Dr. Robert E. Moran, Bradley Case File.
11. Depositions of Dr. Henry B. Moor and Dr. Bert S. Jeremiah, Pawtucket, RI, June 28, 1950, and Affidavit of Alexander Szumita, June 7, 1951, Szumita Case File; Szumita Interview.
12. Deposition of Dr. Robert E. Bruner, Kansas City, MO, September 15, 1950, 11, 22–30, and Affidavit of R. E. Bruner, MD, March 7, 1953, 1–2, Timberlake Case File.
13. Deposition of Dr. Floyd Riggs, 41, 43, Cizek Case File.
14. Children who had heterogeneous grafts included Bradley, Caparco, Cizek, Giacomarro, Izzo, Lockhart, Peterson, Szumita, and Timberlake.
15. Lockhart Interview.

16. Deposition of Dr. Floyd Riggs, 35–39, Cizek Case File; "Both Legs Amputated in Fight to Save Girl," *News* (Saginaw, MI), August 17, 1944, 17; Izzo Interview; Baragona Interview; Deposition of Dr. Jack Savran, 21–27, Caparco Case File; Testimony of Dr. Ernest E. Arnheim, 202, McCormack Record on Appeal.
17. Burnett and Caswell, "Severe Burns from Inflammable Cowboy Pants," 935–36.
18. Habina Interview.
19. Baragona Interview.
20. Deposition of Dr. Floyd Riggs, 37–39, Cizek Case File.
21. Deposition of Dr. Robert E. Moran, 24–27, Bradley Case File.
22. Deposition Dr. Philip Caulfield, 10, Greatorex Case File.
23. Burnett and Caswell, "Severe Burns from Inflammable Cowboy Pants," 935–36.
24. Deposition of Dr. Philip Caulfield, 10, Greatorex Case File.
25. Affidavit of Alexander Szumita, June 7, 1951, 2, Szumita Case File.
26. The photographs of Perry Caparco show the scars from all of these techniques (pp. 128, 597). See also Photographs, February 1, 1950, Cizek Case File; Photographs, March 31, 1949, Baker Case File.
27. Henry N. Harkins, *The Treatment of Burns* (C. C. Thomas, 1942), 290–316; Burnett and Caswell, "Severe Burns from Inflammable Cowboy Pants," 935–36.
28. Affidavit of Alexander Szumita, June 7, 1951, 4, Szumita Case File; Szumita Interview.
29. Warnick Case Summary, Bradley Case File. Edmond Butler represented a number of families whose cases were consolidated by Judge Knox for "trial" (settlement) in spring 1948. In each of those cases, he prepared a brief case summary (Bradley, Burke, Cumberledge, Flesher, Gates, Jones, King, Stultz, Tetla, and Warnick), all of which are in the Bradley case file. For another description of a flap graft, see Lucy Grealy, *Autobiography of a Face* (Harper Perennial, 1994), 153–54.
30. Deposition of Dr. Philip Caulfield, Washington, DC, December 30, 1947, 5–11; Deposition of Arthur A. Cumberledge, San Diego, CA, April 12, 1948, 123; Deposition of Mary Louise Cumberledge, 69–72. All in Cumberledge Case File.
31. Deposition of Dr. Philip Caulfield, 5–11, Cumberledge Case File.
32. Deposition of Dr. Philip Caulfield, 5–11, and Deposition of Mary Louise Cumberledge, 69–70, Cumberledge Case File; Answer to Interrogatories, February 11, 1948, Baer Case File; on time in hospital for Toby Cumberledge and Lawrence Gates, see Cumberledge and Gates case summaries prepared by Edmond Butler, ca. May 1948, Bradley Case File; Petition for Authority to Settle Cause of Action, October 24, 1950, 2, Ikner Case File.
33. Cecil Warnick Case Summary, Bradley Case File; Edward Bradley Case Summary, Bradley Case File; Habina Interview; Affidavit of Fred Cizek, January 21, 1950, Cizek Case File.
34. Deposition of Mary Louise Cumberledge, 79, and Deposition of Arthur Albert Cumberledge, 120, Cumberledge Case File.
35. Deposition of Laura C. Bradley, Washington, DC, December 4, 1947, 14, Bradley Case File.
36. See, e.g., Affidavit of Bill of Particulars/Answer to Interrogatories, August 18, 1949, Cizek Case File; Affidavit of Charles L. Shafer, MD, October 26, 1948, 1–2, Devens Case File; Affidavit of Alexander Szumita, June 7, 1951, 2, Szumita Case File;

"Fire Victim, 7, Is Hopeful on Birthday Eve," *Daily News* (Springfield, MA), July 27, 1948 (news clipping); Szumita Interview.

37. Baragona Interview.
38. Correspondence from Superintendent Mills and Sister Celeste in author's possession; Baragona Interview.
39. See, e.g., "D. C. Parents Warned: Inflammable Cowboy Suits Kill One Child Here, Burn 7"; "Fuzzy 'Chaps' Flare Like Torches; Stores Are Notified, Probe Launched," *Times-Herald* (Washington, DC), April 8, 1945, A1, A3 (photos of Edward Bradley, Arthur Cumberledge, and Lawrence Gates); Roland Nicholson and Spence Drummond, "Cowboy Suit Tragedies Under Police Scrutiny," *Times-Herald* (Washington, DC), April 9, 1945, 1 (photo of Calvin Lee Sibley).
40. "Death Lurks in Boys' Play Suits," *Herald-News* (Passaic, NJ), June 25, 1946, 1 (photo of Joseph Intelisano).
41. Deposition of Arthur A. Cumberledge, 123–24, Cumberledge Case File.
42. "Young Victims of Chap Fires Show Patience," *Cumberland Evening Times*, February 13, 1946, 1 (Bobby Flesher); "Fire Victim, 7, Is Hopeful on Birthday Eve," *Daily News* (Springfield, MA), July 27, 1949 (Richard Szumita) (news clipping from Szumita family), Szumita Interview.
43. Chuck Baragona to his parents while in Shriners' Hospital (in author's possession), Baragona Interview.
44. Habina Interview.
45. Elizabeth Mills to Sister Catherine, October 20, 1947 (in author's possession), Baragona Interview.
46. Staff photo by Langston McEachern, *Shreveport Times*, kept by Baragona family (in author's possession), Baragona Interview.
47. On Autry's appearance at McCrory's, see *Shreveport Times*, January 8, 1948, 1, 10.
48. Roland Nicholson, "LaGuardia Asks Full Report on Cowboy Suits Made in N.Y." and "Maker of Inflammable Togs 'Out' to Reporters," *Times-Herald* (Washington, DC), April 11, 1945, 17 (photo of Robert F. Viands).
49. Photo with caption heading "Steady Customer," *Journal Times* (Racine, WI), February 3, 1950, 1 (photo of Jack Jacobs).
50. "Pilots Brighten David's Day with Surprise Hospital Visit"; "Westbrook Boy, Bedridden 14 Months with Burns, Promises Speedy Recovery," *Portland Press Herald*, June 25, 1947, 1.
51. "Westbrook News"; "David Goes to Parade This Year, Instead of Parade Going to Him," *Portland Press Herald*, May 31, 1949, 14.
52. Stephen A. Barney, W. A. Lewis, J. A. Beach, and Oliver Berghof, eds. and trans., *The Etymologies of Isidore of Seville* (Cambridge University Press, 2006), 5.35.1–3.
53. See also photograph of Richard Szumita in hospital bed, outside, with his brother Bob and mother Margaret (in author's possession), Szumita Interview.
54. Baragona Interview; Habina Interview; Peterson Interview; Lockhart Interview. All those I interviewed spoke to the dread of the ether and surgeries.
55. Charles Baragona Jr. to his mother, January 22, 1948, with note from Supt. Elizabeth Mills (in author's possession), Baragona Interview.
56. Habina Interview.
57. Izzo Interview.

58. Izzo Interview.
59. Elizabeth Mills to Mr. Charles Baragona, March 8, 1948 (in author's possession), Baragona Interview.
60. "Victim of Cowboy Suit Burns Home"; "Cecil D. Warnick, 9, Returns from Baltimore Hospital," *Cumberland Evening Times*, November 22, 1947, 18.
61. Petition for Authority to Settle Claim, March 30, 1949, 1, Izzo Probate Court Record; Izzo Interview.
62. Izzo Interview.

chapter ten: an academic marketplace

1. Teaching Division, Columbia University Placement Bureau, "Columbia Assistance in Your Search for a Teaching Position," May 1958, 9, carton 1, folder 17 Columbia Employment File, 1965–1967, Papers of Gerda Lerner, 75-37-96-M8, Schlesinger (hereafter Gerda Lerner Papers).
2. "Slave Market," *New Yorker*, January 14, 1961, 24–25, box 690, folder Committee on the Professional Register: 1964–1966, AHA Papers (LoC).
3. Shafer conditioned his acceptance of the position on the AHA joining other professional societies in providing some system of placement for its members. See Boyd C. Shafer to Robert Clendenen, November 1960, container 668, folder Committee on the Job Register—1960, AHA Papers (LoC).
4. Professional societies looked to one another, as well as to university placement offices, for models. For a survey of professional societies' placement services, see Office of Education, US Department of Health, Education, and Welfare, *Placement Services for Personnel in Higher Education*, report no. OE-53013 (Government Printing Office, 1961). See also David G. Brown, *Placement Services for College Teachers: A Report to Be Submitted to the Office of Manpower, Automation, and Training* (US Department of Labor, September 1965); and David Brown, *The Market for College Teachers: An Economic Analysis of Career Patterns Among Southeastern Social Scientists* (University of North Carolina Press, 1965).
5. APSA, Placement Service, "Biographical and Professional Data," ca. 1956 (2 p. placement service form), box 477, folder AHA Job Register Corres. (1956); and [Boyd Shafer], "New York Trip. Jan. 20, 1956," box 475, folder Committee on the Job Register [1956], both in AHA Papers (LoC); Lanora G. Lewis, *Placement Services for Personnel in Higher Education* (Government Printing Office, 1961).
6. See, e.g., Frederick G. Heymann to AHA, October 17, 1956 ("I presume you use forms"); Gordon H. Torrey to Boyd C. Shafer, April 4, 1956 ("the blanks"); Floyd L. Warne to AHA, November 30, 1956 ("the necessary application blanks"); Theodore R. Crane to executive secretary, AHA, October 29, 1956; Thomas S. Colehan to AHA, January 23, 1956 ("the necessary job application forms"); James V. Geisendorfer to AHA, March 16, 1956 ("employment application form"), all in box 477, folder AHA Job Register Correspondence (1956), AHA Papers (LoC).
7. See, e.g., Boyd C. Shafer to Gerrit P. Judd IV, February 11, 1957, box 482, folder AHA Job Register [1957], AHA Papers (LoC).
8. Shafer to Judd, February 11, 1957; Boyd C. Shafer to Kerney M. Adams, Decem-

ber 14, 1960, box 668, folder Job Register—Employers—1960, AHA Papers (LoC); "Instruction Sheet for Those Working in the Job Register at the Annual Meeting," 1959, box 666, folder AHA Forms for ADVTing, Exhibits, Job Register, Council Agenda, Etc., AHA Papers (LoC).

9. The example here is from 1960, but the same applied for other years. See, e.g., reply of Boyd C. Shafer to Hilmar C. Krueger, December 16, 1960, box 668, folder Job Register—Employers—1960, AHA Papers (LoC).

10. See, e.g., Wesley M. Gewehr to Boyd Shafer, September 23, 1957, box 482, folder AHA Job Register, AHA Papers (LoC). See Brown, *Placement Services for College Teachers*, 87–88.

11. See, e.g., American Institute of Physics, *Registrants' Qualification Book, First Quarter*, January 1, 1963, series I, AIP Career Services Miscellaneous, 1960–1998 (AR 451), box 1, folder 6, AIP Papers. A list of "companies" that had paid for the Qualification Book for the 1956 meeting, was, as its heading suggested, dominated by industry (e.g., RCA, Westinghouse, Lockheed Aircraft, McDonnel Aircraft, Honeywell, Dow Chemical, and so on). Only a few universities were on the list, including, for example, University of Michigan, Bradley University (Peoria, IL), and North Texas University. See American Institute of Physics, "These Companies Have Paid for the Booklet," American Institute of Physics, Placement Service Records, 1960–1978 (AR 205), box 2 of 4 (unprocessed), folder 25th Anniversary Meeting [January 1956], AIP Papers.

12. Folder Fan Mail (1962–1970), box 4 (unprocessed), Placement Service Records, 1960–1978, AIP Papers.

13. Roderic H. Davison to Boyd C. Shafer, "Re: Operation of the Job Register at the 1956 Annual Meeting," January 1, 1956, box 475, folder Committee on the Job Register [1956], AHA Papers (LoC).

14. Davison to Shafer, "Re: Operation of the Job Register."

15. See "Instructions for Those Working in the Job Register at the Annual Meeting," 1960, box 666, folder AHA Forms for ADVTing, Exhibits, Job Register, Council Agenda, etc., AHA Papers (LoC).

16. *AHA Newsletter* 1, no. 1 (December 1962), AHA Papers (headquarters).

17. "Vacancies Reported" first appeared in the AAUP *Bulletin* in March 1929. In that issue and through the 1930s, the few institutions that advertised vacancies appeared not by name but using general descriptions of geography and institution type. See, e.g., "Appointment Service Announcements," *Bulletin of the AAUP* 15, no. 3 (March 1929): 260–62; *Bulletin of the AAUP* 17, no. 3 (March 1931): 280–82; *Bulletin of the AAUP* 20, no. 3 (March 1934): 213–14; *Bulletin of the AAUP* 22, no. 3 (March 1936): 220. The rare exception proved the rule. See two advertisements by the University of Dubuque for positions in biology/home economics and English, with "college experience desirable but not necessary," *Bulletin of the AAUP* 25, no. 2 (April 1939): 255.

18. See, e.g., *American Economic Review* 40, no. 1 (March 1950); *American Economic Review* 45, no. 1 (March 1955); APSA, *Personnel Newsletter* 2, no. 5 (May 6, 1952), box 6, folder APSA, 1952, 1953, 1954, William Anderson Papers, UA, UMN; Supplement to American Sociological Review, *Employment Bulletin* 24, no. 1 (February 1959), and 24, no. 2 (April 1959), box 662, folder Job Register, Committee on

1959, AHA Papers (LoC). For the rationale, see APSA, "Executive Committee Meeting (Washington, D.C.)," December 7, 1954, n.p., box 6, folder APSA, 1952, 1953, 1954, William Anderson Papers (UAR 0360), UA, UMN.

19. "Professional Register," *AHA Newsletter* 1, no. 1 (December 1962): 2–3, AHA Papers (headquarters); "Professional Register," *AHA Newsletter* 1, no. 2 (February 1963): 10; "Professional Register," *AHA Newsletter* 2, no. 4 (April 1964): 2–3.
20. APSA, *Newsletter* (May 1966), box 690, folder Committee on the Professional Register: 1964–1966, AHA Papers (LoC).
21. APSA, *Personnel Newsletter* 3, no. 2 (March 20, 1953): 1 and APSA, *Personnel Newsletter* 2 (February 7, 1955): 1, box 6, folder APSA, 1952, 1953, 1954, William Anderson Papers (UAR 0360), UA, UMN.
22. See, e.g., American Sociological Society, *Employment Bulletin* 49 (November 1956): 1, AHA Papers, box 477, folder AHA Job Register Correspondence (1956); and Supplement to American Sociological Review, *Employment Bulletin* 24, no. 1 (February 1959): 1, box 662, folder Job Register, Committee on, 1959, AHA Papers (LoC).
23. *AHA Newsletter* 1, no. 1 (December 1962), AHA Papers (headquarters).
24. The language and association's position remained the same across the decades. See, e.g., "Back Matter: Vacancies and Applications," *American Economic Review* 29, no. 4 (December 1939); *American Economic Review* 37, no. 1 (March 1947); *American Economic Review* 45, no. 1 (March 1955); *American Economic Review* 51, no. 5 (December 1961).
25. "Roundtable Conference on the Market for Economists: Demand and Supply Aspects," Papers and Proceedings of the Seventy-First Annual Meeting of the American Economic Association, *American Economic Review* 49, no. 2 (May 1959): 581–93.
26. Boyd C. Shafer to the Committee on the Job Register of the American Historical Association, October 11, 1960, box 668, folder Committee on the Job Register–1960, AHA Papers (LoC).
27. Shafer to the Committee on the Job Register, October 11, 1960.
28. Stanley N. Katz, interview by Barbara Y. Welke, Princeton, NJ, April 25 and May 3, 2019 (hereafter Katz Interview).
29. Cf. Morton Keller, *My Times and Life: A Historian's Progress Through a Contentious Age* (Hoover University Press, 2010), 55, 66–67 (those seen as potentially notable historians were nurtured; others were "left to shift for themselves. . . . I was not a hot property.").
30. Katz Interview. But in both student admissions and faculty hiring, antisemitism had not disappeared. See Morton and Phyllis Keller, *Making Harvard Modern: The Rise of America's University* (Oxford University Press, 2001).
31. Katz Interview.
32. US Bureau of the Census, "Series H 766–787: Number of Doctorates, by Field: 1920 to 1970," in *Historical Statistics of the United States, from Colonial Times to 1970, Bicentennial Edition, Part I* (Government Printing Office, 1975), 387–88. The following fields are included in the table: physics-astronomy, chemistry, earth sciences, mathematics, engineering, basic medical sciences, medical sciences, agricultural sciences, other biological sciences, psychology, economics, anthropology

and sociology, political science, other social sciences, history, English and American language and literature, foreign language and literature, other arts and humanities, professional fields, education, and other and unspecified fields.

33. Columbia University, for example, awarded 276 doctorates in 1956, 299 in 1957, and 356 in 1958. See Jacques Barzun, *Graduate Study at Columbia: The Report of the Dean of the Graduate Faculties for 1958* (Columbia University, 1958), 3. The most important shift that occurred in the 1950s (1955–1956) was that public institutions outstripped private ones in the number of doctorates awarded. See US Office of Education, *Biennial Survey of Education in the United States 1954–56* (Government Printing Office, 1960), 91.
34. *Doctoral Dissertations Accepted by American Universities, 1947–1948* (no. 15), compiled for the Association of Research Libraries (H. W. Wilson Company, 1948), iii; US Office of Education, "Table XXXVI.—Earned Degrees Conferred, by Level, Sex of Recipient, and Field of Study: Aggregate United States, 1955–56," in *Biennial Survey of Education, 1954–56*, 96.
35. James M. Banner Jr., "Historian, Improvised," in *Becoming Historians*, eds. James M. Banner and John R. Gillis (University of Chicago Press, 2009), 273, 276.
36. My brief description of Lerner is drawn from her autobiography focused on her life from childhood through completing her PhD. See Gerda Lerner, *Fireweed: A Political Autobiography* (Temple University Press, 2002), 151–72, 365–68. On the long suspicion in US immigration policy that women immigrating alone were or would become prostitutes and barring them on these grounds, see Martha Gardner, *The Qualities of a Citizen: Women, Immigration, and Citizenship, 1870–1965* (Princeton University Press, 2005); Eithne Luibheid, *Entry Denied: Controlling Sexuality at the Border* (University of Minnesota Press, 2002); Sucheng Chan, "The Exclusion of Chinese Women, 1870–1943," in *Entry Denied: Exclusion and The Chinese Community in America, 1882–1943*, ed. Sucheng Chan (Temple University Press, 1991), 94–146.
37. Although she was from Austria, Lerner's passport was German because she emigrated after the *Anschluss*.
38. Lerner, *Fireweed*, 366–67; Rosalind Rosenberg, *Changing the Subject: How the Women of Columbia Shaped the Way We Think About Sex and Politics* (Columbia University Press, 2004), 229–32.
39. The other two were the University of Illinois and the University of Michigan. See Brown, *Placement Services for College Teachers*, 34–72.
40. *Columbia University Bulletin* (June 1898): 247–48, box 269, folder 5 Appointments Office—Clippings, 1910s–1930s, Historical Subject Files, CUA.
41. "University Placement Bureau Organizational Chart–Nov. 1, 1956," box 433, folder 17, Central Files, CUA. Before 1956, the Columbia University Placement office also handled placement of law graduates. That year law placement was turned over to the Law School. See John A. Krout to Sam Beach, July 17, 1956, box 433, folder 13, Central Files, CUA.
42. Office of University Placement and Career Planning, "Columbia Career Notes," February 1966, 8 ("Academic Placement Notes"), box 634, folder 24, Central Files, CUA.
43. Teaching Division, Columbia University Placement Bureau, "Columbia Assistance in Your Search for a Teaching Position."

44. I follow Lerner's terminology here, which I expect reflects the way she had encountered the document in her adult life outside academia before beginning graduate school.
45. See, e.g., Gerda Lerner to Dorothy Fowler, April 12, 1965, carton 1, folder 17, Gerda Lerner Papers.
46. Lerner wasn't a member of the AHA in 1965. On a draft of the form for Columbia's Office of University Placement, Lerner responded to the question "To what clubs or societies do you belong?" with "AAUN, NAACP" and then, handwritten in pencil, "MVHA." "AAUN" refers to the American Association for the United Nations (AAUN). That Lerner began her list with memberships reflecting her personal and political commitments, adding her membership in the Mississippi Valley Historical Association (later the Organization of American Historians) as something of an afterthought, said something about her individually but also about her professionalization. On the finalized, fully typed version of the form dated April 1, 1965, Lerner added a second professional organization at the end of her list: "American Studies Association."
47. Thomas Stirton to Mrs. Gerda Lerner, April 27, 1965, carton 1, folder 20, Gerda Lerner Papers.
48. Dean, Long Island University Brooklyn Center to Gerda Lerner, June 11, 1965, carton 1, folder 20, Gerda Lerner Papers.
49. Banner, "Historian, Improvised," 279. See also James S. Coleman, "Columbia in the 1950s," on the field of sociology, in Bennett M. Berger, *Authors of Their Own Lives: Intellectual Autobiographies by Twenty American Sociologists* (University of California Press, 1990), 75–103.
50. "Slave Market," *New Yorker* (January 14, 1961), 24–25, box 690, folder Committee on the Professional Register: 1964–1966, AHA Papers (LoC).
51. "Academic Vacancies and Teachers Available," back matter, *AAUP Bulletin* 50, no. 4 (December 1964): 373–80.
52. Between 1940 and 1970, faculty at all institutions of higher education grew from 110,000 to over 500,000. See US Bureau of the Census, *Historical Statistics of the United States, from Colonial Times to 1970, Bicentennial Edition, Part I*, 382. It's important to remember in thinking about these numbers that far from all faculty held PhDs. In 1955, 40 percent of faculty held a PhD or its equivalent. That percentage had risen by 1970 but was nowhere close to 100 percent. Moreover, there was huge growth in the number of junior colleges (456 in 1940; 886 in 1970) that had lower degree requirements for faculty. See F. W. Strothmann, on behalf of the Committee of Fifteen, *The Graduate School, Today and Tomorrow; Reflections for the Profession's Consideration* (Fund for the Advancement of Education, 1955), 7 (re: percentage of faculty with PhDs); Richard M. Freeland, *Academia's Golden Age: Universities in Massachusetts 1945–1970* (Oxford University Press, 1992), 94.
53. Robert L. Zangrando, executive secretary, "The Professional Register," container 683, folder Annual Meeting 1966 Professional Placement Session, AHA Papers (LoC). For Zangrando's biography, see Martin Chasin, "In Memoriam: Robert L. Zangrando (1932–2019)," *Perspectives on History* (July 16, 2020): 45, https://www.historians.org/publications-and-directories/perspectives-on-history/september-2020/robert-l-zangrando-(1932%E2%80%932019).

54. The American Economic Association, for example, reported 2,359 job openings in 1966. See "Report of the Secretary for the Year 1967," Papers and Proceedings of the Eightieth Annual Meeting of the American Economic Association, *American Economic Review* 58, no. 2 (May 1968): 691. The American Institute for Physics' February 1966 "Summary of Academic Openings" ran twenty-one pages listing multiple hundreds of appointments. And here too the same absences: no listings from the top physics departments. See American Institute of Physics, Placement Service, "Summary of Academic Openings," February 1966, box 2 (unprocessed), American Institute of Physics Placement Service Records, 1960–1978 (AR205), AIP Papers.
55. "Finding Employment in the Mathematical Sciences," *Mathematical Sciences Employment Register* (1965): 9.
56. Compare "Professional Register," *AHA Newsletter* 3, no. 3 (February 1965): 10–13, with *AHA Newsletter* 4, no. 3 (February 1966): 19–31, AHA (headquarters).
57. "Professional Register," *AHA Newsletter* 4, no. 2 (December 1965): 13, AHA Papers (headquarters).
58. See "Professional Register," *AHA Newsletter* 3, no. 4 (April 1965) through "Professional Register," *AHA Newsletter* 7, no. 2 (December 1968), AHA Papers (headquarters).
59. See ch. 15, "to be 'judged on our capabilities alone,'" and ch. 17, "on our traditional basis of quality alone."
60. William M. Tuttle Jr., curriculum vitae, box 3, folder 16 Jobs—1960s, Tuttle Collection, Kenneth Spencer Research Library, University of Kansas, Lawrence, KS.
61. William M. Tuttle Jr., interview by Barbara Y. Welke, Lawrence, KS, January 24, 2019 (hereafter Tuttle Interview); William M. Tuttle Jr., *Daddy's Gone to War: The Second World War in the Lives of America's Children* (Oxford University Press, 1993).
62. Katz Interview. See also "Department of History, University of Wisconsin, with the Collaboration of Irvin G. Wylie, Department Chairman," in Brown, *Placement Services for College Teachers*, 73–83.
63. "Department of History, University of Wisconsin, with the Collaboration of Irvin G. Wylie, Department Chairman," in Brown, *Placement Services for College Teachers*, 73–83.
64. Bogue's typewritten note to Tuttle dated October 28, 1966, appears under a brief letter Tuttle had written to Bogue on October 18, 1966, asking him to complete the recommendation form for him for the Teacher Placement Bureau. See box 3, folder 16 Jobs—1960s, Tuttle Collection.
65. For the correspondence from the departments of history at Stanford, the University of Connecticut, and NYU, see box 3, folder 16 Jobs—1960s, Tuttle Collection.
66. US Office of Education, *Biennial Survey of Education in the United States 1954–1956*, 91.
67. See, e.g., Linda Gordon, "History Constructs a Historian," and Temma Kaplan, "My Way," both in *Becoming Historians*, eds. James M. Banner Jr. and John R. Gillis (University of Chicago Press, 2009), 76–100, 204–28.
68. Tuttle Interview.
69. For the correspondence described in this paragraph, see box 3, folder 16 Jobs—1960s, Tuttle Collection.

70. See, e.g., Elbert K. Fretwell Jr., dean for academic development, CUNY, to William M. Tuttle, December 16, 1966 (thanking Tuttle for his letter and noting, "I am sharing copies of your vita with the appropriate people here at the university with the suggestion that they get in touch with you if there are any likely vacancies. The nature of your dissertation sounds exciting. I hope we will have the chance to become acquainted before too long"), box 3, folder 16 Jobs—1960s, Tuttle Collection; Eleanor E. Reilly, executive assistant to the dean of the faculties, Hunter College, to Willam M. Tuttle Jr., December 22, 1966 (noting that she had received Tuttle's vita from Dean Fretwell and had forwarded it to Professor Dorothy Fowler, chairman of the Department of History), box 3, folder 16 Jobs—1960s, Tuttle Collection.
71. See box 3, folder 16 Jobs—1960s, Tuttle Collection.
72. Tuttle Interview.
73. See box 3, folder 22 K.U., 1967–1972, Tuttle Collection.
74. Teaching Division, Columbia University Placement Bureau, "Columbia Assistance in Your Search for a Teaching Position." In 1958, the statement fit professional norms. By 1965, it didn't. But Columbia continued to use the booklet. See Brown, *Placement Services for College Teachers*, 64–65 (quoting from the booklet in his discussion of the Teaching Division of the Columbia University Placement Bureau).
75. "Professional Register," *AHA Newsletter* 4, no. 1 (October 1965): 5, AHA Papers (headquarters).
76. APSA, *Newsletter* (May 1966): 7, box 690, Committee on the Professional Register, 1964–1966, AHA Papers (LoC). Physics came closest to inviting candidates to correspond directly with hiring institutions. At least as early as 1962, the AIP's "Summary of Academic Openings" listed institutions by name and directed candidates, "For more detailed information, please write to the Physics Departments (or unless other specified) of the Universities or to the [AIP Placement Service.]" But note that the language was about inquiring for more information, not an invitation to apply for a position. Nonetheless, the early identification of academic institutions by name reflected the different world of physics (and also chemistry) in which academia competed with industry and government for PhDs. See, e.g., American Institute of Physics, Placement Service, "Summary of Academic Openings," May 1, 1962, 7, box 2 (unprocessed), American Institute of Physics Placement Service Records, 1960–1978 (AR205), AIP Papers.

chapter eleven: family portraits

1. Viands Interview.
2. "Veteran Who Spent 18 Months Overseas Dies First Day Home," *Washington Evening Star*, December 27, 1945, 1.
3. An autopsy revealed that his cause of death was listed as "acute congestive heart failure due to cardio vascular disease." See Richard Moore Viands, Certificate of Death, no. 460335, District of Columbia Health Department, Bureau of Vital Statistics (in author's possession), Viands Interview.
4. "Veteran of 18 Months Overseas Dies First Day Home."

5. Viands Interview. As I discovered, the photograph appeared with a story entitled "LaGuardia Asks Full Report on Cowboy Suits Made in N.Y.," *Times-Herald* (Washington, DC), April 11, 1945, 17.
6. Viands Interview.
7. Complaint, February 25, 1946, Viands Case File.
8. Complaint, February 25, 1946, Viands Case File, 2; Richard M. Viands, Enlisted Record and Report of Separation, Honorable Discharge (date of separation October 31, 1945) (in author's possession); Viands Interview.
9. "Veteran of 18 Months Overseas Dies First Day Home," *Washington Evening Star*, December 27, 1945, A-1, A-2. (The *Evening Star* had multiple editions. In the paper saved by the Viands, the story appeared on 1, 4.).
10. Viands Interview.
11. The collective portrait presented in this chapter rests on extensive genealogical research, including US census, birth, marital, death, immigration, and military records, relating to 123 families who had a child burned in a Gene Autry cowboy suit, as well as legal case files for seventy-five families and extensive newspaper research. On the 1940 census and the data censuses produce, see Dan Bouk, *Democracy's Data: The Hidden Stories in the U. S. Census and How to Read Them* (MCD, 2022). More generally, see Paul Schor, *Counting Americans: How the U.S. Census Classified the Nation* (Oxford University Press, 2017); and Margo J. Anderson, *The American Census: A Social History*, 2nd ed. (Yale University Press, 2015).
12. Charles Baragona Jr.'s mother was born in West Monroe, Louisiana, his father in St. Joseph (Baragona Interview).
13. Baragona Interview; Charles J. Baragona Sr., 1940 US Manuscript Census, Hodge, Jackson, LA, ED 25-3, 13A, in US Census Bureau, *Sixteenth Census of the United States: 1940* (Government Printing Office, 1942), https://catalog.archives.gov/id/16660414.
14. Baragona Interview.
15. The evidence for this claim comes from multiple points: Milton Henry's testimony in McCormack on where the suit was sold; the locations of McCrory stores, one of the largest chains that sold the suit; and the cities in which families of children burned in cowboy suits lived and the retailers those families bought the cowboy suit from. See Testimony of Milton A. Henry, 409, McCormack Record on Appeal; and Milton A. Henry, Answers to Interrogatories ("Shipments to McCrory Stores," 1942, 1943), November 7, 1947, Habina Case File.
16. Affidavit of Elliot B. Paley, October 31, 1949, 4–5, Baragona Case File.
17. Complaint, October 25, 1947, 2, Felton Case File (action against retailer); Felton Interview.
18. Deposition of Elwyn Jones, Pottsville, PA, October 14, 1947, 1a, Jones Case File; John Elwyn Jones, 1940 US Manuscript Census, Pottsville, Schuylkill, PA, ED 54-106, 8B, in US Census Bureau, *Sixteenth Census of the United States*; "Son of Atty. Elwyn Jones Is Seriously Burned," *Republican* (Pottsville, PA), February 26, 1945, 4.
19. "Burns Fatal," *Cincinnati Enquirer*, November 5, 1942, 18; Herbert Lonneman, 1940 US Manuscript Census, Cincinnati, Hamilton, OH, ED 91-244, 22A, in US Census Bureau, *Sixteenth Census of the United States*.

20. Cumberledge Interview; Deposition of Arthur A. Cumberledge, San Diego, CA, December 30, 1947, 115, and Deposition of Mary Louise Cumberledge, San Diego, CA, December 30, 1947, 63, Cumberledge Case File.
21. Deposition of Ben C. Hamilton (managing/salesman at Sayre and Company), Terre Haute, IN, September 12, 1949, 23, Cizek Case File.
22. Answering Interrogatories, Hassie Watley Strong, October 29, 1952, Strong Case File.
23. Thomas Hoyt Felton (lawyer), 1940 US Manuscript Census, Moscow, Latah, ID, ED 29-7, 61A; Lawrence M. Gates (manager), 1940 US Manuscript Census, Arlington, Arlington, VA, ED 7-32, 12B; Edward Johnson (teacher), 1940 US Manuscript Census, Wilkes-Barre, Lucerne, PA, ED 40-308, 62B; Elwyn Jones (lawyer), 1940 US Manuscript Census, Pottsville, Schuylkill, PA, ED 54-106, 8B; William Augustus Strong Jr. (lawyer), 1940 US Manuscript Census, Louisville, Winston, MS, ED 80-2, 3B; Harry E. Tortenson (bank cashier), 1940 US Manuscript Census, Yonkers, Westchester, NY, ED 68-94, 11A; Joseph C. Ulick (chemist), 1940 US Manuscript Census, LA, CA, ED 60-175, 4A, all in US Census Bureau, *Sixteenth Census of the United States*; "Burns Fatal," 18 (noting that the dead child's father was treasurer of the Wittenborg Toy Company); "Yonkers Bank Promotes Ten," *New York Times*, January 13, 1950, 43; William E. Pritchard Sr. (electrical engineer), Allentown, PA, City Directory listing, 1945, *Ancestry.com*.
24. David M. Kennedy, *Freedom from Fear: The American People in Depression and War, 1929–1945* (Oxford University Press, 1999), 287.
25. Cf. Timberlakes (Kansas City, MO, pop. 399,178); Baers (Akron, OH, pop. 244,791); and Weinsteins (Yonkers, NY, pop. 142,598).
26. See, e.g., Michael Blessington Sr. (stonecutter, eighth-grade education), 1940 US Manuscript Census, NY, Queens, NY, ED 41-1294. 2B; Jacob Hizny (coal miner, fifth-grade education), 1940 US Manuscript Census, West Wyoming, Luzerne, PA, ED 40-276, 5B; Joseph Intelisano (foreman clothing manufacturer, one year high school), 1940 US Manuscript Census, Passaic, NJ, ED 16-90, 6B; Intelisano Interview; George Marszalek (laborer, third-grade education), 1940 US Manuscript Census, Ransom, Lackawanna, PA, ED 35-119, 5A; all in US Census Bureau, *Sixteenth Census of the United States*.
27. See *Low-Income Families: Hearings Before the United States Joint Committee on the Economic Report, Eighty-First Congress, First Session, on Dec. 12–17, 19–22, 1949* (Government Printing Office, 1949), 1 (in the hearings, families with earnings under $2,000 in 1948 were defined as "low-income"); US Department of Labor, Bureau of Labor Statistics, Workers' Budgets in the United States: City Families and Single Persons, 1946 and 1947, bulletin no. 927 (Government Printing Office, 1948), 1–2.
28. Samuel Gorab—Syria, immigrated 1911; Lockhart—both parents immigrated from Scotland; Piechota—parents Polish immigrants; Caparco—Italian—but I could not specifically identify this family in the 1940 census; Gerber—father from Austria/mother from Poland; Izzo—father's parents Italian immigrants; Javinsky—mother immigrated from Czechoslovakia; Moore—both parents Irish immigrants; Blessington—both parents Irish immigrants; McCormack—both parents Irish immigrants; Jones—father born in Wales; Flesher—mother born

in Germany; Krau—both parents born in Germany; Szumita—father born to Polish parents; mother born in Scotland; Gidlund—both parents born in Sweden; Wrobbel—father's mother from Germany; Intelisano—parents from Italy; Tetla—father's parents born in Poland; Ulich—father born in Kiev, Russia/mother in Germany; McMaster—Irish heritage; Baragona—father's parents from Italy; Gagnon—father born in French Canada.

29. "Inflammable Cowboy Suits Kill One Child Here, Burn 7," *Times-Herald* (Washington, DC), April 8, 1945, A-1, A-3 ("Willie Wilks, Jr., 9, Negro").
30. In 1910, immigrants made up over 14 percent of the US population, and in many cities immigrants made up half or more of the population. See Paul R. Spickard *Almost All Aliens: Immigration, Race, and Colonialism in American History and Identity* (Routledge, 2007), app. B.
31. Lockhart Interview; John Lockhart, Michigan, registration city: Wayne, roll 2032601, Draft Board 21, *Ancestry.com*; John Lockhart and Euphemia Greer, marriage certificate, June 1, 1922, *Ancestry.com*; John Lockhart Sr., 1940 US Manuscript Census, Royal Oak, Oakland, MI, roll T627_1802, 18B, ED 63-140, in US Census Bureau, *Sixteenth Census of the United States.*
32. George Marszalek, petition for naturalization, March 26, 1920, Naturalization Petitions of the US Circuit and District Courts of the Middle District of Pennsylvania, 1906–1930, microfilm roll 70, microfilm serial M1626, US Naturalization Records 1840–1957, National Archives and Records Administration, Washington, DC, *Ancestry.com.*
33. George Marszalek, 1940 US Manuscript Census, Ransom, Lackawanna, PA, ED 35-119, 5A, in US Census Bureau, *Sixteenth Census of the United States.*
34. George Marszalek, [Selective Service] registration card, April 27, 1942, *Ancestry .com.*
35. Daniel Marszalek was burned on June 23, 1945, and died two days later on June 25, 1945. See "Burns Prove Fatal to Daniel Marszalek, 6," *Scranton Times*, June 25, 1945, 11.
36. James McCormack, Petitions for Naturalization from the US District Court for the Southern District of New York, 1897–1944, series M1972, roll 979, New York Naturalization Records, 1882–1944, National Archives and Records Administration, Washington, DC, *Ancestry*.com; James McCormack, 1940 US Manuscript Census, NY, NY, ED 31-1662, 10A, in US Census Bureau, *Sixteenth Census of the United States: 1940* (Government Printing Office, 1942), https://catalog.archives .gov/id/16660414; Testimony of James McCormack, 75, McCormack Record on Appeal; Michael J. Blessington Sr., 1940 US Manuscript Census, NY, Queens, NY, ED 41-1294, 2B, in US Census Bureau, *Sixteenth Census of the United States.* His wife's brother had no children of his own; he worked as a laborer for the New York City Park Department with earnings in 1939 of $1,500.
37. See Brooke Depenbusch, "Down and Out in the U.S.A.: General Relief and the Politics of Precarity in the Shadow of the Welfare State, 1935–1964" (PhD diss., University of Minnesota, 2019), https://conservancy.umn.edu/items/327ade26 -d78f-4fa7-8b0b-ef146be48065; Laura McEnaney, *Postwar: Waging Peace in Chicago* (University of Pennsylvania Press, 2018); Susan Porter Benson, *Household Accounts: Working-Class Family Economies in the Interwar United States* (Cornell

University Press, 2007); Meg Jacobs, *Pocketbook Politics: Economic Citizenship in Twentieth-Century America* (Princeton University Press, 2005); Lizabeth Cohen, *A Consumers' Republic: The Politics of Mass Consumption in Postwar America* (Alfred A. Knopf, 2003); Lizabeth Cohen, *Making a New Deal*, 2nd ed. (Cambridge University Press, 2008).

38. Benson, *Household Accounts*, 10–11.
39. "Hospital Treats 3 for Serious Burns," news clipping from Peterson family (in author's possession), Peterson Interview. Like many families who clipped news stories about their child's injuries and treatment, Pat Peterson's mother did not note either the date or newspaper name, clipping only the story.
40. "So, Far, So Good; Father Provides Skin Graft for Burned Son, Age Six"; "Burned Boy Has Gallant Aides in Fight to Health" (news clippings in author's possession), Peterson Interview.
41. "Burned Boy in Hospital Faces Long Fight Ahead" (news clipping in author's possession), Peterson Interview.
42. "Elks Give $50 To Aid Boy Here," [newspaper unknown], April 18, 1946; "Fund for Boy Given 10 Dollars," *Tampa Bay Times* (St. Petersburg, FL), April 19, 1946; "Elks Collect $344 to Help Burned Child," *Sunday Tribune* (Tampa, FL), April 28, 1946; "Fund for Boy Reaches $583," *Tampa Bay Times* (St. Petersburg, FL), May 3, 1946; "Fund to Help Burned Child Is Increasing," *Tampa Tribune*, May 5, 1946; "Fund to Help Burned Child Reaches $1200" (undated news clipping in author's possession), Peterson Interview. All of these stories would have been from the Tampa *Bay Times* or *Tribune*.
43. "Elks' Fund Reaches Goal for Aid to Burned Child"; "Burned Child Given $1500" (news clippings in author's possession), Peterson Interview.
44. "Burned Child Leaves Hospital (photo)," *Tampa Tribune*, ca. August 15, 1946; "Today in Tampa," *Tampa Bay Times* (St. Petersburg, FL), August 15, 1946, and "Burned Boy Can Now Walk," *Tampa Bay Times* (St. Petersburg, FL), October 23, 1946 (news clippings in author's possession); Peterson Interview.
45. The home, operated by the Florida State Elks Association, opened in 1933. See "Elks Open Campaign to Help Crippled Children" (undated news clipping in author's possession), Peterson Interview. On disability and charitable fundraising, see Paul Longmore, *Telethons: Spectacle, Disability, and the Business of Charity* (Oxford University Press, 2016).
46. Lockhart Interview. The news clipping Jack Lockhart's mother had torn out of the newspaper was one of several notices in the *Daily Tribune* (Royal Oak, MI), March 24, 1947.
47. "Two Izzo Shows Loom Necessary," *Saginaw News*, February 22, 1948; "Tickets Still Left for Jacqueline Izzo Show Here Sunday," *Saginaw News*, February 27, 1948; "Plans Readied for Two Izzo Benefit Shows," *Saginaw News*, February 28, 1948, 14; "Variety Show Cast Warms Up at Percy Jones," *Saginaw News*, February 23, 1948.
48. "Jackie Attends Benefit with Her Proven Friends," *Saginaw News*, March 1, 1948, 11.
49. Bill of Particulars, January 5, 1949, 2–3, Peterson Case File.
50. James Sparrow, *Warfare State: World War II Americans and the Age of Big Government* (Oxford University Press, 2013); Kennedy, *Freedom from Fear*.
51. That Caparco had been in the shipbuilding industry in the war years likely explains

his having health insurance coverage. As both Paul Starr and Jennifer Klein note, the war provided a strong push for health insurance as an employee benefit. See Paul Starr, *The Social Transformation of American Medicine* (Basic Books, 1982), 290–310 ("The Birth of the Blues"); Jennifer Klein, *For All These Rights: Business, Labor and the Shaping of America's Public-Private Welfare State* (Princeton University Press, 2010), 162–203. Most of these families, like most Americans, did not have health insurance.

52. Affidavit of Michael Caparco, April 14, 1950, 1–3, Petition of Michael Caparco, January 26, 1951, 4–5, Caparco Case File.
53. The exact dollar figure for their medical expenses was $1,216.25. See Answers to Interrogatories, Rachel Johnson Bodie (Chesley Franklin Johnson's mother), January 9, 1950, 3, Chesley Franklin Johnson Case File.
54. Testimony of Stella Urban (Casimir and Stanley Krzeczkowski's mother), Stenographer's Minutes, Hearing before Hon. John C. Knox, February 3, 1950, 2–10, Casimir Kresokowski Case File.
55. Testimony of Catherine McCormack, 251, McCormack Record on Appeal.
56. Petition of Alexander Szumita, June 7, 1951, 1–4; Affidavit of Alexander Szumita, April 10, 1950, 1–2; Deposition of Ross Donaldson, controller of Memorial Hospital, Pawtucket, RI, June 22, 1950, 23, Szumita Case File; Szumita Interview.
57. On the emotional burden of miscarriages, stillbirths, and infant and child mortality, see Judith Walzer Leavitt, *Brought to Bed: Childbearing in America, 1750–1950* (Oxford University Press, 1986), 18, 267–68; Robert Woods, *Death Before Birth: Fetal Health and Mortality in Historical Perspective* (Oxford University Press, 2009). On the effort to reduce infant mortality, see Susan Pearson, *The Birth Certificate: An American History* (University of North Carolina Press, 2021); Samuel H. Preston and Michael R. Haines, *Fatal Years: Child Mortality in Late Nineteenth-Century America* (Princeton University Press, 1991); and Richard A. Meckel, *"Save the Babies": Public Health Reform and the Prevention of Infant Mortality, 1850–1929* (Johns Hopkins University Press, 1990).
58. On the uneven burden of infant mortality, see Pearson, *Birth Certificate*, 23–58.
59. James Szumita death, April 19, 1937, age zero; Edward Szumita death, March 12, 1938, age zero. See "RI Deaths and Burials, 1802–1950," James Szumita, April 19, 1937, Pawtucket, RI, ref. CN 18, FHL microfilm 1,954,395, and Edward Szumita, March 12, 1938, Pawtucket RI, ref. CN 18, FHL microfilm 1, 954,623, *FamilySearch*; Margaret Szumita, Rhode Island State Census, 1935, Providence, FHL microfilm 1, 682,893, *FamilySearch*.
60. Szumita Interview. William McMaster, burned at age five, had been afflicted with polio at age two, and was only able to walk with a full brace on one of his legs (McMaster Interview).
61. Eleanor and Thomas Felton's first child, a son they had named after his father and her father, Thomas Hoyt Felton, died less than two months after birth in 1938. See Thomas Hoyt Felton death certificate, December 15, 1938, Moscow, Latah, ID, certificate no. 112228, in "Idaho, Death Certificates, 1938–1961," *Family Search.com*.
62. William M. Tuttle Jr., *Daddy's Gone to War: The Second World War in the Lives of America's Children* (Oxford University Press, 1993), 31.

63. See, e.g., the case of William August Tormollen, who arrived home from service in the US Naval Reserves on March 19, 1945; his son William Jr. was burned at age four on October 14, 1947. Donald G. Frazer had been in the US Navy in 1946; his son Donald was burned in 1949. Robert Swalwell served in WWII from late 1944 to early 1946; his son Robert Jr. was burned on November 1, 1947, at age five and died the next day. See William August Tormollen, 1945, Arrival: NY, NY, microfilm roll 6928, microfilm serial T715, 1897–1957, line 40, 124, *Ancestry.com*; Donald G. Frazer (Fraser), Nutley, NJ, 1946 (occupation: "in U. S. Navy"), "US City Directories, 1822–1995," *Ancestry.com*; Robert D. Swalwell Jr. death certificate, November 2, 1947, McKeesport, Allegheny, PA, certificate no. 95198, *Ancestry.com*; Robert Depaul Swalwell, PA, WWII Veterans Compensation Applications, ca. 1950s, Records of the Department of Military and Veterans Affairs, RG 19, series 19.92, PA Historical and Museum Commission, Harrisburg, PA, *Ancestry.com*.

chapter twelve: "married, two children"

1. Gerda Lerner, resume, ca. 1965, carton 1, folder 17, Papers of Gerda Lerner, 75-37-96-M8, Schlesinger (hereafter Gerda Lerner Papers).
2. *The New Shorter Oxford English Dictionary* (Clarendon, 1993), under "form."
3. Gerda Lerner, resume, ca. 1965, carton 1, folder 17, Gerda Lerner Papers; William M. Tuttle Jr., curriculum vitae, ca. 1966, box 3, folder 16, KSRL, William M. Tuttle Jr. Collection, University Archives, PP 478, UKansas.
4. For a parallel phenomenon in insurance, see Dan Bouk, *How Our Days Became Numbered: Risk and the Rise of the Statistical Individual* (University of Chicago Press, 2015), 62–63, incl. n. 24; Caley Horan, *Insurance Era: Risk, Governance, and the Privatization of Security in Postwar America* (University of Chicago Press, 2021).
5. Thomas L. Haskell, *The Emergence of Professional Social Science: The American Social Science Association and the Nineteenth-Century Crisis of Authority* (University of Illinois Press, 1977), 236–37.
6. David Reisman, *Constraint and Variety in American Education* (University of Nebraska Press, 1956), 103–5.
7. Initially, only some ads specified sex in listing qualifications. See, e.g., "Vacancies," *Bulletin of the AAUP* 17, no. 2 (February 1931): 194 (6 of 15). Men's and women's colleges and universities in this era made hiring by sex normal. But whereas all-male institutions never hired women, women's colleges often did hire men, and coeducational institutions were as likely to specify "man" as single-sex men's institutions were. But beginning in 1932, ads almost uniformly specified sex. See, for example, "Appointment Service Announcements: Vacancies Reported," *Bulletin of the AAUP* 19, no. 2 (February 1933): 155 (all but one, a women's college, specified "man").
8. See "Personnel Exchange," *American Journal of Sociology* 38, no. 1 (July 1932): 109. In 1935, the following appeared: "Information of value to appointing officials includes: age, sex, marital status and size of family, extent of professional training, length of service in sociology, and information concerning nonacademic experience which may be of value." See "News and Notes: Personnel Exchange," *American*

Journal of Sociology 41, no. 3 (November 1935): 362. In subsequent issues, as though completing a registration blank, ads followed the journals' advice. See, e.g., "News and Notes: Personnel Exchange," *American Journal of Sociology* 41, no. 5 (March 1936): 669–70.

9. Every ad followed the same template: field, sex, age, marital status, highest degree, year, institution (or degree working toward), teaching experience, other experience, date of availability. See, e.g., "Back Matter: Academic Vacancies and Applications," *American Economic Review* 29, no. 4 (December 1939): n.p.; "Back Matter: Academic Vacancies and Applications," *American Economic Review* 30, no. 1 (March 1940): n.p.
10. William M. Tuttle Jr., curriculum vitae, ca. 1966, box 3, folder 16, KSRL, William M. Tuttle Jr. Collection, University Archives, PP 478, UKansas. See also Herbert Gutman, curriculum vitae, ca. 1965–1968; Morton Keller, curriculum vitae, 1965; and Peter Novick, curriculum vitae, ca. 1968–1969, all in box 106, folder 17, Allen G. Debus Papers, UChicago; Peter Rossi, curriculum vitae, March 1961, box 18, folder Job Offers & Inquiries, 1961–1967, Alice S. Rossi Papers, 1927–2009, MC 670, Schlesinger.
11. Names themselves could be self-fashioned. Immigrants "Americanizing" their names had long understood this. But as the example of the prominent Columbia sociologist Robert K. Merton suggests, the original motivation for taking a new name could later serve other ends. See ch. 19, "the road to preferment."
12. See, e.g., box 11, folder 23 (A–I), folder 24 (J–Z), Department of Near Eastern Studies Records, PUA; box 106, folder 17, Allen G. Debus Papers, 1948–1998, UChicago.
13. Theodore Caplow and Reece J. McGee, *The Academic Marketplace* (Basic Books, Inc., 1958), 111.
14. Marital and parental status had long been an element of university employment and information forms. See, e.g., Bosch Wolter, Application for Graduate Assistantship, University of Minnesota, Chemistry and Chemical Engineering, December 21, 1928 ("Place of Birth; Date of Birth; Race; Height; Weight; Married; Children"), box 6, folder Chemistry Personnel BO-BU, School of Chemistry Papers, UA, UMN; Form X, "For Recommendations of New Appointments to All Grades" [recommending appointment of Ormond J. Drake to an instructorship], September 23, 1937 ("Birthday; Married; Living Children"), box 3, folder Drake, Department of English Records, PUA; Raymond Dean Cool, Request for Information, University of Minnesota, Office of the President, December 15, 1945 ("5. Married or single; 6. Number of children"), box 11, folder Faculty Candidates with Ph.D. 1945, School of Chemistry Records (UAR 915), UA, UMN; Dinah L. Rozen, vita (form), Queensborough Community College, City University of New York, November 2, 1967 ("Personal: Date of Birth; Place of Birth; Married; Children (age:)"), 15, box 5, folder 5.6, Schlesinger.
15. Supplement to *American Sociological Review Employment Bulletin* 25, no. 1 (February 1960): 1, box 668, folder Committee on the Job Register 1960, AHA Papers (LoC).
16. Clarence H. Weissenstein, "Presenting Yourself in Writing," *Chemical and Engineering News* (January 26, 1959): 3–7; American Institute of Physics, *Registrants'*

Qualification Book, First Quarter, January 1, 1963, series I, AIP Career Services Miscellaneous, 1960–1998 (AR 451), box 1, folder 6, AIP Papers; *Finding Employment in the Mathematical Sciences* (American Mathematical Society, 1965).

17. MLA, Vacancies in College and University Departments of English for 1965–1966 (October 1965): ii–iii; MLA, Vacancies in College and University Departments of English for Fall 1971 (November 1970): iii. PDFs of the MLA *Job Information Lists* from 1960 to 2020, including the two cited here, are available online at https://www.mla.org/Resources/Career/Job-List/PDFs-of-the-MLA-Job-Information-List.
18. Failure to do so was itself worthy of comment. See, e.g., William C. McNeill to Daniel H. Thomas, April 4, 1962, box 38, folder 13, University of Chicago Department of History Records, UChicago.
19. See, e.g., Registration Blank [1914], Harvard University Appointment Office, Student Records: Samuel Flagg Bemis, HUA. The unevenness of change regarding religion is illustrated by New York and Indiana. See "Columbia Bias in Placement Bureau Alleged," *New York Herald Tribune,* June 10, 1946, box 60, folder 5, Historical Subjects Files, CUA; Columbia University Office of University Placement and Career Planning, confidential reference form and Office of University Placement registration form (1965), box 1, folder 7, Gerda Lerner Papers; Indiana University, School of Education, Bureau of Teacher Recommendations, credentials of Joseph Raben (June 4, 1952), box 5, folder 1, Department of English Records, PUA.
20. Gerda Lerner, resume, ca. 1966.
21. As the resume and vita became normalized in American academic life, physical and health data became rare on vitae in the humanities and social sciences but remained common on resumes in fields like chemistry and physics, where an appointment in industry or research was as or more likely than an academic appointment. See, e.g., Thomas P. Pearsall, resume, ca. 1974 (PhD Cornell 1973): "Birth Date: 2 November 1945; Birthplace: Richmond, Virginia; Height: 6'1" Weight: 180 lb. Health: excellent"; Robert I. Boughton Jr., resume, ca. 1974 (PhD OSU 1968): "Personal Information—Born: April 2, 1942 in Columbus, Ohio; Height: 6 ft 2 in; Weight: 190 lbs.; Married with two children; Health: Good," box 2 (unprocessed), folder Sample of Forms Filled out by Placement Service Registrants, 1974, AIP Placement Service Records, 1960–1978 (AR 205), AIP Papers. In industry physical data collected through forms and medical exams were tools for screening out "risks." See Nate Holdren, *Injury Impoverished: Workplace Accidents, Capitalism, and Law in the Progressive Era* (Cambridge University Press, 2021); Dan Bouk, *How Our Days Became Numbered.*
22. Vitae of Peter Novick, Stephan Albert Thernstrom, and Richard E. Ellis, all ca. 1968, all in box 106, folder 17, Allen G. Debus Papers, UChicago.
23. See, e.g., "Curriculum Vitae, 1958–1960," Department of Near Eastern Studies Records, box 11, folder 23 (A–I), folder 24 (J–Z), PUA; box 2 (unprocessed), folder Sample of Forms Filled out by Placement Service Registrants, 1974, AIP Placement Service Records, 1960–1978 (AR 205), AIP Papers.
24. See Dan Bouk, *Democracy's Data: The Hidden Stories in the U.S. Census and How to Read Them* (MCD, 2022), 76–79.
25. On sexuality and work in modern America, see Margot Canaday, *Queer Career*

(Princeton University Press, 2023). On the pressure for normality in family life in the Cold War, see Elaine Tyler May, *Homeward Bound: American Families in the Cold War Era* (Basic Books, 1988). On homophobia in academia and its personal costs more generally, see Regina Kunzel, *In the Shadow of Diagnosis: Psychiatric Power and Queer Life* (University of Chicago Press, 2024); Regina Kunzel, "Placing Newton Arvin in Queer History," *Nathaniel Hawthorne Review* 44, nos. 1–2 (2018): 82–89; Barry Werth, *The Scarlet Professor: Newton Arvin, a Literary Life Shattered by Scandal* (Anchor Books, 2002); and Kathleen Weiler, "The Case of Martha Deane: Sexuality and Power at Cold War UCLA," *History of Education Quarterly* 47, no. 4 (November 2007): 470–96; Paul Robinson, "Becoming a Gay Historian," in *Becoming Historians*, eds. James M. Banner Jr. and John R. Gillis (University of Chicago Press, 2009), 229–58; Martin Duberman, *Cures: A Gay Man's Odyssey* (Dutton, 1991).

26. Social-scientific studies documenting that married men with children were more successful reinforced the reading, conscious or not, of marriage and fatherhood as indicia of stability and later success. See, e.g., Arlie Russell Hochschild, "Inside the Clockwork of Male Careers," in *Women and the Power to Change*, ed. Florence Howe (McGraw-Hill, 1975), 47–80.

27. For the corollary in corporate life to the ministry, military, and diplomatic service, see Nan Enstad, *Cigarettes, Inc.: An Intimate History of the Corporation* (University of Chicago Press, 2018), 106–15; Hanna Papanek, "Family Status Production: The 'Work' and 'Non-Work' of Women," *Signs: Journal of Women in Culture and Society* (1979): 775–81; Papanek, "Men, Women, and Work: Reflections on the Two-Person Career," *American Journal of Sociology* 78 (1973): 852–72.

28. The wording varied little over time. See, e.g., A. C. McLaughlin to George F. Zook, June 30, 1916 ("I might add that he has a charming wife who is, I believe, both intellectually and socially a real asset—a matter which I think is not without value in a college town"), box 15, folder 1, University of Chicago Department of History Records, 1910–1921, UChicago; Robert K. Merton to Paul H. Giddens, February 4, 1957 ("In a way, I believe that I have saved the best for the last. It was only on my recent trip to Haverford that I met Mrs. Gordon. About her, I have only this to say: I would welcome the thought that she might be one of our faculty wives. She is gracious, unobtrusively intelligent and thoughtful of others"), box 107, folder 9, Robert K. Merton Papers, CUA; Robert K. Merton to Baidya Nath Varma, May 24, 1971 ("And Jan, his wife, is both charming and learned, with each quality reinforcing the other"), box 103, folder 3, Robert K. Merton Papers, 1928–2002, CUA.

29. J. Douglas Brown, Office of the Dean of the Faculty to chairmen of departments, interoffice correspondence, "Subject: Request for Information on Departmental Methods of Assisting and Evaluating Junior Teaching Personnel (i.e., Assistant Professor and Below)," February 9, 1949, box 102, folder 2, Office of the Dean of the Faculty Records, PUA.

30. Stanley E. Howard, Department of Economics and Social Institutions, to Dean J. Douglas Brown, interoffice correspondence, "Subject: Oversight of Junior Personnel," February 21, 1949; Donald A. Stauffer, Department of English, to Dean J. Douglas Brown, February 12, 1949; A. F. Buddington, Department of Geology, to Dean J. Douglas Brown, interoffice correspondence, "Subject Information on De-

partmental Methods of Assisting and Evaluating Junior Teaching Personnel," February 14, 1949; George F. Thomas, Department of Religion, to Dean J. D. Brown, interoffice correspondence, n.d., box 102, folder 2, Office of the Dean of the Faculty Records, PUA.

31. John R. Gillis, "Detours," in *Becoming Historians*, eds. Banner and Gillis, 162.
32. See Katherine Turk, "'The Hand that Rocks the Cradle Should Rock the U. of C.': The Faculty Wife and the Feminist Era," *Journal of Women's History* 26, no. 2 (Summer 2014): 114; Alison Cornish Thorne, "Visible and Invisible Women in Land-Grant Colleges, 1890–1940," Faculty Honor Lecture, Utah State University, October 8, 1985, 16; Evelyn Fox Keller, *A Feeling for the Organism: The Life and Work of Barbara McClintock* (Freeman, 1983), 53.
33. Nancy F. Cott, "Giving Character to Our Whole Civil Polity: Marriage and the Public Order in the Late Nineteenth Century," in *U. S. History as Women's History*, eds. Linda K. Kerber, Alice Kessler-Harris, and Kathryn Kish Sklar (University of North Carolina Press, 1995), 111. See also Cott, *Public Vows: A History of Marriage and the Nation* (Harvard University Press, 2000).
34. Margaret W. Rossiter, *Women Scientists in America, Struggles and Strategies to 1940* (Johns Hopkins University Press, 1982).
35. See the exchange between a faculty wife, commenting on the burdens of parenting alone, and the responding letter on the critical importance of a wife's support of her husband's work: Letters, "Progress or Progeny?," *Chemical and Engineering News* (November 18, 1957): 9–10; and Letters, "Chemists Need Good Wives," *Chemical and Engineering News* (March 17, 1958): 10, 11.
36. See, e.g., Ahmad Rafic Haffar, personal statement, ca. 1959–1960; Hussein M. Hamdan, curriculum vitae, ca. 1961; and Farhang Zabech, curriculum vitae, ca. 1960, all in box 11, folder 23 (A–I) and folder 24 (J–Z), Department of Near Eastern Studies Records, PUA. For letters of recommendation commenting on the fact of a foreign-born scholar's American wife or a Jewish scholar's Protestant wife, see, e.g., Ernest W. Burgess to James A. McCain, September 14, 1946, box 17, folder 12, Ernest Watson Burgess Papers, UChicago; Merle Fainsod to George A. Graham, January 15, 1947, box 12, folder 12, Department of Politics Records (AC 166), PUA.
37. David Walter Morgan, curriculum vitae, ca. 1965–1966, box 106, folder 17, Allen G. Debus Papers, UChicago.
38. Though as a matter of law, coverture—the legal subsuming of a married woman's civil identity under her husband's—had been dramatically curtailed by the 1960s, it was not gone—and its underlying assumptions continued to fundamentally shape women's (and men's) lives even after the legal "revolution" in women's rights in the 1960s and 1970s. See Allison Schwartz, "Banking on a Woman's Worth: Personhood and America's New Patriarchy of Debt, 1968–2008" (PhD diss., University of Minnesota, 2022), https://conservancy.umn.edu/items/e939a866-664c-4370-aed9-8deb4095cb5b; Alison Lefkovitz, *Strange Bedfellows: Marriage in the Age of Women's Liberation* (University of Pennsylvania Press, 2018); Cott, *Public Vows*; Linda Kerber, *No Constitutional Right to Be Ladies: Women and the Obligations of Citizenship* (Hill and Wang, 1998).
39. In 1927–1928, 81.4 percent of faculty at land-grant institutions were men; only 18.6 percent were women. Almost 80 percent of male faculty were married, com-

pared to only 10 percent of female faculty. See US Office of Education, *Survey of Land-Grant Colleges and Universities, Bulletin No. 9*, 2 vols. (Government Printing Office, 1930), vol. 1, 585.

40. Barbara Young Welke, *Law and the Borders of Belonging in the Long Nineteenth Century United States* (Cambridge University Press, 2010), 80; Elizabeth Cady Stanton to the National Woman's Rights Convention, November 24, 1856, included in the appendixes of *The History of Woman Suffrage*, vol. 1, eds. Elizabeth Cady Stanton, Susan B. Anthony, and Matilda Joslyn Gage (New York, 1881), 860.
41. See, e.g., "Curriculum Vitae Mary Catherine Bateson (Mrs. J. Barkov M. Kassarjian)," ca. 1966, and "Resume Lewis, Faye B. (Mrs. Herbert B.)," February 4, 1964, both in box 15, folder 12, Everett Cherrington Hughes Papers, UChicago; see also postcard stating intent to make formal application for the Associate Scholar program of the Radcliffe Institute for Independent Study, "signature Maxine W. Kumin" and immediately below "(Mrs. Victor Kumin)," February 20, 1961, box 38, folder Kumin, Maxine, Records of Mary Ingraham Bunting Institute, 1933–2008 (RG XXVIII), Schlesinger.
42. See, e.g., "Curriculum Vitae Mary Catherine Bateson (Mrs. J. Barkov M. Kassarjian)," ca. 1966; "Resume Lewis, Faye B. (Mrs. Herbert B.)," February 4, 1964; "Curriculum Vitae Jean Huleatt Wheeler (Mrs. Joseph Coolidge Wheeler)," ca. 1962, box 39, folder Wheeler, Jean, Records of Mary Ingraham Bunting Institute, 1933–2008 (RG XXVIII), Schlesinger. That identity could extend even after a husband's death. See, e.g., "Resume (Mrs.) Katharine Strelsky" ("status Widow of Professor Nikander Strelsky, founder/chairman of Russian Department Vassar College"), May 1962, box 41, folder Strelsky, Katharine, Schlesinger. The transformation of Barbara Heldt into Mrs. E. W. Monter Jr. is captured in a *New York Times* wedding announcement from June 20, 1963: "Barbara Heldt, Ph.D. Student, Is Bride on L. I.," subhead "Married in Woodmere to E. W. Monter, Jr., a History Professor." A photo of Heldt in her wedding veil was captioned, "Mrs. E. W. Monter, Jr., formerly Barbara Heldt." *New York Times*, June 20, 1963, 22.
43. Thorne, "Visible and Invisible Women in Land-Grant Colleges, 1890–1940," 15.
44. Gerda Lerner to Bert Loewenberg, October 27, 1967, box 1, folder 7, Gerda Lerner Papers.
45. Dorrian Apple Sweetser, personal data sheet, February 4, 1964, box 15, folder 12, Everett Cherrington Hughes Papers, 1922–1982, UChicago.
46. "I. Robert Rozen" (obituary), *New York Times*, November 19, 1966, 33.
47. Tillie Olsen, "Silences: When Writers Don't Write," *Harper's Magazine* (October 1965), 153–61.
48. Gerda Lerner, resume, ca. 1965, carton 1, folder 17, Gerda Lerner Papers. For another example, see Sylvia Clavan, resume ("Personal Data: Married; 2 children (ages 23 and 20)"), ca. 1973, box 10, folder Resumes, Sociologists for Women in Society Records, 1971–2003, 74-203-2004-M15, Schlesinger.
49. Consider the contrast between Hanna H. Gray's curriculum vitae and that of her husband Charles: see Hanna H. Gray, curriculum vitae ("Date of Birth: October 25, 1930; Heidelberg, Germany"; "Marital Status: Married, no children"), ca. 1968; and Charles M. Gray, curriculum vitae ("Born 23 November 1928, Champaign, Illinois"), ca. 1968, both in box 106, folder 17, Allen G. Debus Papers,

UChicago. For other examples, consider, Arlene Kaplan Daniels, PhD, curriculum vitae ("Born: December 10, 1930, New York, New York"; "Marital Status: Married to Richard R. Daniels, no children"), 1973; and Sylvia Fleis Fava, curriculum vitae ("Born: June 1, 1927, New York City. Married, John L. Fava, 1951, No Children"), 1973, both in box 10, folder Resumes, Sociologists for Women in Society Records, 1971–2003, 74-203-2004-M15, Schlesinger.

50. On the Institute, see Maggie Doherty, *The Equivalents: A Story of Art, Female Friendship, and Liberation in the 1960s* (Alfred A. Knopf, 2020); Elaine Yaffe, *Mary Ingraham Bunting: Her Two Lives* (Frederic C. Bell, 2005), 171–86.
51. Maxine W. Kumin, application form, Radcliffe Institute for Independent Study, February 26, 1961, 3; Tillie Olsen, application form, Radcliffe Institute for Independent Study, January 19, 1962, 4, both in Mary Ingraham Bunting Institute Records, RG XXVIII, Schlesinger.
52. Gillis, "Detours," 162. See also Mary Elizabeth Perry, "Clio on the Margins," in *Voices of Women Historians: The Personal, the Political, the Professional*, eds. Eileen Boris and Nupur Chaudhuri (Indiana University Press, 1999), 248–62.
53. Peter H. Rossi to James S. Coleman, June 26, 1961 (Rossi's reply to an inquiry from Coleman about joining them at JHU); S. M. Lipset to Peter Rossi, July 20, 1962, and August 6, 1962 (re: a potential job for Rossi at Berkeley); Philip M. Hauser to Frederick Mosteller, April 5, 1962 (recommending Peter Rossi as a fellow), all in box 18, folder Job Offers and Inquiries, 1961–1967, Alice S. Rossi Papers, 1927–2009, MC 670, Schlesinger.
54. Peter H. Rossi, curriculum vitae, March 1961.
55. Alice S. Rossi, curriculum vitae, ca. 1966–1967, box 1, folder Curriculum Vitae, 1966–1973, 2007, Alice S. Rossi Papers, 1927–2009, MC 670, Schlesinger.
56. Alice S. Rossi, curriculum vitae, ca. 1966–1967.
57. Alice S. Rossi, curriculum vitae, ca. 1966–1967.
58. Rossi to Coleman, June 26, 1961.
59. Alice S. Rossi, "Seasons of a Woman's Life," in Bennett M. Berger, *Authors of Their Own Lives* (University of California Press, 1990), 308.
60. Michael Walzer letter of recommendation, November 14, 1975, Susan Okin dossier, Harvard University Graduate School of Arts and Sciences, Office of Placement Services, box 2, folder 2, Susan Moller Okin Papers, 1966–2004, MC 734, Schlesinger.
61. Susan Moller Okin, curriculum vitae, March 14, 1984, Susan Okin dossier, Harvard University Graduate School of Arts and Sciences, Office of Placement Services, box 2, folder 2, Susan Moller Okin Papers, 1966–2004, MC 734, Schlesinger.
62. Susan Moller Okin, curriculum vitae, February 20, 1985, Susan Okin dossier, Harvard University Graduate School of Arts and Sciences, Office of Placement Services, box 2, folder 2, Susan Moller Okin Papers, 1966–2004, MC 734, Schlesinger.
63. Susan Moller Okin, curriculum vitae, February 20, 1985.
64. Susan Moller Okin, *Justice, Gender, and the Family* (Basic Books, Inc., 1989).
65. Okin, *Justice, Gender, and the Family*, 8–9.
66. Michael Polanyi, *Personal Knowledge: Towards a Post-Critical Philosophy* (University of Chicago Press, 1958). For a thoughtful and very helpful biography of Polanyi, guide to reading *Personal Knowledge*, and reception of the book, see the

foreword by Mary Jo Nye in Polanyi, *Personal Knowledge: Towards a Post-Critical Philosophy*, enlarged ed. with foreword by Mary Jo Nye (University of Chicago Press, 2015); and Mary Jo Nye, "Michael Polanyi: Science as Personal Knowledge and Social Practice," *Angewandte Chemie International Edition* (2017): 3426–33.

67. Polanyi, *Personal Knowledge*, vii–viii.
68. Polanyi, *Personal Knowledge*, 252.
69. On the distinction between the embodied liberty claimed by abolitionists and feminists in the nineteenth century and the political liberty voiced in the Declaration of Independence, see Karen Sanchez-Eppler, *Touching Liberty: Abolition, Feminism, and the Politics of the Body* (University of California Press, 1993); Elizabeth B. Clark, "Self-Ownership and the Political Theory of Elizabeth Cady Stanton," *Connecticut Law Review* 21 (1989): 905–41.

chapter thirteen: verdict

1. This chapter draws primarily on the McCormack Record on Appeal. The jury trial in New York Supreme Court-New York County, Hon. Thomas L. J. Corcoran, was on January 5, 6, 7, 8, 9, 12, 13, 14, 15, 16, 17, 19, and 20, 1948. The Record on Appeal does not note the specific dates for any individual's testimony. Citations from the record include witness and page numbers of testimony.
2. James McCormack, Petitions for Naturalization from the US District Court for the Southern District of New York, 1897–1944, series M1972, roll 979, New York Naturalization Records, 1882–1944, National Archives and Records Administration, Washington, DC, *Ancestry.com*; James McCormack, 1940 US Manuscript Census, NY, NY, ED 31-1662, 10A, in US Census Bureau, *Sixteenth Census of the United States: 1940* (Government Printing Office, 1942), https://catalog.archives.gov/id/16660414; Testimony of James McCormack, 75, McCormack Record on Appeal.
3. The sixteen-story neo-Renaissance building, designed by New York architect Emery Roth, was built in 1930.
4. Mr. Henry's apartment was on 81st Street, with views of Central Park West and the Natural History Museum; James was the doorman on the 81st Street side of the building. See Testimony of Milton A. Henry, 306–7, McCormack Record on Appeal.
5. Testimony of James McCormack, 107–8, McCormack Record on Appeal; Testimony of Milton A. Henry, 306–7, McCormack Record on Appeal.
6. Testimony of James McCormack, 107–8, McCormack Record on Appeal.
7. Testimony of James McCormack, 107–9, McCormack Record on Appeal. James McCormack both retained his job and was paid while he was off. It seems likely that his position was unionized. The BSEIU (Building Service Employees International Union), which began in Chicago as a union of flat (apartment) janitors in the early twentieth century, had expanded by the 1930s to New York City, where it unionized thousands of apartment janitors and elevator operators. The BSEIU changed its name to SEIU in 1968. On the history of the union, see Benjamin L. Peterson, "From Flats to the White House: A Brief History of SEIU, 1910–2010,"

in *The History and Global Impact of SEIU*, eds. Luís LM Aguiar and Joseph A. McMartin (University of Illinois Press, 2023), 17–23; John B. Jentz, "Labor, the Law and Economics: The Organization of the Chicago Flat Janitors' Union, 1902–1917," *Labor History* 38, no. 4 (Fall 1997): 413–31.

8. Testimony of James McCormack, 112–15, McCormack Record on Appeal.
9. Complaint, 10-25, Testimony of James McCormack, 113–16, 120–21, McCormack Record on Appeal.
10. See ch. 14, "finding their way to law."
11. The parties agreed that all testimony (depositions) taken in the Gene Autry cowboy suit cases pending in federal court at the time of the McCormack trial could be used by any of the parties in McCormack. See Stipulation, May 19, 1947, 1148–49, Plaintiff's Exhibit 3, McCormack Record on Appeal.
12. This was true also of other early cases; see, e.g., Complaint and Summons, April 9, 1946, Richard Johnson Case File.
13. Summons and Complaint, January 24, 1946, Weatherell Case File.
14. Summons and Complaint, 9–10, McCormack Record on Appeal. The complaint included in the Record on Appeal is from September 1946. The action was commenced with a summons filed on the Henry Co. and E. F. Timme & Son on May 15, 1945, with the initial complaint served on July 25, 1945. See Statement Under Rule 234, 1, McCormack Record on Appeal.
15. Seven-year-old Tommy McCormack was severely burned over the lower half of his body on January 6, 1945. The trial for his injuries, suffering, and death, and for the injuries to his father's hands, began on January 5, 1948.
16. The two retailers were McCrory's (Cutter) and Lou's Auto Stores (Detrick, Flesher, Warnick). The other suits pending by early January 1948 (listed chronologically by date of incident) were: Lockhart, Greatorex, Gerber, Habina, Detrick, Touhill (but only against the M. A. Henry Co.), Viands, Wilks, Gates, (John Elwyn) Jones, Bradley, Klinck, DiTrapani, Weatherell, Stultz, Cumberledge, King, Wrobbel, (Richard) Johnson, Adams, Flesher, Warnick, Berry, McCarthy, Bates, Baer, McMaster, Tetla, and Griffin. Gene Autry was also named as a defendant in most of these actions. Du Pont was first named as a defendant in 1947 and was subsequently added to actions in many suits that had been filed earlier in which the statute of limitations had not run. For reasons I explain in ch. 14, "finding their way to law," all the legal actions against the defendants involved in the manufacturing chain were brought in either state or federal court in New York state.
17. Unlike many families who faced ongoing medical expenses for their child, there were no continuing medical expenses for Tommy. The hospital, funeral, and burial expenses for Tommy McCormack totaled $1,618.50 (hospital expenses $1,284.50; funeral and burial expenses $334). There had been no separate expenses for doctors or nurses. James McCormack's hospital expenses for a week's stay totaled only $32 with no separate doctor's bills or expenses for medical supplies. He was paid for the weeks he was off work. See Bill of Particulars, January 22, 1946, 61–62; Testimony of James McCormack, 108, McCormack Record on Appeal.
18. At several points in his testimony James McCormack was "overcome by emotion." See Testimony of James McCormack, 76, 93, McCormack Record on Appeal.
19. Elliot Paley (plaintiffs' lawyer), 100–101, McCormack Record on Appeal.

20. Elliot Paley (plaintiffs' lawyer), 101, McCormack Record on Appeal.
21. Testimony of John ("Jackie") McCormack, 122–24; Testimony of Marvin Kramer, 143–60; Testimony of Dr. Ernest E. Arnheim, 199–213; Testimony of Catherine McCormack, 247–51; all in McCormack Record on Appeal.
22. On this point, see also Elaine Scarry, *The Body in Pain: The Making and Unmaking of the World* (Oxford University Press, 1987), 296–307.
23. He read from the pre-trial testimony of Milton Henry, president of the M. A. Henry Co.; of Arthur Robertshaw Jr., manager, vice president, and secretary of Woonsocket Falls Mill, and employed by E. F. Timme & Son in an advisory capacity to William E. Roschen; and of William E. Roschen, the sole general partner in the limited partnership of E. F. Timme & Son and treasurer of Woonsocket Falls Mill. And through their pre-trial testimony, he built the plaintiff's case, establishing these men's positions within their firms, what their firms did, the duration and character of the firms' business relationships, and with it the chain of production of the Gene Autry cowboy suit.
24. The foundation laid, the judge instructed the jury that the fabric samples and the cowboy suit were "now in evidence as to all parties." See Judge Corcoran, 141, 142, McCormack Record on Appeal.
25. Testimony of Marvin Kramer, 143–44, McCormack Record on Appeal.
26. Testimony of Marvin Kramer, 147–48, 154, 155, McCormack Record on Appeal.
27. Bill of Particulars, January 22, 1946, 61, McCormack Record on Appeal.
28. Testimony of Catherine McCormack, 247–51, McCormack Record on Appeal.
29. Testimony of James McCormack, 81–86, 93–94, McCormack Record on Appeal.
30. Testimony of James McCormack, 121, McCormack Record on Appeal.
31. Testimony of James McCormack, 103, McCormack Record on Appeal.
32. Testimony of Catherine McCormack, 249–51, McCormack Record on Appeal.
33. Judge's Charge to the Jury, 1073, 1081, McCormack Record on Appeal.
34. Testimony of James McCormack, 84, McCormack Record on Appeal.
35. Plaintiff's Exhibits 1 and 2 (introduced in testimony of James McCormack), 82, 1144–46, McCormack Record on Appeal.
36. Recall that when news of the hazard broke in early April 1945, Representative John E. Rankin (D-MS) demanded on the House floor that the Department of Justice "see to it that the ones responsible for this criminal practice are vigorously prosecuted" (Congressional Record, 79th Cong., 1st Sess., microfilm reel 252, April 9, 1945, 3227–28). Though criminal charges against officers and employees of enterprises were rare, they were not totally unheard of. Criminal charges had been brought in the 1944 Hartford Circus fire and the 1942 Cocoanut Grove nightclub fire. See Henry S. Cohn and David Bollier, *The Great Hartford Circus Fire: Creative Settlement of Mass Disasters* (Yale University Press, 1991), 11–12, 52–54; "Ten Are Indicted in Night Club Fire: Four Boston Officials Named by Jury with Cocoanut Grove Operators and Employees," *New York Times*, January 1, 1943, 1; "Night Club Owner Guilty in Boston: Convicted of Manslaughter in 19 of the 491 Deaths in the Cocoanut Grove Fire," *New York Times*, April 11, 1943, 28. Those instances differed in their mass character—hundreds injured and killed in a single event—and more importantly, in the public character of the venues, and the fact of state laws requiring flameproof or flame-retardant curtains and furnishings. In

the 1940s, there were no state laws regulating the use of inflammable materials in clothing or home furnishings. Capt. R. A. Warfield, deputy fire marshal in Washington, DC, noted that the absence of legislation limited his actions to alerting the manufacturer and retailers. See "Parents Warned of Flaming Death in Cowboy Togs," *Times-Herald* (Washington, DC), April 8, 1945, A3. In January 1945, California was the first state to adopt a law relating to the sale of flammable fabrics. See "Governor Signs Urgency Bills," *Los Angeles Times*, January 31, 1945, 12.

37. Defendant M. A. Henry Co.'s Exhibit F, 1168, McCormack Record on Appeal.
38. Testimony of William E. Roschen, 764, McCormack Record on Appeal.
39. Defendants Timme and Woonsocket's Exhibit TW4, 1190, McCormack Record on Appeal.
40. Defendants Timme and Woonsocket's Exhibit TW5, 1192–93, McCormack Record on Appeal.
41. Testimony of Milton A. Henry, 403–4, 1180 (Defendant M. A. Henry Co.'s Exhibits Y, Z, AA "omitted pursuant to stipulation"), McCormack Record on Appeal.
42. Testimony of Milton A. Henry, 306–13, McCormack Record on Appeal.
43. Defendants Timme and Woonsocket's Exhibit TW11, 1200, McCormack Record on Appeal.
44. Testimony of William E. Roschen, 715–16, McCormack Record on Appeal.
45. Charge to the Jury, 1077–78, McCormack Record on Appeal.
46. Testimony of William E. Roschen, 713, McCormack Record on Appeal.
47. Charge to the Jury, 1075, McCormack Record on Appeal.
48. *MacPherson v. Buick*, 217 N. Y. 382, 389–90 (1916). On *MacPherson*, see also Sally H. Clarke, "Unmanageable Risks: MacPherson v. Buick and the Emergence of a Mass Consumer Market," *Law and History Review* 23, no. 1 (Spring 2005): 1–52; and Sally H. Clarke, *Trust and Power: Consumers, the Modern Corporation, and the Making of the United States Automobile Market* (Cambridge University Press, 2007), 91–148. Tort was a matter of state law, and so the MacPherson decision was initially binding only on courts in New York. But, over time, the rule in *MacPherson* was adopted by other states. See also Barbara Young Welke, "The Cowboy Suit Tragedy: Spreading Risk, Owning Hazard in the Modern American Consumer Economy," *Journal of American History* 101, no. 1 (June 2014): 97–121.
49. Noone v. Perlberg, 268 A.D. 149, aff'd 294 N. Y. 680 (1944), aff'd w/o op, 294 N.Y. 680, 60 N.E.2d 839 (1945).
50. Charge to the Jury, 1080–81, McCormack Record on Appeal.
51. Charge to the Jury, 1081, McCormack Record on Appeal.
52. Charge to the Jury, 1081, McCormack Record on Appeal.
53. Charge to the Jury, 1082–83, McCormack Record on Appeal.
54. Charge to the Jury, 1083, McCormack Record on Appeal.
55. Charge to the Jury, 1083–84, McCormack Record on Appeal.
56. Charge to the Jury, 1084–85, McCormack Record on Appeal.
57. Charge to the Jury, 1085, McCormack Record on Appeal.
58. Charge to the Jury, 1089–95, McCormack Record on Appeal.
59. Charge to the Jury, 1085–87, McCormack Record on Appeal.
60. For the history of wrongful death statutes, see John Fabian Witt, "From Loss of Services to Loss of Support: The Wrongful Death Statutes, the Origins of Mod-

ern Tort Law, and the Making of the Nineteenth-Century Family," *Law and Social Inquiry* 25 (2000): 717–55; Viviana A. Zelizer, *Pricing the Priceless Child: The Changing Social Value of Children* (Basic Books, 1985), 140–41; Wex S. Malone, "The Genesis of Wrongful Death," *Stanford Law Review* 17 (1965): 1043.

61. Zelizer, *Pricing the Priceless Child*; James D. Schmidt, *Industrial Violence and the Legal Origins of Child Labor* (Cambridge University Press, 2010).
62. Charge to the Jury, 1087, McCormack Record on Appeal. See Zelizer, *Pricing the Priceless Child.*
63. Charge to the Jury, 1088, McCormack Record on Appeal.
64. Charge to the Jury, 1088–89, McCormack Record on Appeal.
65. Charge to the Jury, 1087–88, McCormack Record on Appeal.
66. Charge to the Jury, 1089, McCormack Record on Appeal.
67. The jury began its deliberations at 11:40 a.m. and returned with a verdict at 6:50 p.m. the same day. See Charge to the Jury, 1138–39, McCormack Record on Appeal. The jurors were not individually identified in the record. On the jury including one woman, see Charge to the Jury, 1073 ("Mr. Foreman, Madam, and Gentlemen of the Jury"), Charge to the Jury.
68. To calculate the present value of these numbers, see "CPI Inflation Calculator," US Bureau of Labor Statistics, accessed October 7, 2025, https://www.bls.gov/data/inflation_calculator.htm.
69. Verdict, 1139–41, McCormack Record on Appeal. The McCormacks' case against Milton Henry individually was a hard one from the start. What kind of man would give something as a gift to another man for his children knowing that it might leave them horribly or fatally burned? But there was another way to look at this question. By December 1944, when Milton Henry gave the gift to James McCormack, he had been making and selling the cowboy suit with the fuzzy fabric for almost two years without—if we are to believe him—notice of any injuries. It did not require, in other words, that jurors attribute a callous disregard for the lives of his doorman's children to Milton Henry for them to find that he in fact had been told the fabric was inflammable.
70. Motions to Set Aside Verdict, Motions for Directions of Verdict, 1141–43; Notice of Appeal, 3–8; both in McCormack Record on Appeal.
71. "$64,500 for Death of Boy, Father Wins Suit Over Fatal Burns," *New York Post*, January 21, 1948, 20; "Award $64,500 in Boy's Death," *New York World-Telegram*, January 21, 1948, 1. See also "64,500 Awarded for Boy's Death," *Sun* (New York, NY), January 21, 1948, 17.
72. "Cowboy Suit Death Gets $64,500 Verdict," *New York Times*, January 22, 1948, 29; "$64,500 Is Won by Father in Death of Boy, 8," *New York Herald Tribune*, January 22, 1948, 21.
73. See, e.g., "Jury Gives $64,500 for Death of Boy," *Buffalo Evening News*, January 21, 1948, 1; "Father Awarded $64,500 for Autry Suit Fatality," *Herald-News* (Passaic, NJ), January 21, 1948, 1; "Cowboy Suit Fire Death Brings $64,500 Award," *Philadelphia Inquirer*, January 21, 1948, 1; "Jury Awards $64,500 in Fatal Burning Suit," *Richmond Times-Dispatch*, January 22, 1948, 11; "$64,500 Awarded in 'Cowboy Suit' Death from Fire," *Atlanta Constitution*, January 22, 1948, 19; "Cowboy Suit Makers Blamed in Boy's Death," *Tampa Tribune*, January 22, 1948, 16; "Award

$64,500 in Boy's Death," *Detroit Free Press*, January 22, 1948, 3; "A $64,500 Award in Death," *Kansas City Star*, January 21, 1948, 1; "$64,500 Awarded Father for Son's Fire Death," *Spokesman-Review* (Spokane, WA), January 22, 1948, 3; "$64,500 Award in Boy's Fire Death," *Des Moines Register*, January 22, 1948, 1; "Flaming Chaps Bring Verdict," *Los Angeles Times*, January 22, 1948, 4.

74. "Flaming Chaps Bring Verdict."

chapter fourteen: finding their way to law

1. "Award $64,500 in Boy's Death," *Detroit Free Press*, January 22, 1948, 3.
2. Even today, the vast majority of individuals with a legal claim for injury do not bring suit. See David M. Engel, *The Myth of the Litigious Society: Why We Don't Sue* (University of Chicago Press, 2016); Tom Baker, *The Medical Malpractice Myth* (University of Chicago Press, 2005), 70; William L. F. Felstiner, Richard L. Abel, and Austin Sarat, "The Emergence and Transformation of Disputes: Naming, Blaming, Claiming . . . ," *Law and Society Review* 15 (1980–1981): 631–54.
3. News reports of war casualties and stories of local boys missing, injured, or dead were ubiquitous. See, e.g., "U.S. Casualties Reach 78,235; 12,123 Killed," *Washington Post*, April 25, 1943, M1; "2,184, Americans Killed in Africa; Wounded Tallied 9,437, Missing, Including Prisoners 6,937, in 18,558 Total Casualties," *New York Times*, May 28, 1943, 9; "Navy Reports 63 Casualties; 6 from Illinois," *Chicago Daily Tribune*, August 11, 1943, 7. Those stories sometimes appeared on the same page as stories of a child burned in a cowboy suit. See, e.g., *Chronicle-Telegram* (Elyria, OH), November 5, 1942, 1 ("Burns Fatal to Boy" [David Lonneman] and immediately above it, with a larger headline, "American Merchant Vessel Torpedoed, 31 Lives Lost"); *Freehold (NJ) Transcript*, May 5, 1944, 13 ("Lad, 4 1/2, Fatally Burned Playing in His Kitchen" [Billy Kingston] and "Morganville Man Dead of Injuries in the Pacific" [with photo]); *Bradford (PA) Era*, May 15, 1944, 10 ("Burns Prove Fatal" [Howard Diable] and "11 Crewman Killed in Bomber Crash"); *Herald-News* (Passaic, NJ), November 1, 1944, 13 ("Wallingford Boy Seriously Burned" [Frederick Piechota] and "2 Lyndhurst Men Listed as Wounded").
4. "Polio Grips 40 Counties in VA," *Washington Post*, August 14, 1944, 3; "Polio Epidemic Reports: 2,048 Cases in 1945," *Chicago Daily Tribune*, July 28, 1945, 5; "154 Dead of Polio in U. S. Since Jan. 1: Over 5,600 Cases Reported," *New York Times*, August 10, 1945, 15. See Daniel J. Wilson, "A Crippling Fear: Experiencing Polio in the Era of FDR," *Bulletin of the History of Medicine* 72, no. 3 (Fall 1998): 464–95.
5. Testimony of James McCormack, 116, McCormack Record on Appeal.
6. See ch. 7, "playing with fire."
7. See ch. 13, "verdict."
8. Roland Nicholson, "Fire Marshal in N.Y. to Test Cowboy Suits," *Times-Herald* (Washington, DC), April 11, 1945, 17; Roland Nicholson, "LaGuardia Asks Full Report on Cowboy Suits Made in N.Y.," *Times-Herald* (Washington, DC), April 11, 1945, 17.
9. The children named in the coverage were: Edward Bradley, Arthur Cumberledge Jr., Tony DiTrapani, Lawrence Gates, Billy Greatorex, Elwood Leary Jr., Ronald

King, Arthur Lunsford, William Nelson, James F. Rees, Calvin Lee Sibley, Charles Stultz, Robert Viands, and Willie Wilks Jr. For the coverage, see ch. 7, "playing with fire."

10. Robert E. Lynch was DC counsel for Cumberledge, Bradley, Wilks, Gates, Greatorex, and Stultz.
11. "Booby Traps: Child Burned When Cowboy Pants Ignite," *Cumberland Evening Times*, May 15, 1945, 1 (second section, Bobby Flesher and Cecil Warnick).
12. "Frostburg Klondike Youth Burned at Play: Seven-Year-Old Boy Suffers Severe Burns When Cowboy Pants Catch Fire," *Cumberland Evening Times*, August 22, 1945, 10; "Two Badly Burned Boys Hope to Leave Hospital Here Soon," *Cumberland Evening Times*, September 11, 1945, 1 (second section, Wayne Cutter and James Detrick).
13. "Cowboy Suit Is Blamed in Death of Boy, Linked to Fires Injurious to 2," *Philadelphia Inquirer*, April 12, 1945, 19.
14. W. Emory Burnett and H. Taylor Caswell, "Severe Burns from Inflammable Cowboy Pants," *Journal of the American Medical Association* (April 1946): 935–36.
15. Tommy Habina's family brought suit in fall 1946; Edward Klinck's family brought suit in early 1947. Habina Interview.
16. Petition of Frank Habina, April 1, 1948, 3, Habina Case File; Petition of Edward Klinck Sr., May 28, 1948, 3, Klinck Case File.
17. Lockhart Interview.
18. Lockhart Interview.
19. On contingent fees, see Herbert M. Kritzer, *Risks, Reputations, and Rewards: Contingency Fee Legal Practice in the United States* (Stanford University Press, 2004); Peter Karsten, "Enabling the Poor to Have Their Day in Court: The Sanctioning of Contingency Fee Contracts, a History to 1940," *DePaul Law Review* 47 (1998): 231; Stephen Landsman, "The History of Contingency and the Contingency of History," *DePaul Law Review* 47, no. 2 (1998): 261–66.
20. The highly networked organization of plaintiffs' personal-injury lawyers came just after these cases. See John Fabian Witt, "The King and the Dean: Melvin Belli, Roscoe Pound, and the Common Law Nation," in *Patriots and Cosmopolitans: Hidden Histories of American Law* (Harvard University Press, 2007), 211–78.
21. On lawyers' role in and reasons for refusing to take cases, see Engel, *Myth of the Litigious Society*, 163–68; and Kritzer, *Risks, Reputations, and Rewards*, 84–86.
22. Affidavit of Paul Javinsky, February 26, 1952, Javinsky Case File.
23. Charles J. Baragona Petition, October 14, 1949, 4, Baragona Case File.
24. Complaint, June 19, 1947; Affidavit of John Lockhart Sr., June 11, 1948, 5; both in Lockhart Case File.
25. "Playing with Fire Costs Boy His Life," *Herald-News* (Passaic, NJ), November 2, 1943, 1.
26. "Death Lurks in Boys' Play Suits," *Herald-News* (Passaic, NJ), June 25, 1946, 1, 12.
27. Testimony of Stella Urban, February 3, 1950, 4, Casimir Kresokowski Case File.
28. Testimony of Stella Urban, February 3, 1950, 4, Casimir Kresokowski Case File.
29. Incidents preceding Tommy McCormack's injuries: Gorab, Sondej, Krzeczkowski, Dorsey, Duffy, Janes, Koble, Giacomarro, Caparco, Izzo, Moore, Javinsky, Malone, Zibor, Piechota, La France, and Blessington. Incidents after Tommy McCormack

was injured but before the McCormack verdict: Chesley Franklin Johnson, Weinstein, Sibley, Lee, Baker, Krau, Strong, Ikner, Kropp, Sullivan, Cizek, Gagnon, Devens, Felton, Intelisano, Hummel, Peterson, Palmateer, and Pritchard. The suit by the Giacomarros was one of many in which the child's father explicitly noted that it was only following news of the McCormack verdict that they knew they had a legal claim and filed suit. See Petition of Ralph Giacomarro, January 31, 1951, 2–3, Giacomarro Case File.

30. Docket Sheet (listing complaint and summons as filed on Jun. 24, 1948), Izzo Case File (federal court).

31. Affidavit of Charles J. Baragona, October 24, 1949, 4, Baragona Case File; Affidavit of Elliot B. Paley, October 31, 1949, Baragona Case File; Affidavit of Paul Javinsky, February 26, 1952, Javinsky Case File.

32. Butler represented Bradley, Cumberledge, DiTrapani, Greatorex, King, Stultz, Warnick, and Wilks. Sibley had different DC and local counsel. See case files.

33. Elliot B. Paley of the firm Nemeroff, Jelline, Danzig & Paley represented at least twenty-one families in the cowboy suit litigation, of which I've identified sixteen (Dorsey, Koble, Giacomarro, Malone, Touhill, McCormack, Weinstein, Peterson, Gagnon, Felton, Ulick (Ulich), Baragona, Timberlake, Brunette, Verbonitz, and Hutchinson). See Affidavit of Elliot B. Paley, December 8, 1954, 3, Touhill Case File (referring to representing twenty families in addition to the McCormacks). Edmond Borgio Butler, of the firm O'Connell and Butler, represented at least twenty-four families (Greatorex, Caparco, Chesley Franklin Johnson, Wilks, Gates, John Elwyn Jones, Bradley, DiTrapani, Stultz, Mitchell Gray Lee, Cumberledge, King, Flesher, Warnick, Baker, Strong, Appleby, Cizek, Burke, Tetla, Tormollen, Szumita, Mistretta, Perry).

34. Felton Case File (action against retailer); "Son of Atty. Elwyn Jones is Seriously Burned," *Pottsville (PA) Republican*, February 26, 1945, 4; Strong Case File.

35. Elmer Groefsema represented Lockhart, Adams, Berry, McMaster, and Javinsky. See case files.

36. In addition to examples already noted, consider the Philadelphia firm of Richter, Lord, and Farage using Leo Gitlin as New York counsel. See Habina Interview; Petition of Frank Habina, April 1, 1948, 3, Habina Case File; Petition of Edward Klinck Sr., May 28, 1948, 3, Klinck Case File; Docket Sheet, Moore Case File.

37. Sec. 27. 605 Limitation of personal actions, and 27.607 Same; accrual of cause of action in case of minority, insanity, or imprisonment, in *Michigan Statutes Annotated (1935)*, comp. and ed. by J. M. Henderson (Callaghan and Company, 1938), 456, 481.

38. Sec. 34 Limitation in cases of personal injury, in *Purdon's Pennsylvania Statutes Annotated* (West Publishing Co., 1931), 62.

39. Moore et al. v. Roschen et al., 93 F. Supp. 993 (S.D.N.Y. 1950).

40. *Roschen et al.*, 93 F. Supp. 993. The suit for James Hummel's death too illustrates the inequities differences in state statutes of limitation produced. See M. A. Henry Co., Inc., Motion for Summary Judgment, October 13, 1949; Judgment Dismissing Complaint Against M. A. Henry Co., Inc., April 7, 1952; and Order Dismissing Case, April 7, 1952; all in Hummel Case File.

41. On the heightened risk of death during the war, see ch. 8, "falling out of time."
42. Petition of Alvin A. Dorsey, Buffalo, NY, May 1952, 3, Dorsey Case File. Complaint, Duffy Case File; Amended Complaint, Blessington Record on Appeal (NY Supreme Court), 38–65; Affidavit of Milton A. Henry, October 2, 1949, Blessington Record on Appeal (NY Supreme Court), 8 (re: date Blessington action filed). For the dismissals in Duffy, see Duffy Case File.
43. Sec. 49 Actions to be commenced within three years, and Sec. 60 Certain disabilities excluded from time to commence action, in *Thompson's Laws of New York, 1939* (Edward Thompson Company, 1939), 1625, 1626; Sec. 130 Action by executor or administrator for negligence or wrongful act or default causing death of decedent, in *The Consolidated Laws of New York Annotated, Book 13, Decedent Estate Law, 1938* (Edward Thompson Company, 1939), 429.
44. Duffy v. E. I. Du Pont de Nemours & Company et al., 193 Misc. 175, 81 N.Y.S.2d 630, affd. 274 A.D. 908, 84 N.Y.S.2d 710 (1948); see also Duffy Case File.
45. Affidavit of Thomas F. Frawley Read in Opposition to Motion of Defendant M. A. Henry Co., Inc. to Dismiss, etc., October 18, 1949, 99–135, Blessington Record on Appeal (NY Supreme Court).
46. Blessington v. McCrory Stores Corporation, et al., 198 Misc. 291, 299 (NY 1950).
47. Sec. 60, *Thompson's Laws of New York, 1939*, 1626.
48. Sec. 722 Actions to be brought in six years, and Sec. 738 Saving in favor of those under disability, in *Mississippi Code 1942, Annotated*, vol. 1, eds. Greek L. Rice and George H. Ethridge (Lawyers Co-Operative Publishing Company, 1943), 784, 804; Sec. 1453 Actions for injuries producing death, *Mississippi Code 1942 Annotated*: vol. 2 (Lawyers Co-Operative Publishing Company, 1944), 221–22.
49. Strong Case File.
50. See ch. 13, "verdict," on the history of wrongful death statutes.
51. Answer (Henry Co.), April. 22, 1946; Amended Answer (Henry Co.), October 25, 1946, 3, DiTrapani Case File.
52. "Father Awarded $64,500 For Autry Suit Fatality," *Herald-News* (Passaic, NJ), January 21, 1948, 1, 2; Docket Sheet (Casimir) Kresokowski, Casimir Kresokowski Case File; Docket Sheet (Stanley) Krzeczkowski, Stanley Krzeczkowski Case File.
53. Sec. 2:24-2 Two years; actions for injuries to person by wrongful act; Sec. 2:24-4 Disabilities affecting limitations prescribed by sections 2;24-1, 2:24-2 and 2:24-3; Sec. 2:47-1 When action lies; and Sec. 2:47-3 Limitation of actions, in *New Jersey Statutes Annotated: Permanent Edition* (West Publishing Co., 1939), 36, 42, 227, 241.
54. Blessington v. McCrory Stores Corporation, et al., 305 N.Y. 140 (1953); Duffy v. E. I. Du Pont de Nemours & Co., et al., 193 Misc. 175, 81 NYS2d 630 (1948), aff'd. 274 A.D. 908, 84 NYS2d 710 (1948).
55. Complaint and Docket Sheet, Habina Case File; Sec. 2315 Torts-Liability-Survival of Action, in *Civil Code of the State of Louisiana Revision of 1870*, ed. Benjamin Wall Dart (Bobbs-Merrill Company, 1945), 16; Petition of Charles J. Baragona, October 14, 1949, 1, 3–4, Baragona Case File.
56. Affidavit of John A. Touhill, December 8, 1954, 3–4; Affidavit of Elliot B. Paley, December 9, 1954, 1–2; both in Touhill Case File.

57. Order, January 1, 1949 (order substituting Nemeroff, Jelline, Danzig, and Paley as plaintiffs' counsel); Affidavit of John Touhill, December 8, 1954, 3–4; both in Touhill Case File.
58. Order, June 30, 1948, Supplemental Amended Complaint, Touhill Case File.
59. Memorandum of Plaintiffs in Opposition to Motion for Summary Judgment, November 13, 1952, Touhill Case File.
60. Motion for Summary Judgment, October 8, 1952; Order, March 3, 1953 (granting summary judgment for Autry), Touhill Case File.
61. Argued November 13, 1953; Order, February 13, 1953, Touhill Case File.
62. Judgment, September 1, 1954, Appellate Division, First Department; Order, November 8, 1954; both in Touhill Case File.
63. The phrase "murderously inflammable" is from Paley's affidavit on appeal. See Affidavit of Elliot B. Paley, December 8, 1954, Touhill Case File.
64. Examples include Elwood Leary Jr., Arthur Lunsford, Larry and Wayne Meisner, and Gerald Sukinik.
65. Consider Donald Frederick Yerkes (Geneva, NY), Daniel Fogarty (Baltimore, MD), Billy Kingston (Freehold, NJ), Howard Diable (Pitcairn, PA), and Thomas James Hizny (West Wyoming, PA), all of whom were wearing cowboy suits the pants of which caught fire. They all died the day of their injuries or within a few days. See "Yule Gift Brings Tragedy to Boy, 11," *Democrat and Chronicle* (Rochester, NY), December 28, 1942, 25; "Burns Are Fatal to Boy, 7," *Baltimore Evening Sun*, July 2, 1943, 33; "Cowboy Playsuit Sales Probed," *Baltimore Evening Sun*, February 28, 1946, 29; "Freehold Boy Dies of Burns," *Evening News* (Asbury Park, NJ), May 3, 1944, 1; "W. Wyoming Boy Fatally Burned," *Mauch Chunk (PA) Times-News*, October 30, 1944, 1.
66. See ch. 16, "the price of settlement."
67. Ralph Nader, *Unsafe at Any Speed* (Grossman, 1965).
68. Roland Nicholson and Spence Drummond, "Cowboy Suit Tragedies Under Policy Scrutiny," *Times-Herald* (Washington, DC), April 9, 1945, 1, 17.
69. Expressed as an equation: ninety-eight (the total number of lawsuits I have identified against the principal defendants) divided by eight-twelfths (the fraction of DC families named in the DC news coverage who brought suit) equals 147 (a conservative estimate of the number of children injured or killed). In a brief filed by William M. Blake Jr., argued by Thomas F. Frawley, lawyers for Michael Blessington's family, they listed the number of children burned in Gene Autry cowboy suits as 150. Brief for Plaintiff-Appellant [Michael Blessington], 6, Blessington Record on Appeal on Appeal (NY Supreme Court, App Divn).
70. The data was produced in a case involving a Gene Autry cowboy suit purchased from McCrory's Philadelphia store in 1943. See Milton A. Henry Answers to Interrogatories (list "Shipments to McCrory Stores," 1942, 1943), November 4, 1947, Habina Case File.
71. Engel, *Myth of the Litigious Society*, 24.
72. Milton A. Henry Answers to Interrogatories (list "Shipments to McCrory Stores," 1942, 1943), November 4, 1947, Habina Case File.
73. The reference is from a letter from Gene Autry's lawyer, Bill Martin, to Autry in 1951, but it fits the defendants' words and actions throughout. See Bill Martin to

Gene Autry, September 17, 1951, 2, box 1, Agents & Licensees, T94-45-30, folder M. A. Henry Co.—New York or Leslie Henry Co. (1 of 2) 1950–1951, Autry Collection.

74. "Fire Marshal in N.Y. to Test Cowboy Suits," *Times-Herald* (Washington, DC), April 10, 1945, 17.

chapter fifteen: to be "judged on our capabilities alone"

1. Jo Freeman, "Women on the Social Science Faculties Since 1892" (draft of a speech given at the minority groups workshop of the Political Science Association Conference, the University panel on the status of women at Chicago, and elsewhere), winter 1970, box 1, folder Women's Caucus-ASA-1969, Sociologists for Women in Society Records, 1971–2003, 74-203-2004-M15 (unprocessed), Schlesinger (hereafter SWS Papers).
2. Freeman, "Women on the Social Science Faculties Since 1892."
3. On the dramatic expansion and democratization of access to higher education between 1945 and the 1970s, see Richard M. Freeland, *Academia's Golden Age: Universities in Massachusetts 1945–1970* (Oxford University Press, 1992).
4. Michael V. Metz, *Radicals in the Heartland: The 1960s Student Protest Movement at the University of Illinois* (University of Illinois Press, 2019); Robert Cohen and Reginald E. Zelnik, *The Free Speech Movement: Reflections on Berkeley in the 1960s* (University of California Press, 2002); Todd Gitlin, *The Sixties: Years of Hope, Days of Rage* (Bantam, 1993).
5. Sex, marital and parental status, and age–all of which had particular resonance for women—were givens on vitae in the 1950s and 1960s. That race almost never appeared on vitae, and that in the rare instances in which it did the reference was "white," reflected the racial apartheid that applied in academic life. Historically Black colleges were the only institutions with Black faculty, and their faculty were largely male. This meant that white women in contrast to Blacks and other minorities, male and female, had a foothold—that is, they were present throughout academia and represented a significant percentage of graduate students in the 1960s, which had the impact of giving them a base from which to mobilize. Black women, by virtue of race and sex, were doubly excluded—from both access to advanced degrees and academic appointments—and, further, they lacked access to even the liminal appointments many white women had as "faculty wives." See Deborah Gray White, "Introduction: A Telling History," in *Telling Histories: Black Women Historians in the Ivory Tower*, ed. Deborah Gray White (University of North Carolina Press, 2008), 1–27; August Meier and Elliott Rudwick, *Black History and the Historical Profession, 1915–1980* (University of Illinois Press, 1986); Rosalind Rosenberg, *The Life of Pauli Murray* (Oxford University Press, 2017), 316–32, 345–52.
6. Malcolm Scully, "Women in Higher Education," *Chronicle of Higher Education*, February 9, 1970, 2. See also *Historical Statistics of the United States, Colonial Times to 1970, Bicentennial Edition, Part I, Series H 751–765. Institutions of Higher Education—Degrees Conferred, by Sex: 1870 to 1970* (US Department of Commerce, Bureau of the Census, 1975), 385–86.

7. Women made up to 34 to 42 percent of the faculties of teachers' and junior colleges. See Scully, "Women in Higher Education," 2; Jessie Bernard, *Academic Women* (Pennsylvania State University Press, 1964), 39 (approximately 28 percent). *Historical Statistics of the United States* places the proportion of women in faculty appointments in 1920 at 36 percent (male: 35,807; female: 12,808) and in 1966 at 28.5 percent of faculty appointments (male: 464,000; female 132,400).
8. In 1920, the number of doctorates (PhDs) or equivalent degrees awarded in the United States was hardly over six hundred total. By the late 1960s, the number was over twenty-five thousand annually. See *Historical Statistics of the United States*, 382–83, 385–86.
9. WEAL, "Percentage of Doctorates Awarded to Women in Selected Fields in 1967–68 (Source: Earned Degrees Conferred: Part A—Summary Data, Office of Education, OE-54013-68-A)," Testimony to Green Committee, June 16, 1970, box 10, folder 8, Bernice R. Sandler Papers (MC 558), Schlesinger (hereafter Sandler Papers).
10. As of July 1, 1970, with the creation of the Zemurray-Stone Radcliffe professorship, there was one female professor at Harvard. Radcliffe (in contrast to Barnard at Columbia) did not have its own faculty. Women admitted to Radcliffe took their courses with Harvard faculty. See Caroline Walker Bynum and Janet M. Martin, "The Sad Status of Women Teaching at Harvard, or 'From What You Said I Would Never Have Known You Were a Woman,'" *Radcliffe Quarterly* 54, no. 2 (June 1970): 12–14. For the record at Princeton, see *A Preliminary Report on the Status of Women at Princeton University* (Task Force on Equal Academic Opportunities of the Central New Jersey Chapter of the National Organization for Women, April 1971), box 333, folder 3, Women at Princeton, Status of, subgroup Robert F. Goheen, Office of the President, PUA.
11. In percentages, 4.6 percent. See Women's Faculty Group, *Preliminary Report on the Status of Women at Harvard* (Women's Faculty Group, March 9, 1970), 5, box 55, folder 6 WEAL, FCCE, Harvard University, 1970–1972, Sandler Papers.
12. Women accounted for 16.7 percent of instructors, 15.5 percent of lecturers, 20.5 percent of teaching fellows, 17.5 percent of research associates, and 12.9 percent of research fellows. See Women's Faculty Group, *Preliminary Report on the Status of Women at Harvard.*
13. Rosalind Rosenberg, *Changing the Subject: How the Women of Columbia Shaped the Way We Think About Sex and Politics* (Columbia University Press, 2004), see esp. ch. 6 and 7.
14. Columbia Women's Liberation, *Report from the Committee on Discrimination Against Women Faculty*, 1970, box 54, folder 7, WEAL, FCCE, Columbia University, 1970–1971, Sandler Papers. On the formation of Columbia Women's Liberation, see Rosenberg, *Changing the Subject*, 241–45.
15. In 1938–1939, Berkeley had appeared to be on a different track: 5 percent of associate and full professors and 19 percent of assistant professors at Berkeley had been women. It showed a path not taken.
16. Psychology and sociology, for example, had not hired a woman to the regular faculty ranks since 1925. A study of median percentages of doctorates in the United States obtained by women in nineteen disciplines in the years from 1964 to 1968

showed that women had earned 17.7 percent of PhDs from the "top ten" universities, 15.6 percent from the "top five," and 11.7 percent from Berkeley itself. In those nineteen departments at Berkeley, women did not hold a single faculty appointment. Data from Susan Ervin-Tripp, PhD, professor, UC, Women's Faculty Group, *Women's Status at the University of California, Berkeley* (UC Women's Faculty Group, 1970).

17. Data from Susan Ervin-Tripp, PhD, professor, UC, Women's Faculty Group, *Women's Status at the University of California, Berkeley* (UC Women's Faculty Group, 1970), and tables in *Report of the Senate Subcommittee on the Status of Academic Women* (Senate Subcommittee on the Status of Academic Women, 1970), incorporated in *League of Academic Women and National Organization for Women's Class Action Complaint Against the University of California at Berkeley and the Office of the President of the University of California for Violation of Executive Orders 11246 and 11375, Forbidding Discrimination on the Basis on Sex* (League of Academic Women and National Organization for Women, 1970), box 53, folder 14, WEAL, FCCE, University of California System, 1969–1971, Sandler Papers.
18. Formal complaint against the University of Michigan under EO 11246, filed May 27, 1970, by Ann Arbor FOCUS on Equal Employment for Women, box 56, folder 1, WEAL. FCCE, University of Michigan, 1970–1971, Sandler Papers.
19. Sally G. Kohlstedt and Suzanne M. Fischer, "Unstable Networks Among Women in Academe: The Legal Case of Shyamala Rajender," *Centaurus* 51 (2009): 40.
20. Shyamala Rajender, "Women in Academia: The Plight and Its Perpetuation," *ChemTech* 3 (1973): 475–78. See also Margaret Rossiter, *Women Scientists in America: Before Affirmative Action, 1940–1972* (Johns Hopkins University Press, 1995); Margaret Rossiter, "1970–2000: A Less Than Golden Age for Women in Chemistry," in *Commission on Physical Science, Mathematics and Applications, Women in the Chemical Workforce: A Workshop Report to the Chemical Sciences Roundtable* (National Research Council, 2000).
21. For Ann Scott's study of women's status at SUNY-Buffalo, see "The Half-Eaten Apple: A Look at Sex Discrimination in the University," *Reporter*, May 14, 1970, 3–10, cited in *Discrimination Against Women: Hearings Before the Special Subcommittee on Education of the Committee on Education and Labor, House of Representatives, Ninety-First Congress, Second Session, on Sec. 805 of H. R. 16098, Part I (June 17, 19, 26, 29, 30, 1970)* (Government Printing Office, 1970), 212; on UC Fullerton, see *Discrimination Against Women*, 202–9; and on the University of Pittsburgh, see Mortar Board Society, *The Mortar Board Study: Graduate Educational Opportunities for Women at the University of Pittsburgh*, ca. 1972, in box 56, folder 14 WEAL, FCCE, University of Pittsburgh, 1970–1972, Sandler Papers.
22. The picture was, if anything, starker when one looked across institutions through the lens of a single discipline. For sociology, see Alice S. Rossi and Arlie Hochschild, "Status of Women in Graduate Departments of Sociology, 1968–1969," *American Sociologist* 5, no. 1 (February 1970): 1–12; Michelle Patterson, "Alice in Wonderland: A Study of Women Faculty in Graduate Departments of Sociology," *American Sociologist* 6, no. 3 (August 1971): 226–34. For early reports from other disciplines, see Victoria Schuck, "Women in Political Science: Some Preliminary Observations," *PS* 2, no. 4 (Autumn 1969): 642–53; Ann Fischer and Peggy Goide,

"The Position of Women in Anthropology," *American Anthropologist, New Series* 70, no. 2 (April 1968): 337–44; *Final Report of the Ad Hoc Committee on the Status of Women in the Historical Profession* (University of Virginia, November 9, 1970) (widely known as the *Rose Report* in reference to its chair, Willie Lee Rose), esp. appendix A, "Graduate Departments of History [1959/60–1968/69] (Berkeley, Univ. of Chicago, Columbia, Cornell, Harvard, MI, Princeton, Stanford, Wisconsin, Yale)," box 615, folder Council—Agendas & Rough Minutes, 1963–1971, AHA Papers (LoC); "Minutes of the 85th Business Meeting of the AHA [Dec. 27, 1970]," *AHA Newsletter* 9, no. 2 (March 1971): 24–27, AHA Papers (headquarters).

23. Suzanne Gossett, interview by Barbara Y. Welke, Chicago, IL, November 16 and December 14, 2022 (hereafter Gossett Interview).
24. He had not yet completed his PhD, but when Chicago offered him an appointment as instructor as a result, Philip refused, saying he would only come to Chicago as an assistant professor. Chicago gave in. Gossett Interview.
25. Dr. R. Ferry to Mrs. Philip Gossett, October 23, 1967; Gwin J. Kolb to Mrs. Philip Gossett, October 31, 1967; Robert A. Wiggins to Mrs. Philip Gossett, October 31, 1967; Robert D. Mayo to Mrs. Philip Gossett, November 7, 1967. Nor was it only a matter of male chairs. See Margaret Neville to Mrs. Philip Gossett, February 16, 1968. That a few departments addressed her as "Mrs. Suzanne Gossett" suggests there was an alternative. See R. B. Ogle to Mrs. Suzanne Gossett, October 31, 1967; Michael Hayes to Mrs. Suzanne Gossett, February 23, 1968. All letters in author's possession, courtesy of Suzanne Gossett. Gossett Interview.
26. The Gossetts had both wanted children and later had two healthy sons, both of whom, as Suzanne Gossett told me, were born, with planning and good fortune, in the summer. There was no maternity leave. Gossett Interview.
27. Gossett Interview.
28. For Sandler's story, see Bernice R. Sandler, "'Too Strong for a Woman'—The Five Words That Created Title IX," in Susan Ware, *Title IX: A Brief History with Documents* (Bedford/St. Martin's, 2007), 35–42.
29. On the inclusion of sex as a prohibited category of discrimination in employment in Title VII of the Civil Rights Act of 1964 and the evolution of what counted as sex discrimination, see Katherine Turk, *Equality on Trial: Gender and Rights in the Modern American Workplace* (University of Pennsylvania Press, 2016); Serena Mayeri, *Reasoning from Race: Feminism, Race, and the Civil Rights Revolution* (Harvard University Press, 2014); Nancy MacLean, *Freedom Is Not Enough: The Opening of the American Workplace* (Harvard University Press, 2006); John David Skrentny, *The Minority Rights Revolution* (Belknap Press, 2002); Alice Kessler-Harris, *In Pursuit of Equity: Women, Men, and the Quest for Economic Citizenship in 20th-Century America* (Oxford University Press, 2001); Hugh Davis Graham, *The Civil Rights Era: Origins and Development of National Policy, 1960–1972* (Oxford University Press, 1990).
30. The exemption was in Sec. 702 of the act: "This title shall not apply . . . to an educational institution with respect to the employment of individuals to perform work connected with the educational activities of such institution." The exception was not in the bill passed by the House of Representatives. The exemption was added in the Senate in a version of the bill known as the Dirksen (R. IL)–

Mansfield (D. MT) compromise, for which there is no legislative history or notes. The House agreed to accept the bill as amended by the Senate. See Dr. Kathryn Heath, USOE, "A Legislative History of Equal Employment Opportunity Provisions Directly Related to Education or Training Under Public Law 88-352 (Civil Rights Act of 1964), July 2, 1964, Title VII (Equal Employment Opportunity), at 78 Stat. 253 (422 U. S. C. 200E-2000E-15)," in *Discrimination Against Women: Hearings Before the Special Subcommittee on Education of the Committee on Education and Labor, House of Representatives, Ninety-First Congress, Second Session on Section 805 of H.R. 16098, Part I, Hearings Held in Washington, D.C., June 17, 19, 26, 29, 30, 1970* (Government Printing Office, 1970), 315–21.

31. Title VI applied only to discrimination on the basis of race, color, and national origin.
32. On the development of sex equality jurisprudence in the constitution, see Mayeri, *Reasoning from Race.*
33. "Summary of Executive Order 11246 as Amended by Executive Order 11375, In Relation to Sex Discrimination in Universities and Colleges Which Have Federal Contracts," from NOW, "Academic Discrimination Kit," 1979, box 7, folder 8, Correspondence: Ann Scott, 1970–1975, Sandler Papers; Bernice Sandler, "A Little Help from Our Government: WEAL and Contract Compliance," in *Academic Women on the Move*, eds. Alice S. Rossi and Ann Calderwood (Russell Sage Foundation, 1973), 439–62.
34. The figure is from an NSF report entitled *Federal Support to Universities and Colleges, Fiscal Year 1968*, quoted in Bernice Sandler's June 1970 testimony before the Special Subcommittee on Education. "Statement of Dr. Bernice Sandler Before the Special Subcommittee on Education June 16, 1970, Re: Sec. 805 of H.R. 16098 Concerning Discrimination Against Women in Higher Education," box 10, folder 8, Sandler Papers.
35. On the dramatic increase in federal funding of education following WWII, see Freeland, *Academia's Golden Age*, 89–93.
36. Macalouso joined the Labor Department in 1965 and was charged with overseeing contract compliance in the construction industry. He proved an invaluable resource and ally to women seeking to challenge sex discrimination in universities. For an obituary, see "Vincent Macalouso, Labor Dept. Official" (obituary), *Washington Post*, January 16, 2017. Sandler's handwritten notes from conversations with Macalouso show him providing a tutorial on the executive order's application to universities, how to file an official complaint, and how to make it effective. [Bernice Sandler], "Interview with Vince Macalouso 10 Dec 69," box 52, folder 17 WEAL, FCCE, OFCC, strategy and ideas, 1969–71, Sandler Papers. See also "Suggested Amendments to Title VII and Other Titles of the Civil Rights Act of 1964," May 13, 1969, and Statement of Dr. Bernice Sandler Before the Special Subcommittee on Education, June 16, 1970 [Green Committee], re: Sec. 805 of H.R. 16098 Concerning Discrimination Against Women in Higher Education, box 10, folder 9, Testimony Green Committee, June 16, 1970, Sandler Papers.
37. WEAL, "Sex Discrimination Charged at University of Maryland," press release, February 6, 1970; "Sex Discrimination at the University of Maryland" (part of "class action" filed January 31, 1970); see also *Report Prepared for the Women's Eq-*

uity Action League, fall 1969, box 10, folder 13 WEAL-FCCE-University of Maryland, 1970–1971, Sandler Papers.

38. A collection of reflections and responses compiled by Richard Ohmann following the December 1968 Annual Meeting of the Modern Language Association offers an extraordinary entry to the ferment and emotions of this moment and the disruption and transformation of professional societies. See Richard Ohmann, ed., "MLA 1968: Documents and Responses," *College English* 30, no. 6 (March 1969): 484–507. On Richard Ohmann, see James Wallenstein, "Richard Ohmann: The Radical Professor Who Enraged the Right, 1931–2021," *Politico*, December 27, 2021. One of the authors of the opening document "What Happened at MLA"—Florence Howe, of Goucher College—became a central figure in the movement within the MLA challenging sex inequality in academia. In the field of history, Berenice Carroll was one of the signatories of the petition to the AHA to establish a Committee on the Status of Women in the Profession on October 1969. For her letter to AHA Executive Secretary Paul Ward and the petition, see box 762, folder Committee—Status of Women in the Profession (ad hoc) 1970–1971, AHA Papers (LoC).
39. Linda K. Kerber, "On the Importance of Taking Notes," in *Voices of Women Historians: The Personal, the Political, the Professional*, eds. Eileen Boris and Nupur Chaudhuri (Indiana University Press, 1999), 44–60; Linda K. Kerber, interview by Barbara Y. Welke, Wellfleet, MA, July 13 and 14, 2019 (hereafter Kerber Interview).
40. For example, the complaint against Harvard was filed by the Boston Chapter of NOW, and the complaint against the University of Pittsburgh was filed by the University Committee for Women's Rights at Pittsburgh.
41. Although WEAL did not file every complaint, even complaints filed by other organizations are addressed in Bernice Sandler's papers at the Schlesinger Library, including all those cited here.
42. Remarks by Rep. Martha Griffiths (D-OR), *Congressional Record*, March 9, 1970, 6398–400.
43. *Discrimination Against Women*. Title IX of the Education Amendments Act of 1972 banned discrimination on the basis of sex in any educational program or activity receiving federal financial assistance and was crucial to the opening of graduate and professional education to women and to the field with which it has become most associated: women's sports. See correspondence relating to the various bills between legislative aide Mari Goldman, Senator Mervyn M. Dymally, and Bernice Sandler between June and October 1970 in box 53, folder 14, WEAL, FCCE, University of California, 1969–1974, Sandler Papers; Heather Sigworth, attorney at law, to Bernice Sandler, chairman, Action Committee for Federal Contract Compliance in Education, WEAL, April 13, 1970, box 52, folder 8, WEAL, FCCE, Nepotism, 1970–1973, Sandler Papers.
44. The intensity, emotion, urgency, and sense of possibility of the moment are captured in early women's caucus and committee newsletters. One can see there the organizing, the disciplinary and institutional studies being done, the individual experiences of discrimination, the debates over strategy and priorities, the sharing of news and forming of new networks, the debates as to what a field of study in their

discipline centering women would include, bibliographies, and news of courses related to women in their field. See, e.g., Coordinating Committee on Women in the Historical Profession, *CCWHP Newsletter* 1, no. 2 (Summer 1970), box 761, folder Committee on the Status of Women AHA, AHA Papers (LoC); [ASA] *Women's Caucus Newsletter* 1, no. 1 (October 1970), carton 10, folder SWS Newsletter, SWS Papers.

45. For an example from the sciences, consider Association of Women in Science (AWIS), press release organized April 13, 1971, box 49, folder 11, WEAL, FCCE, Association of Women in Science (1971–1975), Sandler Papers.
46. [ASA] *Women's Caucus Newsletter* 1, no. 1 (October 1970), 5, carton 10, folder SWS Newsletter, SWS Papers.
47. *SWS Newsletter* 1, no. 1 (March 1971), 7, 10 (SWS employment form), carton 10, folder SWS Newsletter, SWS Papers.
48. *SWS Newsletter* 1, no. 2 (May 1971), 6, carton 10, folder SWS Newsletter, SWS Papers.
49. *SWS Newsletter* 1, no. 2 (May 1971), 6–7, carton 10, folder SWS Newsletter, SWS Papers.
50. Coordinating Committee on Women in the Historical Profession, *CCWHP Newsletter* 2, no. 1 (March 1971): 5–6, box 762, folder Status of Women 1971, AHA Papers (LoC).
51. Dorothy Ross, "A Modest Beginning and a Modest Proposal," presentation at the American Council on Education annual meeting, October 6, 1972, Miami, FL, box 765, folder Committee on Women Historians 1971–1972, AHA Papers (LoC).
52. Ross, "Modest Beginning." See also Linda K. Kerber, *Annual Report to the AHA Council Committee on Women Historians* (American Historical Association, December 22, 1972), box 765, folder Committee on Women Historians 1971–1972, AHA Papers (LoC); Kerber Interview. For a description of how the McBee KeySort card system worked, see Ann Sneesby-Koch, "Me and Mr. McBee," National Endowment for the Humanities (blog), January 31, 2013, https://www.neh.gov/divisions/odh/featured-project/me-and-mr-mcbee.
53. See ch. 10, "an academic marketplace," on the proliferation of sex ("male"; "man") as an explicit qualification for academic appointments in advertisements for appointments in the 1930s and the parallel development in "teacher available" ads. Anti-nepotism policies prohibiting the employment of more than one family member in the same department or even same university or state university system also date from the 1930s. The policies were not limited to married couples but had their most common application to them and effectively excluded married women from tenure-track faculty positions. For an example, consider physicists Freda and George Salzman. See George Salzman, "Discrimination at U. Mass: Woman Scientist Fights Back," *Science for the People* 3, no. 2 (May 1971): 18–21; Eileen Zalisk, "Physicist Freda Salzman," radio interview, *Women in Science*, first aired on WBAI (New York, NY), ca. 1979, online at Berkeley Library Audio/Video Digital Collections, https://avplayer.lib.berkeley.edu/Pacifica/b23306718.
54. The only reason that elite universities were not vulnerable to the same charge was that they did not openly advertise positions.
55. See ch. 12, "married, two children." Press coverage and coverage in higher education

and disciplinary journals was critical in generating pressure for action by the federal government and for putting universities and professional societies on notice. See, e.g., Nancy Gruchow, "Discrimination: Women Charge Universities, Colleges with Bias," *Science* 168, no. 3931 (May 1, 1970): 559–61.

56. Linda K. Kerber to Willie Lee Rose, April 23, 1970, carton 762, folder Status of Women—1970–1971, AHA Papers (LoC); Kerber Interview. See also "Memo: To All Concerned Human Beings, From: Berkeley Women's Sociology Caucus," August 1969 ("End discriminatory job placement at the University placement center. No more sex type jobs"), carton 1, SWS Papers.
57. "A.H.A. Meetings, Dec. 1970, Boston," *CCWHP Newsletter* 2, no. 1 (March 1971): 4, carton 762, folder Status of Women 1971, AHA Papers (LoC). For the new "Professional Register Vita Form," see *AHA Newsletter* 9, no. 5 (November 1971), AHA Papers (headquarters).
58. See Registrants' Qualification Book, October 1970, Placement Service, AIP Placement Service Records, 1960–1978, box 1 of 4 (unprocessed), AIP Papers.
59. By 1974, the AIP stood out only in that it continued to act as an intermediary between those looking for positions and those with jobs to fill. The difference was likely related to far more PhDs in physics taking positions in industry and government than in academia.
60. See American Institute of Physics, Placement Service, Placement Service Records, 1960–1978 (AR 205), box 2 (unprocessed), folder Registrants 4700–4849, and folder Sample of Forms Filled out by Placement Service Registrants 1974, AIP Papers.
61. American Institute of Physics, Placement Service, Placement Service Records, 1960–1978 (AR 205), box 2 (unprocessed), folder Registrants 4700–4849, and folder Sample of Forms Filled out by Placement Service Registrants 1974, AIP Papers.
62. See, e.g., Janet Martin, assistant professor of classics, interview by Prof. [Michael] Walzer and Shirley Weitz, December 8, 1970, box 3, folder COSWH Interviews with Full-time Junior Faculty, Records of the Committee on the Status of Women at Harvard, 1969–1971 (MC 172), Schlesinger (hereafter COSWH Records).
63. See, e.g., Gail Pierson, assistant professor of economics, interview by Prof. Vermuele and Shirley Weitz, December 11, 1970; and [no first name listed] Kiley, assistant professor of English through comparative literature department, undated interview by unspecified interviewer, both in box 4, folder 38 COWSH Interviews with Full-time Junior Faculty, COSWH Records.
64. Bynum and Martin, "Sad Status of Women Teaching at Harvard."
65. Bynum and Martin, "Sad Status of Women Teaching at Harvard."
66. Testimony of Phyllis Jones, Open Hearings, Committee on the Status of Women at Harvard, November. 20, 1970, 13, box 3, folder 26, COSWH Records.
67. Thirteen of forty-one did not reply. For the letter and responses, see box 3, folder 28, COSWH Records.
68. The chairmen who penciled in replies on the original letter included those from mathematics, biophysics, statistics, and Sanskrit and Indian studies.
69. Oscar Handlin to Alan Heimert, December 30, 1970, box 3, folder 28, COSWH Records.

70. Commenting on the significance of committee memberships, Alice Rossi noted: "It is younger women who need the visibility and experience of serving in these roles, for they need it as status-validation . . . as one way of impressing on their chairmen that other sociologists consider them 'comers.'" See Alice S. Rossi to Anne-Marie Henshel, June 16, 1970, carton 1, folder Women's Caucus 1969–1970, SWS Papers. Women's mobilization in every professional society included a demand for greater representation of women on committees and other leadership positions. See, e.g., Florence Howe, chairman, "A Report from the Commission on the Status of Women in the Profession," presented to the Business Meeting of the Modern Language Association, December 1969, Denver, CO, reprinted in the Program of the Eighty-Fourth Annual Meeting of the Modern Language Association, *PMLA* 85, no. 4 (September 1970): 647.
71. Women and minority scholars challenged their exclusion from the whole apparatus of academic life: committees and elected positions in professional societies, journal editorships and editorial boards, scientific review committees. For women, vitae were as important in gaining these positions as the positions were in turn for their vitae. SWS offers a representative example. See carton 10, folder "Resumes", SWS Papers. On women's exclusion from scientific review panels and efforts to secure their representation—again requiring collecting and submitting women's vitae—see box 49, folder 9, WEAL, FCCE, [Julia T.] Apter, 1971–1973, Sandler Papers.
72. Rossi to Henshel, June 16, 1970. At that moment, most vitae—including Rossi's, the young scholars' with whom she was corresponding, and those of other women in the movement—included marital and parental status. See carton 10, folder "Resumes", SWS Papers.
73. "Instruction Sheet, American Institute of Physics Employment Referral Service," box 2, folder Registrants 4700–4849, AIP Placement Service Records, 1960–1978, AIP Papers.
74. Two collections of vitae (one from sociology, the other from physics), both from 1974, provide evidence of the shift. See carton 6 (stuffed envelope of "SWS Job Market Committee Employment Forms and vita [1974–75"]) (unprocessed), SWS Papers; box 2 (unprocessed), folder Registrants 4700–4849, folder Sample of Forms Filled Out by Placement Service Registrants, 1974, AIP Placement Service Records, 1960–1978, AIP Papers.
75. The SWS Job Market Committee continued, but by 1973, jobs were listed in the newsletter, and women sent their vitae directly. See carton 2, folder Fall Newsletter 1973, SWS Papers.
76. See Kerber, *Annual Report to the AHA Council Committee on Women Historians.*
77. The numbers here are from a report in the *AHA Newsletter* (September 1972). For the three reports, see "The Committee on Women Historians of the AHA . . ." *AHA Newsletter* 10, no. 4 (September 1972): 15–16 and *AHA Newsletter* 11, no. 2 (May 1973), AHA Papers (headquarters); and Kerber, *Annual Report to the AHA Council Committee on Women Historians.*
78. "Committee on Women Historians of the AHA . . ." See also Kerber, *Annual Report to the AHA Council Committee on Women Historians.*
79. [form] "If You Are a Woman Historian, Please Fill This Out," in "Women's Roster," *AHA Newsletter* 11, no. 4 (November 1973), AHA (headquarters).

80. "Report of Special Assistant, Committee on Women Historians," *AHA Newsletter* 11, no. 2 (May 1973): 14, AHA (headquarters).
81. The major exception was *Academic Women* (1964) by sociologist Jessie Bernard, a rich mine of data documenting women's exclusion and second-class status in academia explained as the result of women's own choices. The mixed reviews reflected the broader conflict over women in academia. Compare those by William M. Kephart, *Annals of the American Academy of Political and Social Science* 359 (May 1965): 214; Irving Dilliard, *American Scholar*, 35, no. 3 (Summer 1966): 580–82; and Joan W. Moore (UC Riverside), *American Journal of Sociology* 72, no. 2 (September 1966): 223–25.

chapter sixteen: the price of settlement

1. Verdict, 1139, McCormack Record on Appeal. See ch. 13, "verdict."
2. Motions for Direction of Verdict and Notice of Appeal, 1141–43, McCormack Record on Appeal.
3. Stenographer's Minutes, March 25, 1949, Izzo Probate Court Record (note: although the hearing was part of the case filed in federal court in New York, the sealing of that file left only the docket sheet in the file. I found the hearing transcript in the Izzo probate court record in Michigan). Using the Bureau of Labor Statistics' Consumer Price Index inflation calculator (https://data.bls.gov/cgi-bin/cpicalc.pl), the settlement in Izzo of $97,500 would be $1,279,511.34 (as of March 2024). Appearing in the hearing for the Izzos were their New York and Michigan lawyers. Appearing for the defendants were lawyers for the M. A. Henry Co., Milton Henry, Peerless Manufacturing (a subsidiary of the Henry company), E. F. Timme & Son, Woonsocket, Gene Autry, and Du Pont.
4. Stenographer's Minutes, March 25, 1949, Izzo Probate Court Record, 20, 26, Frederick Heilman, Heilman & Purcell, counsel for the Izzos.
5. Stenographer's Minutes, March 25, 1949, Izzo Probate Court Record, 13, Russell Stein, lawyer for E. F. Timme & Son.
6. Stenographer's Minutes, March 25, 1949, Izzo Probate Court Record, 29, Frederick Heilman, Heilman & Purcell, lawyer for the Izzos.
7. Stenographer's Minutes, March 25, 1949, Izzo Probate Court Record, 20–21, Russell Stein, lawyer for E. F. Timme & Son.
8. Stenographer's Minutes, March 25, 1949, Izzo Probate Court Record, 31.
9. Charge to the Jury, 1089, McCormack Record on Appeal.
10. See discussion of Lutz, infra.
11. This pattern held true throughout the litigation. That the defendants continued to demand a jury in cases filed after they lost in *McCormack* in January 1948 and after the decision was affirmed on appeal in April 1949 reinforces that they demanded a jury trial for other reasons than wanting a jury. See, e.g., Complaint, January 12, 1949; and Answer (M. A. Henry Co.) to Amended Complaint, July 5, 1949, both in Javinsky Case File.
12. The phrase is from Viviana A. Zelizer, *Pricing the Priceless Child: The Changing Social Value of Children* (Basic Books, 1985).

13. Deposition, Dr. Philip Caulfield, Washington, DC, December 30, 1948, 8, Greatorex Case File; "D. C. Parents Warned: Inflammable Cowboy Suits Kill One Child Here, Burn 7," *Times-Herald* (Washington, DC), April 8, 1945, A1, A3.
14. Final Order, April 6, 1948, Hon. John C. Knox; Affidavit of Edmond B. Butler, March 31, 1948, Greatorex Case File.
15. Final Order, Hon. Kenneth O'Brien, April 5, 1948, Weatherell Case File.
16. Final Order, Hon. John C. Knox, April 27, 1948; and Affidavit of Dr. H. Taylor Caswell, April 5, 1948, Habina Case File.
17. For the transcript in the proceedings before Judge Knox, see Richard Johnson Case File.
18. The consolidated cases: Adams, Bates, Baer, Berry, Bradley, Burke, Cumberledge, Detrick, DiTrapani, Flesher, Gates, Richard Johnson, Jones, King, Klinck, Lockhart, McMaster, Stultz, Tetla, Warnick, and Wilks.
19. John C. Knox, "What Makes a Good Judge," *American Magazine* (November 29, 1949): 125.
20. This was William Martin's memory of what Judge Knox had said. See William Martin to Gene Autry, November 29, 1951, box 1, Agents & Licensees, T94-45-30, folder M. A. Henry Co.—New York or Leslie Henry Co. (1 of 2) 1950–1951, Autry Collection.
21. Stenographer's Minutes, Consolidated Trial, Hon. John C. Knox, DJ, May 17, 1948, 7–11, Richard Johnson Case File.
22. Stenographer's Minutes, Consolidated Trial, Hon. John C. Knox, DJ, May 17, 1948, 129, Richard Johnson Case File. The Bates case settled close to a year later. See Order, March 25, 1949, Bates Case File.
23. Stenographer's Minutes, Consolidated Trial, Hon. John C. Knox, DJ, May 18, 1948, 62 (Watkins, ins. adj. for Standard Accident, Henry's insurer for 1946, discussing the Burke case), Richard Johnson Case File.
24. Stenographer's Minutes, Consolidated Trial, Hon. John C. Knox, DJ, May 24, 1948, 117, Richard Johnson Case File.
25. Two examples illustrate the broader pattern. In the case of Edward Klinck Jr., although the M. A. Henry Co. paid nothing in the settlement—all parties and the court accepting the claim that the company had "no further funds available for the settlement of this or other similar cases"—the Henry Company was nonetheless covered by the general release. See Stenographer's Minutes, Consolidated Trial, Hon. John C. Knox, DJ, May 24, 1948, 116 (Klinck), Richard Johnson Case File; and Edward Klinck Sr. Petition, May 28, 1948, 4, and Order, Hon. John C. Knox, DJ, June 14, 1948, Klinck Case File. But the same also held for Du Pont. Of the cases in the consolidated settlement hearing before Judge Knox in spring 1948, Du Pont was only a principal defendant in Bates, but the Henry Company had impleaded Du Pont as a third-party defendant in the other cases. Du Pont contributed nothing to any of the settlements in the proceedings but was covered by the general releases. See, e.g., Order and Stipulation, May 25, 1948, Warnick Case File.
26. Stenographer's Minutes, Consolidated Trial, Hon. John C. Knox, DJ, May 18, 1948, 56 (Stultz), Richard Johnson Case File.
27. Stenographer's Minutes, Consolidated Trial, Hon. John C. Knox, DJ, May 18, 1948, 58 (Burke), Richard Johnson Case File.

28. Stenographer's Minutes, Consolidated Trial, Hon. John C. Knox, DJ, May 18, 1948, 62–63, 67–68 (Burke), Richard Johnson Case File. On the conservatism of insurance adjustors and their approach to claims as one of hoping to deny a claim or pay as little as possible in settlement, see H. Laurence Ross, *Settled Out of Court: The Social Process of Insurance Claims Adjustments* (Aldine Publishing Company, 1970), 18.
29. The phrase is Tocqueville's, but my meaning is closer to that of plea bargaining in a criminal-law context today. See Alexis De Tocqueville, *Democracy in America* (1834), with an introduction by Alan Ryan (Alfred A. Knopf, 1941), vol. 1, 140. For an example of the negotiations among lawyers and insurance adjustors that took place out of court in these cases, see Affidavit of William W. Heidelberger, April 30, 1948, 1–8, McCarthy Case File.
30. Stenographer's Minutes, Consolidated Trial, Hon. John C. Knox, May 24, 1948, 116 (discussion of Jones settlement), Richard Johnson Case File.
31. See, e.g., Affidavit of Robert Sheller, 10–11, 13, Weatherell Case File (settled for $30,000).
32. See, e.g., Affidavit of Leo Gitlin, 4, Habina Case File (settled April 16, 1948, for $33,000).
33. For contemporary considerations of plaintiffs' personal injury lawyers' conflict of interest in contingent-fee litigation, see Herbert M. Kritzer, *Risks, Reputations, and Rewards: Contingency Fee Legal Practice in the United States* (Stanford University Press, 2004), 140 (and studies he cites); and John Fabian Witt and Karen M. Tani, *Torts: Cases, Principles*, and Institutions, 4th ed. (CALIe Langdell Press, 2019), 9–10.
34. Andrew Javinsky (Muskegon, MI) and Richard La France (Detroit, MI) were both burned in Gene Autry cowboy suits in 1944. Their families did not bring suit until 1949 and 1950, respectively, by which point every defendant's insurance coverage for 1944 had been long since exhausted. See Javinsky Case File and La France Case File.
35. Stenographer's Minutes, Consolidated Trial, Hon. John C. Knox, May 24, 1948, 116 (Klinck settlement), Richard Johnson Case File.
36. Stenographer's Minutes, Consolidated Trial, Hon. John C. Knox, May 24, 1948, 130–32 (re: Detrick), Richard Johnson Case File.
37. Stenographer's Minutes, Consolidated Trial, Hon. John C. Knox, May 24, 1948, 130–36 (re: Detrick, Johnson, King), Richard Johnson Case File.
38. Stenographer's Minutes, Consolidated Trial, Hon. John C. Knox, May 18, 1948, 87–88 (Warnick), Richard Johnson Case File.
39. See, e.g., Petition (John E. Devens and Laura Devens), October 23, 1948, 5, Affidavit of Charles J. Colgan, November 5, 1948, 2–3, Devens Case File; and citations more generally in this chapter.
40. See, e.g., Testimony of Louis P. Lutz, 11–124, Record in Lutz (Warnick, Detrick, Flesher).
41. Even uncovering the facts of a purchase of a Gene Autry cowboy suit from many years before could be challenging. Andrew Javinsky was burned in September 1944. The cowboy suit had been a gift from an older sister, purchased from a small local retailer in Traverse City, Michigan, 153 miles from Muskegon. Purchased for

cash, whatever receipt there might have been was long gone. By 1948, moreover, the retailer was no longer in business and the wife of the couple who had owned the business had died. See Affidavit of Elmer H. Groefsema, March 4, 1952, Javinsky Case File.

42. For an example of a plaintiff's lawyer setting up a claim in warranty, including privity, see, e.g., Deposition of Dorothy Elizabeth Detrick, Ridgely, WV, December 15, 1948, n.p., Record in Lutz.
43. Stenographer's Minutes, Settlement Hearing, Hon. John C. Knox, DJ, February 3, 1950, 6–7, Zibor Case File.
44. Stenographer's Minutes, Consolidated Trial, Hon. John C. Knox, DJ, May 18, 1948, 45, Richard Johnson Case File.
45. Stenographer's Minutes, Consolidated Trial, Hon. John C. Knox, DJ, May 18, 1948, 46–53.
46. Judgment, March 23, 1949, Record in Lutz.
47. Stenographer's Minutes, Settlement Hearing, Hon. John C. Knox, DJ, February 3, 1950, 6–7, Zibor Case File.
48. Stenographer's Minutes, Settlement Hearing, Hon. John C. Knox, DJ, February 3, 1950, 10, Zibor Case File.
49. Stenographer's Minutes, Settlement Hearing, Hon. John C. Knox, DJ, February 3, 1950, 14, Zibor Case File.
50. Exhibit 49, compilation of Du Pont sales of viscose rayon yarn to Woonsocket Falls Mill, 1940–1945, 159–60, Record in Lutz (before Hon. J. Waties Waring).
51. Complaint, October 20, 1947, Bates Case File. One of the many mysteries in the litigation was how few families named Du Pont as a defendant. For other examples, see Complaint, April 21, 1948, Duffy Case File; Complaint, December 1, 1948, Sullivan Case File; Complaint, September 12, 1949, Frazer Case File; Complaint, October 25, 1948, Timberlake Case File.
52. The Henry Company impleaded Du Pont as a third-party defendant in April 1948 in all the cases consolidated by Judge Knox. See, e.g., Motion (by M. A. Henry Company) to Implead E. I. Du Pont de Nemours and Company as a Third-Party Defendant, April 29, 1948, Warnick Case File. In cases in which Du Pont was a third-party defendant brought into the case by the Henry Company, Du Pont would only be liable if the Henry Company were found liable. As a principal defendant, if Du Pont were found liable, it would be jointly and severally liable with the other defendants found liable.
53. "Appearances," May 17, 1948, 3 (listing Cravath, Swaine & Moore, Esqrs.), Stenographer's Minutes, Consolidated Trial, Hon. John C. Knox, DJ, May 18, 1948, 53, Richard Johnson Case File.
54. See discussion of releases and related endnotes throughout this chapter.
55. Du Pont was initially brought into the Lutz case by the Henry Company as a third-party defendant, but with the permission of the court, the plaintiffs made Du Pont a principal defendant. See Final Judgment in favor of E. I. Du Pont de Nemours & Company, Hon. J. Waties Waring, DJ, March 21, 1949, Record in Lutz.
56. "I think that we were brought in more in the way of hope than anything else," he added. See Stenographer's Minutes, Settlement Hearing, Hon. Vincent L. Leibell, DJ, March 25, 1949, 32–33, Izzo Case File.

57. Stenographer's Minutes, Settlement Hearing, Hon. Vincent L. Leibell, DJ, March 25, 1949, 32, Izzo Case File.
58. Stenographer's Minutes, Settlement Hearing, Hon. Vincent L. Leibell, DJ, March 25, 1949, 33, Izzo Case File.
59. In one of the few cases in which Du Pont was named as a defendant from the start, the family's lawyer bracketed Du Pont in justifying the settlement on grounds that the defendants' resources were quickly being exhausted. Seeking the court's approval of the settlement, the Bates's lawyer recited the same litany related to soon-to-be-exhausted insurance policy limits and the number of other lawsuits pending as justification for settling now for the amount offered by the defendants: "The financial resources of the defendants, other than Dupont, are not limitless," he said. Du Pont did not contribute to the settlement. In the same affidavit, the lawyer noted, "There is some question in affiant's mind whether Dupont is in any way responsible since the yarn they sold was to be used by the mill and that it took on its dangerous propensities only after manufacture. For this reason deponent feels that the action against Dupont should be discontinued." See Affidavit of William V. Marcus, March 11, 1949, 11–12, Bates Case File.
60. Stenographer's Minutes, Consolidated Trial, Hon. John C. Knox, DJ, May 18, 1948, 78–79, Richard Johnson Case File.
61. Stenographer's Minutes, Consolidated Trial, Hon. John C. Knox, DJ, May 18, 1948, 100–102, Richard Johnson Case File.
62. Other cases in which the plaintiffs sought a preference to move the case up on the trial calendar, and the defendants resisted the motion: Cizek, Szumita, Sondej, Mitchell Gray, Tormollen, Baker, Mischetta, Appleby, Weinstein, Brunette, Timberlake, Verbonitz.
63. Affidavit of Eugene L. Bondy, Bondy & Schloss (Attorneys for Timme and Woonsocket), in Opposition to Motion for Preference, April. 26, 1950, Caparco Case File.
64. Affidavit of Edmond Butler, April 28, 1950, 7, Caparco Case File.
65. William C. Martin to Mitchell J. Hamilburg, November 25, 1949, 2, 3 (using this calculus to distinguish the Blessington case, in which the child had died, from the Caparco case, in which the child was alive but horribly burned), box 1, Agents & Licensees, T94-45-30, folder M. A. Henry Co., 1949–1950, Autry Collection.
66. Stenographer's Minutes, Consolidated Trial, Hon. John C. Knox, DJ, May 18, 1948, 53 (discussing Stultz case), Richard Johnson Case File.
67. William C. Martin to Mitchell J. Hamilburg, April 19, 1949, 1 ("GA" handwritten on p. 1), box 1, Agents & Licensees, T94-45-30, folder M. A. Henry Co., Autry Collection.
68. "Damage Suit Ends in Sealed Pact," *Lansing State Journal*, March 31, 1949, 15. See also "Sealed Verdict Is Filed in Suit of Saginaw Girl," *Battle Creek (MI) Enquirer*, April 6, 1949, 9. But, as the defendants feared, the seal was not airtight. Five months later, the headline of a front-page story was "Jacqueline Izzo Gets $97,500, It's Revealed," *Saginaw News*, August 25, 1949, 1.
69. The actions of the businesses involved here were not exceptional. See, e.g., Allan M. Brandt, *Cigarette Century: The Rise, Fall, and Deadly Persistence of the Prod-*

uct that Defined America (Basic Books, 2007); and Gerald Markowitz and David Rosner, *Deceit and Denial: The Deadly Politics of Industrial Pollution* (University of California Press, 2002).

70. Sealed state court files: Baker, Brunette, Caparco, Cizek, Dorsey, Gagnon, Giacomarro, Ormerod, Szumita, Timberlake, Touhill, and Weinstein. Sealed federal court files (final order only): Detrick, Donahue, Gorab, Izzo (full record), Richard Johnson, King, and Casimir Kresokowski.
71. Sealing records in product injury cases was common practice in the 1940s, 1950s, and well beyond. In the 1980s, the plaintiffs' bar, with limited success, began to press for legislation requiring courts to consider whether there was a public interest at stake in publicity. On New York, see George F. Carpinello, "Public Access to Court Records in Civil Proceedings: The New York Approach," *Albany Law Review* 54 (1989–1990): 93–121; and George F. Carpinello, "Public Access to Court Records in New York: The Experience Under Uniform Rule 216.1 and the Rule's Future in a World of Electronic Filing," *Albany Law Review* 66 (2002–2003): 1089–116. See also Laurie Kratky Dore, "Settlement, Secrecy, and Judicial Discretion: South Carolina's New Rules Governing the Sealing of Settlements," *South Carolina Law Review* 791, no. 55 (2004): 791–827; Laurie Kratky Dore, "Secrecy by Consent: The Use and Limits of Confidentiality in the Pursuit of Settlement," *Notre Dame Law Review* 74 (1999): 283–402; Arthur R. Miller, "Confidentiality, Protective Orders, and Public Access to the Courts," *Harvard Law Review* 105 (1991): 427–502; Anne-Thérèse Bechamps, "Sealed Out-of-Court Settlements: When Does the Public Have a Right to Know?," *Notre Dame Law Review* 66 (1990): 117–57.
72. William F. Martin to Mitchell J. Hamilburg, April 19, 1949, 4–5, box 1, Agents & Licenses, T94-45-30, folder M. A. Henry Co. 1949–1950, Autry Collection.
73. At least thirty-five cases were settled from Greatorex to Izzo before the appellate decision in McCormack. For examples of this argument as a ground for settlement, see Stenographer's Minutes, Settlement Hearing, Hon. Vincent L. Leibell, DJ, March 25, 1949, 5, Izzo Case File; Affidavit of Frank Habina, April 1948, 5, Habina Case File. On the impact of the appellate decision, see Martin to Hamilburg, April 19, 1949, 4–5.
74. Martin to Hamilburg, April 19, 1949, 4.
75. Stipulation and Petition to Compromise, November 30, 1948, Pritchard Case File. As Pritchard illustrates, even cases settled outside New York sometimes ended up in the news. See "Court Approves $40,000 Settlement of Action Brought by Parents of Boy Severely in Cowboy Suit Fire," *Morning Call* (Allentown, PA), December 8, 1948, 5, 21; "Boy Awarded $40,000 for Burns," *Courier-News* (Bridgewater, NJ), December 8, 1948, 29; "$40,000 Award for Parents and Boy in Cowboy Suit Blaze," *News* (Paterson, NJ), December 9, 1948, 44; "Autry Cowboy Suit Catches Fire; Award Boy, Parents $40,000," *Chicago Daily Tribune*, December 8, 1948, 22; "Injured Boy Wins in Damage Suit," *Billings Gazette*, December 9, 1948, 12. Headlines of settlements did not reflect the amount that went to the lawyers and so spread a sort of false news with corrosive effects for families who were seen as having received much more than they in fact had.

76. Deposition of Helen C. DiTrapani, Washington, DC, July 11, 1946, 2–24, DiTrapani Case File; Amended Answer, M. A. Henry Co., Inc., October 24, 1946, 3, DiTrapani Case File.
77. Stenographer's Minutes, Consolidated Trial, Hon. John C. Knox, May 17, 1948, 14–16, 20, 21, Richard Johnson Case File.
78. Robert E. Kopp to William Martin, September 21, 1950 (cc. Mr. Gene Autry, Mr. Mitchell J. Hamilburg, Mr. Beverly S. Clendenin), box 1, Agents & Licensees, T94-45-30, folder M. A. Henry Co., 1949–1950, Autry Collection.
79. On the history of photographs as evidence, see Jennifer L. Mnookin, "The Image of Truth: Photographic Evidence and the Power of Analogy," *Yale Journal of Law and the Humanities* 10 (1998): 1–74; Thomas Thurston, "Hearsay of the Sun: Photography, Identity, and the Law of Evidence," Roy Rosenzweig Center for History and New Media, accessed October 13, 2025, http://chnm.gmu.edu/aq/photos/index.htm; Lorraine Daston and Peter Galison, "The Image of Objectivity," *Representations* 40 (Fall 1992): 81–128. For the first treatise, see Charles C. Scott, *Photographic Evidence: Preparation and Presentation* (Vernon Law Book Co., 1942). See also Kenneth B. Hughes and Benjamin J. Cantor, *Photographs in Civil Litigation* (Bobbs-Merrill Company, Inc., 1973).
80. Paul K. Longmore, *Telethons: Spectacle, Disability, and the Business of Charity*, ed. Catherine Kudlick (Oxford University Press, 2016).
81. Bill of Particulars, Exhibit A (photographs of Roy Cizek), October 11, 1949, Cizek Case File.
82. Cases in which photographs were filed with the court include Baker, Caparco, Cizek, Cumberledge, Javinsky, Perry, Szumita, Timberlake, Tormollen, and Weinstein. See case files.
83. Stenographer's Minutes, Consolidated Trial, Hon. John C. Knox, May 24, 1948, 116 (Klinck), Richard Johnson Case File.
84. Stenographer's Minutes, Consolidated Trial, Hon. John C. Knox, May 18, 1948, 64, 66 (Burke), Richard Johnson Case File.
85. Stenographer's Minutes, Consolidated Trial, Hon. John C. Knox, May 18, 1948, 85–91 (Warnick), Richard Johnson Case File.
86. Stenographer's Minutes, Consolidated Trial, Hon. John C. Knox, May 18, 1948, 85–91; May 19, 1948, 102–9 (Warnick), Richard Johnson Case File.
87. Lockhart Interview.
88. Bates Interview.
89. See, e.g., Final Order, Hon. James B. M. McNally, January 31, 1950, Cizek Record; Final Order, Hon. Edward R. Koch, October 17, 1949, Peterson Case File.
90. Re: "cheap settlement" negotiated by Timme in Ormerod, see William F. Martin to Gene Autry, April 26, 1950, 3, box 1, Agents & Licenses, T94-45-30, folder M. A. Henry Co., 1949–1950, Autry Collection.
91. The cowboy suit litigation might be read as carrying the work that Viviana A. Zelizer began in *Pricing the Priceless Child* out of courts and into the domain of settlement. Children retained their "priceless" character by the 1940s, but in settlements out of court, the sentimental value of children held little sway in the calculation of the price of a case. See Zelizer, *Pricing the Priceless Child*, 15–21.

92. The average settlement in death cases was $15,600. This average is from a database I have compiled that includes settlement data for eighty-eight cases.
93. William F. Martin to Gene Autry, September 17, 1951 (Timberlake), box 1, Agents & Licensees, T94-45-30, folder M. A. Henry Co.—New York or Leslie Henry Co. (1 of 2) 1950–1951, Autry Collection; Stenographer's Minutes, Hon. Vincent L. Leibell, DJ, March 25, 1949, 3, Izzo Case File; Petition, Affidavit and Consent and Order, October 17, 1949, Caparco Case File; Order of Compromise, Hon. James B. M. McNally, February 1, 1950, Cizek Case File.
94. The average is based on a database I have compiled that includes settlement data for eighty-eight cases.
95. Stenographer's Minutes, Consolidated Trial, Hon. John C. Knox, DJ, May 17, 18, 19, and 24, 1948, Richard Johnson Case File. $3,600 (Wilks) to $58,000 (Bradley and Jones).
96. Order, Hon. Vincent L. Leibell, November 9, 1950, Ikner Case File. In so ordering, Judge Leibell overruled the same probate court judge in Saginaw, Michigan, who approved the 50 percent contingent fee in Izzo. Order, John P. Murphy, Judge of Probate, State of Michigan, Probate Court for the County of Saginaw, November 6, 1950.
97. See, e.g., Stenographer's Minutes, Consolidated Trial, Hon. John C. Knox, DJ, May 24, 1948, 115–16, Richard Johnson Case File (Klink); Affidavit of Edward Klinck Sr., Philadelphia, PA, May 28, 1948, 5 (contingent fee reduced from 50 percent to 33 percent plus expenses), Klinck Case File; Order, Hon. John C. Knox, DJ, March 8, 1952, and Affidavit of Paul Javinsky, Muskegon, MI, January 4, 1952, 2–3 (contingent fee reduced from 50 percent to 40 percent plus expenses), Javinsky Case File.
98. Final Order, Hon. John C. Knox, April 27, 1948, Habina Case File. The examples here are from Adams, Cumberledge, Intelisano, and Gorab. See Order Approving Settlement ($15,000 settlement; $2,712. 26 to father; $6,967.92 to child; $5,320.82 to attorneys), June 11, 1948, Adams Case File; Order Approving Settlement ($11,000 settlement; $3,500 to father; $7,500 to child; but after attorney's fees, Art Jr.'s portion of the settlement was reduced to $5,000), June 25, 1948, Cumberledge Case File; Order of Compromise ($8,000 settlement for Joseph Intelisano, but after attorney's fees, he received $4,800), February 14, 1949, Intelisano Case File. For an inflation calculator for these awards, see "CPI Inflation Calculator," Bureau of Labor Statistics, accessed October 13, 2025, https://www.bls.gov/data/inflation_calculator.htm.

chapter seventeen: "on our traditional basis of quality alone"

1. For example, when representatives of the Women's Faculty Group at Harvard met with Harvard President Nathan Pusey in January 1970, asking that he establish a committee on the status of women faculty at Harvard, he directed them to document (in a memo) that the status of women in the university "is a problem," including providing comparative data from other universities. See "Agenda for the

Steering Committee—January 26 [1970]," box 1, folder 1, Records of the Committee on the Status of Women at Harvard, 1969–1971 (MC 172), Schlesinger. See also Ann Sutherland Harris to Caroline Bynum, February 24, 1970, and March 17, 1970, re: the resistance of the Columbia University administration to establishing a committee on the status of women, box 4, folder 51, Records of the Committee on the Status of Women at Harvard, 1969–1971 (MC 172), Schlesinger.

2. See box 55, folder 6, and box 56, folder 1, Bernice R. Sandler Papers (MC558), Schlesinger (hereafter Sandler Papers).
3. [news clipping] "Sex Bias Charges at 11 Other Schools Delay U. S. Grants" (noting hold on grants to Michigan, Harvard, and eleven other universities), box 56, folder 1, Sandler Papers. See, e.g., Memorandum of Understanding between the Office for Civil Rights, HEW, and the University of California, Berkeley, box 321, folder 8, Office of the President Records, Subgroup Robert F. Goheen, UA, PUA.
4. See Bernice Sandler to Hon. William G. Millikin, February 24, 1971, box 56, folder 1, Sandler Papers.
5. John G. Bynoc to Nathan M. Pusey, December 31, 1970, box 55, folder 6, Sandler Papers. A federal contract compliance review had been underway at Harvard when the complaint alleging sex discrimination was filed. It became the first institution reviewed by HEW for sex discrimination. Harvard's responses and tactics proved typical in many respects.
6. Nathan M. Pusey to John G. Bynoc, October 16, 1970, 1, box 55, folder 6, Sandler Papers.
7. On the relative authority of department heads, deans, and central administrations, see Richard M. Freeland, *Academia's Golden Age: Universities in Massachusetts 1945–1970* (Oxford University Press, 1992); Rebecca S. Lowen, *Creating the Cold War University: The Transformation of Stanford* (University of California Press, 1997). Harvard was not alone in making the argument about departmental autonomy. See, e.g., Committee of the Council of the University Senate, "Equal Employment Opportunity: Affirmative Action Fifth Annual Report," *University of Chicago Record* 8, no. 6 (September 28, 1974): 154–55, box 6, folder 2, Committee on University Women Records, UChicago.
8. The University of Michigan and Princeton University offer two such examples. See R. W. Fleming to Richard A. Lester, April 19, 1972 (describing the standoff between MI and HEW on this point); Ellen E. Morgan to William R. Valentine, April 4, 1972 (objecting to Princeton's affirmative-action plan, which set hiring goals by division rather than departments); Robert F. Goheen to William R. Valentine, January 13, 1972, 3; and Richard A. Lester, "The Difficulties with Application of Numerical Goals by Academic Department in Affirmative Action Plans for Universities," April 10, 1972 (statement drafted by Dean Lester and sent to President Robert F. Goheen and Provost William G. Bowen), all in box 321, folder 8, Robert. F. Goheen Subgroup, Office of the President Records, PUA.
9. See, e.g., Committee of the Council of the University Senate, "Equal Employment Opportunity: Affirmative Action Fifth Annual Report," 156–57. Other elite universities made versions of the same argument. See, e.g., Goheen to Valentine, January 13, 1972, 3.
10. Goheen to Valentine, January 13, 1972. See also Lester, "Difficulties with Applica-

tion of Numerical Goals by Academic Department in Affirmative Action Plans for Universities."

11. Robert F. Goheen to William R. Valentine, March 3, 1972, box 321, folder 8, Robert F. Goheen Subgroup, Office of the President Records, PUA.
12. See, e.g., Nathan M. Pusey to John G. Bynoc, October 16, 1970, 1, box 55, folder 6, Sandler Papers. For the experience at Columbia, see Rosalind Rosenberg, *Changing the Subject: How the Women of Columbia Shaped the Way We Think About Sex and Politics* (Columbia University Press, 2004), 245–57.
13. See, e.g., "Equal Employment Opportunity: Affirmative Action Fifth Annual Report," *University of Chicago Record* 8, no. 6 (Sept. 28, 1974): 153, box 6, folder 2, Committee on University Women Records, Committee of the Council of the University Senate, UChicago.
14. Richard A. Lester to chairmen of departments, interoffice correspondence, "Subject: Recruitment of Female Faculty," December 15, 1969, box 321, folder 8, subgroup Robert F. Goheen, Office of the President Records, PUA.
15. Richard A. Lester to chairmen of departments, interoffice correspondence, "Subject: Experience with Recruiting Female Faculty and Research Staff," April 15, 1971, box 321, folder 8, subgroup Robert F. Goheen, Office of the President Records, PUA. Both this memo and Lester's memo from December 15, 1969, were included in the appendices to Princeton's Affirmative Action Plan—as evidence of its ongoing efforts to increase the ratio and numbers of female faculty.
16. Richard A. Lester to chairmen of academic departments and programs, interoffice correspondence, "Subject: Implementation of Equal Employment Opportunity Policy in Recruitment Communications for Faculty and in Recommendations to Fill Faculty Vacancies in the Three Professorial Ranks," November 1, 1971, box 333, folder 3, subgroup Robert F. Goheen, Office of the President Records, PUA.
17. Ellen E. Morgan to William R. Valentine, April 4, 1972, 3, box 321, folder 8, subgroup Robert F. Goheen, Office of the President Records, PUA.
18. "Draft, Faculty Form EEO," in Richard A. Lester to department chairmen, interoffice correspondence, "Subject: Record of Recruitment and Department Selection in Filling Faculty Positions in the Three Professorial Ranks or Positions Leading to Appointment in Those Ranks," April 6, 1972, box 321, folder 8, subgroup Robert F. Goheen, Office of the President Records, PUA.
19. Other internal correspondence also highlighted increasing pressure to prove compliance and to advertise open positions as one tool to that end. See, e.g., A. J. Maruca to Dean Richard Lester, inter-university correspondence, "Subject: Dartmouth's Affirmative Action Plan," May 1, 1972, box 321, folder 8, subgroup Robert F. Goheen, Office of the President Records, PUA.
20. WEAL filed a formal complaint of sex discrimination against the University of Chicago under Executive Order 11246 on November 23, 1970. For the complaint, see box 54, folder 5, Sandler Papers. The minutes from the department interviews are all in box 157, folder 4, Office of the President, Levi Administration Records, UChicago.
21. John T. Wilson, provost, to academic deans, memorandum, May 2, 1972, box 157, folder 4, Office of the President, Levi Administration Records, UChicago.
22. William B. Cannon to academic deans, intra-university correspondence, "Re: Af-

firmative Action—Academic Units," June 7, 1972, box 157, folder 4, Office of the President, Levi Administration Records, UChicago.

23. Robert McCormick Adams to department chairmen, intra-university correspondence, June 9, 1972, box 157, folder 4, Office of the President, Levi Administration Records, UChicago.
24. *Federal Grants and Contracts at the University of Chicago: Report of an Ad Hoc Committee Appointed by Presidents George W. Beadle and Edward H. Levi*, 1969, 4, 5, 11, box 166, folder 9, Office of the President, Levi Administration Records, UChicago.
25. See, e.g., AHA *Employment Information Bulletin* 4, no. 1 (October 1974), and 4, no. 2 (November 1974) (including advertisements for positions in history at Berkeley, Chicago, Columbia, Cornell, Harvard, Michigan, Penn, Princeton, Stanford, UVA, and Yale), AHA (headquarters); Committee of the Council of the University Senate, "Equal Employment Opportunity: Affirmative Action Fifth Annual Report," 156–73 (for departmental reports, see, e.g., Biochemistry Department—advertised position in *Chemical and Engineering News*; Biophysics and Theoretical Biology Department and Pharmacological and Physiological Sciences Department—advertised in *Science*; Classical Languages and Literatures Department—advertised in American Philological Association, *Positions for Classicists*; Philosophy Department—advertised in *Jobs in Philosophy*; Anthropology Department—advertised in *Nature*, *Science*, and the American Anthropological Association's *Newsletter*; History Department—advertised in AHA *Employment Information Bulletin*; Political Science Department—advertised in the APSA *Newsletter*).
26. AHA *Employment Information Bulletin* 4, no. 2 (November 1974), AHA (headquarters).
27. "Draft, Faculty Form EEO." Princeton's plan highlighted the collection of vitae as evidence of its good-faith efforts at expanding the representation of women on the faculty. See Princeton University, *An Affirmative Action Report and Affirmative Action Plan for 1972–73 and 1973–74* (Princeton University, March 1972), 97, appendix B, "Efforts to Increase the Proportion of Women on the Faculty, the Professional Research and Technical Staff, and the Library, Especially in High Level Positions, 1969–70 to 1971–72," box 321, folder 8, subgroup Robert F. Goheen, Office of the President Records, PUA.
28. Stuart A. Rice to Albert Crewe, intra-university correspondence, June 14, 1972; and Stuart A. Rice to Cedric L. Chernick, memorandum, June 12, 1972, both in box 157, folder 4, Office of the President, Levi Administration Records, UChicago.
29. On "creditworthiness" and other sex and marriage-based strategies for denying women financial independence, see Allison Schwartz, "Banking on a Woman's Worth: Personhood and America's New Patriarchy of Debt, 1968–2008" (PhD diss., University of Minnesota, 2022), https://conservancy.umn.edu/items/e939a866-664c-4370-aed9-8deb4095cb5b.
30. Stuart A. Rice to Albert Crewe, intra-university correspondence, June 13, 1972, box 157, folder 4, Office of the President, Levi Administration Records, UChicago; and Rice to Chernick, memorandum, June 12, 1972.
31. Chairman, Department of Statistics, to Albert Crewe, intra-university correspon-

dence, June 13, 1972, box 157, folder 4, Office of the President, Levi Administration Records, UChicago; and Rice to Chernick, memorandum, June 12, 1972.

32. Karl F. Morrison to William B. Cannon, intra-university correspondence, June 15, 1972, box 157, folder 4, Office of the President, Levi Administration Records, UChicago.
33. Hanna Holborn Gray, *An Academic Life: A Memoir* (Princeton University Press, 2018), 23–64.
34. Gray, *Academic Life*, 136.
35. Gray, *Academic Life*, 155.
36. Gray, *Academic Life*, 172. On the distinction between "the college" and the university at the University of Chicago, see John W. Boyer, *The University of Chicago: A History* (University of Chicago Press, 2015).
37. Gray, *Academic Life*, 184.
38. The record of Marlene Dixon's case and the protests related to her dismissal on which I have drawn here are in box 108, folders 8–12, and box 109, folders 1–2, Lloyd and Susanne Rudolph Papers, UChicago (hereafter Rudolph Papers).
39. The Committee on Human Development was established in 1938 as an interdisciplinary, degree-granting unit within the Division of Social Sciences.
40. Like most vitae from the mid-1960s, Dixon's began with personal data, including date and place of birth and "married, nine years, no children." The UCLA Department chairman's letter too mentioned marriage: "Her husband is in the music field, and will definitely locate wherever it serves her career best."
41. William E. Henry to D. Gale Johnson, March 7, 1966 ("Recommendation for appointment: Mrs. Marlene D. Dixon"), box 108, folder 9 Dixon Case, Rudolph Papers.
42. D. Gale Johnson to Edward H. Levi, provost, March 8, 1966 ("Re: Offer of appointment to Marlene Dixon as Assistant Professor, Committee on Human Development"), enclosing: memorandum of W. E. Henry; letter of recommendation from Ralph H. Turner, UCLA; Marlene Dixon's vita; and parts 1 and 2 of Marlene Dixon's "Professionalism in Engineering," all in box 108, folder 9 Dixon Case, Rudolph Papers.
43. D. Gale Johnson to John T. Wilson, December 12, 1968, box 108, folder 9 Dixon Case, Rudolph Papers.
44. For Gray's comments on the Dixon case in her memoir, see Gray, *Academic Life*, 188–93.
45. *Report of the Faculty Committee to Review the Decision with Regard to the Reappointment of Assistant Professor Marlene Dixon* [n.d.], box 108, folder 10, Rudolph Papers. The Gray committee speaks to (at least) two other points. First, university administrators do not appoint committees that they think will be hostile to them. As here, universities may establish committees under pressure, but in staffing them they work to create a "friendly" committee. Second, the fallacy that "sisterhood is powerful." Three of the seven members of the "Gray committee" were women: Hanna Gray, associate professor of history; Susanne Hoeber Rudolph, professor of political science; and Helen Harris Perlman, professor of social work. Their appointment was not a boon to Dixon. I do not know Perlman beyond her field, but Gray and Rudolph shared common family backgrounds, training, and professional lives that led them to share the elitism of the University of Chicago—and both

had joined the Chicago faculty through hires of their husbands and felt "grateful" to the university. On their backgrounds and Gray's low estimation of Dixon's qualifications, see Gray, *Academic Life*, 69, 98–99, 184, 191. For other examples of women in sex and race discrimination actions finding themselves isolated, with other women faculty and administrators taking the viewpoint of administration or remaining silent, see Sally G. Kohlstedt and Suzanne M. Fischer, "Unstable Networks Among Women in Academe: The Legal Case of Shyamala Rajender," *Centaurus* 51 (2009): 37–62; and Carolyn Chalmers, *They Don't Want Her There: Fighting Sexual and Racial Harassment in the American University* (University of Iowa Press, 2022), re: Jean Jew. For the Rudolphs' vitae, see box 109, folder 6, Rudolph Papers.

46. I say "male" here—and he was. But it is important to remember that every member of the faculty in the Department of Sociology other than Marlene Dixon was male.

47. Richard Flacks, assistant professor of sociology, "A Response to the Sociology Faculty," (February 10, 1969), box 127, folder 4, Office of the President, Levi Administration Records, UChicago.

48. Another case against the University of Chicago from the early 1970s is especially telling because it fits so damningly the narrative Jo Freeman traced in her "simple sex census." Barbara Heldt Monter, a University of Chicago PhD, was hailed as "the best" of the department's students in literature in 1967 when appointed as an instructor and, a year later when appointed assistant professor, as "an excellent addition to our Russian literature program." But in 1971, despite her publication record, she was denied reappointment. In the same year that she had been appointed as an instructor, a male PhD candidate at Columbia was hired as an assistant professor. She had completed her degree; he had not. His reappointment sailed through without the department taking a formal vote, though her scholarly credentials were stronger. The initial findings of HEW were against the university, finding sex discrimination in the rank of her initial appointment, in her salary, and in the denial of reappointment. The university challenged the findings, gathering the credentials of every individual who had taught in the department from 1967 to 1971. At the end of a five-year battle, all that was left was the case of salary discrimination. The cost to the university (not counting legal fees) was just over $4,000. Heldt's career was very nearly destroyed, and she and her husband, a professor at Northwestern, divorced. She faced searching for a job in a market where there were very few positions in her field, with no assistance from Chicago. The department chair refused her request for an open letter of recommendation. Even the explanation of that request was expressed in sexist terms. As the dean described in a memo to the provost, the chair "thinks it frivolous and unprofessional for an academic applicant to expect to have her credentials under her direct control—like a Victorian housemaid carrying her 'character' testimonials from house to house." Years later, a dean at the University of Western Ontario, where Heldt found a position after three years of searching, showed her a letter warning that she "was trouble." In a 2015 article in the AWSS (Association for Women in Slavic Studies) newsletter *Women East-West*, Heldt shared the story of meeting in 2013 the young HEW lawyer who had been sent to Chicago to investigate her case. As he told her, when he had walked into the office of University of Chicago President Edward Levi, who

was surrounded by a "phalanx" of lawyers, Levi's first words were, "What does that f*ing bitch want now?" See Barbara Heldt, "Founding Mothers: Barbara Heldt on Women in Slavic Studies and the AWSS," *AWSS Women East-West Newsletter* 4, no. 1 (June 2015). The records of Barbara Heldt Monter's legal challenge against the University of Chicago can be found in box 165, folders 5–7, Office of the President, Levi Administration Records, UChicago.

49. Shyamala Rajender's suit against the Department of Chemistry and the University of Minnesota offers a powerful example of the costs of even a "winning" case. Rajender's suit became the first sex discrimination (Title VII) class action in academia and led to a consent decree to which the University of Minnesota was subject for over a decade (1980–1992). Over three hundred women brought claims under that decree, 180 of whom received monetary or appointment settlements. But there were high personal, economic, and professional costs. Rajender's career in chemistry was destroyed. She had been on one-year assistant-professor appointments at the university (1968–1971), and after she brought a formal grievance, the department did not offer her another contract. "Branded as a 'troublemaker,'" doors elsewhere were closed to her. Though the case ended with a settlement, the judge rejected the university's claim that even if Rajender had been a white male she would not have been qualified for the position, and he issued a finding that she was qualified. But the settlement of $100,000 did not cover her legal costs, and, closed out of chemistry, Rajender was forced to find a new profession. She earned a JD and became a patent lawyer. Women who made claims under the decree found their credentials denigrated, and both they and those who supported their claims lost valuable time for research and other professional activities. See Kohlstedt and Fischer, "Unstable Networks Among Women in Academe," 37–62; Debra Hartley, "Strength, Spirit, and Shattered Illusions in the Making of Social Change: A History of the Faculty Advisory Committee for Women at the University of Minnesota," Special Collections, Anderson Library, UMN; Laura J. Cooper, J. Stewart, and Mario Thomas, McClendon Professor in Law and Alternative Dispute Resolution, University of Minnesota Law School, interview by Barbara Young Welke, University of Minnesota Law School, 2017, Law Library Archives, UMN. Carolyn Chalmers also briefly refers to her work on the Rajender case in Chalmers, *They Don't Want Her There.*

50. The full history of Dinah Moché's challenge against sex discrimination is documented in her papers held at the Schlesinger Library. Moché was a meticulous record-keeper. Her papers include her detailed documentation of her credentials, all exchanges with the P&B Committee, Physics Department Chairman Joseph Shaffer, QCC President Kurt R. Schmeller, and all files relating to the formal grievance process. I have concentrated on her battle for promotion and the university's grievance procedures. See folder 5.6 [Dinah Moché] initial hiring, promotions, vita, 1965–1976, and folder 5.7 [Dinah Moché] initial hiring, promotions, vita, 1977–1979, Dinah L. Moché Papers, 1966–1995 (MC 799), Schlesinger.

51. See ch. 12, "married, two children."

52. Helen Astin, *The Woman Doctorate in America: Origins, Career, and Family* (Russell Sage Foundation, 1969); Alan E. Bayer and Helen S. Astin, "Sex Differences in Academic Rank and Salary Among Science Doctorates in Teaching," *Journal of*

Human Resources 3, no. 2 (Spring 1968). Astin's research was drawn on repeatedly in the challenge against sex discrimination in academia: in Bernice Sandler's files as she prepared her case to file formal complaints against universities under Executive Order 11246; in Martha Griffith's statement before Congress on March 9, 1970; and in the hearings held by Representative Edith Green in summer 1970. See box 51, folder 1, Sandler Papers; Rep. Martha Griffiths, "The Federal Government Violates National Policy, as well as the President's Executive Orders, by Providing Billions of Dollars of Federal Contracts to Universities Which Discriminate Against Women," *Congressional Record*, March 9, 1970, 6399, Sandler Papers; *Discrimination Against Women: Hearings Before the Special Subcommittee on Education of the Committee on Education and Labor, House of Representatives, Ninety-First Congress, Second Session on Section 805 of H.R. 16098, Part I, Hearings Held in Washington, D.C., June 17, 19, 26, 29, 30, 1970* (Government Printing Office, 1970), 244, 311, 312.

53. Pursuing a legal claim was expensive, and without dedicated funds, organizations could do little more than write to universities on the women's behalf seeking reconsideration or fund-raising campaigns among members. The AAUP, NOW, and—following Natalie Allon's tragic accident—SWS and others established legal defense funds to help support women's legal challenges, but they could not cover the cost. Many women who brought suit spent their life's savings. For examples of professional societies writing on women's behalf, raising funds, and providing advice on the legal avenues open to them, see, e.g., Nona Glazer to James Stuart [*sic*], July 17, 1977, carton 8, folder Discrimination-Affirmative Action, SWS Papers; Anne Briscoe to members, April 25, 1975 (fundraising appeal in support of Sharon Johnson's sex discrimination suit against the University of Pittsburgh), box 49, folder 11, Sandler Papers; Correspondence between Janet Emig (denied tenure in the University of Chicago Department of Education, 1969), Bernice Sandler, and Florence Howe, on legal steps Emig might take, in box 54, folder WEAL, FCCE, University of Chicago, sex discrimination, 1969–1971, Sandler Papers.
54. In a letter to Nona Glazer, president of SWS, on July 9, 1977, two weeks after the decision denying her tenure, Allon wrote, "Any kind word would be great or any advice," and signed her handwritten note "Scared + angry, Natalie." For documents in Allon's case, see carton 8, folder Discrimination-Affirmative Action, SWS Papers.
55. Judith Lorber, "Natalie Allon (1941–2001)" (obituary) *Footnotes* 30, no. 1 (January 2002): 14, https://www.asanet.org/wp-content/uploads/january_2002.pdf; Jeffery Sobal, "Group Dieting, the Stigma of Obesity, and Overweight Adolescents: Contributions of Natalie Allon to the Sociology of Obesity," *Marriage and Family Review* 7, no. 1–2 (1984): 9–20; David J. Kallen and Marvin B. Sussman, "Dedication," *Marriage and Family Review* 7, no. 1–2 (1984): 3. An interview with Natalie Allon by Terry Gross on *Fresh Air* in April 1979 offers the opportunity to hear Allon speak about her research and book *Urban Lifestyles* (1979) in her own voice; see https://freshairarchive.org/segments/natalie-allon-discusses-me-generation.
56. Richard A. Lester, *Antibias Regulation of Universities: Faculty Problems and Their Solutions* (McGraw-Hill, 1974). Even as the high tide of affirmative action passed, EO 11246 remained an important tool against discrimination. On January 21, 2025, President Trump, by executive order (14173), revoked it.
57. For a parallel story of resistance and procedural reform, see Karen M. Tani, *States*

of Dependency: Welfare, Rights, and American Governance, 1935–1972 (Cambridge University Press, 2016).

58. On the term "individual" and women's struggle in the nineteenth century, see Linda K. Kerber, "Can a Woman Be an Individual? The Discourse of Self Reliance," in Kerber, *Toward an Intellectual History of Women* (UNC Press, 1997), 200–23.
59. Katherine Turk, *Equality on Trial: Gender and Rights in the Modern American Workplace* (University of Pennsylvania Press, 2016), 76–177, 191, but see generally ch. 7 and the conclusion.
60. Katherine Turk, "'The Hand That Rocks the Cradle Should Rock the U. of C.': The Faculty Wife and the Feminist Era," *Journal of Women's History* 26, no. 2 (Summer 2014): 129.
61. Important accommodations such as maternity leaves and tenure clock extensions, intensely fought for, slow and uneven in their adoption and terms, did not prove the great equalizing forces that had been imagined. Women increasingly pushed motherhood back after grad school, after tenure, had fewer children than they desired, and still faced costs to their careers for pregnancy and motherhood. The University of Minnesota did not adopt a maternity leave policy until the late 1980s. Laura Cooper, hired in 1974 and in 1979 the first woman to receive tenure at the University of Minnesota Law School, waited until after getting tenure to have a child. As she explained to me, "I certainly had a feeling on the faculty here that one [a woman] should not have a child before seeking tenure, that your chances of seeking tenure would be greatly diminished, if you did." Laura J. Cooper, J. Stewart, and Mario Thomas, McClendon Professor in Law and Alternative Dispute Resolution, University of Minnesota Law School, interview by Barbara Young Welke, University of Minnesota Law School, 2017, Law Library Archives, UMN. On the pregnancy and baby penalty in higher education, consider Aurélie Vialette, "Colleges' Sexist Scandal: Too Many Institutions Have No Maternity Leave," *Chronicle of Higher Education*, August 18, 2020, https://www.chronicle.com/article/colleges-sexist-scandal; Joan C. Williams and Jessica Lee, "Is It Time to Stop Stopping the Clock? No, but It May Be Time to Redraft Our Poorly Defined Policies," *Chronicle of Higher Education*, August 9, 2016, https://www.chronicle.com/article/is-it-time-to-stop-stopping-the-clock/; Mary Ann Mason, "The Baby Penalty," *Chronicle of Higher Education*, August 5, 2013, https://www.chronicle.com/article/the-baby-penalty/; and Mary Ann Mason, "Title IX and Babies: The New Frontier," *Chronicle of Higher Education*, November 29, 2012, https://www.chronicle.com/article/title-ix-and-babies-the-new-frontier/. See also Serena Mayeri, *Marital Privilege: Marriage, Inequality, and the Transformation of American Law* (Yale University Press, 2025), 178, 317–18; and Jennifer Bennett Shinall, "The Pregnancy Penalty," *Minnesota Law Review* 103, no. 2 (2019): 749–842. Other accommodations—part-time and shared faculty appointments—remain exceptional.

chapter eighteen: "public cowboy no. 1"

The chapter title is from the 1937 Republic Pictures film *Public Cowboy No. 1*, directed by Joseph Kane and starring Gene Autry. See also Holly George-Warren, *Public Cowboy No. 1: The Life and Times of Gene Autry* (Oxford University Press, 2007).

1. Mitchell J. Hamilburg to William Martin, November 23, 1949, box 1, Agents & Licensees, T94-45-30, folder Mitchell Hamilburg 1949–1950 (2 of 3), Autry Collection. On other correspondence related to the cowboy suit litigation, Autry was cc'd, and even on correspondence relating to the cases not addressed to him, his handwritten initials at the top indicate that he followed the litigation closely throughout. For letters cc'd to Autry, see, e.g., Mitchell J. Hamilburg to Milton Henry (re: Philip Warren Hooper case), March 21, 1949, and Martin Gang to William F. Martin (re: the Izzo case), March 23, 1949. For examples of letters not addressed to Autry, but which his handwritten initials at the top show that he had seen, see, e.g., William F. Martin to Mitchell Hamilburg, April 19, 1949 (re: Izzo) and William F. Martin to Mitchell Hamilburg, November 25, 1949 (providing an accounting of cases to date). This series of letters all appears in box 1, Agents & Licensees, T94-45-30, folder M. A. Henry Co., 1949–1950, Autry Collection, but the point holds more generally.
2. Mitchell J. Hamilburg to Huston E. Turpin, November 30, 1949, box 1, Agents & Licensees, T94-45-30, folder Mitchell Hamilburg, 1949–1950 (2 of 3), Autry Collection.
3. Du Pont's sales of viscose rayon thread to Timme from 1940–1945 totaled 3,325,207. Defendant's Exhibit 49, 160, Record in Lutz. See David A. Hounshell and John Kenly Smith Jr., *Science and Corporate Strategy: Du Pont R&D, 1902–1980* (Cambridge University Press, 1988), 386.
4. Gene Autry Licensees, April 20, 1950, box 1, Agents & Licensees, T94-45-30, folder Mitchell Hamilburg 1949–1950 (2 of 3), Autry Collection.
5. Affidavit of Joseph Rosenberg, Nemeroff, Jelline, Danzig & Paley (Peterson family's lawyer), June 24, 1949, 3–4, Peterson Case File. For a complaint, see Complaint, October 18, 1946, 2–6, Greatorex Case File.
6. Deposition of Gene Autry, NY, NY, October 29, 1947 (Weatherell case), 8, Peterson Case File; Deposition of Gene Autry, NY, NY, October 1949 (Peterson case), 5, box 1, Agents & Licensees, T94-45-30, folder M. A. Henry Legal 1948–1949, Autry Collection. Autry was deposed (sworn testimony) twice in the cowboy suit litigation (Weatherell in 1947 and Peterson in 1949). That neither deposition was filed with the case in which it was taken reflects Autry's consistent distancing of himself from the litigation. Nonetheless, for the deposition in Weatherell, see Peterson Case File; for the deposition in Peterson, see Autry Collection.
7. William F. Martin to Mitchell J. Hamilburg, April 19, 1949, 4, 2, box 1, Agents & Licenses, T94-45-30, folder M. A. Henry Co. 1949–1950, Autry Collection.
8. See ch. 7, "playing with fire."
9. Deposition of Gene Autry (in Weatherell), October 29, 1947, 10, Peterson Case File.
10. In the 1949 deposition in Peterson, Autry was specifically asked a series of questions about his actions after he learned in March 1945 of the fire hazard the fabric on chaps presented: Had he examined the Henry Company's books to ascertain the names of retailers and jobbers to whom Henry had sold the suit or asked the Henry Company for the names of such retailers and jobbers? Had he requested any Henry Company customers to stop selling the suit? Had he made any statement

about the hazard the suit posed in his radio or other appearances, or to newspapers, or other periodicals? The answer to each of these questions was no. See Deposition of Gene Autry, October 1949 (Peterson case), 5, Autry Collection. On Autry and Hamilburg only having notified Henry orally, not in writing, to discontinue sales of the cowboy suit, and continuing to receive royalties on sales for months after being notified of the hazard, see William F. Martin to Gene Autry, September 17, 1951, 3, box 1, Agents & Licensees, T94-45-30, folder M. A. Henry Co.—New York or Leslie Henry Co. (1 of 2) 1950–1951, Autry Collection.

11. Author conversation with Marva Felchlin, director of the Autry Library, December 28, 2005. The fire is also referenced in a description of the Autry papers. See "Gene Autry Personal Papers and Business Archives [Manuscript Materials] 1900–2002," ArchiveGrid, accessed April 21, 2025, https://researchworks.oclc.org/archivegrid/collection/data/829119082.
12. See, e.g., Autry's touring schedule listed in Mitchell J. Hamilburg Agency, Gene Autry Enterprises, bulletin no. 2, December 1, 1949, 2, box 1, Agents & Licensees, T94-45-30, folder Mitchell Hamilburg, 1949–1950 (2 of 3), Autry Collection.
13. Just as families brought suit independently against some retailers, they could have done the same with Autry. But I suspect that lawyers working on a contingent fee basis with ready access to the other defendants would not have been anxious to pursue such a case. So, even as Martin raised the risk of such a suit on more than one occasion, Autry's distance from New York provided protection.
14. Madison Square Garden Rodeo appearances between 1945–1950: 1946, 1947, 1948, 1949. See "Gene Autry / Time Spent in New York State from December 27, 1944—March 2, 1950," box 1, Agents & Licensees, T94-45-30, folder Mitchell Hamilburg 1949–1950 (2 of 3), Autry Collection. On skipping the 1951 rodeo, see William F. Martin, NY, NY, to Mitchell J. Hamilburg, Hollywood, CA, October 5, 1951, 4, box 1, Agents & Licensees, T94-45-30, folder M. A. Henry Co.—New York or Leslie Henry Co. (1 of 2) 1950–1951, Autry Collection.
15. Martin to Hamilburg, April 19, 1949. For similar examples, see William F. Martin to Messrs. Seidman and Seidman, May 18, 1949, 1, Autry Collection; William F. Martin to Mitchell J. Hamilburg, November 25, 1949, box 1, Agents & Licensees, T94-45-30, folder M. A. Henry Co., 1949–1950, Autry Collection.
16. Martin to Hamilburg, April 19, 1949, 5.
17. William F. Martin to Gene Autry, September 6, 1949 (re: Tormollen, case settled for $43T), box 1, Agents & Licensees, T94-45-30, folder M. A. Henry Company, 1949–1950, Autry Collection.
18. See, e.g., William F. Martin to Gene Autry, April 26, 1950, 4 (noting settlements in at least eight cases in which Autry had not been served in which Martin had faced pressure to nonetheless contribute to settlements, had refused, and the settlements had gone through with no contribution from Autry), box 1, Agents & Licensees, T94-45-30, folder M. A. Henry Co., 1949–1950, Autry Collection.
19. Martin to Hamilburg, April 19, 1949, 4.
20. William F. Martin to Gene Autry, August 8, 1951, 2–3, box 1, Agents & Licensees, T94-45-30, folder M. A. Henry Co.—New York or Leslie Henry Co. (2 of 2) 1950–1951, Autry Collection.

21. William F. Martin to Mitchell J. Hamilburg, October 5, 1951, 4, box 1, Agents & Licensees, T94-45-30, folder M. A. Henry Co.—New York or Leslie Henry Co. (1 of 2) 1950–1951, Autry Collection.
22. Mitchell J. Hamilburg to S. E. Kane, March 7, 1949; Mitchell J. Hamilburg to Gene Autry, Hollywood, CA, March 7, 1949 (noting first letter as a copy of the letter Hamilburg had sent to all licensees), box 1, Agents & Licensees, T94-45-30, folder Mitchell Hamilburg, 1949–1950 (3 of 3), Autry Collection.
23. Mitchell J. Hamilburg Agency, Gene Autry Enterprises, bulletin no. 6, June 1950, 3, box 1, Agents & Licensees, T-94-45-30, folder Mitchell Hamilburg, Jan. 1951, Autry Collection.
24. Mitchell J. Hamilburg Agency, Gene Autry Enterprises, bulletin no. 6, June 1950, 6.
25. See, e.g., Mitchell J. Hamilburg to O'Melveny and Myers, March 29, 1949; March 30, 1949; and April 21, 1949, box 1, Agents & Licensees, T94-45-30, folder Mitchell Hamilburg, 1949–1950 (3 of 3), Autry Collection.
26. Mitchell J. Hamilburg to licensees, October 1950, box 1, Agents & Licensees, T-94-45-30, folder Mitchell Hamilburg, 1949–1950, Autry Collection.
27. See, e.g., Norman R. Tyre to Gene Autry, September 27, 1949, 1, 3, box 1, Agents & Licensees, T-94-45-30, folder M. A. Henry Company, 1949–1950, Autry Collection; Martin to Hamilburg, November 25, 1949, 1, 3 (w/ "GA 1/2/49" handwritten in on the first page).
28. Tyre to Autry, September 27, 1949, 1.
29. Affidavit of John J. De Luca, Martin and Clearwater, June 22, 1949, 4, Peterson Case File.
30. Affidavit of Joseph Rosenberg, Nemeroff, Jelline, Danzig and Paley (Peterson family's lawyer), June 24, 1949, 3–4, Peterson Case File.
31. Martin to Hamilburg, April 19, 1949.
32. Gene Autry to William F. Martin, January 4, 1950, box 1, Agents & Licenses, T94-45-30, folder M. A. Henry Co. 1949–1950, Autry Collection.
33. William F. Martin to Messrs. Seidman and Seidman (cc'd to Gene Autry), May 18, 1949, 2; William F. Martin to Gene Autry, May 18, 1949 ("GA" handwritten signature on page 1), box 1, Agents & Licenses, T94-45-30, folder M. A. Henry Co., 1949–1950, Autry Collection.
34. Martin to Autry, April 26, 1950, encl. "Summary of Amounts Paid by Gene Autry in Connection with Henry Cases as of April 26, 1950."
35. Martin to Hamilburg, April 19, 1949, 2–3, 5.
36. William F. Martin to Gene Autry, November 29, 1951, 3—following up on Martin to Autry, August 8, 1951; Martin to Hamilburg, October 5, 1951, 4; Martin to Autry, November 29, 1951, 3, box 1, Agents & Licensees, T94-45-30, folder M. A. Henry Co.—New York or Leslie Henry Co. (1 of 2) 1950–1951, Autry Collection.
37. Gene Autry to William F. Martin, November 28, 1951, box 1, Agents & Licensees, T94-45-30, folder M. A. Henry Co.—New York or Leslie Henry Co. (1 of 2) 1950–1951, Autry Collection.
38. Percy Knauth, "Gene Autry, Inc.," *Life Magazine*, June 28, 1948, 89–90.
39. Knauth, "Gene Autry, Inc."
40. Licensees Comparison Statement, 1949–1950 (incl. Leslie Henry Co. and M.A.

Henry Co.-Canada), bx 1 Agents & Licensees, T-94-45-30, folder Mitchell Hamilburg, Jan. 1951, Autry Collection.

41. Royalty statements from April 1941 to November 1948 from the Henry Co. sent as an enclosure in a letter to Martin in October 1949 were not filed with the letter in Autry's correspondence. See Louise Heising to William F. Martin, October 7, 1949, box 1, Agents & Licensees, T-94-45-30, folder M. A. Henry Company, 1949–1950, Autry Collection. Forbes estimated Autry's net worth in 1998 at $320M. George-Warren, *Public Cowboy No. 1*, 302.
42. $11,092.63 (1949); $32,796.23 (1950). See Licensees Comparison Statement, 1949–1950, box 1, Agents & Licensees, T-94-45-30, folder Mitchell Hamilburg, Jan. 1951, Autry Collection.
43. Individual Licensee Payment Records, 1952–1957, box 1, Agents & Licensees, T-94-45-30, folder Mitchell Hamilburg, Jan. 1951, Autry Collection. Disputes over Henry's failure to pay royalties as provided under the contract dogged the relationship. See, e.g., Mitchell J. Hamilburg to Milton Henry, March 28, 1950, box 1, Agents & Licensee, T-94-45-30, folder M. A. Henry Co., 1949–1950, Autry Collection.
44. James Ikner Jr. (Saginaw, MI), December 30, 1945; John Devens (Center Moreland, PA), April 29, 1946 (Goodyear wholesaler); Michael Felton (Lewiston, ID), May 11, 1946; Hans Patrick Peterson (Tampa, FL), November 2, 1946; Gerald Palmateer (Alexandria, VA), November 15, 1946.
45. Affidavit of Elliot B. Paley, November 20, 1951, 3–4, Timberlake Case File.
46. Martin to Autry, August 8, 1951.
47. Martin to Autry, September 17, 1951.
48. Martin to Autry, September 17, 1951. On Autry's claimed conversations with Henry, see Deposition of Gene Autry, October 1949 (Peterson case), 3, 8, 9, Autry Collection.
49. Martin to Autry, September 17, 1951.
50. Martin to Autry, September 17, 1951. On Autry's claimed conversations with Henry, see Deposition of Gene Autry, October 1949 (Peterson case), 3, 8, 9, Autry Collection.
51. William F. Martin to Gene Autry, October 5, 1951, box 1, Agents & Licensees, T94-45-30, folder M. A. Henry Co.—New York or Leslie Henry Co. (1 of 2) 1950–1951, Autry Collection. See also Mitchell J. Hamilburg to Gene Autry, October 3, 1951, box 1, Agents & Licensees, T-94-45-30, folder Mitchell Hamilburg, Jan. 1951, Autry Collection. For earlier correspondence on the issue of liability of licensors, see William F. Martin to Robert E. Kopp, August 7, 1950, 2, box 1, Agents & Licensees, T-94-45-30, folder M. A. Henry Co., 1949–1950, Autry Collection; Note, "Liability of Advertising Endorsers," *Stanford Law Review* 2, no. 3 (1950): 496–514.
52. Martin to Hamilburg, October 5, 1951, 4.
53. Mrs. John Grosch Jr. to Gene Autry, June 8, 1951, box 1, Agents & Licensees, T94-45-30, folder M. A. Henry Co.—New York or Leslie Henry Co. (1 of 2) 1950–1951, Autry Collection.
54. Virginia MacPhail to William F. Martin, June 16, 1951, box 1, Agents & Licensees, T94-45-30, folder M. A. Henry Co.—New York or Leslie Henry Co. (1 of 2) 1950–1951, Autry Collection.
55. William F. Martin to Virginia MacPhail, June 18, 1951, box 1, Agents & Licens-

ees, T94-45-30, folder M. A. Henry Co.—New York or Leslie Henry Co. (1 of 2) 1950–1951, Autry Collection.

56. Gene Autry to Bobby Grosch, June 21, 1951, box 1, Agents & Licensees, T94-45-30, folder M. A. Henry Co.—New York or Leslie Henry Co. (1 of 2) 1950–1951, Autry Collection.
57. Gene Autry to Mrs. John Grosch Jr., June 21, 1951, box 1, Agents & Licensees, T94-45-30, folder M. A. Henry Co.—New York or Leslie Henry Co. (1 of 2) 1950–1951, Autry Collection.
58. Investigator's Report, Case no. 4779, June 21, 1951, box 1, Agents & Licensees, T94-45-30, folder M. A. Henry Co.—New York or Leslie Henry Co. (1 of 2) 1950–1951, Autry Collection.
59. Martin to Autry, November 29, 1951.
60. Martin to Autry, November 29, 1951.
61. Gene Autry to William F. Martin, December 4, 1951. The case settled for $22,500 with a $1000 contribution from Autry. See William F. Martin to Gene Autry, December 18, 1951; both letters are in box 1, Agents & Licensees, T94-45-30, folder M. A. Henry Co.—New York or Leslie Henry Co. (1 of 2) 1950–1951, Autry Collection.
62. Quoted in George-Warren, *Public Cowboy No. 1*, 277. George-Warren gives three paragraphs to discussion of the events, offering a sympathetic portrayal of Autry. My accounts here and in a 2014 article are the first full considerations. See Barbara Young Welke, "The Cowboy Suit Tragedy: Spreading Risk, Owning Hazard in the Modern American Consumer Economy," *Journal of American History* 101 (June 2014): 97–121.
63. The name of the new company likely came from Milton Henry's sister Gloria's married name. Gloria had been a salesperson in the M. A. Henry Company Broadway showroom. In 1926, she married Nathan Leslie. For Gloria Henry's marriage (June 15, 1926, Bronx, NY, certificate number 3235), see New York, New York, Extracted Marriage Index, 1866–1937, *Ancestry.com.*
64. Mitchell J. Hamilburg to O'Melveny and Myers, May 6, 1949, box 1, Agents & Licensees, T94-45-30, folder Mitchell Hamilburg 1949–1950 (3 of 3), Autry Collection. 1949 proof-of-coverage insurance certificates from licensees showed insurance of $100T per product. See Manufacturers Casualty Insurance Company, Certificate of Insurance, "Insured the Leslie Henry Co., Inc., Mt Vernon, NY: Proof of Coverage," July 18, 1949 (showing bodily injury liability of $100,000 for each person and $300,000 for each accident), box 1, Agents & Licensees, T94-45-30, folder M. A. Henry Co., 1949–1950, Autry Collection.
65. Timme incorporated sometime between May 1950 and April 1951, well before the litigation had concluded. See "Fabrics in Daytime and House Dress Merchandising: Van Schalscha Joins E. F. Timme & Son as Asst. General Mgr.," *Women's Wear Daily*, May 8, 1950, 26 (referring to "E. F. Timme & Son"); "Pile Fabric Output at New Timme Plant to Start in 6 Weeks," *Women's Wear Daily*, April 10, 1951, 6 (referring to "Timme Corp.").
66. See, e.g., "Pile Fabric Output at New Timme Plant to Start in 6 Weeks," 6; "Timme to Expand," *Women's Wear Daily*, July 19, 1956, 15; "New President of E. F. Timme,"

Women's Wear Daily, December 21, 1959, 17; "Timme Expansion Set at Million Dollars," *Women's Wear Daily*, November 7, 1966, 37; "Timme Corp. to Build Mill," *Women's Wear Daily*, February 7, 1969, 31.

67. See, e.g., "Social Activities in New York and Elsewhere," *New York Times*, October 26, 1941, 40; "Three Girls Who Have Become Affiances and Three Debutantes," *New York Times*, December 23, 1953, 18; "Cotillion Plans Completed at Tea," *New York Times*, November 18, 1955, 28; "Susan A. Brown, Marymount Ex-Student Engaged to William Edward Roschen, Jr.," *New York Times*, February 18, 1956, 12; "Susan Ann Brown Is Married Here; Bride of William Roschen Jr., Trinity Student, in Church of St. Ignatius Loyola," *New York Times*, August 26, 1956, 99; "W. J. Buff 3d Weds Cynthia A. Roschen," *New York Times*, November 2, 1958, 93.
68. "William E. Roschen" (obit.), *New York Times*, August 3, 1963, 17. Other executives in Timme and Woonsocket also had flourishing careers. See, e.g., "Robertshaw Named Timme President," *Women's Wear Daily*, January 7, 1960, 14.
69. Bergamini was named vice president of Timme Corp. in 1952 and executive vice president in 1959, and he succeeded Arthur Robertshaw Jr. as president in 1967. See "Bergamini Elected Timme Corp. Head," *Women's Wear Daily*, December 19, 1967, 26.
70. "E. F. Timme & Son Promotes Two," *Women's Wear Daily*, July 7, 1964, 29.
71. "Five Women Who Can Easily Afford Any Fur Coat in the World Tell Why They're Proudly Wearing Fakes" (E. F. Timme & Son advertisement), *New York Times Sunday Magazine*, August 22, 1971, 33. See also the E. F. Timme & Son tiger coat advertisement in *Women's Wear Daily*, June 4, 1970, 37–40; and "Does the International Beauty Who Bought the Bengal Tiger Coat Know That There May Now Be Less Than 600 Bengal Tigers Left?" (E. F. Timme & Son advertisement), *New York Times*, August 30, 1970, 67. For commentary on the campaign, see, e.g., "Timme Ads Hit at Real Fur Use," *Women's Wear Daily*, April 15, 1970, 2; "Furriers Cry Foul, Claim Ad's Facts Are Also Fake," *Women's Wear Daily*, June 5, 1970, 1, 80; "Say Timme's Fake Fur Ads in Bad Taste," *Women's Wear Daily*, July 19, 1971, 28; "Timme Ad in *Times* Rubs the Wrong Way," *Women's Wear Daily*, August 16, 1971, 133.
72. In 1945, the FTC had slapped Timme with a cease-and-desist order for representing its rayon fabrics as having been made from fur. Timme faced several lawsuits over the 1970 ad campaign. See, e.g., "Emba Suit Hits Timme Ads," *Women's Wear Daily*, August 18, 1971, 35; "Emba, Timme Settle Suit over Advertising Campaign," *Women's Wear Daily*, February 2, 1972, 8; "Judge Finds 2 Timme Ads Bear False Innuendos," *Women's Wear Daily*, September 26, 1973, 20; "Supreme Court Refuses to Hear E. F. Timme Case," *Women's Wear Daily*, November 19, 1974, 7; Fur Information and Fashion Council, Inc., et al., v. E. F. Timme & Son, Inc., 364 F. Supp. 16 (1973), aff'd Fur Information and Fashion Council v. E. F. Timme & Son, Inc., 501 F. 2d 1048 (2nd Cir. 1974). In 1977, Timme was acquired by a Belgian manufacturer of carpeting and velvets. See "In Brief: Depoortere Freres Acquires Timme," *Women's Wear Daily*, May 6, 1977, 9.
73. The company's overall sales in 1946 were $648.7 million; by 1970, the company's sales had increased to $3.6 billion. See Regina Lee Blaszczyk, "Styling Synthetics:

Du Pont's Marketing of Fabrics and Fashions in Postwar America," *Business History Review* 80, no. 3 (Autumn 2006): 527; Hounshell and Smith, *Science and Corporate Strategy*, 328, 504, 538.

74. D. F. Holmes, *History of the Du Pont Company's Textile Fibers Department* (E. I. du Pont de Nemours and Co., 1983), Hagley Library and Archives (Wilmington, DE), 16 (chart 2); Hounshell and Smith, *Science and Corporate Strategy*, 182, 250, 258.

75. Holmes, *History of the Du Pont Company's Textile Fibers Department*, 46–49. Whether the inflammability of rayon for high-pile fabrics played a role in Du Pont's decision to leave the rayon field, we are unlikely to ever know. Holmes's internal corporate report on the "History of the Textile Fibers Department" from 1974 does not mention inflammability in charting the history of rayon. Holmes, *History of the Du Pont Company's Textile Fibers Department*, 26, 260. The privacy of corporate records, as well as corporate practices of culling records, when set against the accessibility of this "internal" corporate history, has led scholars to rely heavily on Du Pont's carefully manicured account of its own history. Neither Hounshell and Smith in *Science and Corporate Strategy* nor Blaszczyk in "Styling Synthetics" mentions inflammability.

76. Others who had worked closely with Timme and Woonsocket and who died before age sixty included Waldemar Kuenzel (fifty-three) and Manfred Keller (fifty-five). See "Philip F. Brown, Rayon Pioneer, DuPont Executive," *Women's Wear Daily*, March 25, 1953, 36; "Philip F. Brown," *New York Times*, March 25, 1953, 31; "Waldemar Kuenzel, Textile Executive," *New York Times*, October. 5, 1957, 17; "Rites Tomorrow for W. H. Charch," *Women's Wear Daily*, July 28, 1958, 10; "Manfred Keller," *New York Times*, June 20, 1959, 21; "Manfred Keller," *Women's Wear Daily*, June 22, 1959, 11. Nothing in the coverage of these men's deaths identified them as caused by their work—and the era presented other major health hazards, especially among men, most obviously cigarette smoking—but Du Pont and others were aware of the hazards in the production of rayon and ignored them. See Paul David Blanc, *Fake Silk: The Lethal History of Viscose Rayon* (Yale University Press, 2016).

77. Testimony of Lester S. Sinness, director, Rayon Research Section, Du Pont, 176–88, Record in Lutz.

78. "Du Pont Makes Staff Changes in Rayon Department," *Women's Wear Daily*, March 27, 1950, 21; "Du Pont Reassigns Executive Staff in Rayon Department," *Women's Wear Daily*, December 3, 1951, 18; "Emphasis on Merchandising: Du Pont Textile Fiber Sales Revamped on End-Use Basis," *Women's Wear Daily*, December 3, 1954, 1, 12; "Du Pont Promotes Sinness," *New York Times*, October 7, 1961, 30; Robert Cole, "The Boss is Expert at Getting Raises," *New York Times*, May 11, 1969, F1; "Average Pay for Top Executives in U.S. Rose $35,031 in 1968," *Minneapolis Tribune*, May 12, 1969, 11; "Du Pont Promotes Lester S. Sinness," *Women's Wear Daily*, January 22, 1963, 31; Du Pont Annual Report (1971), 36 (accessible through ProQuest Historical Annual Reports).

79. *The Playthings Directory, 1954* (McCready Publishing Company, 1954), 421.

80. "550 Will Be Employed at Former Hess Goldsmith Plant After Jan. 1," *Wilkes-Barre Record*, October 2, 1961, 11. Children burned in Gene Autry cowboy suits in

the Wilkes-Barre area included Thomas James Hizny (seven, West Wyoming, PA, burned and died on October 28, 1944), Richard Johnson (six, Wilkes Barre, PA, burned March 30, 1945, died August 25, 1945), John Devens (six, Center Moreland, PA, burned April 29, 1946), Nelson Hoxie (six, Osterhout, PA, burned January 1, 1949, died January 31, 1949), Thomas Purcell (four, Minersville, PA, burned and died October 10, 1952). See "Lantern Ignites Halloween Suit; Boy Fatally Burned," *Star-Gazette* (Elmira, NY), October 30, 1944, 11; "Son of Meyers Coach Is Seriously Burned at Play," *Wilkes-Barre Record*, March 31, 1945, 11; "'Cowboy,' 6, Badly Burned," *Wilkes-Barre Record*, April 30, 1946, 1; "Cowboy Suit Fire Is Fatal," *Wilkes-Barre Record*, February 1, 1949, 12; "Cowboy Suit Catches Fire; Boy, 4, Dies," *Wilkes-Barre Times Leader*, October 11, 1952, 13.

81. See, e.g., "Gould Denies Army Charges of Conspiracy: Ex-Fight Manager Accused of Influencing Contract Awards," *Brooklyn Citizen*, October 31, 1944; "Joe Gould's Witness Hints Others Involved," *Daily News* (New York, NY), November 3, 1944, 495; "Denies $18,000 Was Paid to Gould," *News* (Paterson, NJ), November 3, 1944, 24; "Gould Gets 3 Years; Fired; Fined $12,000," *Daily American* (Somerset, PA), November 14, 1944, 8; "2 Persons Killed and 12 Burned When Explosions Wreck Toy Factory," *Wilkes-Barre Record*, March 14, 1961, 1, 20. His personal life too showed a pattern of failure and new attempts. Henry married twice, maybe three times. His first two marriages ended in divorce.
82. See Kim Lunman, "Stores Check Safety Worry," *Calgary Herald*, August 30, 1995, B3 (injuries to children from plastic slides manufactured by M.A. Henry, Ltd., established by Milton Henry in 1948); David Akin, "Toy Maker M. A. Henry Gets Credit Protection," *Hamilton (ON) Spectator*, June 25, 1997, C1; John Burman, "M.A. Henry in Toyland Again After Court OK," *Hamilton (ON) Spectator*, October 21, 1997, D7; Susan Clairmont, "A Broken Toy Story: M. A. Henry Files for Bankruptcy, in Trustee's Hands," *Hamilton (ON) Spectator*, February 14, 1998, D9; John Burman, "Dundas Toymaker in Trouble: Henry Ltd. In Receivership," *Hamilton (ON) Spectator*, September 24, 1998, D8.
83. On Autry's struggles with alcohol beginning in the mid-1940s and its negative impact on his performing career, see George-Warren, *Public Cowboy No. 1*, 223, 245–46, 273, 276, 282–86, 288, 291–92, 295.
84. George-Warren, *Public Cowboy No. 1*, 272–302 (the final quote is from 302).
85. Legal Department to Executive Committee, *Annual Report*, February. 11, 1955, 3, Du Pont Legal (accession no. 1729), Du Pont Collection.
86. J. Richard Burns to Gene Autry, February 7, 1955, box 1, Agents & Licensees, T94-45-30, folder M. A. Henry Co., 1952–1956, Autry Collection.
87. Burns to Autry, February 7, 1955.

chapter nineteen: "the road to preferment"

1. Richard M. Freeland, *Academia's Golden Age: Universities in Massachusetts, 1945—1970* (Oxford University Press, 1992), 106–7.
2. Dan Kevles, "Cold War and Hot Physics: Science, Security, and the American State, 1945–56," *Historical Studies in the Physical and Biological Sciences* 20, no. 2

(1990): 239–64; Daniel Kevles, *The Physicists: The History of a Scientific Community in Modern America* (Harvard University Press, 1995).

3. R. C. Lewontin, "The Cold War and the Transformation of the Academy," in *The Cold War and the University: Toward an Intellectual History*, eds. Noam Chomsky, Richard C. Lewontin, and Ira Katznelson (New Press, 1997), 12–13.
4. Vannevar Bush, director of the Office of Scientific Research and Development, *Science: The Endless Frontier*, report to the president (Government Printing Office, July 1945), vii–viii; Freeland, *Academia's Golden Age*, 71–72; A. Hunter Dupree, "The Great Instauration of 1940: The Organization of Scientific Research for War," in *The Twentieth-Century Sciences: Studies in the Biography of Ideas*, ed. Gerald Holton (W. W. Norton and Company, Inc., 1972), 443–67; Kevles, *Physicists*, 293–301.
5. *Science: The Endless Frontier*.
6. That support provided the foundation for what Richard Freeland calls "academia's Golden Age," and it is especially because of his focus on a broad range of institutions (Harvard, MIT, Brandeis, Tufts, Boston University, Boston College, Northeastern, and the University of Massachusetts) that one can see the transformative impact across institutions of federal funding. See Freeland, *Academia's Golden Age*.
7. Nathan Pusey, *American Higher Education, 1945–1970: A Personal Report* (Harvard University Press, 1978), 78–79. At the University of Minnesota, for example, the total expenditure for research in 1939–1940 was $500,000. By 1953–1954, that figure was $6.9 million. And whereas in 1939 there were no federal research contracts, in 1953, federal contracts accounted for 63 percent of the total research spending at the university. See University of Minnesota Self Survey, Research (University of Minnesota, 1956), 55–62, box 2, 00316, UA, UMN.
8. Pusey, *American Higher Education*, 78–79.
9. Clark Kerr, *The Uses of the University* (Harvard University Press, 1963), 46–49.
10. Kerr, *Uses of the University*, 50, 69. Kerr acknowledged, as the source for the limerick, Don K. Price, *Government and Science: Their Dynamic Relation in American Democracy*, James Stokes Lectureship on Politics (New York University Press, 1954), 87.
11. University Development Plan Committee's Subcommittee on Academic Eminence, *Columbia's Academic Eminence* (University Development Plan Committee, January 27, 1953), box 258, folder 2 Sti, 1952–1953, Central Files, CUA. See also University of Minnesota Self Survey, Research (1956), 1, box 2, UA00316, UA, UMN.
12. Freeland, *Academia's Golden Age*, 144.
13. They got a cut from every contract for "overhead." By 1969, for example, federal funds made up about one-third of the operating expenditures of the University of Chicago. See *Federal Grants and Contracts at the University of Chicago*, report of an ad hoc committee appointed by Presidents George W. Beadle and Edward H. Levi (University of Chicago, 1969), 1918–75, box 166, folder 9, Office of the President, Levi Administration Records, UChicago. See also Freeland, *Academia's Golden Age*, 146.
14. Kerr, *Uses of the University*, 54–55. A. Hunter Dupree describes the "research contract" in "The *Great Instauration* of 1940: The Organization of Scientific Research

for War," in *The Twentieth-Century Sciences: Studies in the Biography of Ideas* ed. Gerald Holton (W. W. Norton and Company, Inc., 1972), 457–59. See also Larry Owens, "MIT and the Federal 'Angel': Academic R & D and Federal-Private Cooperation Before World War II," *Isis* 81, no. 2 (June 1990): 188–213.

15. Kerr, *Uses of the University*, 57. Although legally the money was/is given to the academic institutions in which the investigators work, in practice that control was fiscal, not substantive.
16. William G. Bowen, *The Federal Government and Princeton University: A Report on the Effects of Princeton's Involvements with the Federal Government on the Operations of the University* (Princeton University Press, 1962), v. For the other reports, see Charles G. Dobbins, ed., *Higher Education and the Federal Government: Programs and Problems* (American Council on Education, 1963): The ACOE study was based on twenty-three universities, including Harvard and Princeton; Harold Orlans, *The Effects of Federal Programs on Higher Education: A Study of 36 Universities and Colleges* (Brookings Institution, 1962); *Harvard and the Federal Government: A Report to the Faculties and Governing Boards of Harvard University* (Harvard University, September 1961).
17. Kerr, *Uses of the University*, 53; Lewontin, "Cold War and the Transformation of the Academy," 24–25.
18. Freeland, *Academia's Golden Age*, 147. See Samuel Z. Klausner and Victor M. Lidz, eds., *The Nationalization of the Social Sciences* (University of Pennsylvania Press, 1986); Immanuel Wallerstein, "The Unintended Consequences of Cold War Area Studies," in *Cold War and the University*, eds. Chomsky et al., 195–231.
19. Robert Nisbet, *The Degradation of the Academic Dogma: The University in America, 1945–1970*, John Dewey Society Lecture no. 12 (Basic Books, Inc., 1971), 72. "Academic dogma" referred to universities as sites dedicated to the pursuit of knowledge for its own sake and to sharing that knowledge through teaching. The post-WWII critique that universities had drifted from their central mission was not the first such challenge. Consider Thorstein Veblen's searing critique of the corrosive power of the pursuit of money in diverting universities from what he argued was their "primary mission": "the disinterested pursuit of knowledge." See Thorstein Veblen, *The Higher Learning in America* (B. W. Huebsch, 1918), edited and with annotations and an introduction by Richard F. Teichgraeber III (Johns Hopkins University Press, 2015). See also see Laurence R. Veysey, *The Emergence of the American University* (University of Chicago Press, 1965), 302–17, 346–56.
20. Nisbet, *Degradation of the Academic Dogma*, ch. 5, 6, and 7.
21. Freeland, *Academia's Golden Age*, 106–7.
22. Robert K. Merton, "The Unanticipated Consequences of Purposive Social Action," *American Sociological Review* 1, no. 6 (December 1936): 894–904.
23. Consider the difference between Nisbet, *Degradation of the Academic Dogma* (1971), and Richard Lewontin, "Cold War and the Transformation of the Academy" (1997). Other critical voices include Ian Hacking, "Weapons Research and the Form of Scientific Knowledge," *Canadian Journal of Philosophy*, supp. 12 (1986): 237–60; Stuart W. Leslie, *The Cold War and American Science* (Columbia University Press, 1993); Laura Nader, "The Phantom Factor: Impact of the Cold War on Anthropology," in *Cold War and the University*, eds. Chomsky et al., 107–

46; and Ellen Herman, "Project Camelot and the Career of Cold War Psychology," in *Universities and Empire: Money and Politics in the Social Sciences During the Cold War*, ed. Christopher Simpson (New Press, 1998), 97–133.

24. Robert K. Merton, vita, box 347, folder 12, Robert K. Merton Papers, CUA.
25. Robert K. Merton, *A Life of Learning*, Charles Homer Haskins Lecture, ACLS Occasional Paper no. 25 (American Council of Learned Societies, 1994), 1–7.
26. Merton, *Life of Learning*, 8–9.
27. Craig Calhoun, ed., *Robert K. Merton: Sociology of Science and Sociology as Science* (Columbia University Press, 2010), 6.
28. Ruth W. Schultz, "The Improbable Adventures of an American Scholar," *Temple Review* 47, no. 1 (Spring 1995): 11.
29. The society was named the American Sociological Society (ASS) at the time Merton was president (1957) but was changed to American Sociological Association (ASA) in 1959.
30. Merton's works include *Science, Technology & Society in Seventeenth Century England* (1938 [1st American ed.] H. Fertig, 1970); *Mass Persuasion; The Social Psychology of a War Bond Drive* (Harper, 1946); *Social Theory and Social Structure* (1949, rev. and enl. ed., Free Press 1957); Robert K. Merton, ed., *Studies in the Scope and Method of "The American Soldier"* (Free Press, 1950); *The Focused Interview: A Manual of Problems and Procedures* (Free Press, 1956); Richard Peter McKeon, Walter Gellhorn, Robert K. Merton, The *Freedom to Read: Perspective and Program* (R. R. Bowker Co., 1957); Robert K. Merton, ed., *Contemporary Social Problems* (Harcourt, Brace and World, 1961); and *On the Shoulders of Giants: A Shandean Postscript* (Free Press, 1965).
31. Merton, vita.
32. See Calhoun, *Robert K. Merton*, 1–31; Schultz, "Improbable Adventures of an American Scholar," 8–13; Merton, *Life of Learning*; Morton M. Hunt, "How Does It Come to Be So? Robert K. Merton," *New Yorker*, June 28, 1961, 39–63; Paul F. Lazarsfeld, "An Episode in the History of Social Research: A Memoir," in *The Intellectual Migration: Europe and America, 1930–1960*, eds. Donald Fleming and Bernard Bailyn (Belknap Press of Harvard University Press, 1969), 270–337; Allen H. Barton, "Paul Lazarsfeld and Applied Social Research: Invention of the University Applied Social Research Institute," *Social Science History* 3, no. 3/4 (1979): 4–44; and James S. Coleman, "Columbia in the 1950s" (on the field of Sociology and the department at Columbia) in *Authors of Their Own Lives: Intellectual Autobiographies by Twenty American Sociologists*, ed. Bennett M. Berger (University of California Press, 1990), 75–103.
33. Allen H. Barton, the author of "Paul Lazarsfeld and Applied Social Research," was himself an example of the impact centers had in the postwar era in the development of research scholars.
34. Robert K. Merton, "The Matthew Effect in Science, II: Cumulative Advantage and the Symbolism of Intellectual Property," *Isis* 79, no. 4 (December 1988): 619.
35. Robert K. Merton, "Priorities in Scientific Discovery: A Chapter in the Sociology of Science," *American Sociological Review* 22, no. 6 (December 1957): 635–59.
36. Merton, "Priorities in Scientific Discovery," 636, 640.
37. Robert K. Merton, "The Matthew Effect in Science," *Science, New Series* 159, no.

3810 (January 5, 1968): 59; Harriet Anne Zuckerman, "Nobel Laureates: Sociological Studies of Scientific Collaboration" (PhD diss., Columbia University, 1965).

38. Robert K. Merton, "The Matthew Effect in Science," in *Robert K. Merton, The Sociology of Science: Theoretical and Empirical Investigations*, ed. and intro. Norman W. Storer (University of Chicago Press, 1973), 439. See also Robert K. Merton, "The Matthew Effect in Science, II," 607, n. 2. Merton's belated mea culpa did not change who received scholarly recognition for "the Matthew effect." Nor did it change authorship of the original article. Search for "The Matthew Effect in Science" on JSTOR and the article it will pull up lists as sole author Robert K. Merton. See Merton, "Matthew Effect in Science," *Science, New Series* 159, 56–63. The Merton/Zuckerman example reflects a broader pattern of women's intellectual work not being appropriately credited. See Margaret W. Rossiter, "The Matthew/Matilda Effect in Science," *Social Studies of Science* 23, no. 2 (1993): 325–41. For Zuckerman's book (based on her 1965 dissertation), see Harriet Zuckerman, *Scientific Elite: Nobel Laureates in the United States* (Free Press, 1977).
39. Merton, "Matthew Effect in Science," *Science, New Series* 159, 57.
40. On the proliferation of journals since the late 1940s, see Carol Tenopir and Donald W. King, "The Growth of Journals Publishing," in *The Future of the Academic Journal*, 2nd ed., eds. Bill Cope and Angus Phillips (Elsevier/Chandos, 2014), 59–178; Carol Tenopir and Donald W. King, "Trends in Scientific Scholarly Journal Publishing in the United States," *Journal of Scholarly Publishing* 23 (2000): 135–70; D. A. Kronick, *A History of Scientific and Technical Periodicals: The Origins and Development of the Scientific and Technological Press, 1665–1790*, 2nd ed. (Scarecrow Press, 1978); B. Houghton, *Scientific Periodicals: Their Historical Development, Characteristics and Control* (Clife Bingley/Linnet Books, 1975).
41. D. J. de Solla Price, *Little Science, Big Science* (Columbia University Press, 1963); Price, *Science Since Babylon*, enlarged ed. (Yale University Press, 1975), 169. See Carol Tenopir and Donald King, in the preceding note, for more recent data on the proliferation of journals.
42. Merton pointed to two studies on journal readership. A 1958 study in chemistry showed that "only about half of 1 percent of the articles published in journals of chemistry are read by any one chemist." And a 1963 study in psychology, the results of which were basically the same, showed that "about one-half of the research reports in 'core' journals will be read [or skimmed] by 1% or less of a random sample of psychologists." See Merton, "Matthew Effect in Science," *Science, New Series* 159, 59.
43. Allen G. Debus to David C. Lindberg, March 2, 1984 (re: Bill Coleman), box 18, folder 19, Allen G. Debus Papers, UChicago.
44. Calhoun, *Robert K. Merton*, 1–31. Consider also Norbert Weiner, *I Am a Mathematician* (Doubleday, 1956), 87, quoted in Merton, "Priorities in Scientific Discovery," 649, n. 51.
45. Zuckerman, *Scientific Elite.*
46. Joel Best, "Prize Proliferation," *Sociological Forum* 23, no. 1 (March 2008): 1–2.
47. Harriet Zuckerman, "The Proliferation of Prizes: Nobel Complements and Nobel Surrogates in the Reward System of Science," *Theoretical Medicine* 13 (1992): 217. On the Nobel Prize, see Zuckerman, *Scientific Elite.*

48. Paul Wasserman, ed., *Awards, Honors and Prizes: A Directory and Source Book*, 1st ed. (Gale Research Company, 1969).
49. Paul Wasserman, ed., *Awards, Honors and Prizes*, vol. 1, 5th ed. (Gale Research, 1982), vii. International and foreign prizes were listed in a second volume.
50. Donna Batten, ed., *Awards, Honors and Prizes*, vol. 1: *United States and Canada*, 13th ed. (Gale Research, 1997), vii.
51. James F. English, *The Economy of Prestige: Prizes, Awards, and the Circulation of Cultural Value* (Harvard University Press, 2005); Joel Best, *Everyone's a Winner: Life in Our Congratulatory Culture* (University of California Press, 2011), 3.
52. Steven Ruggles, vita, December 1983, in author's possession.
53. Steven Ruggles, "Curriculum Vitae," February 1997, *umn.edu*, archived February 5, 1998, at https://web.archive.org/web/19980205153831/http://www.hist.umn.edu/~ruggles/vitaf97.html.
54. Best, "Prize Proliferation," 13–15.
55. Zuckerman, "Proliferation of Prizes," 228.
56. Consider, for example: By 1997, the American Physical Society had forty awards, honors, and prizes, twenty-eight of which were named for a particular scholar in the field. For the full listing, see Batten, ed., *Awards, Honors and Prizes*, vol. 1, 188–90. Similarly, consider two early recognitions Ruggles received: the ASA William J. Goode Distinguished Book Award, Family Section, named for a former president of the ASA and distinguished scholar of the family (see "ASA Family Section: Past Recipients," *Sociology of the Family*, accessed November 3, 2025, http://www.asafamilysection.com/william-j-goode-book-award-recipients.html); and the SSHA Allan Sharlin Memorial Award, named for a promising young population historian, an assistant professor of sociology at Berkeley who died of cancer in 1985 at the age of thirty-three. Friends and family established the award in his name. His life and promise would in a sense be carried forward by others, his name appearing on their vitae. See "Allan Sharlin Memorial Book Award," Social Science History Association, accessed November 3, 2025, https://ssha.org/awards-and-prizes/sharlin-memorial-book-prize/.
57. Even if one did not have to be a member of a society to receive a particular award, membership surely helped in a culture in which society members selected prize recipients. And having received a prize awarded by a given society, one likely felt a greater affinity toward it.
58. Or a traveling trophy room, with its "concentrated aroma of achievement" or—at least—striving. See E. B. White, "Good-Bye to Forty-Eighth Street" (1957), in *Essays of E. B. White* (Harper Perennial, 1992 [1979]), 5.
59. "Steven Ruggles," vita, August 2022, archived at https://web.archive.org/web/20221010222252/https://users.pop.umn.edu/~ruggles/vita_ruggles.pdf. Many vitae were much longer. As Jim Grossman, executive director of the American Historical Association, former vice president of research and education at the Newberry Library, and before that a faculty member in history at the University of Chicago, wrote in an email exchange with me in early 2023, "I will never forget the first time I saw a 98 page c.v., [in] a fellowship proposal at the Newberry." James (Jim) Grossman to Barbara Welke, January 15, 2023, email (quoted with permission from Grossman).

60. Ruggles's publications on his August 2022 vita include one book; close to one hundred articles and chapters, more than half of which—reflecting the character of his field—had multiple authors; reports; "miscellaneous publications"; software; and book reviews. "Steven Ruggles," vita, August 2022.
61. Steven Ruggles, email exchange with Barbara Y. Welke, February 14, 2023.
62. In fiscal year 2023, for example, the University of Minnesota received $1.125 billion in sponsored research; see *2023 Annual Financial Report* (University of Minnesota, 2023), 19, https://drive.google.com/file/d/1I-M_ZBDskhAbMA-vII7TP8yZ4sOQILtS/view. By 2023, there were more than three hundred centers at the University of Minnesota.
63. Going forward, departments might elect to require that PhD candidates append curriculum vitae to their dissertations, but it was no longer a university requirement for the PhD.
64. Before 1945, the University of Minnesota had had no comprehensive written regulations relating to faculty tenure. The Board of Regents adopted regulations concerning academic tenure, establishing seven years as the point at which one gained permanent tenure, on February 9, 1945. See William Anderson, "The Academic Tenure Regulations," University of Minnesota, December 3, 1946, box 172, folder Staff Tenure 1945–67, Office of the President Central Files, UA, UMN.
65. William Anderson, professor of political science and chair of Subcommittee of Senate Committee on Education, to all department chairs and deans, September 19, 1947, box 172, folder Staff Tenure 1945–67, Office of the President Central Files, UA, UMN.
66. James B. Conant, *My Several Lives: Memoirs of a Social Inventor* (Harper and Row, Publishers, 1970), 175.
67. *Report of Committee on Appointment and Promotion Procedures* ("Stigler Report"), January 27, 1953, 2, box 258, folder 2, Central Files, 1895–1971, CUA.
68. *Report of Committee on Appointment and Promotion Procedures*, 3, 9.
69. The Faculty Handbook of Columbia University 1959, 31, 35, CUA.
70. Jack H. Schuster and Martin J. Finkelstein, *The American Faculty: The Restructuring of Academic Work and Careers* (Johns Hopkins University Press, 2006).
71. Robert K. Merton offers a representative example. See, e.g., S. N. Eisenstadt to R. K. Merton, May 21, 1960, box 109, folder 1, Robert K. Merton Papers, CUA (hereafter Merton Papers); W. R. Scott to Robert Merton, October 17, 1973, letter and reply (November 12, 1973), box 104, folder 3, Merton Papers.
72. *UMN Department of Psychology Self-Survey Report*, May 1975, appendix A, Graduate School Program Reviews Collection (unprocessed), UA, UMN. The curriculum vitae of the twenty-seven full-time faculty of the Department of Psychology at the University of Minnesota were attached as an appendix to the department's 1975 self-survey.
73. That marital status was included as one of the categories for vitae in a 1975 departmental self-survey suggests the challenge in uprooting this norm. Every faculty member but two responded to the question; one of those was the only woman in the department.
74. For example, Marvin D. Dunnette, curriculum vitae ("4. September 30, 1926. Austin, Minnesota"; "5. married"), in *UMN Department of Psychology Self Survey Re-*

port, 1975, appendix A, Graduate School Program Reviews Collection (unprocessed), UA, UMN.

75. Michael Chibnik, *Scholarship, Money, Prose: Behind the Scenes at an Academic Journal* (University of Pennsylvania Press, 2020), ch. 3.
76. "Oppenheimer: No. 1 Thinker on Atomic Energy" (cover featuring J. Robert Oppenheimer), *Life Magazine*, October 10, 1949; "Men of the Year: U.S. Scientists," (cover featuring geneticist George Beadle; astronauticist Charles Draper; virologist John Enders; physicist Donald Glaser; geneticist Joshua Lederberg; chemist Willard Libby; chemist Linus Pauling; physicist Edward Purcell; physicist I. I. Rabi; physicist Emilin Segre; transistor co-inventor William Shockley; physicist Edward Teller; physicist Charles Townes; physicist James Van Allen; and chemist Robert Woodward, *Time Magazine*, January 2, 1961); "Toward an Artificial Heart: Surgeon Michael DeBakey," (cover featuring Michael DeBakey), *Time Magazine*, May 28, 1965.
77. Hunt, "How Does It Come to Be So?"
78. That development depended on the invention of browsers and search tools. The first web browser, Mosaic, was created in 1994; Netscape followed in 1996 and Google in 1998.
79. Steven Ruggles, "Steven Ruggles," *umn.edu*, archived December 7, 1998, https://web.archive.org/web/19981207041146/http://www.hist.umn.edu/~ruggles/.
80. Steven Ruggles, email exchange with Barbara Y. Welke, March 11, 2023.
81. Consider, for example, the faculty bios of the Chemistry Department at the University of Michigan in 1997. Their bios, all narrative descriptions of their research, highlight another aspect of the web: It offered an ideal medium for the description of group research. The (re)turn to narrative grew more pronounced with time. See "Mark M. Banaszak Holl," *umich.edu*, archived August 11, 1997, https://web.archive.org/web/19970811114559/http://www.umich.edu/~michchem/faculty/banaszakholl/; "Brian P. Coppola," *umich.edu*, archived December 23, 1996, https://web.archive.org/web/19961223173516/http://www.umich.edu:80/~michchem/faculty/coppola/; and "Raoul Kopelman," *umich.edu*, archived August 11, 1997, https://web.archive.org/web/19970811113329/http://www.umich.edu/~michchem/faculty/kopelman/.
82. Sarah E. Igo, *The Known Citizen: A History of Privacy in Modern America* (Harvard University Press, 2018), 307–9.
83. See the title essay in Ruth Behar, *The Vulnerable Observer: Anthropology That Breaks Your Heart* (Beacon Press, 1996), 1–33.
84. Ruth Behar, *Translated Woman: Crossing the Border with Esperanza's Story* (Beacon Press, 1993).
85. Behar, *Vulnerable Observer*, 15.
86. Behar, *Translated Woman*, 338, 339–40, quoting from Mary John, "Postcolonial Feminists in the Western Intellectual Field: Anthropologists and Native Informants?" *Inscriptions* 5 (1989): 49–73. As Behar notes, the term "sanctioned ignorances" is from Gayatri Spivak.
87. "Ruth Behar," *www-personal.umich.edu*, archived August 29, 2000, https://web.archive.org/web/20000829085934/http://www-personal.umich.edu/~rbehar/, noting that the site was designed by David Frye on February 20, 1998.

88. Behar, *Translated Woman*, 235.

89. A. Hunter Dupree, "The *Great Instauration* of 1940: The Organization of Scientific Research for War," in *The Twentieth-Century Sciences: Studies in the Biography of Ideas*, ed. Gerald Holton (W. W. Norton and Company, Inc., 1972), 457–58. "Instauration" meaning restoration, renewal, renovation. Dupree took his title from Francis Bacon, who used it in the seventeenth century to refer to a great renewal of the arts and sciences. See also A. Hunter Dupree, *Science in the Federal Government: A History of Policies and Activities to 1940* (Belknap Press of Harvard University Press, 1957).

90. Berkeley (www.berkeley.edu) seems to have been the first university URL captured by the Wayback Machine: October 30, 1996. The first captures of Columbia (www.columbia.edu), Michigan (www.umich.edu), Princeton (www.princeton .edu), Minnesota (www.umn.edu), Wisconsin (www.wisc.edu), and Stanford (www.stanford.edu) followed in November and December 1996. Harvard (www .harvard.edu), Yale (www.yale.edu), and the University of Chicago (www.uchicago .edu) were first captured in 1997. All are archived at the Wayback Machine (https:// web.archive.org). Evidence of the life of the web among academics before the Wayback Machine—or at least anticipation of the web's potential—is clear in references noting "last modified" dates that significantly predate the earliest captures. For example, Stanford University's School of Engineering was first captured by the Wayback Machine on January 29, 1997, but many of the specific faculty links include the following: "Last modified by angwin on September 20, 1994"—in other words, more than two years before the first capture. The Stanford School of Engineering faculty postings also highlight two other aspects of the web that were true from the start. First, the "angwin" reference appears in many of the 1996 School of Engineering posts and shows that posting was clearly done by a staff member or graduate student very possibly working from faculty vitae. Second, "last modified" references highlight that, just as in vitae that bear a date, there was an expectation from the start not only that websites would be updated but that research lives were in motion and forward looking—and so a reader should know when the information dated from. I began from the first capture year, date, time of www.stanford .edu (December 29, 1996, at 18:10:22) and drilled down from there to the School of Engineering faculty (http://www-soe.stanford.edu/facultyindex.html). Clicking on any individual faculty member (each of whom has a specific URL), the capture date again shifts—some earlier and some later.

91. See, e.g., "Faculty and Senior Lecturers," *law.uchicago.edu*, archived February 13, 2001, https://web.archive.org/web/20010213235059/http://www.law.uchicago .edu/faculty/index-faculty.html; "Faculty Members," *law.upenn.edu*, archived November 11, 2001, https://web.archive.org/web/20011111022745/http://www.law .upenn.edu/.

92. John Gilliom and Torin Monahan, *SuperVision: An Introduction to the Surveillance Society* (University of Chicago Press, 2013), 51 (emphasis in original); Julia Angwin, *Dragnet Nation: A Quest for Privacy, Security, and Freedom in a World of Relentless Surveillance* (Times Books, 2014), 154, both quoted in Igo, *Known Citizen*, 344.

93. "Barbara Y. Welke, Curriculum Vitae," hist.umn.edu, archived September 1, 2006, https://web.archive.org/web/20060901101357/http://www.hist.umn.edu

/faculty/Welke%20cv%202005.pdf. And for an earlier "capture," see "Barbara Y. Welke," hist.umn.edu, archived March 3, 2001, https://web.archive.org/web/20010303171923/http://www.hist.umn.edu/Faculty/welke.html.

chapter twenty: "for the rest of his natural life"

The chapter title is from an affidavit by Fred L. Timberlake, Scott's Timberlake's father, noting that "the infant plaintiff will remain a custodial case for the rest of his natural life." See Affidavit of Fred L. Timberlake, November 6, 1951, Timberlake Case File.

1. Bates Interview.
2. Lockhart Interview. Art Cumberledge Jr. said something very similar. "I'm sure it had a big impact," Art Cumberledge reflected, "because it disrupted the whole family; it disrupted everything." Cumberledge Interview.
3. Bill of Particulars (incl. photographs of Scott Timberlake), April. 3, 1950; Affidavit of Fred L. Timberlake (Scott's father), May 24, 1950; Deposition of Robert E. Bruner, MD, Kansas City, MO, September 15, 1950, 8–11, 14; Deposition of Ruth S. Miller, Kansas City, MO, September 15, 1950, 91–105; Deposition of Kathryn Timberlake, Kansas City, MO, September 15, 1950, 273–74; Affidavit of Fred L. Timberlake, November 6, 1951, Timberlake Case File.
4. "Victim of Fire Well, Home from Hospital," *Tampa Bay Times*, May 8, 1947 (np., clipping from Peterson album).
5. Peterson Interview.
6. Affidavit of C. A. Rudisill, MD, October 1, 1949, Peterson Case File.
7. Peterson Interview.
8. Lockhart Interview.
9. Lockhart Interview.
10. Lockhart Interview.
11. Lockhart Interview. John Sansbury said something very similar in my conversation with him. Sansbury Interview.
12. Izzo Interview.
13. Bates Interview.
14. Felton Interview.
15. Izzo Interview.
16. Lockhart Interview.
17. "Once Near Death by Burns, Boy Wins Eagle Scout Rank," *Tampa Morning Tribune*, September 17, 1955 (n.p., clipping from Peterson album). See also Peterson Interview.
18. Habina Interview.
19. Hearing before Hon. John C. Knox, February 3, 1950, 2, Casimir Kresokowski Case File.
20. For example, of five grafts done in August 1952, when Casimir was sixteen, only three took, requiring another surgery with deeper grafts for the two that hadn't taken the first time. See Michael I. Lewin, MD, to M. Norman, Esq., October 16, 1952, Casimir Kresokowski Case File; Michael I. Lewin to M. Norman, October 7, 1953, Casimir Kresokowski Case File.

21. Izzo Interview.
22. Anonymous Interview; Sansbury Interview; Affidavit of Fred Cizek (Roy's father), January 2, 1950, 3, Cizek Case File.
23. Affidavit of Eugene P. McManamy (physician who treated David Gagnon), January 16, 1950, and Affidavit of Elliot B. Paley, January 26, 1950, 10–11, both in Gagnon Case File.
24. Izzo Interview.
25. Bates Interview.
26. Viands Interview.
27. Deposition of Kathryn Timberlake, Kansas City, MO, September 15, 1950, 302–3, Timberlake Case File; Timberlake Interview; "State UCP Founder Is Heart Attack Victim" (with photo of Fred L. Timberlake and detailing his long work since 1950 in establishing and leading United Cerebral Palsy of Greater Kansas City), *CLASP* 14, no. 4 (June–July 1967): 1 (in author's possession).
28. Timberlake Interview (with Kay Bryant, sister of Scott Timberlake).
29. Lockhart Interview.
30. Bates Interview.
31. Felton Interview.
32. I have high school/college yearbook photos for twenty-seven men. Four are of individuals (or their family members) I interviewed (Baragona, Felton, Sansbury, Szumita). The yearbooks are posted on "U.S., School Yearbooks, 1880–2012," *Ancestry.com*.
33. "Once Near Death by Burns, Boy Wins Eagle Scout Rank," *Tampa Morning Tribune*, September 17, 1955 (news clipping, Peterson photo album).
34. Habina Interview; Petition of Stella Kresokowski, New York, NY, December 7, 1951, Casimir Kresokowski Case File.
35. Gerald Palmateer, *Theodore Roosevelt High School Yearbook* (Washington, DC, 1957), Rifle Team photo, "U.S., School Yearbooks, 1880–2012," *Ancestry.com*.
36. Gerald Woodrow Palmateer, Certificate of Death, April 25, 1958, file no. 58-016960, State Board of Health, Florida Bureau of Vital Statistics.
37. Casimir Krzeczkowski Jr. was burned in 1943 at age seven; by 1950, when the legal case his mother had brought settled, he was thirteen. $16,273 of the $34,000 settlement was designated for Casimir Jr.
38. Petition (Stella Kresokowski, guardian), December 7, 1951 (request for funds to purchase television set among other things); Order, December 12, 1951; both in Casimir Kresokowski Case File.
39. Petition of Stella Kresokowski, October 20, 1953; Affidavit of Casimir Kresokowski, October 20, 1955; Order, October 20, 1955; Petition of Stella Kresokowski, February 1, 1957; Affidavit of Casimir Kresokowski, February 1, 1957; Order, February 5, 1957; all in Casimir Kresokowski Case File.
40. See, e.g., Order, April 1, 1952, Record in Bates (approving withdrawal of $2,250 for medical expenses); Petition (Sam Gorab, guardian), September 28, 1950; Order, October 2, 1950 (typewriter and desk), all in Gorab Case File; Habina Interview (seashore summer rental); Annual Account (Bessie Izzo, guardian), September 9, 1955 (July 15, 1955, $280 Cold Au Sable Resort Cottage); Annual Account (Bessie Izzo, guardian), August 7, 1954 (July 10, 1954, $90), Izzo Probate Court Record.

41. In states with probate courts, the local court was ostensibly responsible for protecting the minor's interests. That might mean court authorization was required for any expenditures while the child remained a minor, but it was as likely to mean some form of annual accounting of expenditures on behalf of the infant by the guardian, or something less. See, e.g., Order (Hon. Julius Miller), November 3, 1948, n.p., Gerber Case File; Order (Hon. James B. M. McNally), April 2, 1951, Weinstein Case File; Order (Hon. Henry W. Goddard), February 14, 1949, Intelisana Case File.
42. Final Order (Hon. John C. Knox), June 14, 1948, McMaster Case File. The total settlement was $30,000.
43. McMaster Interview.
44. Peterson Interview.
45. Author phone conversation with Charles F. Baragona Jr., November 11, 2016. The settlement in Baragona's case had been $33,000, $22,000 of which was set aside for him. See Order (Hon. Joseph A. Gavagan), November 3, 1949, Baragona Case File.
46. Answer to Petition, Heilman and Purcell, June 19, 1950, Probate Court, County of Saginaw, Izzo Record on Appeal.
47. Supplemental Order (Hon. John P. Murphy), June 27, 1949; Order Denying Motion for Rehearing (Hon. John P. Murphy), October 16, 1951, In the Matter of the Estate of Jacqueline L. Izzo, Probate Record in Izzo.
48. Izzo Interview.
49. Proceedings before Hon. Timothy C. Quinn, circuit judge, 40th Judicial Circuit of MI, presiding in the 10th Judicial Circuit, Saginaw, MI, January 8, 1954, 38, 51, Izzo Record on Appeal (fees dispute).
50. *In re Izzo v. Purcell*, 358 MI 101, 99 N.W.2d 625 (1959).
51. Izzo Interview.
52. Petition for Authority to Invest Funds of Minor's Estate, October 23, 1950; Order for Authority to Invest Funds of Minor's Estate (Hon. John P. Murphy), October 30, 1950, Probate Court, Saginaw County, MI, Izzo Probate Court Record.
53. See, e.g., Annual Account (Bessie Izzo, guardian), October 14, 1953; Annual Account (Bessie Izzo, guardian), August 7, 1954; Annual Account (Bessie Izzo, guardian), September 9, 1955, Izzo Probate Court Record.
54. Izzo Interview.
55. Felton Interview.
56. Habina Interview.
57. Final Order (Hon. John J. Knox), April 27, 1948, Habina Case File; Habina Interview.
58. Order (Hon. John M. Cashin), April 27, 1962; Petition, April 6, 1962; both in Bates Case File.
59. Bates Interview. But then his business went belly up—"bang," as he described it. Others too used the settlements to buy or pay for a substantial portion of their first house. Lockhart Interview; Cumberledge Interview.
60. Baragona Interview.
61. Herbert Ulick, Michael Felton, William Pritchard Jr., and John Sansbury were among those whose parents had college degrees and who themselves in turn graduated from college. Those who completed college although neither of their par-

ents had gone to college included Charles Baragona Jr., Roy Cizek, John Devens, Robert Gorab, Joseph Intelisano Jr., William McMaster Jr., Richard Szumita, and William Weatherell Jr.

62. See ch. 10, "an academic marketplace," and ch. 15, "to be 'judged on our capabilities alone.'"
63. Fred and Florence Cizek, 1940 US census, Terre Haute, Vigo, Indiana, roll T627_1104, 8A, ED: 8435, *Ancestry.com*; Affidavit of Fred Cizek, September 16, 1949, Cizek Case File; "Florence Cizek Dance Studio," *Terre Haute Tribune*, March 8, 1951, 23; Fred Cizek, Terre Haute, IN, City Directory, 1959.
64. For biographical data on Roy Cizek, see 1976 Cizek Audio Systems information, at "Roy F. Cizek," *Stereonomomono*, accessed May 19, 2025, http://stereonomono.blogspot.com/2012/09/roy-f-cizek.html; "Biography," *Cizekspeaker*, accessed May 19, 2025, http://cizekspeaker.weebly.com/biography.html.
65. "Big Day for Richard Szumita: Man Battles Handicaps to Earn URI Degree," ca. May 1969, news clipping shared by Szumita family, in author's possession. Szumita Interview.
66. Affidavit of Alexander Szumita, April 10, 1950, Szumita Case File; Richard Szumita, *Grist 1969*, yearbook (University of Rhode Island, 1969), 374, archived at https://archive.org/stream/YEARBOOK1969/YEARBOOK_1969_djvu.txt.
67. Szumita Interview.
68. "James Ikner Dies in Crash," *Ludington (MI) Daily News*, August 31, 1964, 3; "James C. Ikner in US Marines," *Ludington (MI) Daily News*, July 25, 1956, 3; James Ikner, Arthur Hill High School, Saginaw, MI, 1955, "U.S., School Yearbooks, 1880–2012," *Ancestry.com*.
69. "James Baer Killed as Auto Hits Tree," *Akron Beacon Journal*, February 25, 1966, 1–2.
70. The NHTSA (National Highway Traffic Safety Administration) was established by Congress in 1970. Ralph Nader's 1965 book *Unsafe at Any Speed: The Designed-In Dangers of the American Automobile* (Grossman, 1965) was an important pressure point. See Michael Pertschuk, *Revolt Against Regulation: The Rise and Pause of the Consumer Movement* (University of California Press, 1982).
71. Felton Interview.
72. Lockhart Interview.
73. Habina Interview.
74. Sansbury Interview.
75. Felton Interview.
76. Viands Interview.
77. Viands Interview. There were other families who lost children. Thomas and Eleanor Felton lost their first child, a boy named Thomas Hoyt Felton, at just under two months. Born on October 19, 1938, he died December 15, 1938. Thomas Hoyt Felton, Certificate no. 112228, Idaho Death Certificates, 1938–1961, *Ancestry.com*; Felton Interview.
78. Habina Interview. As Tom Habina noted, as he got older, he felt bad about not having gone in the water with his children when they were little.
79. Szumita Interview.
80. Viands Interview.

81. There is much that is personal in this account, but I have chosen not to include some of the specifics that individuals shared with me in these conversations.
82. William McMaster, Jack Lockhart, Charles Baragona, Joseph Intelisano, and Art Cumberledge all divorced, some after only a few years, some longer. McMaster Interview; Lockhart Interview; Baragona Interview; Intelisano Interview; Cumberledge Interview.
83. "Circuit Court," *Logansport (IN) Pharos Tribune*, March 21, 1966, 11.
84. "Circuit Court," *Logansport (IN) Pharos Tribune*, March 21, 1966; "Biography," *Cizekspeaker*; Roy Cizek (obit), *Tribune* (Terra Haute, IN), June 3, 1993, 2; Cathy Cizek (obit), *Kokomo (IN) Tribune*, July 18, 2002, 2; Michelle Day (stepdaughter of Roy Cizek's second marriage), forum post, September 30, 2009 on *Audiocircuit.com* (accessed January 6, 2016).
85. See Alison Lefkovitz, *Strange Bedfellows: Marriage in the Age of Women's Liberation* (University of Pennsylvania Press, 2018), 11 and ch. 2 more generally; Stephanie Coontz, *The Way We Never Were: American Families and the Nostalgia Trap* (Basic Books, 1992), 14–16, 166–67.
86. King Interview. See also McMaster Interview.
87. Lockhart Interview.
88. Goffman's path on the road to preferment and his prominence in the fields of sociology and social psychology began with the publication in 1956 of his first book, *The Presentation of Self in Everyday Life*, based on ideas from his University of Chicago dissertation. A revised edition in 1959 was awarded the American Sociological Association's 1961 MacIver Award.
89. See Nate Holdren, *Injury Impoverished: Workplace Accidents, Capitalism, and Law in the Progressive Era* (Cambridge University Press, 2020); Karen M. Tani, "After 504: Training the Citizen-Enforcers of Disability Rights," *Disability Studies Quarterly* 42, no. 3–4 (2023); Paul K. Longmore, "The Disability Rights Movement, Activism in the 1970s and Beyond," in Longmore, *Why I Burned My Book and Other Essays on Disability* (Temple University Press, 2003), 102–15.
90. Habina Interview.
91. Habina Interview.
92. On the role of physicians and pre-employment screening—what Nate Holdren describes as "human weeding"—to avoid employment of those with disabilities or other medical conditions, see Holdren, *Injury Impoverished*, 218–52.
93. Izzo Interview.
94. Felton Interview.
95. King Interview.
96. See biography of Roy Cizek at *Cizekspeaker*.
97. Lockhart Interview. See also McMaster Interview.
98. Lockhart Interview.
99. McMaster Interview.
100. Felton Interview.
101. Lockhart Interview.
102. Lockhart Interview; Felton Interview.
103. Edward B. Bradley (May 1975), US Social Security Death Index database, *Fam-*

ily Search; Casimir Krzeczkowski Jr. (February 1981), US Social Security Applications and Claims Index, 1936–2007, *Ancestry.com*; Herbert Ulick, California Death Index, 1940–1997, *Ancestry.com*; Richard W. Szumita (December 1991), US Social Security Death Index database, 1935–2014, *Ancestry.com*. Joseph R. Powell's date of death is in an obituary for his wife Alice (Hartshorn) Chichester. The couple married in 1959 and had four daughters. Given his injuries as a child, it is interesting that she was in nursing school when the couple married and returned to complete her nursing degree and work as a nurse after their daughters were raised (copy of obit in author's possession). Additional records are at Roy Cizek (obit), *Terre Haute (IN) Tribune*, June 3, 1993, 2; and William E. Pritchard, US Social Security Applications and Claims Index, 1936–2007, *Ancestry.com*.

104. Szumita Interview. Richard Szumita died of a brain tumor.
105. "Chesapeake Honors William E. Pritchard," *Sun* (Baltimore, OH), December 20, 1993, 8C. William Pritchard died of cancer.
106. Peterson Interview.
107. Peterson Interview.
108. On Cizek, see note 64 above.
109. "John Devens, Valdez Mayor During Exxon Spill, Dies at 74," *New York Times*, June 19, 2014, B18.

chapter twenty-one: the vita of precarity

1. My thinking on precarity in academia and its relationship to preferment is indebted to Margot Canaday's work on "gay labor" in the Fordist economy and Brooke Depenbusch's on the working poor and general relief in the same period. See Margot Canaday, *Queer Career: Sexuality and Work in Modern America* (Princeton University Press, 2023); and Brooke Depenbusch, "Down and Out in the USA: General Relief and the Politics of Precarity in the Shadow of the Welfare State, 1935–1964" (PhD diss., University of Minnesota, 2019), https://conservancy.umn.edu/items/327ade26-d78f-4fa7-8b0b-ef146be48065.
2. John J. Rumbarger, assistant executive secretary, "Annual Report on the Professional Register, 1969," box 759, folder Committee on the Professional Register, 1961–70, AHA Papers (LoC). For the "seller's market" quote, see Robert L. Zangrando, executive secretary, "The Professional Register," 1966, container 683, folder Annual Meeting 1966 Professional Placement Session, AHA Papers (LOC).
3. Zangrando, "Professional Register," 3.
4. "Association Items" [April 1972 AHA Council Meeting], *AHA Newsletter* 10, no. 4 (September 1972): 11, AHA Papers (headquarters).
5. Henry Bryant Avery to "Prof. Potter," February 14, 1971, box 759, folder Professional Register (standing), 1971, AHA Papers (LoC).
6. Avery to Potter, February 14, 1971.
7. Allan M. Cartter, *Ph.D.'s and the Academic Labor Market: A Report Prepared for The Carnegie Commission on Higher Education* (McGraw-Hill Book Company, 1977), 21.

8. Between 1950 and 1970, American universities awarded 233,274 doctorates. Between 1948 and 1970, the *annual* number of PhDs awarded in the United States increased from roughly four thousand to thirty thousand. See Richard M. Freeland, *Academia's Golden Age: Universities in Massachusetts, 1945–1970* (Oxford University Press, 1992), 94; Modern Language Association, *A Guide for Job Candidates and Department Chairmen in English and Foreign Languages* (MLA, 1973), 4.
9. US Bureau of the Census, "Series H 766–787: Number of Doctorates, by Field: 1920 to 1970," in *Bicentennial Edition: Historical Statistics of the United States, from Colonial Times to 1970, Part I* (Government Printing Office, 1975), 387–88.
10. See Cartter, *Ph.D.'s and the Academic Labor Market*, 83 (table 5-5), 129 (figure 7-1).
11. *AHA Newsletter* 10, no. 4 (September 1972): 8–11, AHA Papers (headquarters).
12. MLA, *Job Information List* (October 1971): ii–iii, http://www.mla.org/Resources/Career/Job-List/PDFs-of-the-MLA-Job-Information-List. For other professional societies' response to the employment crisis, see, e.g., "Report of Committee on Placement," *Proceedings and Addresses of the American Philosophical Association* 1970, no. 43 (1969–1970): 128–29; "The Employment Register," *American Mathematical Monthly* 67, no. 9 (November 1960): 951–52; "Arrangements, Entertainment, and Recreation," *American Mathematical Monthly* 82, no. 5 (May 1975): 575.
13. The end of society registers like the AHA's did not eliminate the indignity. Many institutions continued to hold the interviews they had scheduled in the space provided by professional societies, others in hotel rooms with candidates and interviewers seated on hotel beds.
14. Jane W. Ferrar to Robert Merton, October 31, 1973, box 106, folder 10, Robert K. Merton Papers, CUA.
15. See ch. 12, "married, two children," and ch. 15, "to be 'judged on our own capabilities.
16. Jessie Bernard, *Academic Women* (Penn State University Press, 1964), 100.
17. Vicki Schultz, "Life's Work," *Columbia Law Review* 100 (2000): 1919. On the explosion in precarity in the US and globally, see Alison Pugh, *The Tumbleweed Society: Working and Caring in an Age of Insecurity* (Oxford University Press, 2015); Robert O. Self, *All in the Family: The Realignment of American Democracy Since the 1960s* (Hill and Wang, 2012); Jacob Hacker, *The Great Risk Shift: The New Economic Insecurity and the Decline of the American Dream* (Oxford University Press, 2006); David Harvey, *The Condition of Postmodernity: An Enquiry into the Origins of Cultural Change* (Blackwell, 1990). On academia, see Adrianna Kezar, Tom DePaola, and Daniel T. Scott, *The Gig Academy: Mapping Labor in the Neoliberal University* (Johns Hopkins University Press, 2019); Marc Bousquet, *How the University Works: Higher Education and the Low-Wage Nation* (NYU Press, 2008), 186–210; Jack H. Schuster and Martin J. Finkelstein, *The American Faculty: The Restructuring of Academic Work and Careers* (Johns Hopkins University Press, 2006), ch. 3 and ch. 7; Sheila Slaughter and Gary Rhodes, *Academic Capitalism and the New Economy* (Johns Hopkins University Press, 2004), 181–206; Judith M. Gappa and David W. Leslie, *The Invisible Faculty: Improving the Status of Part-Timers in Higher Education* (Jossey-Bass Publishers, 1993).
18. See MLA, *Job Information List*; AHA Professional Register, *Employment Informa-*

tion Bulletin 1, no. 1 (December 1971); ASA, *Employment Bulletin* 2, no. 10 (October 1977).

19. The MLA *Job Information List* was first available in electronic form in 1997.
20. See, e.g., the entry for English vacancies at Bowdoin College, Brunswick, ME, in the MLA *Job Information List* (October 1971), 6, https://www.mla.org/content/download/10464/file/jil_eng_1971_12.pdf?inLanguage=eng-US&version=1.
21. See, e.g., the entry for English vacancies at Tufts University, Medford, MA, in the MLA *Job Information List* (October 1971), 4.
22. "We hope," "At most we might" (Yale University, English, 9); "if circumstances allow" (Fairfield University, Fairfield, CT, English, 9); "possibility of" (Stockton College, Pomona, NJ, English and comparative literature, 11); "may eventually have openings for" (Queens College, CUNY, English, 14), all in the MLA *Job Information List* (October 1971).
23. Hamilton College, English vacancy listing, MLA *Job Information List* (October 1971), 16.
24. See, e.g., Grove City College, Grove City, PA, English vacancy listing, MLA *Job Information List* (October 1971), 19.
25. AHA Professional Register, *Employment Information Bulletin* 1, no. 1 (December 1971), AHA Papers (headquarters). The "no-vacancy" sort of listing examples are from UC Davis and Southern Colorado State College Pueblo.
26. AHA Professional Register, *Employment Information Bulletin* 2, no. 4 (May 1973), AHA Papers (headquarters).
27. AHA Professional Register, *Employment Information Bulletin* 3, no. 4 (May 1974), AHA Papers (headquarters); AHA Professional Register, *Employment Information Bulletin* 4, no. 1 (October 1974), AHA Papers (headquarters).
28. The shortfall in positions for new PhDs appeared first in physics and mathematics beginning in 1967 and 1968. The contraction of federal research and development between 1971 and 1973 brought the full impact of the imbalance between the supply of new PhDs and the demand home to the sciences more generally. See Cartter, *Ph.D.'s and the Academic Labor Market*.
29. "Summary, Placement Service Register, The American Physical Society—American Association of Physics Teachers Annual Joint Meeting, Feb. 3–6, 1969, New York City" (loose), box 1, AIP Placement Service Records, 1960–1978 (AR 205, unprocessed), AIP Papers; "Summary, Placement Service Register, The American Physical Society—American Association of Physics Teachers Annual Joint Meeting, Jan. 26–29, 1970, Chicago, Illinois," (loose), box 1, AIP Placement Service Records, 1960–1978 (AR 205, unprocessed), AIP Papers.
30. "Correspondence Placement Service 1971," box 3, AIP Placement Service Records, 1960–1978 (AR 205, unprocessed), AIP Papers. Given the source and date of these materials, I have elected not to include full names of specific letter writers. I list the letters in the order in which I have included them in the paragraph: Bortz, December 4, 1971; Burba, May 18, 1971; Hobart, April 19, 1971.
31. Hicks, resume, 1974, box 2 of 4, folder Registrants 4700–4849 [1974], American Institute for Physics Placement Service Records, 1960–1978 (AR 205, unprocessed), AIP Papers.

32. Raymond W. Sears to [Miss Martha Dickinson], October 15, 1971, box 3, folder Correspondence Placement Service 1971, American Institute for Physics Placement Service Records, 1960–1978 (AR 205, unprocessed), AIP Papers.
33. MLA, *Job Information List* (October 1971): ii–iii. For similar warnings issued by other societies, see "Professional Register," *AHA Newsletter* 4, no. 1 (October, 1965): 5; *APSA Newsletter* (May 1966): 7, box 690, folder Committee on the Professional Register, 1964–1966, AHA Papers (LoC).
34. AHA, *Employment Information Bulletin* (May 1974).
35. MLA, *A Guide for Job Candidates and Department Chairmen in English and Foreign Languages* (MLA, 1973), 8.
36. For example, the AIP had revised its system in hopes of attracting employers who were reluctant to publicize positions because of the flood of applicants that would result.
37. Mary Jean Cornish to Robert K. Merton, August 7, 1973, box 105, folder 5, Robert K. Merton Papers, CUA.
38. Bryant Avery, Bill and Nancy Doub, Jon Livingston, and Joe Moore, "Speaking Truth to Power: Editors' Perspectives on the First Twenty Years of the *Bulletin of Concerned Asian Scholars*," *Critical Asian Studies* 50, no. 2 (2018): 278–93. The details in this paragraph are drawn from Bryant Avery's portion of the article, 279–83, 293.
39. The MLA spoke for many disciplines in noting in 1973 the widespread sense of alienation. See MLA, *A Guide for Job Candidates and Department Chairmen in English and Foreign Languages* (MLA, 1973), 14.
40. Avery et al., "Speaking Truth to Power," 279–83, 293. Avery became managing editor of the *Bulletin of Concerned Asian Scholars* and in 1981 moved to Edmonton, Canada, where he spent the remainder of his working career as an editor of one of the city's major dailies.
41. Freeland, *Academia's Golden Age*, 93–97.
42. Canaday, *Queer Career*, 258–60; Harvey, *Condition of Postmodernity*, 150.
43. AAUP, "Statement: On the Imposition of Tenure Quotas" (October 1973), *AAUP Bulletin* 59, no. 4 (December 1973): 428–30; AAUP, "Report: On Full-Time Non-Tenure-Track Appointments" (June 1978), *AAUP Bulletin* 64, no. 3 (September 1978): 267–73.
44. AAUP, *The Status of Part-Time Faculty* (AAUP, November 1980), https://www.aaup.org/report/status-part-time-faculty.
45. AAUP, *Status of Part-Time Faculty*. The AAUP's 1940 "Statement of Principles on Academic Freedom and Tenure" referred only to full-time service "in defining the probationary years preceding the attainment of tenure." For the AAUP's 1940 statement, see *AAUP Policy Documents and Reports* (AAUP, January 1977), https://files.eric.ed.gov/fulltext/ED136646.pdf.
46. "Modern Language Association Statement on the Use of Part-Time Faculty," MLA *Job Information List*, English ed. (October 1982), iii. The statement was included three years later in English Showalter, ed., *A Career Guide for PhDs and PhD Candidates in English and Foreign Languages* (MLA, 1985), 58–59.
47. MLA, "Statement on the Use of Part-Time and Full-Time Adjunct Faculty," MLA *Job Information List*, English ed. (October 1995), viii.

48. On departments' use of budget constraints to explain their failure to hire women and other minorities, see ch. 15, "to be 'judged on our capabilities alone.'"
49. See ch. 17, "on our traditional basis of quality alone."
50. On professional societies that had long listed candidates' sex in candidate available listings and had directed candidates to include age, sex, and marital and parental status on vitae, dropping those practices in the early 1970s, see ch. 15, "to be 'judged on our capabilities alone.'"
51. Showalter, ed., *Career Guide for PhDs and PhD Candidates in English and Foreign Languages*, 17.
52. Showalter, ed., *Career Guide for PhDs and PhD Candidates in English and Foreign Languages*.
53. English Showalter, "The Academic Job Search," in *MLA Career Guide for PhDs and PhD Candidates in English and Foreign Languages*, ed. English Showalter (MLA. 1996), 24–25.
54. Showalter, "Academic Job Search," 16–17.
55. There was a running commentary in the pages of *The Chronicle of Higher Education* about academia's "lost generation." But who it included and whether they had been "lost" was disputed, even as there were calls that they offered institutions an untapped pool of qualified teachers. See, e.g., Scott Heller, "The Expected Turnaround in the Faculty Job Market May Come Too Late for 'Lost Generation' of Scholars" (May 23, 1990); "Voices from the 'Lost Generation' of Scholars" (June 13, 1990); "'Lost Generation' Made Important Contributions" (July 4, 1990); Constance B. Bouchard, "The 'Lost Generation' of Scholars Can Help Colleges Avoid the Looming Faculty Shortage" (November 21, 1990); Scott Heller, "Scholar of American Poetry Ends His Long Odyssey" (April 15, 1992); "Hope for Academe's 'Lost Generation'" (May 20, 1992); Alison Schneider, "Persistence Paid Off for 'Lost Generation' of English Ph.D.'s, Study Finds" (September 3, 1999); Jennifer Howard, "MLA Panel Finds No 'Lost Generation of Scholars' from the Tenure Track" (December 15, 2006).
56. Michael Seadle, letter to the editor, in "'Lost Generation' Made Important Contributions," *Chronicle of Higher Education* (July 4, 1990).
57. "People: Ph.D. Students," *cs.columbia.edu*, archived January 2, 1997, https://web.archive.org/web/19970606191651/http://www.cs.columbia.edu/home/people/people.html#phd.
58. "Grad CSE Students with Home Pages," *cs.umich.edu*, archived October 22, 1997, https://web.archive.org/web/19980210132700/http://www.eecs.umich.edu/home/people/students/g_cse_students.html.
59. "This page contains a list of students on the job market in the Fall-Winter 1998–1999. Additional information (including a packet of CV's) can be requested from Julie Less [link], the Student Affair Administrator. . . . You can also contact the students directly via the email addresses provided. Some students also have a web page with additional information" ("Job Market Candidates," *spc.uchicago.edu*, archived December 1, 1998, https://web.archive.org/web/19981203044018/http://www.spc.uchicago.edu/Economics/).
60. See, e.g., the list of student bios in history and physics that Yale sent to other universities (here University of Chicago and Princeton) in 1931 and 1933, in E. S. Fur-

niss to "Mr. Dodd" (chairman, Department of History, University of Chicago), December 9, 1931 (with enclosure "Graduate School—Yale University: Candidates for the Ph.D. Degree in History"), box 7, Applications for Faculty Positions, 1914–48, folder 1 1914–1931, University of Chicago, Department of History Records, UChicago; and Anna M. Hanson to "Prof. Adams" (chair, Department of Physics, Princeton University), December 9, 1933 (with enclosure "Confidential Information Concerning a Selected Group of Candidates for Teaching Positions in Physics—1934–1935"), box 13, folder 1, Department of Physics (AC 133), Asst. Chairman Adams, E.P., 1931–1934, PUA.

61. Mary Morris Heiberger and Julie Miller Vick, "Do I Need My Own Web Page?" *Chronicle of Higher Education*, August 28, 1998. The authors of the article were the authors of *The Academic Job Search Handbook* (University of Pennsylvania Press, 1996). A note at the end of the article states: "'They have provided career services for thousands of graduate and professional students since 1985. Ms. Heiberger is associate director and Ms. Vick is a graduate career counselor at the Career Services office of the University of Pennsylvania."
62. "Carolyn Fischer," *econ.lsa.umich.edu*, archived October 24, 1997, https://web.archive.org/web/19971024130556/http://www.econ.lsa.umich.edu/~cfischer/.
63. "Carolyn Fischer."
64. The linked CV was completely professional and devoid of the personal information and emotion on her home page. See Carolyn Fischer, "CV," *econ.lsa.umich.edu*, archived October 24, 1997, https://web.archive.org/web/19971024133109/http://www.econ.lsa.umich.edu/~cfischer/resume.htm.
65. "John Bakija," *econ.lsa.umich.edu*, archived October24, 1997, https://web.archive.org/web/19971024130532/http://www.econ.lsa.umich.edu/~jbakija/.
66. Heiberger and Vick, "Do I Need My Own Web Page?"
67. "Home Page: Andrew Wong," *gsb.uchicago.edu*, archived November 28, 2001, https://web.archive.org/web/20011128021001/http://home.uchicago.edu/~awong/Bschool/bschool.htm. Note that the capture date for the home page leading to Wong's vita (April 14, 2001) is earlier than date for the vita itself (November 11, 2001). In a capture of Wong's home page on November 28, 2001, he had revised the statement accompanying his CV to read, "My life compacted into a three page document." Captures on the Wayback Machine are complicated. Often the capture date on which one initially clicks does not apply to every element of that site. So, for example, here, the capture date for the GSB at the University of Chicago I clicked on was December 19, 2000. But clicking on the link for Faculty and then PhD Candidate Resumes, the date that showed when the page appeared was several weeks earlier (December 3, 2000), and clicking on Andrew Wong (one of the students listed) showed a date of April 14, 2001. Screenshots of the full screen are key to keeping track of when a given internal element of a URL or document was actually captured.
68. "Home Page: Andrew Wong."
69. Elizabeth Martin, "My First Invitation to the Dance" (August 10, 2001); Elizabeth Martin, "The End of the Academic Affair" (May 11, 2001); Arthur Athelstand, "On the Market: To Rule in Hell or Serve in Heaven" (February 2, 2001), all in *Chronicle of Higher Education*. See also Elizabeth Martin, "On the Market: Wasting Time

Learning to Teach" (November 24, 2000); Elizabeth Martin, "On the Market with a Second- and a Third-Body Problem" (February 9, 2001); Elizabeth Athelstand, "The Endless Trade-Offs of an Academic Marriage" (June 8, 2001), all again in *Chronicle of Higher Education.*

70. For Daniel Kowalsky's posts in *The Chronicle of Higher Education*, see "On the Market: Diary of a Would-Be Historian" (October 20, 2000); "What I Saw at the Job Conference" (February 16, 2001); "My Narrow Escape from a Life Without Letterhead" (June 15, 2001); and "Next Stop: Cairo" (July 3, 2002).
71. The reference to *A Chorus Line* was so much truer than I expect even Daniel Kowalsky realized. See *AAUP Contingent Faculty Index: 2006* (AAUP, 2006), https://www.aaup.org/sites/default/files/files/AAUPContingentFacultyIndex2006.pdf.
72. For Kowalsky's personal profile and the broader, international focus on metrics documenting productivity, see "Daniel Kowalsky," Queens University Belfast, accessed April 10, 2024, https://pure.qub.ac.uk/en/persons/daniel-kowalsky.
73. For data on contingent faculty, see "Resources on Contingent Positions," AAUP, accessed November 7, 2025, https://www.aaup.org/issues/contingent-faculty-positions/resources-contingent-positions. See also Schuster and Finkelstein, *American Faculty.*
74. The University of Akron's dismissal of ninety-six faculty members in 2022 is just one example. See "'An Assassination of Our Careers': How Faculty Layoffs Have Forever Changed the University of Akron," *Chronicle of Higher Education*, August 9, 2022.
75. Erving Goffman, *Stigma: Notes on the Management of Spoiled Identity* (New York, 1963), 4–5 ("an individual who might have been received easily in ordinary social intercourse possesses a trait that can obtrude itself upon attention and turn those of us whom he meets away from him, breaking the claim that his other attributes have on us"). Consider the following from *The Chronicle of Higher Education*: "To the Editor: The Discouraging Job Market in Academe" (May 18, 1994); Robin Wilson, "Scholars Off the Tenure Track Wonder if They'll Ever Get On" (June 7, 1996); "To the Editor: Discrimination Against Part-Timers" (April 10, 1998); W. T. Pfefferle, "A Former Adjunct Professor Comes (Mostly) Clean" (August 6, 1999); Marc Bousquet, "Downwardly Mobile" (August 26, 2008).
76. The soundtrack to the 1975 musical *A Chorus Line*, including the opening number, "I Hope I Get It," can be accessed through iTunes, under *A Chorus Line—40th Anniversary Celebration (Original Cast Recording)*, Masterworks, 2015.

chapter twenty-two: growing old

1. Bates Interview.
2. *Spiral Jetty*'s location, shape, and history are powerfully symbolic of the course of a life. There are also parallels in Smithson's life to those burned in Gene Autry cowboy suits. Like a number of the victims, Smithson was born in Passaic, New Jersey—where the Gene Autry cowboy suit was made—in 1938, making him also of the same generation as children burned in Gene Autry cowboy suits. He died in 1973 at the age of thirty-five in an airplane accident in Texas, the site of a new

earthwork sculpture he was overseeing. On Smithson, see Michael Kimmelman, "Sculpture from the Earth, but Never Limited by It," *New York Times*, June 24, 2005, https://www.nytimes.com/2005/06/24/arts/design/sculpture-from-the-earth-but-never-limited-by-it.html.

3. King Interview.
4. Izzo Interview.
5. Bates Interview.
6. Lockhart Interview.
7. Lockhart Interview.
8. Lockhart Interview.
9. Habina Interview.
10. Izzo Interview.
11. King Interview.
12. Viands Interview.
13. Izzo Interview.
14. McMaster Interview.
15. On this point, see Emmanuel Carrere's memoir *Lives Other Than My Own*, trans. Linda Coverdale (Picador, 2009).
16. Lockhart Interview.
17. Izzo Interview.
18. Izzo Interview.
19. Felton Interview.
20. Sansbury Interview.
21. Bates Interview.
22. Lockhart Interview.
23. Arthur Cumberledge Jr. shared the scrapbook with me when we met. It remains in his possession. Cumberledge Interview.
24. Cumberledge Interview.
25. Baragona Interview.
26. For later articles, see "Congressman Convinced: Priest Wants Law to Insure Against Flammable Textile" and "Victims of Autry Playsuits Shake Hands with Their Hero," *Times-Herald* (Washington, DC), April 21, 1945, 17; "Saved Lad, 8, from Burning in Play Suit," *Times-Herald* (Washington, DC) April 22, 1945, B-1.
27. [Full front-page photo of Franklin D. Roosevelt], "Born Jan. 30 1882: Died April 12, 1945," *Times-Herald* (Washington, DC), April 13, 1945, 1; "Body of Roosevelt Enroute Here: Truman Will Address Congress," *Washington Evening Star*, April 13, 1945, 1.
28. The neatness of the arc captured there was a mistaken one: the legislation effectively written by the textile industry, thousands of children burned in cotton flannelette in the 1950s and 1960s, leading to another round of legislation, then to flame-resistant chemicals that were themselves hazardous. For a glimpse of the longer, darker arc of this history, see Barbara Young Welke, "Owning Hazard: A Tragedy," *UC Irvine Law Review* 1, no. 3 (2011): 693–771.
29. Cumberledge Scrapbook, Cumberledge Interview.
30. Lockhart Interview.
31. Family photo album made by Pat Peterson's mother for her son. Peterson Interview.

32. Peterson Interview.
33. Jayne (Cumberledge) Borberg to Gene Autry, December 22, 1997 (copy in author's possession); Cumberledge Interview.
34. Maxine Hansen to Ms. Jayne B. Borberg, March 4, 1998 (copy in author's possession); Cumberledge Interview.
35. Cumberledge Interview.
36. Cumberledge Interview.
37. Lockhart Interview.
38. Welke, "Owning Hazard: A Tragedy"; Barbara Young Welke, "The Cowboy Suit Tragedy: Spreading Risk, Owning Hazard in the Modern American Consumer Economy," *Journal of American History* 97 (June 2014): 97–121.
39. Izzo Interview.
40. Consider Lisel Mueller, "Curriculum Vitae" (1992), in *Alive Together: New and Selected Poems* (Louisiana State University Press, 1996), 5–6.

note on methods and sources

1. One case, Pritchard, was filed in the Court of Common Pleas, Lehigh, PA, for settlement purposes only. In several other late cases, the defendants settled without the plaintiffs having filed suit.
2. George F. Carpinello, "Public Access to Court Records in Civil Proceedings: The New York Approach," *Albany Law Review* 54 (1989–1990): 93–121, 106–7, 115.

cowboy suit case files, published legal opinions, and oral histories

cowboy suit case files

U. S. DIST. CT., SDNY, NARA NORTHEAST REGION–NEW YORK (NY, NY)

Adams Case File. Robert Adams, an infant, by his guardian ad litem, Mary Adams and Wilfred Adams, individually v. M. A. Henry Co., Inc., et al., Civ. 34-759.

Baer Case File. James F. Baer, an infant, by Russell Baer, his guardian ad litem, and Russell Baer v. Gene Autry, et al., Civ. 41-30.

Bates Case File. Gaither Bates, Jr., by his guardian ad litem, Gaither Bates, Sr., and Gaither Bates, Sr., individually v. Gene Autry, et al., Civ. 43-669.

Berry Case File. David I. Berry, an infant, by his guardian ad litem, Ivan Eugene Berry, and Ivan Eugene Berry, individually v. M. A. Henry Co., Inc., et al., Civ. 43-660.

Bradley Case File. Edward B. Bradley, an infant, by his mother and next friend, Laura C. Bradley, and Laura C. Bradley, individually v. Gene Autry, et al., Civ. 38-282.

Burke Case File. Richard Burke, an infant, by his father and next friend Jack Burke, and Jack Burke, individually v. Gene Autry, et al., Civ. 44-588.

Cumberledge Case File. Arthur A. Cumberledge, Jr., an infant, by his father and next friend, Arthur A. Cumberledge, and Arthur A. Cumberledge, individually v. Gene Autry, et al., Civ. 38-280.

Cutter Case File. (Wayne Cutter). General Accident Fire & Life Assurance Corporation, Ltd. v. M. A. Henry Co., Inc., et al., Civ. 42-611.

Detrick Case File. James Edmund Detrick, an infant by his guardian ad litem, W. Philip Van Kirk v. M.A. Henry Co., Inc., et al., Civ. 39-558.

Devens Case File. John S. Devens, a minor, by his father and next friend, John E. Devens, and John E. Devens and Laura Devens v. M. A. Henry Co., Inc., et al., Civ. 45-518.

DiTrapani Case File. Helen C. DiTrapani, administrator of the estate of Marco Antonio DiTrapani, deceased, and Vito DiTrapani v. M.A. Henry Co., Inc., et al., Civ. 35-386.

Donahue Case File. Willis B. Donahue, an infant, by his guardian ad litem, Willis J. Donahue, and Willis J. Donahue, individually v. M. A. Henry Co., Inc., et al., Civ. 45-163.

Flesher Case File. The State of Maryland to the use of Floyd I. Flesher, and Frances C. Flesher, and Floyd I. Flesher, individually and as administrator of the estate of Robert H. Flesher, deceased v. Gene Autry, et al., Civ. 44-428.

Frazer Case File. Donald G. Frazer, by his guardian ad litem, George E. Frazer, and George E. Frazer, individually v. Gene Autry, et al., Civ. 52-112.

Gates Case File. Lawrence E. Gates, an infant, by his mother and next friend, Dorothy J. Gates, and Dorothy J. Gates, individually v. Gene Autry, et al., Civ. 43-569.

Gorab Case File. Robert Gorab, by his next friend Sam Gorab, and Sam Gorab, individually v. M. A. Henry Co., Inc., et al., Civ. 45-272.

Greatorex Case File. William F. Greatorex, an infant, by his father and next friend, William H. Greatorex, and William H. Greatorex, individually v. Gene Autry, et al., Civ. 38-279.

Habina Case File. Thomas Habina, a minor by his father and next friend, Frank Habina, and Frank Habina v. M. A. Henry Co., Inc., et al., Civ. 38-237.

Hummel Case File. Albert E. Hummel and Alverda E. Hummel, in their own right as parents of James Hummel, deceased, and Albert E. Hummel and Alverda E. Hummel, administrators of the estate of James Hummel, deceased v. William E. Roschen, Martha E. Sultan, Carola Terwilliger, and Ilse Bischoff, individually and as co-partners doing business in the name and style of E. F. Timme & Son, et al., Civ. 48-659.

Intelisana Case File. Joseph Intelisana, Jr., an infant under the age of 14 years by Joseph Intelisana, Sr., his guardian ad litem, and Joseph Intelisana, Sr. v. Woonsocket Falls Mill, Inc., et al., Civ. 46-504.

Izzo Case File. Bessie Izzo, as guardian of the person and estate of Jacqueline L. Izzo, a minor v. Gene Autry, et al., Civ. 46-439.

Richard Johnson Case File. Edward Johnson, administrator of the estate of Richard Johnson, deceased, and Edward Johnson and Laura Johnson v. M. A. Henry Co., Inc., et al., Civ. 35-454.

Chesley Franklin Johnson Case File. Rachel Johnson Bodie, individually, and as administratrix of the estate of Chesley Franklin Johnson, deceased v. M. A. Henry Co., Inc., et al., Civ. 62-386.

Jones Case File. John Elwyn Jones, an infant by his father and next friend, Elwyn Jones, and Elwyn Jones, individually v. Gene Autry, et al., Civ. 40-357.

Ikner Case File. Ann Ikner, as guardian of the person and estate of James Ikner, Jr., a minor vs. Gene Autry, et al., Civ. 50-192.

Javinsky Case File. Andrew Javinsky, an infant, by his guardian ad litem, Paul Javinsky, and Paul Javinsky, individually v. M. A. Henry Co., Inc., Civ. 48-622.

King Case File. William Ronald King, an infant by his father and next friend, William A. King, and William A. King, individually v. Gene Autry, et al., Civ. 40-35.

Klinck Case File. Edward Klinck, Jr., a minor, by his father and next friend, Edward Klinck, Sr., and Edward Klinck, Sr. v. M. A. Henry Co., Inc., et al., Civ. 40-402.

Stanley Krzeczkowski Case File. Stella Urban (formerly Stella Krzeczkowski) and Casimir Krzeczkowski, as administrators of presequendum of Stanley Krzeczkowski, deceased v. M. A. Henry Co., Inc., et al., Civ. 47-289.

Casimir Kresokowski Case File. Casimir Kresokowski, by his next friend, Stella Kresokowski, and Stella Kresokowski, individually v. M. A. Henry Co., Inc., Civ. 45-274.

La France Case File. Richard Joseph LaFrance, an infant, by his guardian ad litem George La France v. M. A. Henry Co., Inc., et al., Civ. 55-274.

Lockhart Case File. John Lockhart, Jr., an infant by his guardian ad litem, John Lockhart, Sr., and John Lockhart, Sr., individually v. M. A. Henry Co., Inc., et al., Civ. 42-201.

Lutz Case File. Louis P. Lutz and Ida K. Lutz, co-partners doing business under the name and style of Lou's Auto Stores v. M. A. Henry Co., Inc., et al., Civ. 40-283.

McMaster Case File. William K. McMaster, Jr., an infant, by his guardian ad litem, William McMaster, Sr., and William McMaster, Sr., individually v. M. A. Henry Co., Inc., et al., Civ. 40-710.

Moore Case File. Samuel Moore and Elizabeth Moore, in their own right as parents of Joseph Moore, and Joseph Moore, a minor, by his father and natural guardian, Samuel Moore v. William E. Roschen, Martha E. Sultan, Carola Terwilliger and Ilsa Bischoff, individually and as co-partners doing business in the name and style of E. F. Timme & Son, et al., Civ. 48-658.

Palmateer Case File. Gerald W. Palmateer, an infant, by his next friend, Harry W. Palmateer, and Harry Palmateer, individually v. Gene Autry, et al., Civ. 48-264.

Perry Case File. Virgil Perry, individually, and as guardian ad litem of John Perry, an infant under the age of fourteen years v. M. A. Henry Co., Inc., et al., Civ. 66-42.

Russell Case File. John C. Russell, a minor, by his father, John S. Russell v. Woonsocket Falls Mill, et al., Civ. 59-160.

Strong Case File. William Augustus, Jr., individually, and as administrator of the estate of William Augustus Strong, III, deceased v. M. A. Henry Co., Inc., et al., Civ. 70-298.

Stultz Case File. Charles William Stultz, Jr., an infant, by his father and next friend, Charles William Stultz, and Charles William Stultz, individually v. Gene Autry, et al., Civ. 40-36.

Sullivan Case File. Charles William Sullivan, by his next of kin and father, Charles Lester Sullivan, and Charles Lester Sullivan, individually v. McCrory Stores Corporation, et al., Civ. 48-265.

Tetla Case File. Wallace Tetla, an infant, by his father and next friend, Walter Tetla, and Walter Tetla, individually v. Gene Autry, et al., Civ. 43-633.

Warnick Case File. Cecil D'Wayne Warnick, an infant, by his father and next friend, Cecil D. Warnick, and Cecil D. Warnick, individually v. Gene Autry, et al., Civ. 38-281.

Wilks Case File. Willie B. Wilks, individually, and as administrator of the estate of Willie B. Wilks, Jr., deceased v. M. A. Henry Co., Inc., et al., Civ. 36-249.

Zibor Case File. John Zibor, Jr., by his next friend, John Zibor, and John Zibor, individually v. M. A. Henry Co., Inc., et al., Civ 45-273.

NEW YORK SUPREME COURT, NEW YORK COUNTY (NY, NY)

Baker Case File. George E. Baker, an infant, by George B. Baker, Jr., his guardian ad litem, and George B. Baker, Jr., individually v. M. A. Henry Co., Inc., et al., index no. 10341/1949.

Baragona Case File. Charles J. Baragona, as guardian ad litem of Charles J. Baragona, Jr., an infant, and Charles J. Baragona v. M. A. Henry Co., Inc., et al., index no. 19216/1949.

Blessington Record on Appeal (NY Supreme Court, App Divn). Michael Blessington, as administrator of the goods, chattels and credits which were of Michael Blessington, Jr., deceased v. McCrory Stores Corp., et al., Papers on Appeal from Judgments and Orders, NY Supreme Court, Appellate Division—Second Department, State Law Library (Albany, NY).

Blessington Record on Appeal (NY Ct of Appeals). Michael Blessington, as administrator of the goods, chattels and credits which were of Michael Blessington, Jr., deceased v. McCrory Stores Corp., et al., 140–47, Record on Appeal, NY Ct of Appeals, State Law Library (Albany, NY).

Brunette Case File. Joseph Brunette, as guardian ad litem of John Brunette, an infant, and Joseph Brunette v. M. A. Henry Co., Inc., et al., index no. 7176/1950.

Caparco Case File. Perry Caparco, by Michael Caparco, his guardian ad litem, and Michael Caparco, individually v. M. A. Henry Co., Inc., et al., index no. 21897/1949.

Cizek Case File. Roy Cizek, an infant, by Fred Cizek, his guardian ad litem, and Fred Cizek v. M.A. Henry Co., Inc., et al., index no. 8141/1949.

Dorsey Case File. Alvin A. Dorsey, as guardian ad litem of Richard LaVerne Dorsey, an infant, and Alvin A. Dorsey, individually v. M. A. Henry Co., Inc., et al., index no. 6714/1950.

Duffy Case File. Dennis A. Duffy, as administrator of the goods, chattels, and credits of Dennis Duffy, Jr. v. E.I. DuPont de Nemours & Company, et al., index no. 08560/1948.

Gagnon Case File. Armand J. Gagnon, as guardian ad litem of David Gagnon, an infant, and Armand J. Gagnon v. M. A. Henry Co., Inc., et al., index no. 28294/1948.

Gerber Case File. Melvin Gerber, Jr., an infant under age 14, by his guardian ad litem, Dorothy Gerber and Charles Gerber v. M. A. Henry Co., Inc., et al., index no. 34268/1946.

Giacomarro Case File. Ralph Giacomarro, as guardian ad litem of Ralph Giacomarro, Jr., an infant, and Ralph Giacomarro v. M. A. Henry Co., Inc., et al., index no. 15284/1948.

McCormack Record on Appeal. James McCormack, administrator of the goods, chattels and credits of Thomas McCormack, deceased, and James McCormack v. M. A. Henry Co., Inc., et al., Supreme Court, New York Cty, Case on Appeal, NY Supreme Court, Appellate Division—First Department, New York State Library (Albany, NY).

Ormerod Case File. Marion J. Ormerod, an infant, by Walter Ormerod, her guardian ad litem, and Walter Ormerod v. Gene Autry, et al., index no. 1777/1950.

Peterson Case File. Richard Peterson, as guardian ad litem of Hans Patrick Peterson, an infant, and Richard A. Peterson v. M. A. Henry Co., Inc., et al., index no. 5999/1948.

Piechota Case File. Frederick Piechota, by his guardian ad litem Leon Piechota, and Leon Piechota, individually v. M. A. Henry Co., Inc., index no. 46-398.

Sondej Case File. John Sondej, by his guardian ad litem, Joseph Sondej, and Joseph Sondej v. M. A. Henry Co., Inc., et al., index no. 765/1949.

Szumita Case File. Richard Szumita, an infant, by Alexander Szumita, his guardian ad litem, and Alexander Szumita, individually v. M. A. Henry Co., Inc., et al., index no. 15168/1949.

Timberlake Case File. Fred L. Timberlake, as guardian ad litem of Scott Timberlake, an infant, and Fred L. Timberlake v. M. A. Henry Co., Inc., index no. 31289/1948.

Tormollen Case File. William A. Tormollen, Jr., an infant, by William A. Tormollen, Sr., his guardian ad litem, and William A. Tormollen, Sr., individually v. M. A. Henry Co., Inc., et al., index no. 32331/1949.

Touhill Case File. William Touhill, an infant, by John A. Touhill, his guardian ad litem, and John A. Touhill v. M. A. Henry Co., Inc., et al., index no. 38082/1946.

Weatherell Case File. William Weatherell Jr., an infant, by William Weatherell, his guardian ad litem, and William Weatherell v. Gene Autry, et al., index no. 31089/1945.

Weinstein Case File. Maurice Weinstein, as guardian ad litem of Arnold Weinstein, an infant, and Maurice Weinstein, individually v. M. A. Henry Co., Inc., et al., index no. 7986/1949.

OTHER COURTS

Felton Case File.

(action against retailer). Michael Felton, a minor, by his father and guardian ad litem, Tom Felton, Tom Felton, and Eleanor Felton v. The Goodyear Tire & Rubber Co., Inc., Civ. 1704, U. S. Dist. Ct., ID, Central Divn, RG 21, box 13, file 1704, National Archives–Pacific Alaska Region (Seattle, WA).

(state court). Tom Felton, as guardian ad litem of Michael Felton, an infant, and Tom Felton v. M. A. Henry Co., Inc. et al., Civ. _____/1949, M. A. Henry Co. Legal 1948–1949, box 1, Agents & Licensees, T94-45-30, Autry Collection.

Izzo Case File.

Izzo Case File (federal court). Bessie Izzo, as guardian of the person and estate of Jacqueline L. Izzo, a minor v. Gene Autry, et al., Civ. 46-439, U. S. Dist. Ct., SDNY, NARA Northeast Region–New York (NY, NY) (docket sheet only).

Izzo Probate Court Record (probate court). In the Matter of the Estate of Jacqueline Izzo, minor, docket no. 43003, MI Probate Court (Saginaw, MI).

Izzo Record on Appeal (fees dispute). *In re Izzo*, 358 Mich. 101 (1959), Record on Appeal, MI Supreme Court docket no. 46,596, University of Michigan Law School (Ann Arbor, MI).

Krau Case File. In the Matter of the Appointment of a Guardian ad Litem for Ralph Manfried Krau, NY Supreme Court, Erie County, Buffalo, NY.

McCarthy Case File. Dennis McCarthy, by his guardian ad litem, Lawrence McCarthy and Lawrence McCarthy, individually v. Gene Autry, et al., index no. 15403/1947, New York Supreme Court, Kings County (NY, NY).

Sibley Case File.

(action against retailer). Calvin Lee Sibley, an infant, by his mother and next friend, Violet Sibley Slawson, and Violet Sibley Slawson, individually v. The Hecht Company, Civ. 34,509, U. S. Dist. Ct. District of Columbia, National Archives at Kansas City (KC, MO).

(federal court). Calvin Lee Sibley, an infant, by his next friend, Violet Sibley Slawson, and Violet Sibley Slawson, individually v. Gene Autry, et al., Civ. 45-161, U. S. Dist. Ct., SDNY, NARA Northeast Region–New York (NY, NY).

Viands Case File. Robert Franklin Viands, an infant, by his mother and next friend, Anne Louise Viands, and Anne Louise Viands, individually v. The Hecht Co., Civ. 33,367 and 34,509, U. S. Dist. Ct. District of Columbia, NARA at Kansas City (KC, MO).

Wrobbel Case File. John Wrobbel, an infant, by Walter W. Wrobbel, his guardian ad litem, and Walter W. Wrobbel, individually v. M. A. Henry Co., Inc., et al., docket no. A-97401, New York Supreme Court, Erie County (Buffalo, NY).

SETTLED WITHOUT FORMALLY FILING SUIT

Grosch Case File. Box 1, Agents & Licensees, T94-45-30, folder M. A. Henry Co.—New York or Leslie Henry Co. (1 of 2) 1950–1951, Autry Collection.

Hooper Case File. M. A. Henry Co. Legal 1948–1949, box 1, Agents & Licenses, T94-45-30, Autry Collection.

(appointment of guardian; request for court authorization to settle; bond). Frank E. Hooper, as legal guardian of Philip Warren Hooper, an infant, v. Philip Warren Hooper, petition no. 13909, Circuit Court of Harrison County, WVA.

(release of defendants from liability).

Pritchard Case File. William E. Pritchard, Jr., a minor, by William E. Pritchard, Sr. and Helen S. Pritchard, father and mother and natural guardians of the said minor, and William E. Pritchard, Sr. and Helen S. Pritchard, in their own right v. M. A. Henry Co., Inc., et al., no. 216 Jan. Term, 1949, Court of Common Pleas, Lehigh City, PA (Allentown, PA).

cowboy suit published opinions

Blessington v. McCrory Stores Corporation, et al., 195 Misc. 710, 91 NYS2d 73 (1949).

Blessington v. McCrory Stores Corporation, et al., 198 Misc. 291, 95 NYS2d 414 (1950), affd 279 AD 806 (1952), affd 305 NY 140, 111 NE2d 421 (1953).

Blessington v. Autry, 105 NYS2d 953 (1951).

Devens et al. v. M. A. Henry Co., Inc., et al., 8 FRD 368 (1948).

Di Trapani et al. v. M. A. Henry Co., Inc. et al., Wilks v. Same, Johnson et al. v. Same, 7 FRD 123 (1946).

Donahue et al. v. M. A. Henry Co., Inc. et al., 78 F Supp. 91 (SD NY1948).
Duffy v. E. I. Du Pont de Nemours & Company et al., 193 Misc. 175, 81 NYS2d 630 (1948), affd, 274 AD 908, 84 NYS2d 710 (1948).
Habina et al. v. M. A. Henry Co., Inc. et al., 8 FRD 52 (1948).
In re Izzo, 358 Mich. 101, 99 NW2d 625 (1959).
McCormack v. M. A. Henry Co., Inc., et al., 275 AD 758, 88 NYS2d 890 (1949).
Malone et al. v. M.A. Henry Co., Inc., et al., 85 NYS2d 393 (1948).
Moore et al. v. Roschen et al., 93 F Supp. (SD NY 1950).
Timberlake v. M. A. Henry Co., Inc. et al., 104 NYS2d 284 (1951).

cowboy suit oral histories

Anonymous Interview. Mansfield, OH, November 21, 2016.
Baragona Interview. Charles J. Baragona Jr. and Rebecca Griffiths (daughter), Lake Mary, FL, December 7, 2016.
Bates Interview. Gaither R. Bates Jr., Hawthorne, NJ, November 30, 2016.
Cumberledge Interview. Arthur Cumberledge Jr. and Jenny Cumberledge (wife), Ventura, CA, March 28, 2017.
Felton Interview. Michael Felton and Judy Felton (wife), Buhl, ID, March 23, 2017.
Habina Interview. Thomas F. Habina and Dorothy Habina (wife), Winterhaven, FL, December 5, 2016.
Intelisano Interview. Camille Intelisano and Pat Intelisano-Cerrigone (sisters of Joseph Intelisano), Verona, NJ, May 31, 2017.
Izzo Interview. Jacqueline ("Jackie") Izzo, Saginaw, MI, December 14, 2016.
King Interview. Rosanne King (widow of William R. King), Boca Raton, FL, February 21, 2017.
Lockhart Interview. John (Jack) Lockhart Jr. and Angela Lockhart (wife), Spring Hill, FL, August 14, 2015.
McMaster Interview. William K. McMaster, Ypsilanti, MI, December 15, 2016.
Peterson Interview. Ellen Theresa Peterson (widow of Hans Patrick Peterson), Zephyr Hills, FL, February 20, 2017.
Sansbury Interview. John R. Sansbury and Kristen (Kris) Sansbury (wife), Tucson, AZ, March 29, 2017.
Szumita Interview. Bruce Szumita (youngest brother of Richard Szumita), Denise Szumita (Bruce's wife), Ken Szumita (Richard's second-youngest brother), Andrew Szumita (Richard's third son), and Lisa Szumita (Andrew's wife), Raynham, MA, November 28, 2016.
Timberlake Interview. Kay Bryant (sister of Scott Timberlake), Thousand Oaks, CA, March 27, 2017.
Viands Interview. Robert F. Viands and Sarah Catherine Viands (wife), Graham, NC, November 29, 2016.

list of illustrations

Index

Page numbers in italics refer to photographs.